Thieme

Knee Surgery

Tricks of the Trade

James P. Stannard, MD
Medical Director
Missouri Orthopaedic Institute;
Hansjörg Wyss Distinguished Professor of Orthopaedic Surgery;
Chair
Department of Orthopaedic Surgery
University of Missouri
Columbia, Missouri, USA

Andrew Schmidt, MD
Professor
Department of Orthopaedics
University of Minnesota;
Chief
Department of Orthopaedic Surgery
Hennepin County Medical Center
Minneapolis, Minnesota, USA

Mauricio Kfuri, MD, PhD
Director
Orthopaedic Residency Program;
James P. Stannard, MD, and Carolyn A. Stannard Distinguished Professor in Orthopaedic Surgery
University of Missouri;
Missouri Orthopaedic Institute
Columbia, Missouri, USA

367 illustrations

Thieme
New York • Stuttgart • Delhi • Rio de Janeiro

Library of Congress Cataloging-in-Publication Data is available from the publisher.

Illustrations: Stacy Turpin Cheavens, Missouri, USA

Important note: Medicine is an ever-changing science undergoing continual development. Research and clinical experience are continually expanding our knowledge, in particular our knowledge of proper treatment and drug therapy. Insofar as this book mentions any dosage or application, readers may rest assured that the authors, editors, and publishers have made every effort to ensure that such references are in accordance with **the state of knowledge at the time of production of the book.**

Nevertheless, this does not involve, imply, or express any guarantee or responsibility on the part of the publishers in respect to any dosage instructions and forms of applications stated in the book. **Every user is requested to examine carefully** the manufacturers' leaflets accompanying each drug and to check, if necessary in consultation with a physician or specialist, whether the dosage schedules mentioned therein or the contraindications stated by the manufacturers differ from the statements made in the present book. Such examination is particularly important with drugs that are either rarely used or have been newly released on the market. Every dosage schedule or every form of application used is entirely at the user's own risk and responsibility. The authors and publishers request every user to report to the publishers any discrepancies or inaccuracies noticed. If errors in this work are found after publication, errata will be posted at www.thieme.com on the product description page.

Some of the product names, patents, and registered designs referred to in this book are in fact registered trademarks or proprietary names even though specific reference to this fact is not always made in the text. Therefore, the appearance of a name without designation as proprietary is not to be construed as a representation by the publisher that it is in the public domain.

Thieme addresses people of all gender identities equally. We encourage our authors to use gender-neutral or gender-equal expressions wherever the context allows.

Thieme Medical Publishers, Inc.
333 Seventh Avenue, 18th Floor,
New York, NY 10001, USA
www.thieme.com
+1 800 782 3488,
customerservice@thieme.com

Cover design: © Thieme
Cover Image source: © Thieme/Stacy Turpin Cheavens
Typesetting by TNQ Technologies, India

Printed in Germany by Beltz Grafische Betriebe 5 4 3 2 1

ISBN: 978-1-62623-541-0

Also available as e-book:
eISBN (PDF): 978-1-62623-542-7
eISBN (epub): 978-1-63853-481-5

Contents

Section II: Sports Medicine

Section III: Adult Reconstruction

Videos

Video 4.1: Tibial plateau fractures case in the coronal plane

Video 22.1: Quadriceps tendon ACL reconstruction including graft harvest

Video 27.1: Preparation of the antero-lateral (AL) PCL femoral tunnel insertion site. Note that the meniscofemoral ligament (MPFL) has been preserved

Video 27.2: Final preparation and marking for the k-wire for the AL femoral tunnel drilling. Note the proximity of the medial femoral articular cartilage to the AL insertion site

Video 27.3: Graft passage has occurred. This is the view of the quad tendon autograft insertion into the AL PCL insertion site

Video 27.4: The postero-medial portal is established (viewed with 70 degree arthroscope from the antero-lateral portal). This is followed by placing a 30-degree arthroscope into the posterior medial portal. The insertion site is to your right an angled PCL curette is used to further mark the PCL tibial insertion site approximately 102 cm below the medial joint line (to be confirmed with intra op fluoroscopy)

Video 27.5: PCL tibial tunnel insertion site is identified, and the PCL tibial guide is brought from the antero-medial portal. Note the location of the posterior horn of the medial meniscus to the right. The guide is placed well distal to the body of the medial meniscus

Video 27.6: The PCL tibial tunnel is marked with a k wire and intra op fluoroscopy is obtained to check the position on a lateral x-ray. If acceptable the tunnel is drilled, and a protective PCL guide is used to protect the posterior neurovascular structures.

Video 30.1: Posterolateral corner reconstruction

Video 33.1: Lateral lengthening

Video 38.1: Medial meniscus transplant

Video 38.2: Lateral meniscus transplant

Video 38.1: Opening wedge distal femur osteotomy – valgus knee

Preface

Knee Surgery: Tricks of the Trade is a book designed to help orthopaedic surgeons in the operating room. It is a concise book that presents expert opinions and surgical tips from a superb international group of authors. It is not designed to have references or detailed history of treatment, but rather to provide expert guidance on successful surgical treatment of a wide variety of knee problems, spanning the disciplines of trauma, sports medicine, and arthroplasty/reconstruction.

We hope the readers will find this a helpful book of surgical tips and tricks that they can look at prior to heading into the operating room to treat their patients.

James P. Stannard, MD
Andrew Schmidt, MD
Mauricio Kfuri, MD, PhD

Acknowledgment

I would like to thank my wonderful wife Carolyn and our children for putting up with me doing yet another book project. Their patience, love, and support are what keep me going. This is the last one—I promise!

James P. Stannard, MD

I dedicate this book first to my wife Jamie and my children, Michael and Katherine, whose love, support, and friendship mean more than anything to me, and secondly I would like to acknowledge my partners at Hennepin Healthcare for their dedication to their patients, their resilience, and their teamwork. It is an honor and a privilege to work with such incredible people. I would also like to thank the Thieme staff who assisted us in the development and production of this book.

Andrew Schmidt, MD

I dedicate this book to you, who is passionate about the knee and interested in understanding the multiple facets of this complex joint. At first, I would like to thank and especially acknowledge my wife, Glaucia, and our children, Pedro and Julia, whose love and support allowed me to commit time to this project. You are phenomenal and the main drive to all my actions. I have been inspired by my mentors, Cleber Paccola and Joseph Schatzker, and by my residents and fellows, who probably have offered me more than they received in return. Finally, I dedicate this book to my patients, individuals that have honored me with their trust and whom I feel privileged to serve.

Mauricio Kfuri, MD, PhD

Contributors

Rene Jorge Abdalla, MD, PhD
Full Professor;
Head of the Knee Institute – Hcor;
Professor of the Translational Surgery Post-Graduation Program;
Department of Orthopedics and Traumatology
Paulista School of Medicine - Federal University of São Paulo
São Paulo, Brazil

John D. Adams Jr, MD
Orthopaedic Surgeon
Prisma Health
University of South Carolina SOM- Greenville
Greenville, South Carolina, USA

Ajay Aggarwal, MD
Orthopaedic Surgeon
Department of Orthopedic Surgery
University of Missouri
Columbia, Missouri, USA

Marcio Albers, MD
Orthopedic Surgeon;
Resident Physician
Department of Radiology
University of Pittsburgh
Pittsburgh, Pennsylvania, USA

Rodrigo Satamini Pires E Albuquerque, MD, PhD
Orthopaedic Surgeon
Department of General and Specialized Surgery
Fluminense Federal University (UFF)
Niterói, Brazil;
National Institute of Traumatology and Orthopedics
Rio de Janeiro, Brazil

Zachary S. Aman, MD
Medical Student
Sidney Kimmel Medical College
Philadelphia, Pennsylvania, USA

Elizabeth A. Arendt, MD
Professor and Vice Chair
Department of Orthopedic Surgery
University of Minnesota
Minneapolis, Minnesota, USA

Diego da Costa Astur, MD
Affiliated Professor and Post-Doctorate in Translational Surgery
Department of Orthopedics and Traumatology
Escola Paulista de Medicina / Federal University of São Paulo;
Head
Knee Group of the Discipline of Sports Medicine
Department of Orthopedics and Traumatology
EPM/UNIFESP
São Paulo, Brazil

Suthorn Bavonratanavech, MD
Chief of Orthopedic and Trauma Network;
Senior Director
Bangkok Orthopedic Center
Bangkok International Hospital
Huaykwang, Bangkok, Thailand

Stefano A. Bini, MD
Professor of Clinical Orthopaedics;
Chief Technology Officer
Department of Orthopaedic Surgery
University of California San Francisco (UCSF);
Founder and Chair, UCSF Digital Orthopedics Conference (DOCSF)
San Francisco, California, USA

Jordan A. Bley, MPH
Department of Orthopaedic Surgery
Vanderbilt University
Nashville, Tennessee, USA

William D. Bugbee, MD
Department of Orthopaedic Surgery
Scripps Clinic
La Jolla, California, USA

Jeremy M. Burnham, MD
Orthopedic and Sports Medicine Surgeon;
Medical Director of Sports Medicine;
Orthopedic Surgery Department Head
Ochsner Health – Baton Rouge
Baton Rouge, Louisiana, USA

John Byron, DO
Orthopedic Spine Surgeon
Florida Orthopedic Institute
Florida, Miami, USA

Gilberto Luis Camanho, MD, PhD
Full Professor
Department of Orthopedics and Traumatology
University of São Paulo School of Medicine
São Paulo, Brazil

Moises Cohen, MD
Full Professor of Orthopedics, Traumatology and Sports Medicine
Federal University of São Paulo- Brazil;
Head of Cohen Orthopedic and Sports Medicine Institute
Hospital Israelita Albert Einstein
São Paulo, Brazil

Juan Manuel Concha, MD
Professor of Orthopedics and Traumatology
University of Cauca;
Susana López Hospital in Valencia
Popayán, Colombia, Bogotá

Corey Cook, MA
Clinical Research Coordinator
Columbia Orthopaedic Group
Columbia, Missouri, USA

Brett D. Crist, MD, FAAOS, FACS, FAOA
Professor
Vice-Chairman of Business Development;
Director Orthopaedic Trauma Service;
Director Orthopaedic Trauma Fellowship;
Co-Director Limb Preservation Center;
Surgery of the Hip and Orthopaedic Trauma
Department of Orthopaedic Surgery
University of Missouri
Columbia, Missouri, USA

Marco Kawamura Demange MD, PhD
Associate Professor
Department of Orthopedics and Traumatology
University of São Paulo School of Medicine
São Paulo, Brazil

Vishal S. Desai, MD
Resident Physician
Department of Orthopedic Surgery
State University of New York Upstate
Syracuse, New York, USA

Lars Engebretsen, MD, PhD
Professor
Division of Orthopedic Surgery
University of Oslo
Oslo, Norway

Igor A. Escalante Elguezabal, MD
Attending professor of Orthopaedic Surgery
Universidad Central de Venezuela
Hospital Universitario de Caracas
Caracas, Venezuela

George C. Fanelli, MD
Orthopaedic Surgeon
Geisinger Woodbine - Orthopaedics and Sports Medicine
Danville, Pennsylvania, USA

Matthew G. Fanelli, MD
Orthopaedic Surgeon
Geisinger Woodbine - Orthopaedics and Sports Medicine
Danville, Pennsylvania, USA

Fabricio Fogagnolo, MD
Head of Knee Surgery and Orthopaedic Trauma
Department of Orthopaedics and Anesthesiology
Hospital das Clínicas
University of São Paulo
São Paulo, Brazil

Carlos Eduardo Franciozi, MD, PhD
Affiliate Professor;
Head of the Orthopedic Surgery Residency Program;
Professor of the Post-Graduation Orthopedics - Radiology Program;
Department of Orthopedics and Traumatology
Paulista School of Medicine - Federal University of São Paulo
Knee Institute - HCor
São Paulo, Brazil

Freddie Fu, MD
Chair
Department of Orthopaedic Surgery;
David Silver Professor of Orthopaedic Surgery
University of Pittsburgh School of Medicine
Pittsburgh, Pennsylvania, USA

Nicholas P. Gannon, MD
Orthopedic Surgeon Resident
Department of Orthopaedic Surgery
University of Minnesota
Minneapolis, Minnesota, USA

Andrew J. Garrone, MD
Professor
Department of Orthopaedics
The Ohio State University
Columbus, Ohio, USA

Alan Getgood, MD, FRCS (Tr and Orth), Dip SEM
Assistant Professor
Schulich School of Medicine & Dentistry;
Fowler Kennedy Sport Medicine Clinic
3M Centre, University of Western Ontario
London, Ontario, Canada

Vincenzo Giordano, MD, PhD, FBCS
Orthopaedic Trauma Surgeon
Orthopedics and Traumatology Service Professor
Nova Monteiro
Miguel Couto Municipal Hospital;
Orthopaedic Trauma Surgeon
Clínica São Vicente
Rio de Janeiro, Brazil

Riccardo Gobbi, MD, PhD
Associate Professor
Hospital das Clínicas
Institute of Orthopedics and Traumatology
Faculty of Medicine
University of São Paulo
São Paulo, Brazil

Jan S. Grudziak, MD, PhD
Assistant Professor
Department of Orthopaedic Surgery
University of Pittsburgh
Pittsburgh, Pennsylvania, USA

Benjamin Hansen, MD
Orthopaedic Surgeon
Department of Orthopedic Surgery
Kirk Kerkorian School of Medicine
University of Nevada Las Vegas
Las Vegas, Nevada, USA

George Hanson, MD
George Hanson, MD
Orthopaedic Surgeon
Hennepin Healthcare System
Minneapolis, Minnesota, USA

Arlen D. Hanssen, MD
Orthopedic Surgeon
Department of Orthopedic Surgery
Mayo Clinic
Rochester, Minnesota, USA

Christopher D. Harner, MD, FAOA, FAAOS
Orthopaedic Surgeon
Pittsburgh, Pennsylvania, USA

Jörg Harrer
Orthopaedic Surgeon
Department of Orthopedics and Traumatology
Regiomed Klinikum Lichtenfels
Lichtenfels, Germany

Steven F. Harwin, MD, FAAOS
Chief of Advanced Technology of Total Hip and Knee Arthroplasty
Mount Sinai West;
Professor of Orthopaedic Surgery
Icahn School of Medicine at Mount Sinai
New York, New York, USA

Betina B Hinckel, MD, PhD
Assistant Professor
Oakland University
Rochester, Minnesota, USA;
Department of Orthopaedic Surgery
William Beaumont Hospital
Royal Oak, Michigan, USA

Patrick Horst, MD
Assistant Professor
Department of Orthopedic Surgery
Medical School, University of Minnesota
Minneapolis, Minnesota, USA

David Hubbard, MD
Chief
Orthopaedic Trauma Service;
Professor
Department of Orthopaedics
School of Medicine
West Virginia University
Morgantown, West Virginia, USA

Felix Hüttner, MD
Orthopaedic Surgeon
Department of Orthopaedics and Traumatology
Regiomed Klinikum Lichtenfels
Lichtenfels, Germany

Sheila J. McNeill Ingham, MD, PhD
Affiliate
Department of Orthopedics and Traumatology
Escola Paulista de Medicina - Universidade Federal de São Paulo
São Paulo, Brazil

Eli Kamara, MD
Assistant Professor of Orthopaedic Surgery
Albert Einstein College of Medicine
Bronx, New York, USA

James Keeney
Chief, Adult Reconstruction Service;
Associate Professor
Department of Orthopaedic Surgery
University of Missouri
Columbia, Missouri, USA

Mitchell I. Kennedy, MD
Research Coordinator II
Eastside Research Associates
Seattle, Washington, USA

Peter Kloen, MD, PhD
Professor of Orthopaedic Traumatology
Amsterdam University Medical Center
Amsterdam, The Netherlands

Christian Krettek, FRACS, FRCSEd
Professor
Medizinische Hochschule Hannover (MHH)
Hannover, Germany

Robert F. LaPrade MD, PhD
Complex Knee and Sports Medicine Surgeon
Twin Cities Orthopedics;
Adjunct Professor
Department of Orthopaedic Surgery
University of Minnesota
Minneapolis, Minnesota, USA

Samantha L. LaPrade MD
Resident Physician
Department of Otolaryngology
Medical College of Wisconsin
Milwaukee, Wisconsin, USA

Mark A. Lee, MD, FACS
Professor and Vice Chair of Education;
Chief, Orthopaedic Trauma Service;
Director, Orthopaedic Trauma Fellowship
Department of Orthopaedic Surgery
UC Davis Health
Sacramento, California, USA

Frank A. Liporace, M.D.
Chief
Division of Orthopaedic Trauma & Adult Reconstruction
Department of Orthopaedic Surgery
Saint Barnabas Medical Center
Livingston, New Jersey, USA

Robert Longstaffe, MD, FRCSC
Fowler Kennedy Sport Medicine Clinic
3M Centre, University of Western Ontario
London, Ontario

Philipp Lobenhoffer, MD, PhD
Professor, Orthopedic and Trauma Surgery
Go: h Joint Surgery Orthopedics Hanover
Lobenhoffer, Agneskirchner, Tröger GbR
Hanover, Germany

Walter R. Lowe, MD
Ed T Smith Professor and Chair
University of Texas McGovern Medical School
Houston, Texas, USA

Congfeng Luo, MD
Orthopaedic Surgeon
Department of Orthopaedic Surgery
Shanghai Sixth People's hospital
Shanghai Jiaotong University
Shanghai, China

Richard Ma, MD
Gregory L. and Ann L. Hummel Distinguished Professor
Department of Orthopaedic Surgery;
Chief, Division of Sports Medicine
Missouri Orthopaedic Institute
University of Missouri – Columbia
Columbia, Missouri, USA

Sven Märdian, MD
Chief Senior Physician
Head of the Traumatology and Musculoskeletal Tumor Surgery Section
Center for Musculoskeletal Surgery (CMSC)
Campus Virchow Klinikum
Charité - University Medicine Berlin
Berlin, Germany

Chatchanin Mayurasakorn, MD
Orthopaedic Trauma Surgeon
Bangkok International Hospital
Bangkok, Thailand

Wilson Mello Jr, MD
Research and Study Center
Wilson Mello Institute;
Pontifical Catholic University Hospital of Campinas
Campinas, Brazil

Rory McHardy, ATC
Program Director - Ochsner Sports
Medicine Institute SMA Residency
Ochsner Health – Baton Rouge
Baton Rouge, Louisiana, USA

Conor I. Murphy, MD
Orthopedic Surgeon
Department of Orthopaedic Surgery
University of Pittsburgh
Pittsburgh, Pennsylvania, USA

Volker Musahl, MD
Department of Orthopaedic Surgery
UPMC Freddie Fu Sports Medicine Center
University of Pittsburgh
Pittsburgh, Pennsylvania, USA

Douglas D.R. Naudie, MD, FRCSC
Professor
Department of Surgery (Division of Orthopaedic Surgery)
Schulich School of Medicine
Western University;
Consultant Orthopaedic Surgeon
London Health Sciences Center
Joint Replacement Institute
University Hospital
London, Ontario, Canada

Julio César Palacio-Villegas, MD
Professor of Orthopaedic Surgery
Javeriana University;
Chief of the Hip and Knee Reconstruction Group;
Coordinator of The Fellowship Program in Hip and
Knee Reconstruction Surgery
Clínica Imbanaco Grupo QuirónSalud.
Cali, Colombia, Bogotá

Idemar Monteiro da Palma, MD
Orthopaedic Surgeon
Montese Medical Center
Resende - RJ
Rios D'Or Hospital
Rio de Janeiro, Brazil

Kevin I. Perry, M.D.
Orthopedic Surgeon
Department of Orthopedic Surgery
Mayo Clinic
Rochester, Minnesota, USA

Robinson Esteves Pires, MD, PhD
Professor of Orthopaedic Surgery;
Chief of the Department of the Locomotor Apparatus
Federal University of Minas Gerais;
Director of the Orthopaedic Trauma Division
Felicio Rocho Hospital and Orizonti Institute
Belo Horizonte, Minas Gerais, Brazil

Joshua Pratt, MS, LAT, ATC, OTC, PES
Sports Medicine Assistant Resident
Ochsner Health – Baton Rouge
Baton Rouge, Louisiana, USA

J. Spence Reid, MD
Orthopaedic Surgeon
Penn State University College of Medicine
Milton S. Hershey Medical Center
Hershey, Pennsylvania, USA

Rodrigo Salim, MD, PhD
Knee Surgeon Orthopedist
Foundation for Support of Teaching,
Research and Assistance
HCFMRP;
Clinical Hospital of the Faculty of
Medicine of Ribeirão Preto
Ribeirão Preto, Brazil

Dominique Saragaglia, MD
Professor Emeritus
Orthopaedic Unit
Grenoble-Alpes-Voiron University Hospital
Voiron, France

Michael Schuetz, FRACS, FaOrth
Director
Jamieson Trauma Institute;
Professor & Chair of Trauma
Queensland University of Technology;
Department of Orthoapedics and Trauma Service
Royal Brisbane and Women's Hospital
Brisbane, Australia

Seth L. Sherman, MD
Associate Professor of Orthopedic Surgery
Stanford University California, USA

Patrick A. Smith, MD
Columbia Orthopaedic Group
Adjunct Professor of Orthopaedic Surgery;
Co-Director of Sports Medicine Fellowship;
Team Physician
University of Missouri
Columbia, Missouri, USA

Felipe Serrão de Souza, MD
Orthopaedic Trauma Surgeon
Orthopedics and Traumatology Service Professor
Nova Monteiro
Miguel Couto Municipal Hospital;
Rio de Janeiro, Brazil

Matthew Stillwagon, MD
Orthopaedic Surgeon
Mission Hospital
Asheville, North Carolina, USA

Wolf Strecker, MD
Orthopaedic Surgeon
Department of Orthopedics and Traumatology
Klinikum Bamberg
Bamberg, Germany

Michael J. Stuart, MD
Professor
Department of Orthopedic Surgery
Mayo Clinic
Rochester, Minnesota, USA

Luis Eduardo Passarelli Tirico, MD
Knee Surgeon
Orthopedic and Traumatology Institute
Hospital das Clinicas;
Assistant Professor
University of São Paulo Medical School;
São Paulo, Brazil

Elizabeth C. Truelove, MD
Orthopedist
University of Chicago Medical Center
University of Chicago
Chicago, Illinois, USA

David Volgas, MD
Orthopaedic Surgeon
Department of Orthopedic Surgery
University of Missouri Health Care
Columbia, Missouri, USA

André Wajnsztejn, MD, MBA, PhD
Orthopaedic Surgeon
Hospital Israelita Albert Einstein
São Paulo, Brazil

Yukai Wang, MD
Orthopaedic Surgeon
Department of Orthopaedic Surgery
Shanghai Sixth People's hospital
Shanghai Jiaotong University
Shanghai, China

Ryan J. Warth, MD
Director of Operations
REDCap Cloud
Houston, Texas, USA

Jacob Worsham, MD
Assistant Professor
Orthopaedic Surgery - Sports Medicine
University of Texas at Houston
Houston, Texas, USA

Richard S. Yoon, MD
Director of Orthopaedic Research
Department of Orthopaedic Surgery
Division of Orthopaedic Trauma & Adult Reconstruction
Saint Barnabas Medical Center
Livingston, New Jersey, USA

Connor G. Ziegler, MD
Orthopedic Shoulder, Elbow, Hip, and Knee Specialist
New England Orthopedic Surgeons,
Springfield, Massachusetts, USA

Section I

Trauma

I

1 Unilateral Lateral Tibial Plateau Fractures

David Hubbard

1.1 Description

This procedure is intended for use in isolated lateral tibial plateau fractures, which typically are associated with cortical disruption (the split component) and articular impaction (the depression component) (▶ Fig. 1.1). The articular surface is reduced, and fixation applied.

1.2 Key Principles

The lateral tibial plateau is exposed using an extensile lateral surgical approach with direct visualization of the articular surface (if needed) under the lateral meniscus through a submeniscal arthrotomy (▶ Fig. 1.2). This allows evaluation of the lateral meniscus and repair as necessary. Depressed articular fragments are elevated. Metaphyseal defects are filled with bone graft or bone graft substitute (▶ Fig. 1.3). Compression of the intra-articular fracture lines is applied. A buttressing-type implant is applied. This is usually a nonlocking implant. There is no indication for a locking implant other than severe osteoporosis. Many implant companies have specific proximal tibial implants.

1.3 Expectations

The technique provides good visualization of the anterior and central articular surface, but repair of posterior articular impaction is more difficult. Outcomes are generally good when knee alignment and stability are restored, even if there is some residual articular incongruity. The goal is an articular reduction that is stepped off less than 2 millimeters. Despite the high likelihood of associated soft tissue injury to knee ligaments or menisci, late surgery is uncommon, and the risk of posttraumatic arthritis is low.

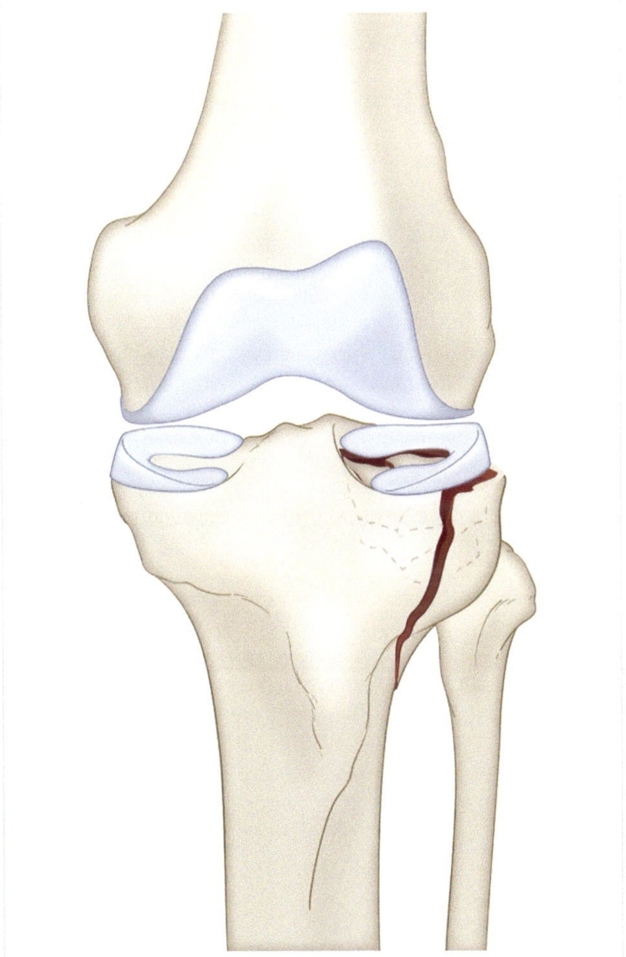

Fig. 1.1 Illustration of a typical split-depression fracture of the lateral tibial plateau.

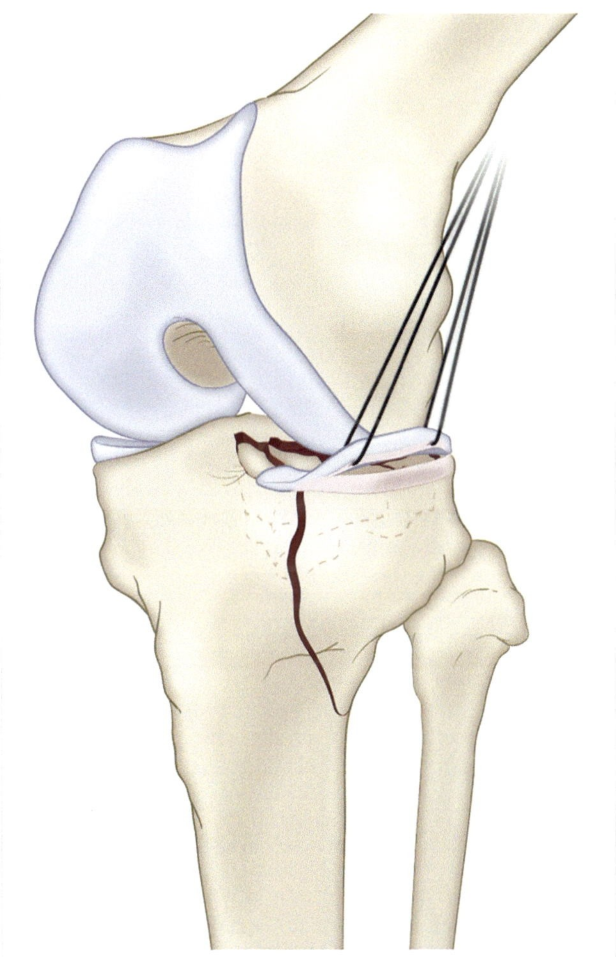

Fig. 1.2 Illustration of the use of a submeniscal arthrotomy to improve intraoperative visualization of the articular fracture.

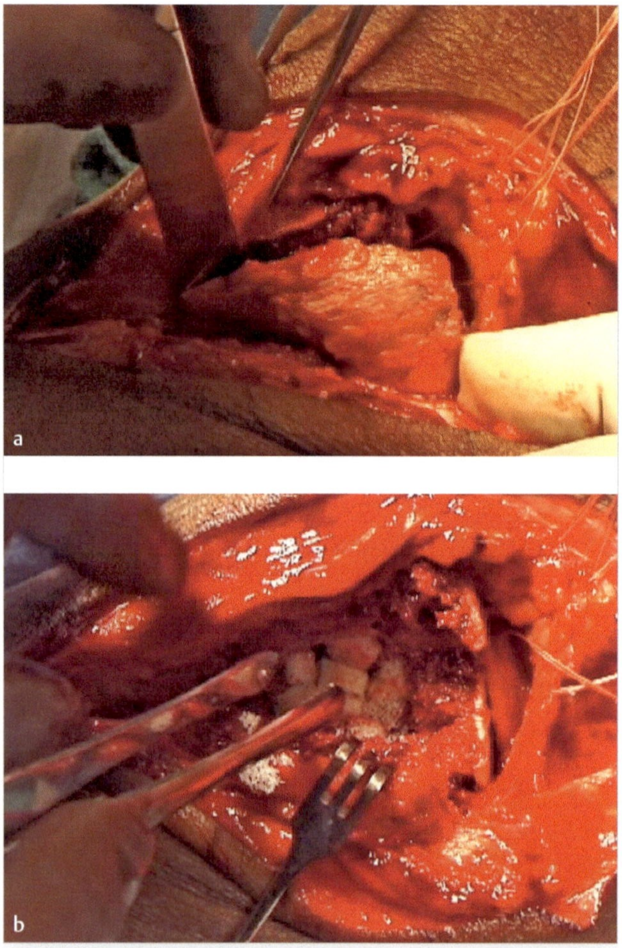

Fig. 1.3 (a,b) Bone graft (in this case cancellous allograft chips) are placed in the metaphyseal defect that is present after elevation of the articular surface.

1.4 Indications

General indications for surgical treatment of a lateral tibial plateau fracture include articular surface step-off and/or depression, joint instability, and/or widening of the proximal tibia relative to the contralateral side.

1.5 Contraindications

Contraindications include soft tissue injury that precludes a safe surgical approach or a medically unstable patient. For example, fracture blisters and/or abrasions should be allowed to resolve, and skin "wrinkles" should be present.

1.6 Special Considerations

Prior to surgery, the three-dimensional anatomy must be completely understood. Most surgeons use computed tomography (CT) to better understand the fracture pattern; however, recently, some surgeons are advocating magnetic resonance imaging (MRI). The other important consideration is the state of the soft tissues. Significant swelling must be allowed to decrease prior to surgery and fracture blisters should be resolved.

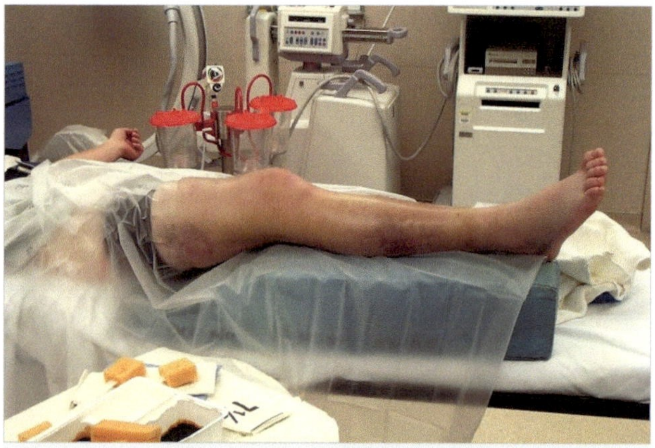

Fig. 1.4 Photo showing intraoperative positioning for surgical repair of a lateral tibial plateau fracture.

Compartment syndrome provides another challenge. Fasciotomies should be performed when indicated. The lateral fasciotomy incision can be aligned such that it is a continuation of the lateral approach incision. Before definitive fixation, the fasciotomy incision should be closed or closeable at that time.

1.7 Special Instructions, Positioning, and Anesthesia

The patient is positioned in the supine position. A bump is placed under the ipsilateral hip to slightly internally rotate the leg. A tourniquet is applied. A foam ramp or stack of blankets is placed under the leg to elevate it above the contralateral leg to make lateral fluoroscopy easier. The C-arm is brought in from the opposite side of the operative field and should be free to rotate between an anteroposterior (AP) view and lateral view. Anesthetic of choice is used but muscle paralysis is necessary (▶ Fig. 1.4).

1.8 Tips, Pearls, and Lessons Learned

1.8.1 Approach

After the skin incision is made, the fascia over the tibialis anterior muscle and the iliotibial band are divided to create one long continuous incision. The tibialis anterior is released off of the tibia as needed for plate fixation, and the iliotibial band may need to be released off of Gerdy tubercle. A submeniscal arthrotomy is then performed between the meniscus and the tibia. Sutures are then placed to provide superior retraction of the meniscus.

1.8.2 Visualization

Use of a universal or femoral distractor allows "opening" of the lateral joint, which is further facilitated by applying varus stress (▶ Fig. 1.5). Use of a headlight allows light to be directed into

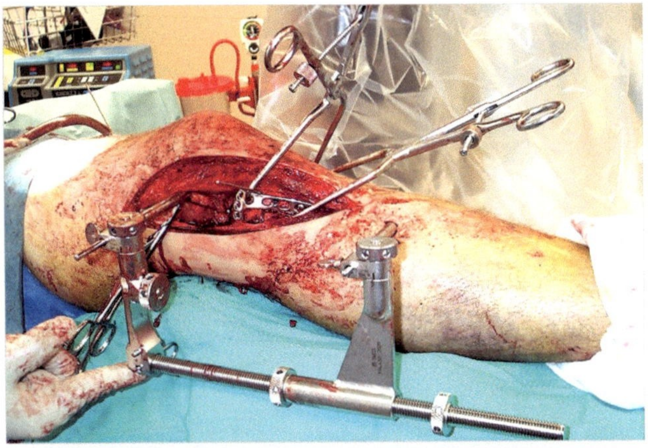

Fig. 1.5 Photo demonstrating the application of a distractor to assist in opening the lateral knee joint in order to facilitate fracture reduction.

the wound for better visualization. The anterior horn of the lateral meniscus can be divided and later repaired to further improve visualization.

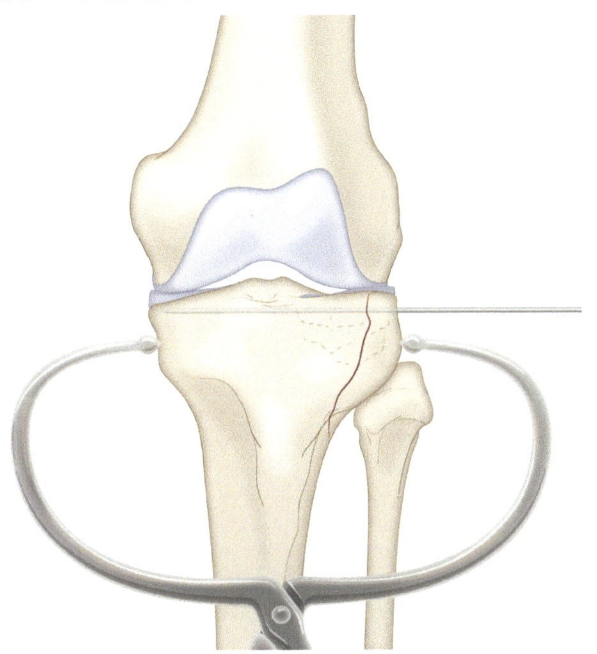

Fig. 1.6 Use of a "c-shaped" periarticular reduction clamp to provide external compression across the reduced metaphysis.

1.8.3 Fracture Reduction

How the fracture is reduced is dictated by whether it is a pure split fracture with no depression vs. a split/depression pattern. A pure split fracture pattern needs compression. After the joint surface is exposed, a large pelvic clamp or a specific periarticular clamp is used to squeeze the fragments together (▶ Fig. 1.6). The joint is visualized throughout the reduction. Once the joint is reduced anatomically, provisional K-wires are placed to maintain the reduction temporarily. This is then replaced by the definitive implant.

A split/depression pattern is reduced in a different fashion. One of two methods is used: the "containment method" or the "open book" method. In the containment method, the depressed area is elevated through a cortical window created with an osteotome (▶ Fig. 1.7). The split component is left until the articular surface is reestablished. This elevation is performed with a tamp or an impactor. The defect is filled with bone graft or bone graft substitute. The articular surface is supported with subchondral K-wires. The articular surface is then compressed with a clamp as above. In the open book method, the split component is hinged open anteriorly. This allows direct visualization of the depressed fragment(s) which is(are) then directly manipulated and reduced to either the lateral fragment or the medial intact joint surface. The defect is again filled with bone graft or substitute (▶ Fig. 1.3). The lateral fragment is then rotated to reduce it while visualizing the joint surface. This is then compressed with a clamp.

In all cases, the reduction is checked visually and with fluoroscopy.

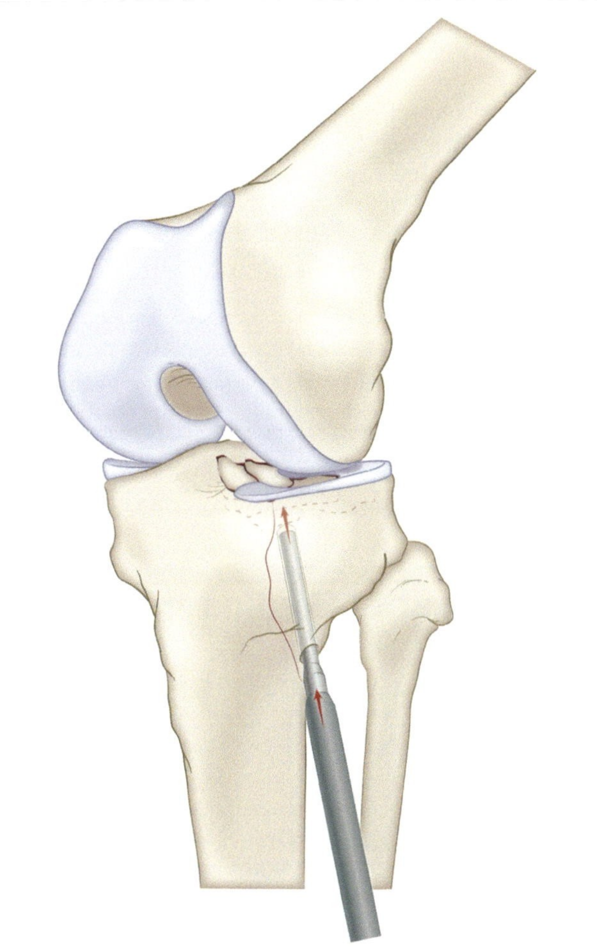

Fig. 1.7 Illustration of the use of a cylindrical bone tamp to elevated depressed articular fragments.

1.8.4 Internal Fixation

By definition, lateral-sided-only tibia plateau fractures need a plate that functions in a buttressing mode. The only exception is a purely depressed fracture which only needs subchondral support. For this reason, the most commonly used plates are nonlocking plates. Locked plates would only be used in the

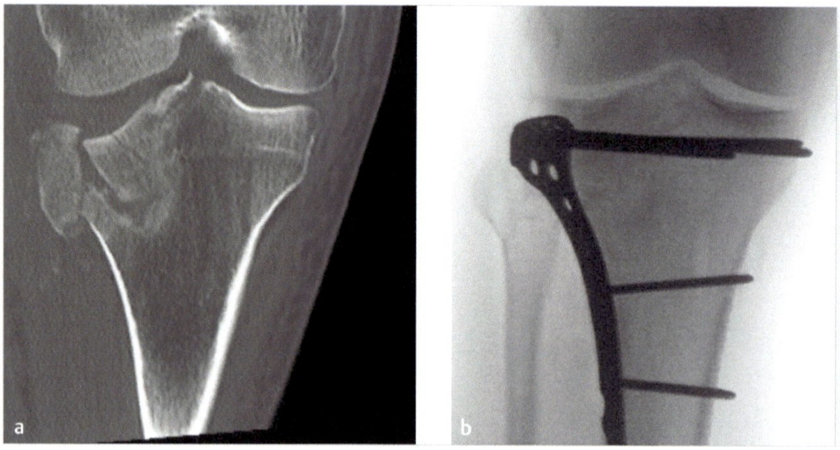

Fig. 1.8 (a,b) Radiographs of a split-depression fracture with large articular fragments stabilized with a precontoured nonlocking lateral tibial buttress plate.

case of poor bone quality. There are many commercially available "proximal tibial" plates. These can be large or small fragment implants.

In the case of a simple split fracture, a buttressing plate is applied after reduction as described above. The plate is positioned laterally; the first screw is placed just distal to the most distal extension of the fracture. Slight overcontouring of the plate will provide compression. Additional screws can then be placed more distally to secure diaphyseal fixation. Next, subchondral lag screws are applied to compress the joint (▶ Fig. 1.8).

In the case of a split/depression fracture, a similar plating technique is used to compress the joint as well. If the fragments are small, K-wires or small diameter screws may be used or left in position to support these fragments. So-called subchondral "raft screws" may also be applied to compress and support these previously depressed fragments (▶ Fig. 1.9).

Ideally, the plate length in any of these cases should allow for three to four screws distal to the most distal extent of the fracture laterally.

1.8.5 Closure

Wound closure is started by closing the submeniscal arthrotomy. The soft tissue on the proximal tibia is often either absent or of poor quality. Some plates provide holes for proximal suture fixation; however, the sutures can also be tied around the plate and/or the screw heads. The skin is closed with atraumatic technique.

1.9 Difficulties Encountered

If the area of articular injury and/or depression is posterior, visualization and fixation may be difficult. Exposure can be increased either by performing a fibular head osteotomy or a lateral epicondyle of the femur osteotomy. Identifying and reducing all impacted fracture fragments is important and facilitated by careful study of preoperative imaging including CT reconstructions. Sometimes, if the split portion of the fracture is incomplete, the vertical fracture can be completed to allow "opening of the book" to better see the metaphyseal cancellous bone. Skin closure problems should be anticipated, and soft tissues handled carefully. Incisions should be carefully planned over fracture lines to minimize the need for skin retraction.

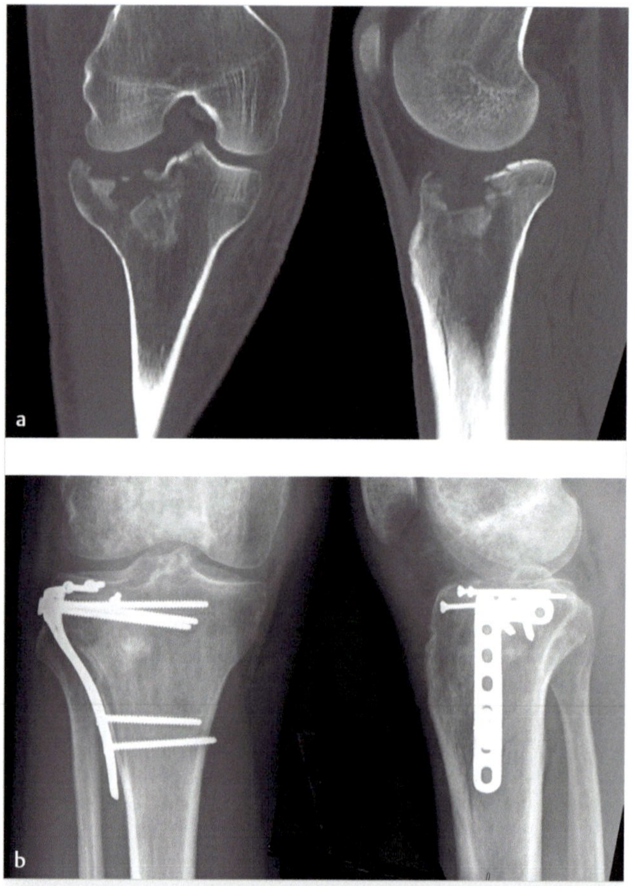

Fig. 1.9 (a,b) Radiographs of a split-depression fracture with comminuted articular fragments stabilized with two subchondral "raft" screws placed proximal to a precontoured lateral tibial buttress plate. In this case, because of fracture orientation, the raft screws are oriented from anterior to posterior in the lateral plateau.

1.10 Key Procedural Steps

- Exposure performed. The meniscus is retracted superiorly.
- Visualization adjuncts are applied as necessary.
  Reduction is judged by both direct visual inspection and fluoroscopy.

- Articular surface is reduced and provisionally held with K-wires. If the fracture pattern is a split/depression, the actual approach for articular reduction can be accomplished in one of two ways: The "containment" method where a cortical window is made and the articular depression is elevated from below with an impactor (▸ Fig. 1.7). The other method is by "opening the book." The split component is hinged open on its posterior aspect and the depressed segment is either reduced to the lateral fragment or the medial fragment and then the "book is closed" (▸ Fig. 1.3). If the posterior aspect is depressed, it can be elevated by a bone impactor and visualized from the anterior aspect. It is difficult to place implants more posterior unless a fibular head osteotomy is used to increase the exposure.
- Any residual bone void is filled with bone graft or bone graft substitute.

Articular fracture lines are compressed and a buttress plate is applied.

1.11 Bailout, Rescue, Salvage Procedures

The surgeon should be aware of methods to increase surgical exposure when needed, such as submeniscal arthrotomy, transection and repair of the anterior horn of the lateral meniscus, epicondylar osteotomy. The use of a joint distractor is rarely needed for lateral plateau fractures but could be of benefit in rare cases. In cases of postop compartment syndrome, immediate fasciotomy is warranted. Early plastic surgery referral for consideration of a gastrocnemius rotation flap should be considered in any case of wound breakdown or infection.

1.12 Pitfalls

One pitfall is failure to recognize or realize the position of a torn lateral meniscus. A tear of the lateral meniscus is almost always a peripheral tear that is seen upon creating the submeniscal arthrotomy. This is easily repaired during closure. However, the meniscus may not be seen in cases of split/depression fractures with severe depression. This is because the torn meniscus is trapped in the fracture site and must be retrieved before reduction can occur.

Another pitfall is failure to recreate the patient's previous alignment because of failure to completely elevate the depressed joint surface. This can be checked by comparing radiographs or fluoroscopic views of the opposite normal knee. You must compare axial alignment as well as the posterior slope of the lateral joint surface.

Finally, joint stability must be checked once fixation and joint closure are complete. This can be performed and visualized with fluoroscopy. Valgus stress is applied to the knee in full extension to check for medial joint line gapping. The posterior and anterior cruciate ligaments should also be checked manually.

2 Unicondylar Medial Tibial Plateau Fractures

Nicholas P. Gannon and Andrew Schmidt

2.1 Description

This procedure addresses unicondylar medial tibial plateau fractures, repair of which may require reconstruction of the articular surface, restoration and containment of the rim of the tibial plateau, and buttress plate fixation of the metaphyseal component of the fracture.

2.2 Key Principles

Unicondylar medial tibial plateau fractures are associated with high-energy trauma and have a high risk of associated soft tissue and neurovascular injury. With large shear-type medial condyle fractures, the tibial shaft and lateral tibial plateau translate laterally from the medial plateau and femur, representing a knee dislocation variant. These fractures usually have gross mechanical instability. A staged treatment approach via temporary knee-spanning external fixator allows assessment and treatment of various injuries at appropriate times.

Medial tibial plateau fractures can be considered as a split wedge wherein the primary fracture plane bisects the tibial plateau rim, exiting at the level of the proximal tibial metaphysis. It is critical to recognize the primary morphology of the main fracture fragment, since it determines the surgical approach. The plane of the fracture is quite variable, and although the sagittal fracture most often comes to mind, in approximately 60% of medial tibial plateau fractures, the main fracture is in the coronal plane (▶ Fig. 2.1, ▶ Fig. 2.2, ▶ Fig. 2.3). In a significant number of the cases, the main fracture plane extends to the lateral tibial plateau and is associated with comminution of the posterolateral aspect of the rim.

In the simple fracture patterns, a buttress plate placed on the metaphysis parallel to the main fracture plane restores the stability of the fracture and the patient's limb alignment. More complex fracture patterns, such as those associated with comminution of the posterolateral tibial plateau, are more difficult to manage due to the limited area available for buttress plate fixation. The surgeon can choose to attempt anatomical reduction of this area, or instead restore containment of the rim of the tibial plateau.

Fractures in the sagittal plane can be approached using a direct medial incision, whereas fractures oriented in the coronal plane require a posteromedial approach. For fractures without articular comminution, reduction of the metaphyseal fracture may be direct with the assumption that an anatomic cortical "read" will result in indirect articular reduction as well (verified using imaging or arthroscopy). For fractures that extend to the lateral tibial plateau, any articular comminution or depression will require direct articular reduction and possible bone grafting. This may be accomplished through the same approach used for the application of the buttress plate, provided it is possible to reduce the fracture using a bone tamp introduced throughout the main fracture plane. Alternatively, extended approaches to the lateral tibial plateau condyle may grant exposure to the posterolateral depressed fragments, allowing for their direct reduction and support with bone grafting. Fixation is typically performed with a nonlocking implant.

2.3 Expectations

This fracture pattern carries the worst prognosis of tibial plateau fractures because of the greater potential morbidity from associated neurovascular injury. Patients generally have favorable outcomes in the absence of neurovascular injury, compartment syndrome, or significant soft tissue compromise and can expect reasonable function and range of motion. Posttraumatic arthritis is uncommon, although slightly higher in those with fracture extension into the intercondylar eminence. Associated injuries to the posterolateral corner of the knee should be documented either with preoperative magnetic resonance imaging (MRI) or physical exam under anesthesia after fixing the medial

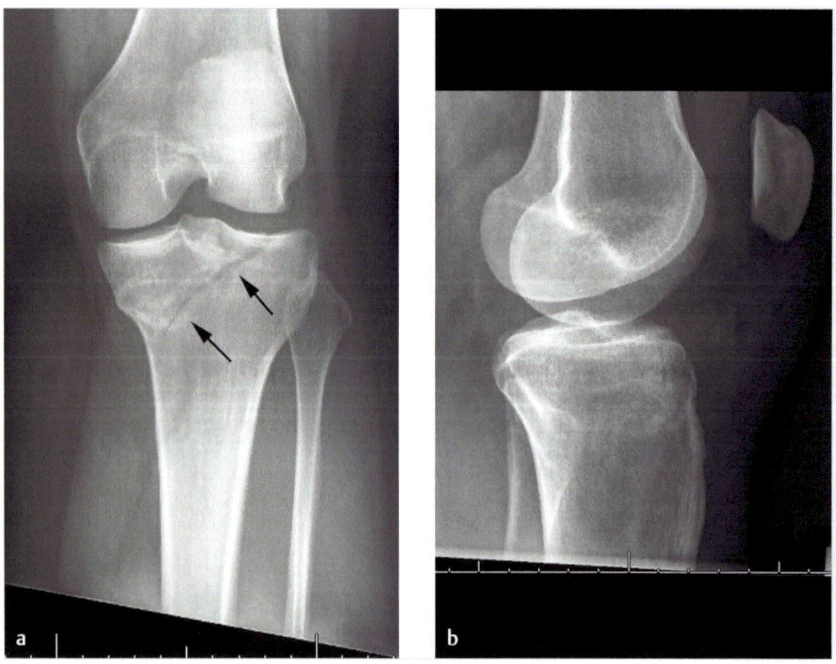

Fig. 2.1 (a,b) Radiographs of a simple sagittal split fracture of the medial tibial plateau: anteroposterior and lateral views.

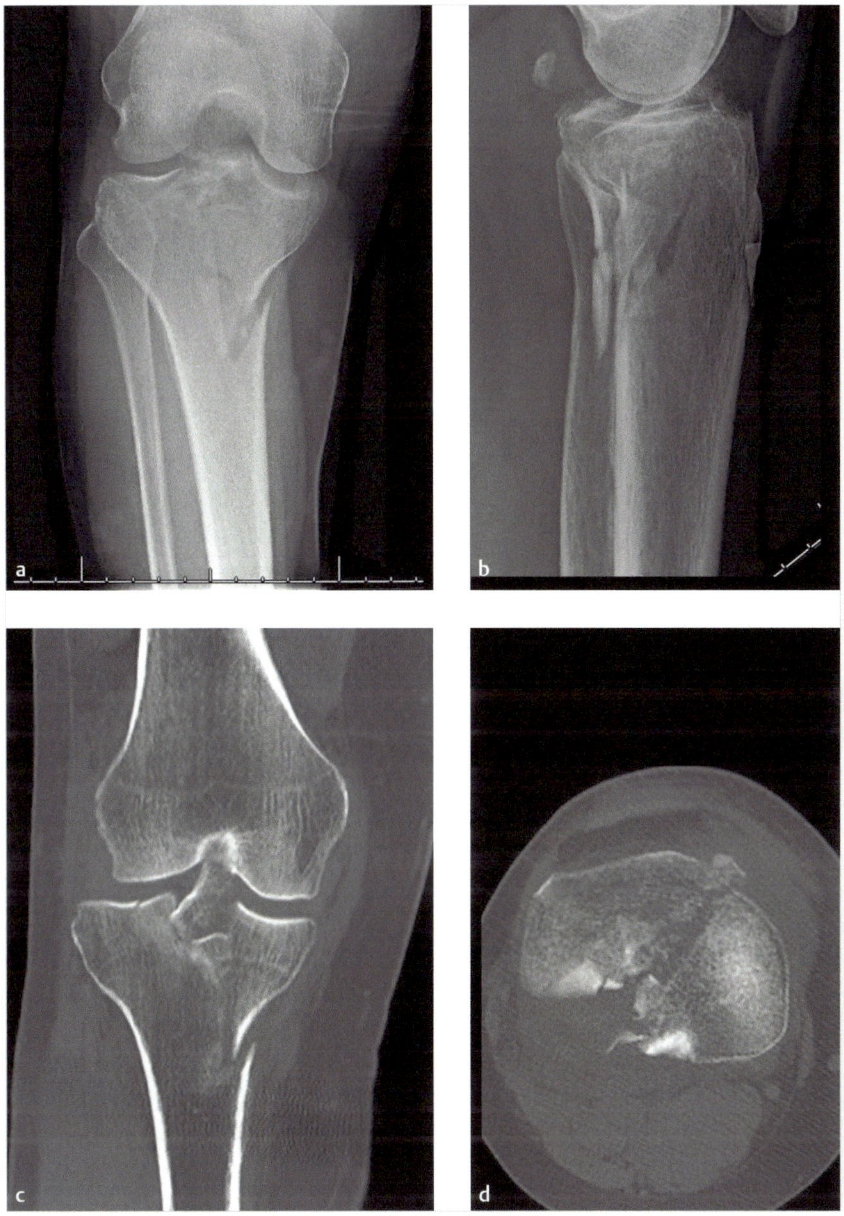

Fig. 2.2 (a-d) Images of a comminuted medial tibial plateau fracture that is largely in the sagittal plane, but with articular and posterior cortical comminution: anteroposterior and lateral radiographs (top panels) and CT images (bottom panels).

tibial plateau. In case of posterolateral instability, a reconstruction of the posterolateral corner should be planned, aiming to avoid secondary failure of the internal fixation.

2.4 Indications

General indications for surgical management include varus angulation of the knee ≥ 5 degrees associated with fracture displacement, articular step-off or gap of ≥ 2 mm, articular impaction of ≥ 5 mm, osseous or ligamentous joint instability, or evidence of complications such as compartment syndrome, vascular injury, or an open fracture.

2.5 Contraindications

Open surgical repair of a medial tibial plateau fracture should not be performed when there is a threatened or compromised soft tissue envelope as evidenced by fracture blisters, contaminated skin abrasions, or deep skin contusion or necrosis. In such cases, "damage control" with placement of a provisional spanning external fixation should be carried out. Special consideration is needed when considering internal fixation of open fractures or fractures complicated by acute compartment syndrome if the wounds will leave exposed hardware. Patients should be appropriately resuscitated prior to surgery and without medical comorbidities precluding safe anesthesia.

2.6 Special Considerations

In high-energy injuries, associated local soft-tissue injury should be assumed and definitive fixation delayed. Medial tibial plateau fractures have increased risk of injury to the popliteal artery and its trifurcation. There is additional risk of injury to soft tissues including the cruciate ligaments (often evidenced by avulsion fractures of the intercondylar eminence), posterolateral corner (popliteus tendon and popliteal fibular ligament), and menisci. With substantial varus displacement of the knee joint, the common peroneal nerve can be susceptible to traction injury.

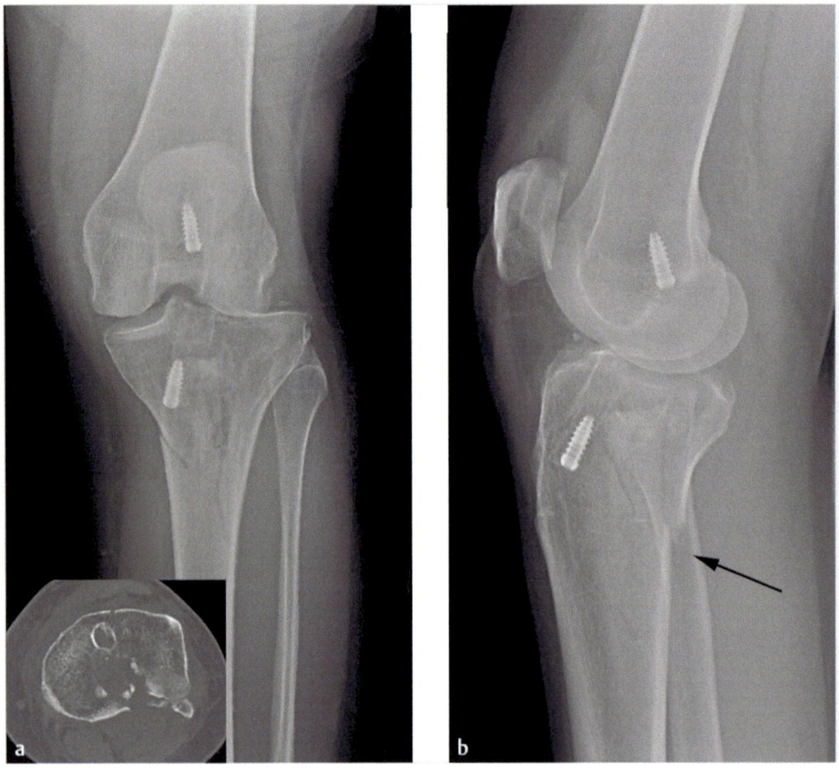

Fig. 2.3 (a,b) Images of a comminuted coronal plane proximal tibia fracture, in a patient with remote history of anterior cruciate ligament (ACL) reconstruction. Anteroposterior and lateral radiographs shown with a cross-section computed tomography (CT) images (inset, lower left).

At presentation, a thorough physical exam should be performed. Patients with vascular injuries should undergo exploration and necessary revascularization. Those with compartment syndrome should undergo immediate fasciotomy. A temporary knee-spanning external fixator provides immediate stability when definitive fixation is contraindicated in the acute setting. Computed tomography after external fixation scans allow better fracture assessment and facilitates preoperative planning. If ligamentous injury is suspected, MRI can be useful, preferably prior to external fixation as this causes artifact.

2.7 Special Instructions, Positioning, and Anesthesia

Patients undergoing fracture repair using a medial approach are positioned supine on a radiolucent table. A posteromedial approach can also be done with the leg supine, but care should be taken to make sure that the patient's ipsilateral hip can abduct and externally rotate in order to provide more access to the posteromedial tibia (▶ Fig. 2.4). A bump can be placed under the contralateral hip to externally rotate the operative extremity to further facilitate the posteromedial approach. If a straight posterior (Lobenhoffer) approach is selected, the patient is positioned prone. A nonsterile tourniquet is placed high on the thigh. Approach is eased with the surgeon positioned contralateral and the C-arm positioned ipsilateral to the injury. For medial approaches, the operative extremity can be placed on a commercially available foam ramp or blanket stack for elevation to optimize lateral fluoroscopy. General anesthesia is typically used with paralysis based on surgeon preference.

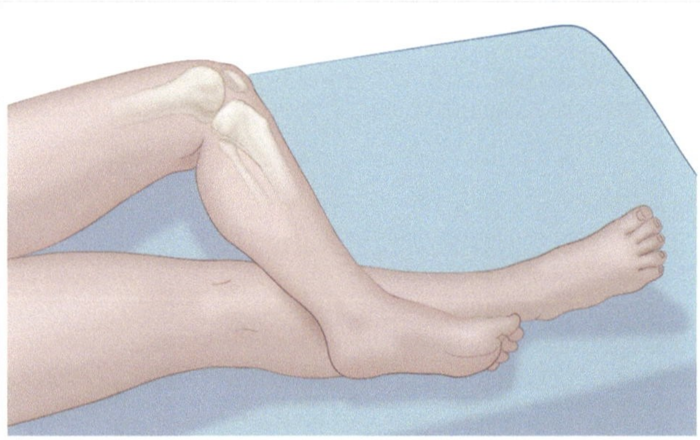

Fig. 2.4 Illustration of patient position for posteromedial approach in the supine position.

2.8 Tips, Pearls, and Lessons Learned

- It is crucial for the surgeon to recognize any associated neurovascular injuries prior to temporization, reduction, and fixation. Medial tibial plateau injuries may be a component of an injury that actually represents a knee fracture-dislocation, and the initial evaluation would demand precise and thorough documentation of motor and sensation in the injured limb, and measurement of ankle-brachial index (ABI). An ABI of 0.9 or less demands vascular surgery consultation.
- Obtain radiographs of the uninjured, contralateral knee for comparison to restore native condylar width and slope.
- In the circumstance of the application of a spanning external fixation, make sure that the knee dislocation is reduced by

obtaining multiple fluoroscopic projections during the procedure.
- Preoperatively plan screw position to allow for possible future ligament reconstruction.
- If fasciotomy is to be performed, plan the fasciotomy incision with consideration for future incisions needed for open reduction internal fixation.
- Headlights can be utilized to direct light into the surgical field.
- A medially placed universal femoral distractor serves to remove the femoral deforming force on the tibial plateau and distract the knee joint. If a knee-spanning external fixator was placed as a temporizing measure it is also used to distract the joint, promoting ligamentotaxis.
- If using a posteromedial approach, retractors should be placed anterior to the popliteus muscle to avoid injury to the popliteal vessels.
- Avoid violation of the deep medial collateral ligament. Don't peel off the medial collateral ligament from the upper tibia in order to expose the metaphyseal area.
- Knee flexion can relax the posterior neurovascular bundle to aid in its protection, and also prevent surgeon's ability to get the fracture reduced because the femoral condyle may push the tibial plateau down. Once safe exposure has been obtained, reduction is best obtained with the knee in extension, secured with K-wires and then the knee may be slightly flexed for the application of a posteromedial buttress plate.
- Preposition K-wires in the medial fragment to use as a joystick and to pass for provisional fixation once reduction is obtained.
- A mildly undercontoured plate can aid in reduction and compression.
- Locked plates offer low utility in this setting, except in the case of severe osteoporosis or poor bone quality.
- Place the first cortical screws immediately distal to the fragment apex.
- Depending on fracture orientation and obliquity to the frontal plane, plate placement may need to be directly medial, posteromedial, or a combination of both. A buttress plate should always be placed parallel to the main fracture plane. The plate will preferably be placed exactly where the surgeon would like to have his/her thumb.
- Percutaneous plate application is efficacious for a fracture with diaphyseal extension.
- In the setting of an open fracture resulting in a soft tissue defect, a rotational flap from the medial head of the gastrocnemius is an excellent option for coverage.
- After definitive fixation, a complete physical exam under anesthesia should be performed to assess ligamentous integrity. If functional instability is indicated, staged ligament reconstruction should occur.

2.9 Difficulties Encountered

Thoroughly interrogate imaging to identify lateral condylar fracture or depression for appropriate surgical planning. Failure to identify associated soft tissue injuries will limit postoperative stability, rehabilitation, and functional outcomes. Carefully plan incisions to obtain adequate fracture exposure, especially in the setting of fasciotomy.

2.10 Key Procedural Steps

2.10.1 Straight Medial Approach

- The patient is positioned supine, and the leg prepped from the upper thigh to the ankle with a tourniquet in place. The knee is kept slightly flexed.
- The incision is directly over the medial tibia, beginning distal to the medial epicondyle of the distal femur and continuing distally toward the tibial crest.
- The superficial dissection is through the sartorius fascia, and the pes anserinus is identified in the proximal and posterior part of the incision. The pes and superficial medial collateral ligament can be divided and repaired. The medial collateral ligament should not be peeled off the tibia. Care should be taken to avoid injury to the deep medial collateral ligament. Beware of the infrapatellar branch of saphenous nerve, the saphenous vein, the medial inferior genicular artery, and the popliteal artery.
- The fracture is exposed and debrided of clot and any soft tissue that is in the fracture site. Direct reduction of the metaphyseal fracture is obtained. Articular reduction is confirmed indirectly using fluoroscopy.
- Kirschner wires are used for provisional fixation. Pointed reduction forceps placed perpendicular to the fracture plane can provide compression. Depending on fracture orientation, a small incision can be made laterally to place reduction forceps.
- A buttress plate is applied direct on the medial surface of the tibia. Depending on the anatomy, the pes tendons can be partially released, but the plate can be placed over the tendons as well (▶ Fig. 2.5).
- Routine skin closure is performed.

2.10.2 Lobenhoffer Posteromedial Approach in the Prone or Supine Position

- Position the patient prone or supine with a bump under the opposite hip to facilitate exposure of the posteromedial leg.
- An 8-cm incision is made along the medial border of the medial head of the gastrocnemius, beginning at the joint line and extending distally. Beware of the small saphenous vein in the proximal aspect of the incision; usually it lies between the two heads of the gastrocnemius.
- Incise the medial gastrocnemius fascia and retract the medial gastrocnemius laterally.
- Identify the pes anserinus tendons and retract them medially or incise them for later repair depending on fracture pattern.
- Fracture access is anterior to the medial head of the gastrocnemius. The popliteus muscle should be elevated from the tibia for further fracture exposure and also to allow proper placement of Hohmann elevator, protecting the neurovascular bundle (▶ Fig. 2.6).
- Reduction is often aided from knee extension, axial traction, valgus force, and slight internal rotation.
- Direct reduction of the metaphyseal fracture is obtained. Articular reduction is confirmed indirectly using fluoroscopy.
- Kirschner wires are used for provisional fixation. Pointed reduction forceps aid for compression perpendicular to the

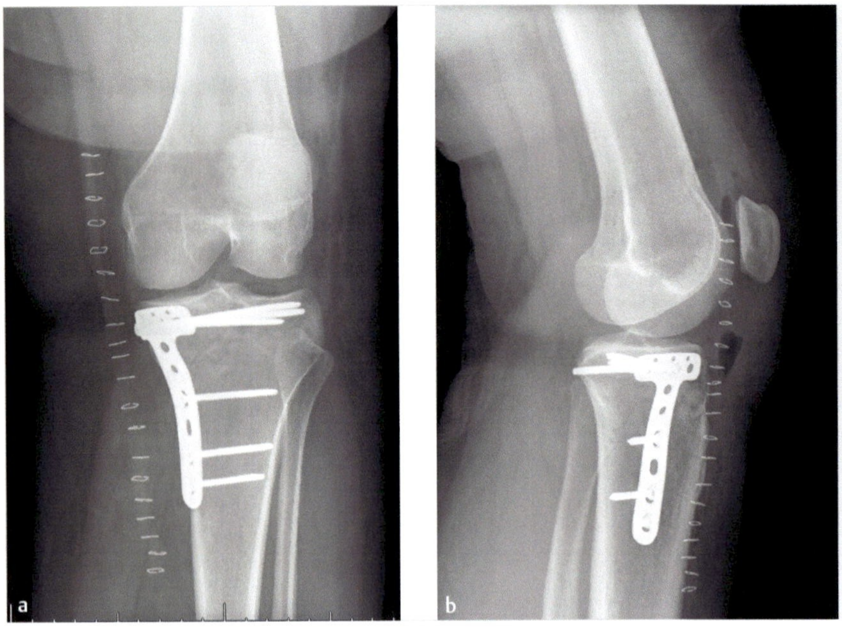

Fig. 2.5 (a,b) Example of a medial buttress plate for a sagittal split fracture of the medial tibial plateau (same case as shown in ▶ Fig. 2.1).

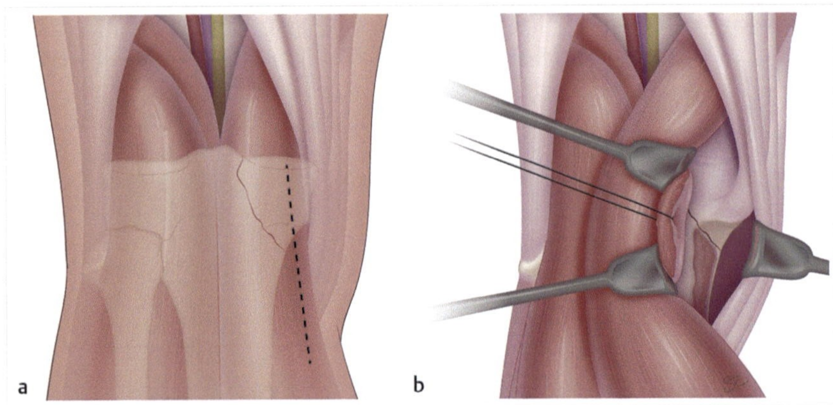

Fig. 2.6 (a,b) Illustration of Lobenhoffer approach to the posteromedial proximal tibia.

fracture plane. Depending on fracture orientation, a small incision can be made laterally to place a reduction forceps.

- A buttress plate is applied underneath the pes tendons and posterior to the superficial medial collateral ligament insertion. Precontoured periarticular plates are commercially available, often 3.5 mm, allowing for shorter OR time without the need to contour intraoperatively (▶ Fig. 2.7).
- If fragment permits, cruciate avulsion fractures should be fixed using small screws or suture-through drill holes.

2.11 Bailout, Rescue, Salvage Procedures

Fracture pattern variation can warrant the need for increased exposure. A medial submeniscal arthrotomy is rarely needed, as articular commination and depression are uncommon. The pes anserinus tendons can be divided longitudinally or tagged and reflected from their insertion, later repaired while closing. The superficial medial collateral ligament may be longitudinally split, but not transversally divided in such an exposure. Subperiosteal elevation of the popliteus from its origin proximally and the soleus from its origin distally on the posteromedial tibia is beneficial to expose the fracture site, and to protect the neurovascular bundle. The medial head of the gastrocnemius can also be released; however, take care to identify and protect the medial inferior genicular artery. In addition, the posteromedial approach can be extensile distally for more complex fractures.

2.12 Pitfalls

- Position the leg in a way to ensure accessible angles to place all screws.
- A midline incision is not recommended for unicondylar medial tibial plateau fractures, as it is quite difficult to place a medial-sided plate secondary to required soft tissue dissection and stripping. An incision placed too anteriorly may place the saphenous nerve and vein at risk of injury in the superficial dissection. Place the incision 1 to 2 cm posterior to the posteromedial edge of the tibial metaphysis.
- During surgical exposure, one may avoid popliteal neurovascular bundle injury by elevating the popliteus muscle from the posterior tibia, keeping the muscle as a buffer between the surgical exposure and the popliteal space.

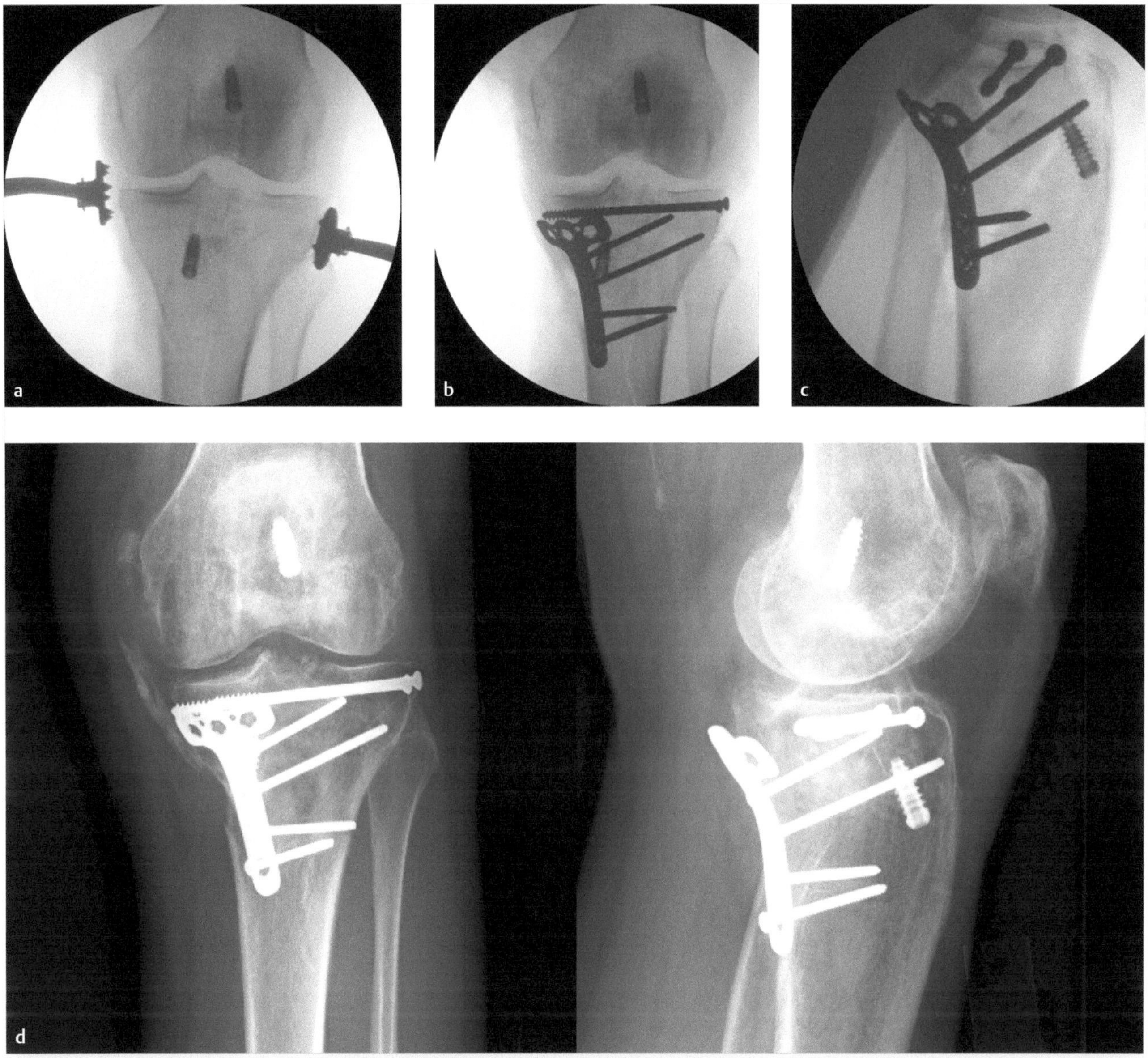

Fig. 2.7 **(a–d)** Example of a posteromedial buttress plate for a coronal split fracture of the medial tibial plateau (same case as shown in ▶ Fig. 2.3). **(a)** Intraoperative fluoroscopic view in the coronal plane showing a reduction clamp used to restore the width of the tibial plateau. **(b)** Intraoperative anteroposterior and **(c)** lateral views of the completed fixation. The lateral–medial lag screws were used to restore the width of the plateau, while a posteromedial plate was used to buttress the posteromedial fracture fragment. **(d)** Final radiographs after healing.

- Subtle fracture malreduction can lead to varus collapse, promoting early posttraumatic arthritis. Once exposure is obtained, reduction of the fracture with the knee in extension can facilitate accurate realignment.
- A perfect reduction "read" at the apex of the fracture may not translate into anatomical reduction of the rim of the tibial plateau because the fracture fragment may be rotated. Taking a proper "plateau view" of the joint (with the image intensifier angled 10 degrees posteriorly) will help to identify a double contour at the level of the joint surface, indicating articular malreduction.
- Percutaneous fixation is not often recommended secondary to fracture pattern instability.
- Locking plates are only indicated for patients with severe osteoporosis, as locked screws may only help secure fixation without providing necessary compression.
- Utilize anesthesia to examine for associated ligamentous injury at the end of the case.
- Postoperative immobilization in a cast or splint will lead to knee stiffness. However, the use of a knee brace while the patient is sleeping could help avoid antalgic flexion contracture of the knee in the postoperative set.

3 Bicondylar Tibial Plateau Fractures

Mark A. Lee

3.1 Description

This procedure addresses the stabilization of bicondylar tibial plateau fractures. Because there is significant variation in the fracture pattern in these injuries, the surgeon must carefully analyze the specific fracture pattern in a given case and be able to adapt the general surgical procedure described to the case at hand.

3.2 Key Principles

3.2.1 Alignment

The most significant goal of surgery is restoration of functional alignment to the fractured limb. Frontal plan malalignment is problematic and easily detected with plain radiography. While alignment is difficult to ascertain in the operative theater, one should always attempt to restore the mechanical frontal plane axis. Sagittal plane malalignment may also be functionally significant and careful posterior buttressing of posterior sagittal fragments is critical to avoid late fracture displacement and dynamic instability.

3.2.2 Buttress

Presurgical analysis of the fracture displacement tendency and fragment position is critical to optimize buttressing efficiency in bicondylar fracture patterns. Surgical exposures must be carefully selected to allow precise application of buttressing implants to the metaphyseal apex of all significant partial articular fracture fragments. A number of different types of plates are frequently utilized for stabilization depending on the size, position, and anticipated load on the fragment requiring stabilization. Careful contouring of implants that optimizes plate bone contact just below the metaphyseal escape site is the most critical part of plate applications.

3.2.3 Articular Exposure

Typically, medial articular injury is absent or of minimal severity, and the medial fracture line may be either coronal or sagittal in orientation. There is more significant variation in the lateral fracture pattern with varying amounts and location of depression. Understanding the fracture pattern is the key to choosing the necessary surgical exposure(s). Multiple approaches to optimizing the surgical viewing of the knee joint are critical for the articular reconstruction of these fractures. Submeniscal arthrotomy verifies adequate articular reduction versus radiographically guided joint restoration. Mechanical joint distraction is extremely helpful in improving the local joint distraction and adds little surgical time or morbidity. More aggressive surgical releases can be performed (epicondylar osteotomies) to maximize joint distraction and allow for more invasive viewing of the more midline and posterior parts of the joint.

3.2.4 Compression of Articular Segment

The major articular fracture lines must be compressed to optimize stability. The joint must be narrowed to native width. Traditional implants that provide plate-bone contact and compression are favored at the joint level to optimize compression. Locking implants have utility in securing fixation in poor quality bone only after the fracture segments have been compressed and the joint has been narrowed to native width.

3.3 Expectations

In the absence of major soft tissue complications (compartment syndrome, surgical site infection, wound dehiscence), outcomes are usually very good. Early hardware instability is unusual and functional return is typically excellent. With few exceptions, patients can expect return to preinjury functional status within 4 to 6 months. Posttraumatic arthritis is rare if limb alignment is restored and the knee is functionally stable.

3.4 Indications

These are complete articular fractures and are treated surgically to restore articular congruity, joint stability, and limb alignment. Specific surgical indications.

- Open fracture:
  - These are uncommon but indicative of high-energy trauma.
- Displaced fracture:
  - Some patterns will have minimal articular displacement but still require articular compression.
- Unstable knee:
  - Joint instability resulting from fracture instability or ligamentous injury is problematic for long-term function and joint longevity.
- Compartment syndrome:
  - Occurs in up to 30% of high-energy tibial plateau fractures and changes sequence/timing of fracture care.

3.5 Contraindications

- Massive soft tissue swelling or major soft tissue injury: In such circumstances, a staged protocol with temporary knee-spanning external fixation may be utilized.
- Severe medical illnesses.
- Active joint infection.

3.6 Special Considerations

Fractures with associated compartment syndrome require specific planning. Optimal management is feasible when the surgeon performing the fasciotomies is the same surgeon performing the articular reconstruction. In this setting, the anticipated surgical incisions can be drawn on the extremity and the fasciotomy incisions can be modified to maintain safe skin bridges. The surgical timing of fixation is controversial and may be done at the time of fasciotomy, the time of fasciotomy closure, or in a delayed fashion. Early fixation of the fracture does not seem to increase risk in this setting, but soft tissue reconstruction may be needed.

3.7 Special Instructions, Position, and Anesthesia

Positioning is dependent on the selected surgical exposure. While many bicondylar patterns can be managed using the supine position (anterolateral and posteromedial incisions), lateral and/or "floating" (floppy lateral) patient positions are typically utilized for extensile lateral, posterolateral, or extensile posteromedial (Reverse-L) approaches. Select the position that optimizes the most challenging exposure and reduction for the case at hand.

Anesthesia is usually general since regional blocks may mask postoperative symptoms of compartment syndrome in select cases. Muscle paralysis is rarely useful, especially when mechanical distraction is utilized.

3.8 Tips, Pearls, and Lessons Learned

- Computed tomography (CT) is indispensable in understanding the position, size, and displacements of the articular fragments in complicated fractures.
- Bicondylar tibial plateau fractures are most typically a result of high-energy trauma; caution and potentially staged protocols are appropriate to avoid soft tissue complications from the multiple surgical approaches that are frequently required to effectively buttress these fractures and restore stable alignment.
- Preoperative fluoroscopic images of the uninjured contralateral limb should be obtained on the fluoroscopy unit.
- Center your incisions on the articular zone so that you are not impeded by soft tissues during exposure.
- Mechanical distraction always improves joint exposure and assists in restoration of alignment in highly comminuted fractures.
- Start reconstructions with the condylar fragment that has a reliable reduction "read." Many times, the medial fracture is simpler in configuration at the metaphyseal exit site, and reduction of that extra-articular spike allows for correct positioning of the whole condylar fragment.

3.9 Difficulties Encountered

Delayed repairs past 3 weeks are particularly difficult, especially when trans-articular distraction has not been maintained. These late fixations should be avoided at all costs.

3.10 Key Procedural Steps

- The fracture must be converted from a bicondylar pattern to a unicondylar pattern by reduction and preliminary fixation of the most intact condylar segment. Almost always this will be the medial condyle or frequently the posteromedial segment

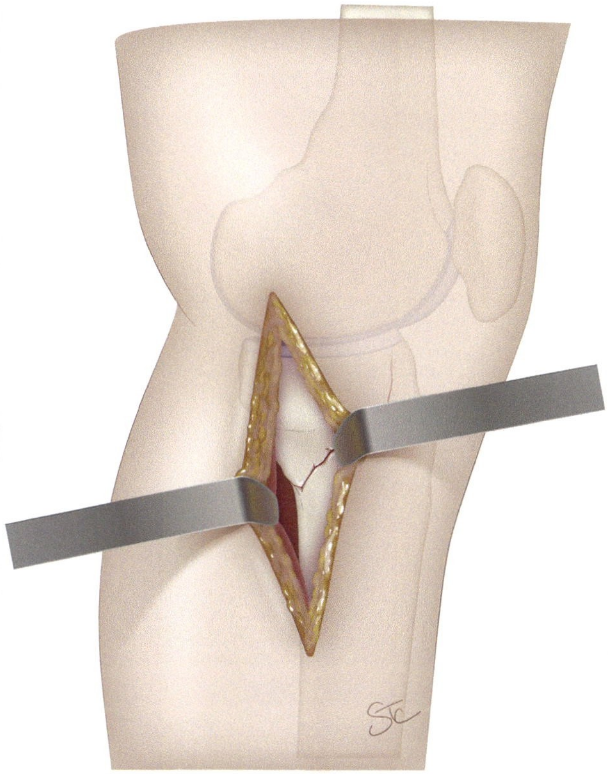

Fig. 3.1 An exposure is selected that provides visualization and plating access to the medial metaphyseal fracture escape site.

of the medial condyle. Identify the metaphyseal apex and provide an efficiently positioned buttressing plate aligned at the apex of the metaphyseal escape site of the fragment. The medial plate may need to be posteromedial or directly medial depending on the location of the fracture apex (▶ Fig. 3.1). Use a plate with some flexibility and undercontour the plate slightly to optimize fragment contact (▶ Fig. 3.2). Mechanical distraction is frequently helpful in achieving this but sometimes the medial fragment reduction requires flexion and mechanical traction is less straightforward.
- Lateral joint reduction requires optimal visualization. Radiographic indirect reduction is not reliable in complicated articular patterns. Perform an aggressive exposure to view the joint surface, utilizing mechanical distraction as needed. Always perform a submeniscal arthrotomy to directly view the articular reduction. Focused lighting (headlight) is very helpful in viewing deeper parts of the joint. A laterally based mechanical distraction device is indispensable in optimizing joint distraction and exposure (▶ Fig. 3.3).
- In multisegment articular injuries, maximize exposure by rotating anterior fragments out of the joint to view the deeper parts of the joint. Consider osteotomy to improve visualization deeper into the joint. Rebuild the joint from the deepest or most medial part out laterally using wire fixation through the medial side of the joint. Wires can be pulled flush to the intra-articular side of the fragment to allow for lateral fragment apposition.
- In addition to articular reduction, you must optimize stability by compressing the articular surface and re-establishing joint

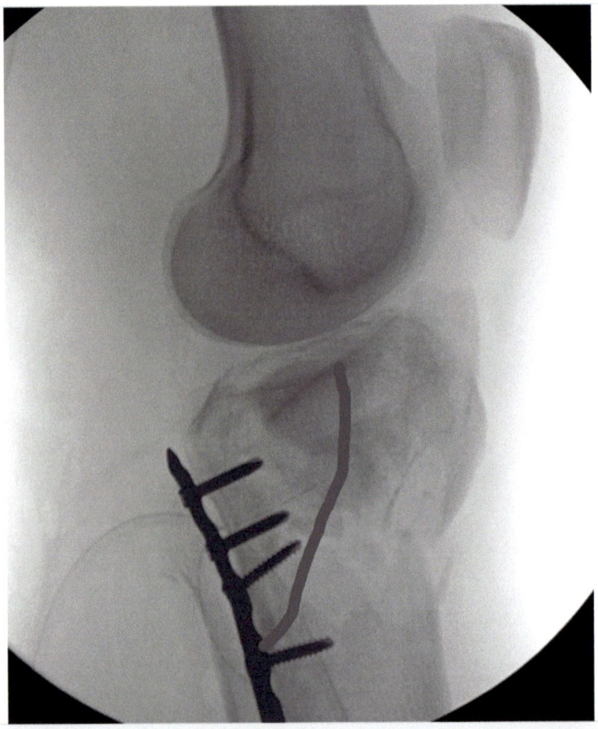

Fig. 3.2 Place buttress plate precisely in the anti-glide position at the apex of the fracture.

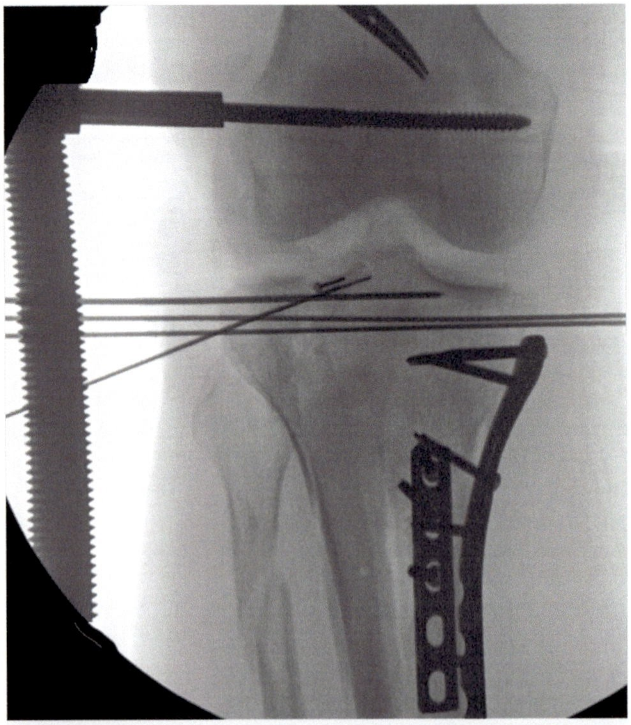

Fig. 3.3 Mechanical distraction is critical to optimize joint viewing and space to work.

width using periarticular clamps (▶ Fig. 3.4). These should ideally be clamped against implants to prevent intrusion and loss of compression strength.

- The joint requires compression for stability both across the articular segment and up from the metaphyseal segments. Avoid the use of locking screws until the compression has been optimized.

3.11 Bailout, Rescue, Salvage Procedures

Restoration of alignment should be prioritized in settings when the articular reduction cannot be optimized due to comminution or cartilage/bone loss. Always restore the stability of the meniscus to the capsule. Greater exposure may be helpful in the most complicated patterns. In this setting, lateral epicondylar osteotomy or tubercle osteotomy can maximize joint exposure; however, these should be reserved for the most complicated, severe articular injuries in younger patients.

Articular allografting is an option for nonreconstructable injuries but should likely be reserved for delayed treatment once soft tissues are optimized and risks for wound complications and infection is minimized.

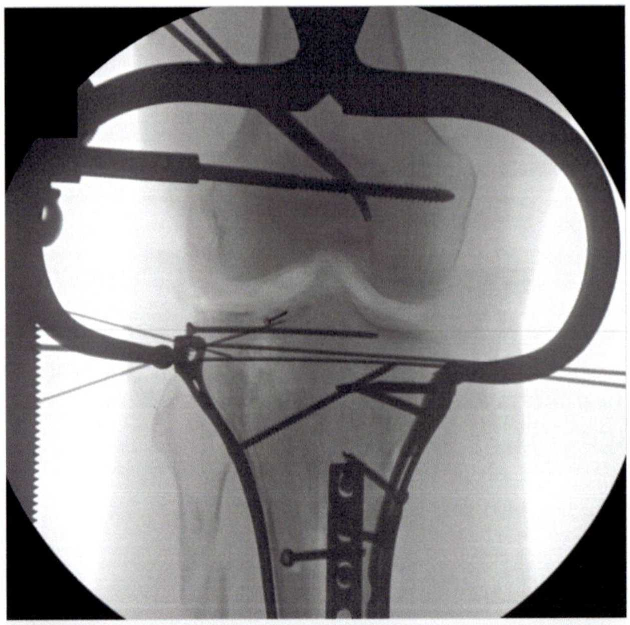

Fig. 3.4 A large peri-articular clamp is used to compress the articular surface to achieve interfragmentary compression and restore joint width.

3.12 Pitfalls

Misidentification of medial fracture dislocation variant as bicondylar facture is a common fixation error. The medial fracture dislocation variant may have a medial or a posteromedial fracture exit site or displacement which needs a specific buttressing approach. There may be a lateral articular injury requiring a separate, specific surgical approach. Most significantly, specific fracture dislocation variants have associated ligamentous injuries that may require repair or treatment.

A posteromedial sagittal fracture is present in a significant number of bicondylar fractures. The approach, reduction, and buttress must be performed through a posteromedial approach. The more anterior condylar fragment may require a separate buttressing implant. The posteromedial fracture fragment must have an optimal plate buttress as well and cannot be well controlled by locking screws from a laterally based implant.

Use of a locking implant that is not compressed to the bone and does not compress the joint back to normal medial to lateral width creates abnormal joint loading. Locking screws may be helpful for securing fixation in poor quality bone but are not helpful in producing desired joint compression.

The posterior approaches are excellent for buttressing posterior partial articular fragments but are not ideal for joint viewing. These approaches will frequently require simultaneous exposures to improve the ability to accurately reduce the articular fracture lines.

4 Tibial Plateau Fractures in the Coronal Plane

Yukai Wang and Congfeng Luo

4.1 Description

This procedure addresses tibial plateau fractures (TPFs) involving the posterior half of the tibial plateau, which require specific surgical approaches to restore knee stability and/or to address posterior articular impaction. The reversed-L approach can be used alone for posterior column fractures and can also be combined with lateral approaches for more complex injuries.

4.2 Key Principles

Surgical planning for posterior column TPFs can be formulated based on the initial "Three Column Classification" and further assessment of injury mechanism (▶ Fig. 4.1a, b). The fracture deformity is a result of the injury mechanism, which consists of two related parts, the position of the knee (flexion/extension) at the time of injury and the direction of the injury force (varus/valgus). Preoperative planning proceeds in step-by-step manner as follows: (1) evaluation of posterior tibial slope angle (pTSA) and medial tibial plateau angle (mTPA) by X-rays and CT images (▶ Fig. 4.2a, b); (2) analysis of injury mechanism via the above radiographic parameters; (3) determination of compression or tension fracture side according to the radiographic parameters (▶ Fig. 4.3); (4) involvement of the articular surface is assessed on computed tomography (CT) scans. Decreased mTPA and pTSA indicate a flexion-varus injury, which have posteromedial and posterolateral fractures in the coronal plane.

4.3 Expectations

Posterior column fractures always fall into either two-column or three-column TPFs and can be divided into flexion-valgus and flexion-varus accordingly. The reversed-L approach is mainly indicated for flexion injuries, which avoids injury to the posterolateral corner complex and the common peroneal nerve.

4.4 Indications

The surgical indications for coronal plane fractures of the posterior tibial plateau are the same as those for TPFs in general, including open fractures, fractures with neurovascular lesions or compartment syndrome, displaced intra-articular fractures, articular depression causing knee instability and fracture dislocations. Knee instability is the most important factor correlating with a need for surgery, and varus/valgus stress testing of the knee at 30-degrees of knee flexion is recommended. One must also look for posterior subluxation of the femur relative to the tibia on the lateral X-ray view.

4.5 Contraindications

- Poor general condition.
- Deep vein thrombosis (DVT) without proper treatment.
- Soft tissue lesions in the surgical field.

4.6 Special Considerations

Detailed preoperative assessment of soft tissues (skin, ligaments, and menisci), osseous, and associated injuries is critical. X-rays and CT scans allow complete understanding of the fracture morphology, and fractures are classified according to the previously reported "Three Column Classification" (▶ Fig. 4.2c–f). The fixation strategy can be developed based on injured columns. Associated

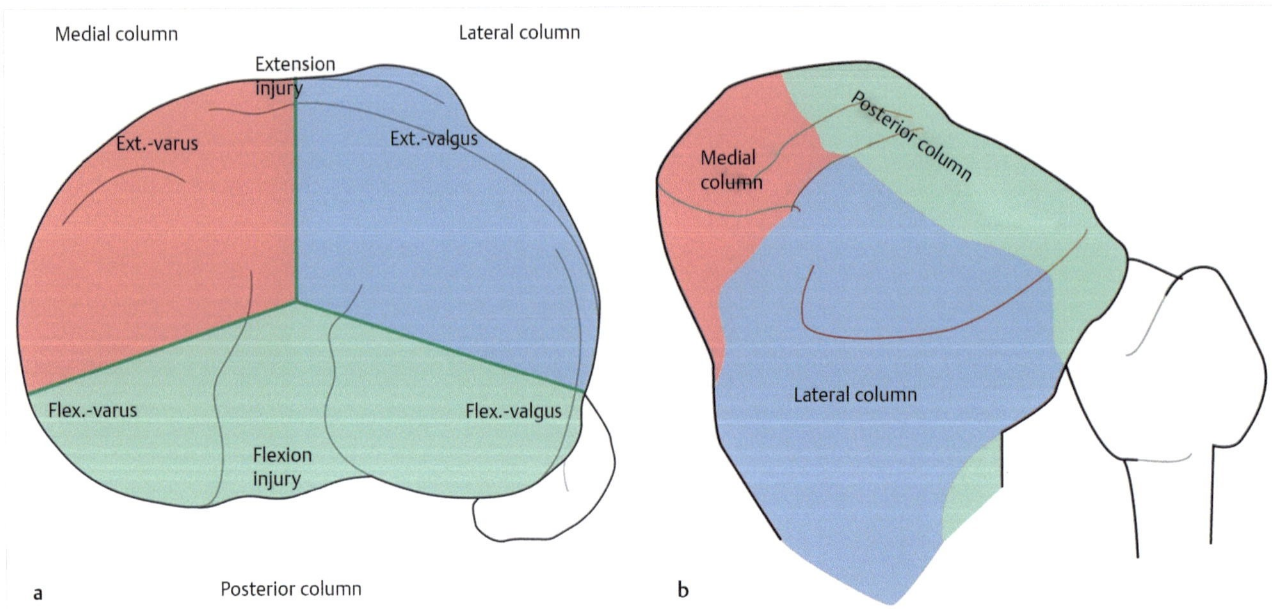

Fig. 4.1 **(a,b)** Three-column classification and injury mechanism.

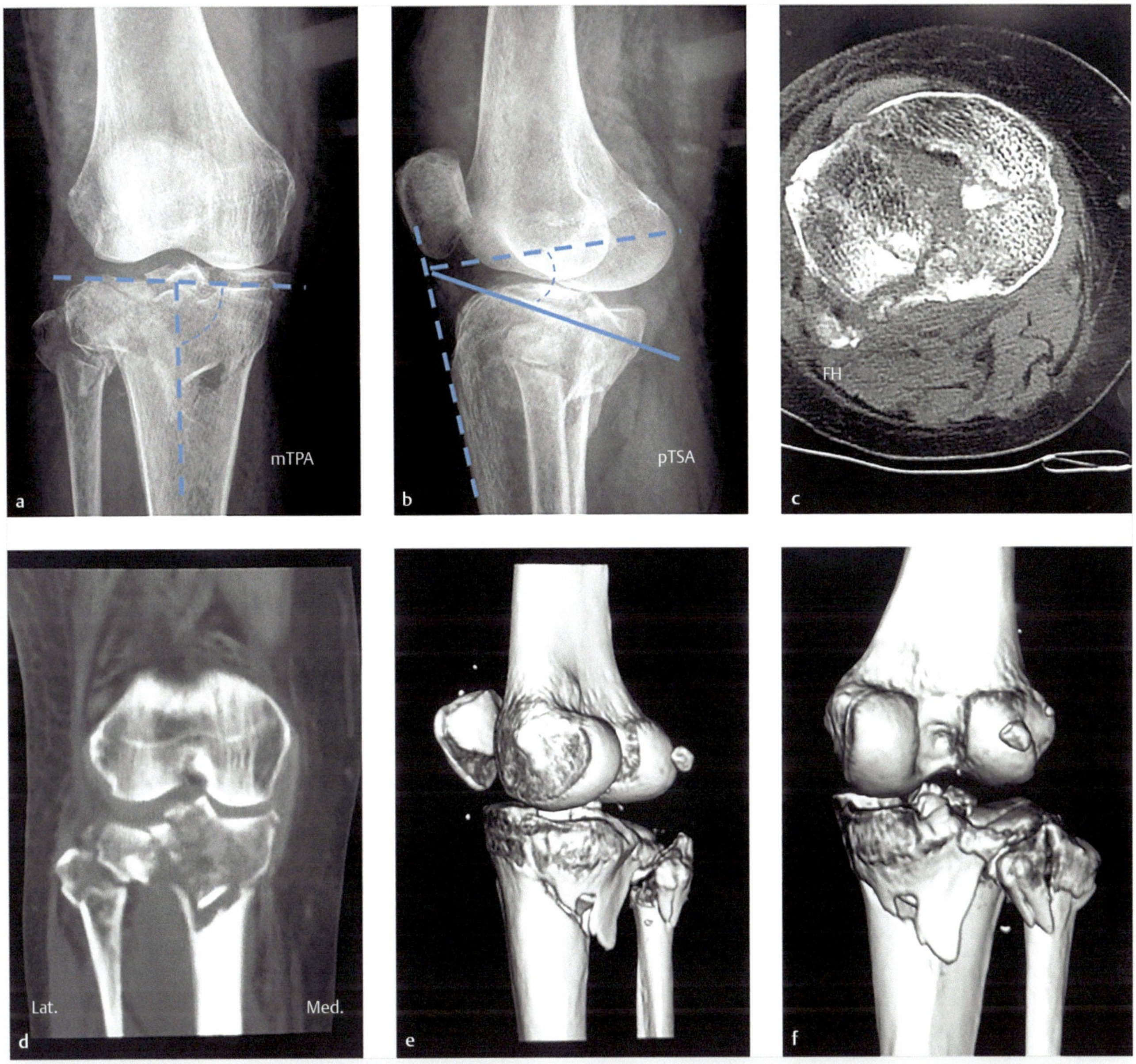

Fig. 4.2 Example of posterior tibial plateau injury. Decreased in medial tibial plateau angle (mTPA) **(a)** and posterior tibial slope angle (pTSA) **(b)**, indicating a flexion-varus injury. There are posteromedial and posterolateral fractures in the coronal plane **(c)**, while the key articular surface lies in the middle of tibial plateau **(d–f)**.

injuries of the soft tissue stabilizers of the knee can be predicted by understanding the mechanism of injury, which can be inferred from the fracture pattern. For example, extension-varus injuries that result in fracture of the anteromedial tibial plateau can also damage the posterior/posterolateral soft tissues, such as the posterior cruciate ligament (PCL) and/or posterolateral complex (PLC). These related injuries often occur on a diagonal line. Similarly, with coronal-plane TPFs, care should be taken to rule out anterior cruciate ligament (ACL), medial collateral ligament (MCL), or lateral capsular ligament injury. Magnetic resonance imaging (MRI) is useful for detailing the type and severity of associated soft tissue injuries.

4.7 Special Instructions, Position, and Anesthesia

The patient is positioned in the so-called "floating position" to provide access to the posterior, medial, or lateral aspects of the knee (▸ Fig. 4.4a).

- The upper body is in the lateral decubitus position, and the lower body is rotated into an almost prone position (▸ Fig. 4.4a).
- A bolster is placed under the axillary fossa.
- Consider intubation instead of laryngeal mask for airway control.

- Consider the use of additional muscle relaxants (e.g., vecuronium bromide) in strong muscular patients for better exposure of the posterior tibial plateau.
- A radiolucent operation table is required, and the one that is able to tilt is preferred.
- A bump is placed under the injured ankle to help keep the knee slightly flexed to facilitate exposure with the reversed-L incision (▶ Fig. 4.4b). However, in some types of flexion injury, the bump should be replaced under the knee after the initial incision and dissection, as the knee must be kept in extension to help reduction and fixation.

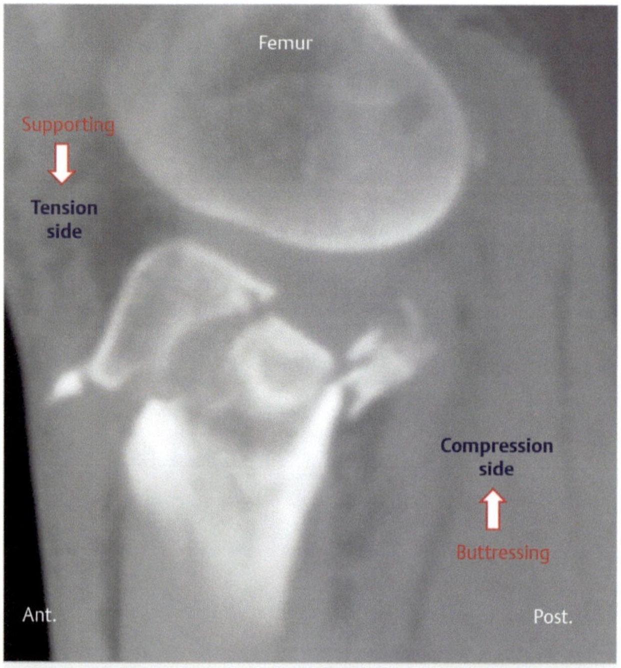

Fig. 4.3 Illustration of the compression and tension sides of a tibial plateau fracture, which relate to injury mechanism and determine fixation strategy. This sagittal computed tomography (CT) view demonstrates the flexion injury of tibial plateau fracture in the coronal plane, which had compression fracture on the posterior side and tension fracture on the anterior side.

- An additional anterolateral approach can be performed by flexing the knee and externally rotating the limb (▶ Fig. 4.4c).

4.8 Tips, Pearls, and Lessons Learned

4.8.1 Exposure and Dissection

During the deep dissection of the reversed-L approach, the pes anserinus tendons should be protected and retracted anteriorly. If iatrogenic injury happens, it should be marked and repaired afterwards.

To avoid injury to the neurovascular bundle in the popliteal space, all the dissection from medial to lateral should be done beneath popliteus muscle in the proximal part.

4.8.2 Reduction Principle

A primary buttress plate which aims to reverse the compressive force on the fracture side is applied first. A secondary supporting plate which aims to hold the reduced articular surface and prevent over-reduction is placed on the tension side. A supporting plate is only indicated when articular comminution is present, or instability remains after primary buttressing.

4.8.3 Intraoperative Fluoroscopy and CT Scans

Oblique views of the knee taken at about 35° from the coronal plane provide the most accurate assessment of the posteromedial and posterolateral tibial plateau. In these two oblique views, either posteromedial or posterolateral articular surface is the largest and has the smallest fibular block.

With the leg in a free-floating position, a bump is placed under the operative limb before taking intraoperative fluoroscopic views. The C-arm should be adjusted according to the direction of joint line, which aims to provide clear tangential views in both anteroposterior (AP) and lateral planes.

When available, intraoperative CT scans can help the surgeon verify the screw length and depth, which avoids intra-articular

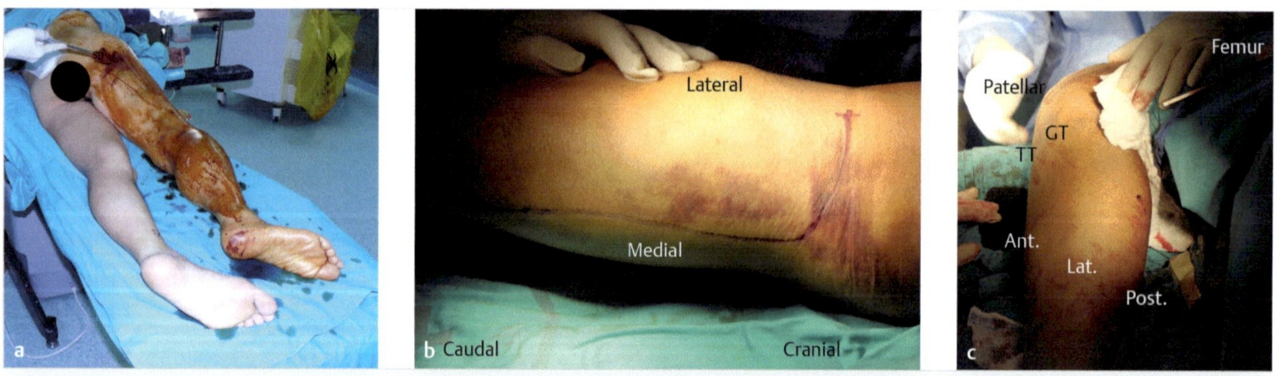

Fig. 4.4 Example of patient positioning. **(a)** The "Floating position," with the upper body in lateral decubitus position while the lower body is nearly prone. **(b)** Reversed-L incision. **(c)** Lateral approach can be undertaken with the patient in the floating position as long as the operation table is tilted toward the unaffected side and the injured leg is flexed with a bump placed beneath. *Abbreviations:* TT, tibial tubercle; GT, Gerdy tubercle.

screw penetration, especially in cases with multiple plates' fixation.

4.8.4 Precontour of the Posterolateral Buttress Plate

Following the anatomic shape of posterolateral tibial plateau, a 3.5-mm buttressing plate (e.g., oblique distal radius plate) is bent either before or during the operation, which is placed in the direction from cranial-lateral to caudal-medial.[1]

4.8.5 Evaluation of the Placement of the Posterolateral Buttressing Plate

It is not recommended to use AP view for evaluation of the height of posterolateral buttressing plate, which is always misleading since the anterior and posterior tibial plateau can overlap. The height of posterolateral buttressing plate is considered proper when it is in line with fibular head in true lateral view.

4.9 Difficulties Encountered

4.9.1 Reduction of Posterolateral Articular Surface

Direct visualization of depressed regions of the posterolateral articular surface using an anterolateral or lateral approach is difficult. However, the depressed articular surface can be observed through (an iatrogenic) fracture window using reversed-L approach with the leg in a free-floating position, and articular elevation through the window can be achieved. The evaluation of fracture reduction is indirect, which requires intraoperative fluoroscopic images.

4.9.2 Fracture Pattern

- In extreme cases, which fall into the category of flexion-varus injury, the major fracture line is in the posterior coronal plane and a minor fracture line exists in the anterior coronal plane. Thus, the medial tibial plateau is separated into three segments: posteromedial, medial, and anteromedial. It can be solved by more anterior exposure through reversed-L approach to access the anteromedial fragment; however, medial and posteromedial fragments can be manipulated as usual. Care must be taken to protect the anterior skin flap.
- In another type of extreme case, which falls into the category of flexion-valgus injury, the anterior fragment is not only displaced but also flipped and compressed, while the posterolateral fragment is comminuted and displaced. Under these circumstances, the anterolateral approach is made first with the leg positioned free (▸ Fig. 4.4c), and the anterolateral fragment is explored and may be opened via the soft tissue hinge. The posterolateral fragments can be explored via the fracture window, and incarcerated meniscus or soft tissue as well as inverted articular surface is taken out in case it prevents posterolateral buttressing.

Next, a posterior reversed-L approach is made to reduce and buttress the posterior column fractures. As the posterior wall of posterolateral is buttressed, the anterolateral or lateral TPFs can then be reduced and stabilized. Otherwise, the reduction of lateral TPFs can displace posteriorly.

4.10 Key Procedural Steps

4.10.1 Fracture Reduction and Internal Fixation

The surgical steps below are based on the illustrative case (▸ Fig. 4.5), which belongs to flexion-varus injury with medial compression and lateral tension fracture. It has major coronal fracture line on the posterior tibial plateau.

- A reversed-L-shaped incision begins at the center of popliteus parallel to Langer lines superiorly and medial. Distally, the incision turns at the medial corner of the popliteal fossa and is carried down to the deep fascia. The incision should be distal to the fracture line. Care must be taken to protect sural nerve and short saphenous vein in superficial dissection[2] (▸ Fig. 4.4b).
- The tendon of the medial head of the gastrocnemius is exposed and retracted laterally. After careful blunt dissection, the popliteus and soleus origin are elevated off the posteromedial aspect of the proximal tibia from medial to lateral. With the help of Hoffman retractor, the fractures in coronal plane are displayed (▸ Fig. 4.5a).
- The posteromedial fragment is accessed first; fracture reduction is achieved via traction and knee extension. A precontoured posteromedial tibial plateau plate (or an undercontoured 3.5-mm locking compression-dynamic compression plate (LC-DCP) or 3.5-mm T-plate) can be placed longitudinally on the posteromedial ridge of tibia, which functions as primary buttress. Note that the screw placed proximally should be inadequately long, in case further reduction and fixation of lateral tibial plateau fragment is interfered with (▸ Fig. 4.5b, c).
- The posterolateral fragment is manipulated next. The articular surface is elevated by working through the "fracture window" by using a periosteum elevator. An oblique posterolateral plate was usually used to buttress the fragment. After placement of distal compression screws through the plate, the proximal screw holes can be spared (▸ Fig. 4.5d, e). Temporary closure of the reversed-L incision is necessary before accessing the lateral approach.
- Finally, an anterolateral approach, where the incision starts at the joint line, curving at the anterior aspect of Gerdy tubercle and continuing distally over the proximal tibia, is used to reduce and stabilize the lateral or anterolateral fragment. An arthrotomy is performed through a submeniscal approach. The articular surface is reduced via the fracture window and lateral periarticular fixation is applied, which acts as a supporting fixation for both lateral and posterolateral fragment (▸ Fig. 4.5 f-h).
- During wound closure, the deep fascia is left open to prevent compartment syndrome. Subcutaneous tissue and skin were closed over suction drainages.

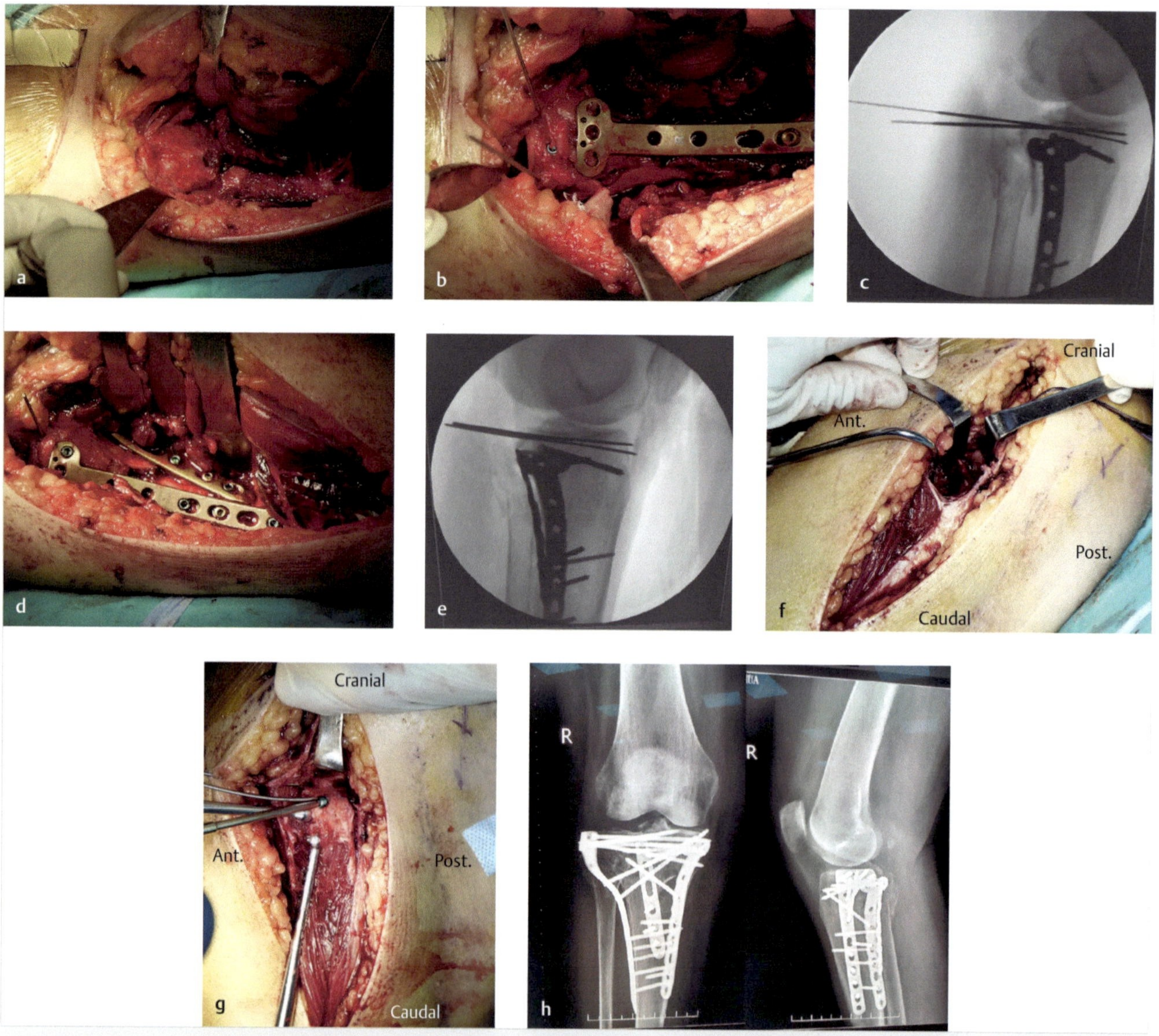

Fig. 4.5 Operative steps. **(a)** Posteromedial fragment is exposed via reversed-L approach. (The same patient displayed in ▸ Fig. 4.2.) **(b)** Primary buttressing fixation of posteromedial fragment after reduction. **(c)** Oblique view (34-degree) of posteromedial tibial plateau after buttressing, noticing the displaced posterolateral fragment. **(d)** After bending the plate, the displaced posterolateral fragment is reduced with the help of this secondary buttressing plate. **(e)** Oblique view (34-degree) of posteromedial tibial plateau showing both fragments in coronal plane are reduced and buttressed. **(f)** Lateral depressed articular surface exposure. **(g)** Rafting screw fixation after key lateral articular surface reduction. **(h)** Immediate postoperative anteroposterior (AP) and lateral X-rays of this case.

4.10.2 Treatment of Associated Injuries

- All ruptured menisci are repaired to the best degree possible.
- Avulsion fracture of the PCL insertion can be found in posterior column fractures. The injured ligament is repaired via the same reversed-L approach for fracture reduction and fixation. Additional screw fixation may be applied for the avulsion fractures.
- ACL injury is commonly seen in posterior column fractures as well. If the insertion is fractured, it can be explored via the anterolateral approach under direct visualization. The remnant of ACL ligament can be repaired using Ethibond sutures and stabilized through the bone tunnel. However, if the body part of ACL is disrupted, reconstruction under arthroscopy may be required in the later stage.
- MCL ruptures are treated nonoperatively in most cases.

4.11 Bailout, Rescue, Salvage Procedures

Although the incidence is very low, the posterior tibial recurrent artery, which is a branch from the proximal part of the anterior tibial artery and bifurcation of the tibial arteries, can be injured by overdissection laterally via reversed-L approach or by K-wire misplacement.[3] The first thing to do is to make sure that the tourniquet is on, and the incision is extended more laterally. The bleeding vessel is explored: if the recurrent branch of tibial artery were injured, it can be ligated; if the bifurcation of tibial artery were injured, immediate repair is required.

4.12 Pitfalls

Clinical studies have demonstrated good radiological and functional results using reversed-L approach with the knee in a free-floating position for complex TPF with posterior fragments. However, the reversed-L approach should be reserved to fracture patterns that cannot be addressed through the traditional approaches. As long as anatomical reduction and stable fixation can be achieved, it is better to choose traditional bilateral approaches in supine position. The traditional approach takes advantage in shorter learning curve, fewer assistants required, less operation time, and easier intraoperative alignment evaluation.

5 Distal Femur Unicondylar Fracture

Vincenzo Giordano, André Wajnsztejn, and Felipe Serrão de Souza

5.1 Description

Displaced partial intra-articular fractures of the distal femur in the sagittal plane are best treated by anatomic reduction and absolute stability. We describe the use of lag screws and/or a buttress plate allowing for a stable fixation and early motion of the joint.

5.2 Key Principles

Unicondylar fractures of the distal femur should be anatomically reduced. It is important to identify the main fracture plane. Lag screws should be placed perpendicular to the plane of the fracture, while buttress plates should be parallel to it. Buttress plates applied parallel to the fracture plane and located over the apex of the fracture have optimal biomechanical properties withstanding shearing forces. If the bone has good density, as observed in young active adults, we use a cortical screw with a metallic washer at the level of the apex of the fracture, instead of a buttress plate. The fixation is then complemented by two other lag screws across the main fracture plane. Nonlocking straight plates 3.5 mm or 4.5 mm are the standard implants used for buttressing. Locking plates should be considered in cases of osteoporotic bones. When using buttress plates, we advocate for the use of two screws proximal to the apex of the fracture, and at least two lag screws across the main fracture plane.

5.3 Expectations

In 33 B1-type shearing fractures, closed reduction and percutaneous fixation under C-arm imaging can be attempted. Open reduction techniques have been adopted for irreducible fractures, for split depression patterns, and for open injuries. For the fractures of the lateral femoral condyle, our preferred approach is the anterolateral.

In 33 B2-type fractures, closed reduction and percutaneous fixation are indicated only when the fracture is completely nondisplaced. In general, open reduction is preferred for most of B2-type distal femur fractures. A direct medial subvastus approach to the distal femur is sufficient to adequately reduce and fix the fracture. More complex fractures involving articular impaction or an associated medial Hoffa component are better exposed with a medial parapatellar approach.

5.4 Indications

Fractures classified according to AO/OTA as 33 B1 (lateral femoral condyle) or 33 B2 (medial femoral condyle) should be treated surgically, allowing for stable fixation and early motion of the knee.

5.5 Contraindications

The absolute contraindication for a surgical fixation of a displaced articular femoral condyle fracture is the presence of acute infection. A relative contraindication would be a nondisplaced fracture in individuals that are nonambulatory and considered too sick for a surgical procedure. Blasting injuries to the femoral condyle with significant osteochondral and/or soft tissues loss may preclude any effort of bone fixation, and may raise consideration for reconstructive procedures of the joint.

5.6 Special Considerations

Detailed preoperative evaluation is critical. A computed tomography (CT) scan is helpful to clarify fracture morphology and the shape of the condylar fragments. Careful assessment of the degree of osteopenia and the amount of comminution is necessary to determine the reduction technique (closed vs. open) and the implant selection (nonlocking vs. locking).

During surgery, a tourniquet can be used when managing more complex fracture patterns. Intraoperative fluoroscopy provides significant information regarding fracture reduction and implant positioning. Reduction tools are critical. Ball spikes, point reduction clamps, periarticular clamps, and collinear clamps should be available for this procedure. In cases of articular depression, the use of bone tamps to reduce the osteochondral impaction and bone void fillers is necessary. Most typically we use autograft from the iliac crest, but we also have used bone substitutes as void fillers in such situations. We favor the use of low-profile implants, especially on the lateral aspect of the femur, aiming to avoid friction of the iliotibial band. The small fragment and the large fragment sets may be considered depending on the size of the patient, the size of the femoral condyle, and fracture pattern. A 3.5-mm implant is preferred, and for the distal femur, it is important to have extralong screws, which are normally available in the pelvic set.

5.7 Special Instructions, Position, and Anesthesia

- Spinal anesthesia associated with intravenous sedation.
- Position patient supine on a radiolucent table.
- Leave a tourniquet on the proximal aspect of the thigh, in case bleeding becomes an issue during the procedure precluding an optimal visualization of the fracture.
- Check for fluoroscopy imaging before draping to ensure proper visualization of the distal femur. It is critical to obtain anteroposterior and lateral fluoroscopic projections of the knee, allowing for optimal control of the fracture reduction and hardware placement.
- The skin over the iliac crest on either side is also prepared in case an autologous bone graft is planned.
- The surgical incision is placed either lateral or medial depending on where the fracture is located.

5.8 Tips, Pearls, and Lessons Learned

5.8.1 Closed Reduction

Fracture is reduced under image intensifier using special clamps. Normally two clamps or a clamp and a ball-spike are necessary to obtain an adequate reduction. A small skin incision is placed over the apex of the fracture either on the lateral or the medial sides of the distal aspect of the thigh, depending on the fracture pattern. A 4.0-mm Steinmann pin is inserted to the apex of the fracture and used to distally manipulate the unicondylar fragment (▶ Fig. 5.1a). A ball-spike—or a pointed reduction clamp—is applied to close the proximal aspect of the fracture. A second small skin incision is made over the projection of the articular component of the fracture. A pointed reduction clamp (or a colinear clamp) is applied to anatomically reduce the articular fracture (▶ Fig. 5.1b). Fluoroscopy imaging is obtained to ensure the quality of reduction (▶ Fig. 5.1c). A temporary 2.5-mm nonthreaded K-wire is used proximally to secure reduction and avoid shear during lag-screwing insertion (▶ Fig. 5.2). A 3.5-mm cortical lag-screw is placed on the anterior third of the femoral condyle while a second 3.5-mm cortical lag-screw is placed on the transition between the mid-third and posterior thirds of the femoral condyle. The fracture is then compressed, and absolute stability is obtained. We recommend the use of metal washers even in the young adult patient to optimize interfragmentary compression (▶ Fig. 5.3). A small-fragment precontoured straight plate is percutaneously inserted through the proximal incision (on the fracture side) and used to buttress the apex of the fracture.

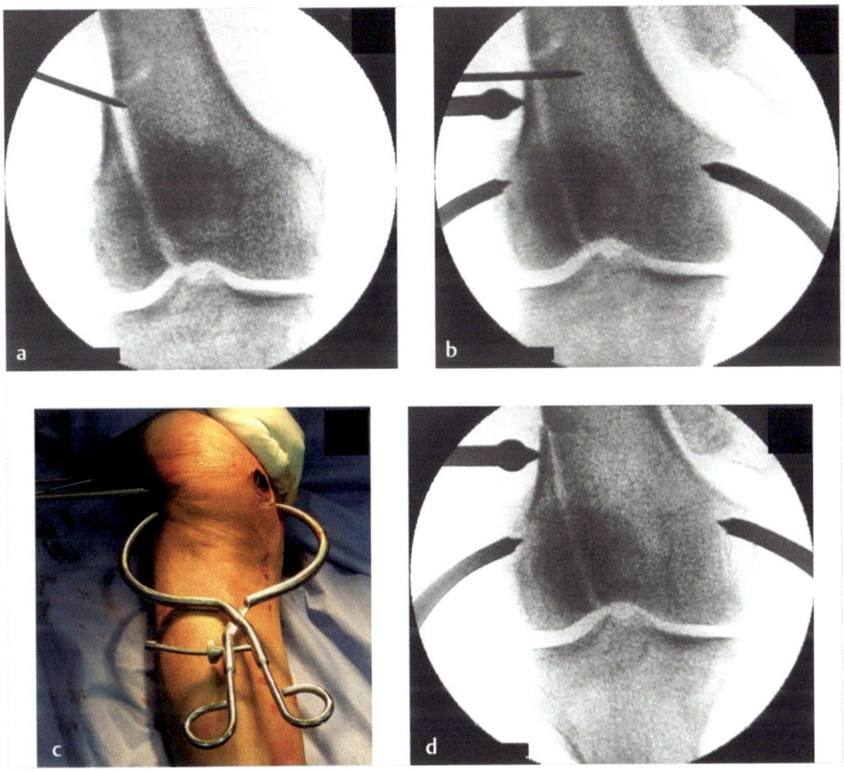

Fig. 5.1 Percutaneous reduction of a B1-type unicondylar distal femur fracture. **(a)** A 3.5-mm Steinmann pin is inserted at the apex of the fracture and used to distally manipulate the unicondylar fragment. **(b)** A ball-spike reduction tool is applied closing the fracture proximally while a pointed reduction clamp is applied to anatomically reduce the articular component of the fracture. **(c)** Intra-operative picture illustrating the combined use of a periarticular clamp and a ball spike; **(d)** Fluoroscopic control revealing a proper reduction of the articular surface.

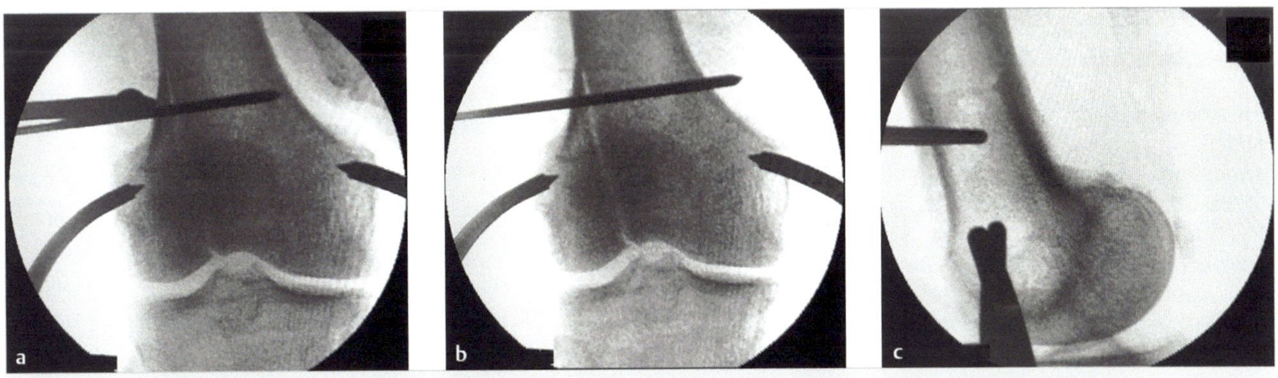

Fig. 5.2 Percutaneous reduction of a B1-type unicondylar distal femur fracture. **(a)** A temporary 2.5-mm nonthreaded K-wire is used proximally to secure the reduction avoiding a proximal shearing at the time of insertion of distal lag screws. **(b)** The ball-spike tool is removed but the periarticular distal femur clamp is still in place, securing the reduction of the articular surface. **(c)** Lateral view of the distal femur revealing anatomic reduction of the femoral condyle.

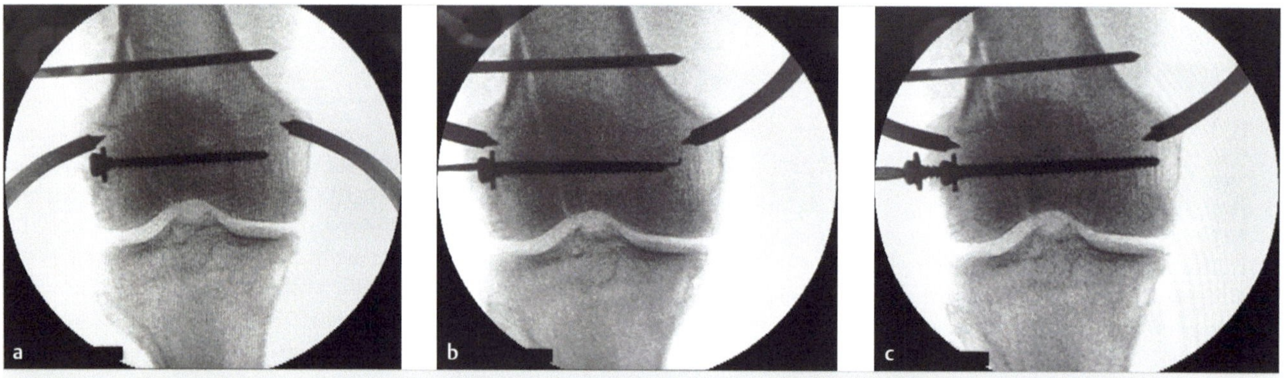

Fig. 5.3 (a-c) Percutaneous fixation of a 33 B1-type unicondylar distal femur fracture. Two lag-screws are inserted, one placed anteriorly and the next one placed posteriorly, both perpendicular to the fracture plane. We favor the use of washers optimizing interfragmentary compression.

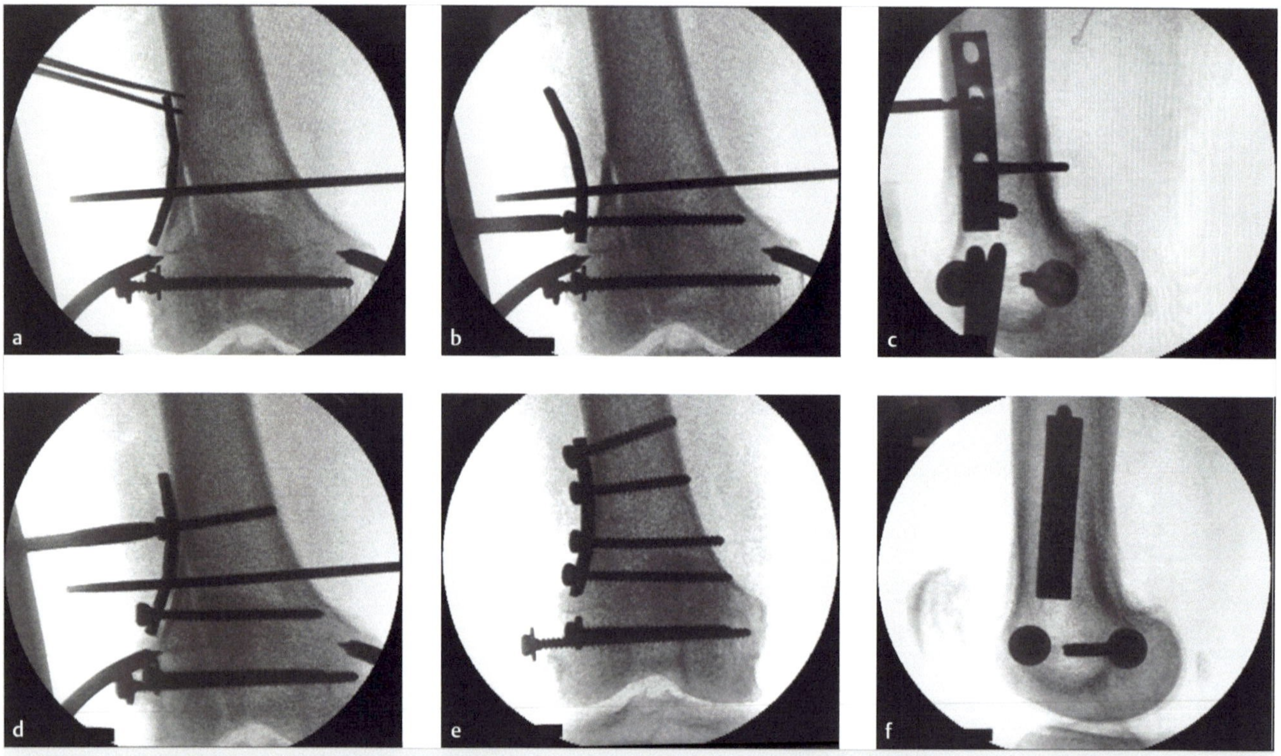

Fig. 5.4 (a-f) Placement of a buttress plate. Once the fracture is reduced and properly compressed, a precontoured one-third tubular four-hole plate is placed parallel to the main fracture plane. Two position screws are applied proximal to the apex of the fracture and two lag-screws are placed through the distal holes of the plate.

It is advisable to place one of the holes of the plate over the Steinmann pin to help positioning the plate. The position of the plate is checked prior to inserting the screws. The first 3.5-mm cortical screw should attach the plate to the distal fragment but should not be tightened completely. A second 3.5-mm cortical screw is inserted just proximal to the apex of the fracture and firmly tightened to compress the plate to the bone surface. The first screw is firmly tightened, and the other cortical screws are inserted (▶ Fig. 5.4). The final position is checked with multiple fluoroscopic views to confirm that proper reduction and hardware placement were achieved. The stab incisions are irrigated, and the skin is closed with nonresorbable sutures.

5.8.2 Open Reduction

Open fractures, nonreducible and/or severe impacted B1-type fractures, and displaced B2-type fractures are best treated by open reduction and internal fixation (ORIF). Open injuries should have the initial management as all open fractures, consisting of irrigation and debridement of the traumatic wound and fixation of the articular fracture. For closed displaced fractures, after the exposure of the fracture site, intra-articular hematoma and debris should be removed to facilitate reduction. The fracture is reduced under direct visualization and temporarily fixed with nonthreaded 2.5-mm K-wires; if subchondral bone graft is planned, it must be packed under the osteochondral elevated fragments before the main fracture is reduced. Minifragment or headless screws can be used to hold small osteochondral pieces in place. The next steps including fixation sequence are exactly the same as described before.

5.9 Difficulties Encountered

During closed reduction, intra-articular hematoma and cartilage debris may prevent anatomical apposition of the fragments, thus making open reduction necessary for direct articular surface visualization. Osteoporotic bone may subside at the time of the application of pointed reduction clamps. The use of spiked discs applied to the tips of pointed reduction clamps increase the contact area of these clamps reducing the risks of cortical subsidence. Inappropriate plate positioning due to incorrect fluoroscopy imaging can lead to loss of reduction. In the distal femur, it is of paramount importance to obtain oblique views ensuring that screws are not too long and proud on the opposite cortex.

During open reduction, impacted articular osteochondral fragments and associated coronal fracture can cause difficulty in the procedure. Adequate preoperative imaging study is critical to understand the fracture morphology and to plan the surgical tactic.

If fracture care is delayed, it may be challenging to reduce an articular fracture. In those cases, an open procedure is mandatory, aiming to remove scar tissue at the fracture site, and allowing for proper reduction and internal fixation of the fracture.

5.10 Key Procedural Steps

5.10.1 Patient Positioning

Patient should be positioned supine on a radiolucent table with a bump under the operated limb, allowing for proper elevation of this leg in relationship to the opposite limb. This positioning facilitates the use of fluoroscopy in multiple projections.

5.10.2 Approaches for ORIF

The anterolateral approach is used for almost any ORIF of 33 B1-types distal femur fracture treatment. It allows for direct exposure of the lateral femoral condyle and articular surface. The skin incision should begin 4.0 cm proximally and about 1.0 cm laterally to the patella, curving anteriorly over the lateral femoral condyle toward the anterior tibial tubercle. The fibers of the iliotibial band are divided longitudinally in line with the skin incision. The vastus lateralis should be retracted laterally ligating the perforating vessels. A lateral arthrotomy is made by incising the capsule over the anterior third of the lateral femoral condyle, thus exposing the articular surface. If a pointed reduction clamp is used for reduction, a medial stab incision must be done to allow for clamp positioning on the medial femoral condyle.

In B2-type fractures, a direct medial approach to the distal femur is generally sufficient to adequately reduce and fix the fracture. The skin incision is centered on the adductor tubercle, beginning proximally in the line of the adductor magnus tendon, curving over the medial side of the patella, and extending distally about 2.0 cm below the articular line. A subvastus approach carefully elevating the vastus medialis from the posterior septum allows for good exposure of the distal medial aspect of the femur. If a pointed reduction clamp is used, a lateral stab incision must be done to allow for clamp positioning.

5.10.3 Fixation

After reduction, temporary fixation may be achieved with non-threaded 2.5-mm K-wires or a periarticular pointed reduction clamp. The K-wire is used proximally to secure reduction and avoid shear during lag-screwing insertion. Two to three 3.5-mm cortical screws with metal washers are placed on the most distal part of the distal femur, compressing the articular component of the unicondylar fracture. Then a small-fragment plate is applied to support the split fragment. Minifragment or headless screws should be considered for the fixation of small osteochondral fragments.

5.11 Bailout, Rescue, and Salvage Procedures

A longer locking plate must be used if there is severe osteoporosis. Augmentation procedures, such as injectable calcium phosphate cement around the tip of the distal screws, generally used in proximal femur and humerus osteoporotic fractures, can increase construct stiffness. In old fractures with fixed angular deformity, we use a femoral distractor for a reconstructive procedure.

5.12 Pitfalls

The use of small-fragment cortical screws to compress the condylar fracture should be associated with a buttress plate. When a 4.5-mm cortical screw with a washer is used to buttress the fracture apex, then it is recommended to use either large-fragment cortical screws or cancellous screws to compress the articular component of the fracture. In osteoporotic bone, a large fragment locking plate is our preference.

Care should be taken not to place the hardware lower to the level of the Blumensaat line. This prevents intra-articular screw placement at the level of the intercondylar notch. We obtain multiple fluoroscopic views including tunnel view, and oblique views of the distal femur confirming adequate placement of the hardware.

Arthrofibrosis and knee stiffness are observed when postoperative rehabilitation is delayed. Early motion should follow stable internal fixation. Patients should have proper pain and rehabilitation management after internal fixation of articular fractures.

Failure to recognize ligamentous and/or meniscal injuries may lead to chronic pain and instability. Meniscal injuries should be acutely repaired when the fracture is fixed. Ligamentous injuries may be treated after fracture healing when the patient has clinical evidence of knee laxity. The use of magnetic resonance imaging (MRI) preoperatively should be considered in cases of severely displaced or comminuted articular fractures of the knee. The MRI allows for a complete understanding of the extent of the injury and a more comprehensive preoperative planning, which may include concomitant approach to soft tissues injuries or staged planned procedures to the knee.

6 Distal Femur Fractures—Bicondylar

Brett D. Crist

6.1 Description

This chapter describes open reduction and internal fixation (ORIF) of bicondylar distal femur fractures, reviewing indications/contraindications for surgical repair, surgical tips and pitfalls, key procedural steps, and bailouts when intraoperative difficulties are encountered.

6.2 Key Principles

- Articular reduction requires rotational correction in all planes and then compression when feasible.
- Avoid coronal and sagittal plane malreduction of the metadiaphyseal segment.
- Decrease risk of nonunion and hardware failure by avoiding use of short plates.

6.3 Expectations

- Anatomical articular reduction is the goal.
- Correct coronal and sagittal plane reduction of the metadiaphyseal segment.
- Construct stability that allows for early range of motion and patient mobilization.
- Outcomes for intra-articular fractures are primarily related to the degree of articular comminution. Most patients can achieve a functional range of motion with at least 90-degrees of knee flexion and a stable knee.

6.4 Indications

A fracture with any articular displacement should be considered for ORIF. Even if the metaphyseal component is minimally displaced, ORIF is beneficial to allow for early knee range of motion and patient mobilization. Therefore, generally all bicondylar intra-articular distal femoral fractures undergo operative management to minimize the consequences of intra-articular displacement, long-term joint immobilization, or limited patient mobility.

6.5 Contraindications

Contraindications to surgery usually include the presence of severe medical comorbidities that make the patient unable to tolerate anesthesia, or when the physiological burden of surgery is too great (such as in a physiologically unstable trauma patient). A relative contraindication to surgery is an unreconstructible articular surface, especially in a geriatric patient with severe comminution and/or poor bone quality. In this setting, ORIF should be avoided due to the high risk of failure, and total knee arthroplasty (TKA) with a distal femur replacement should be considered.

6.6 Special Considerations

6.6.1 Geriatric and Osteoporotic Fractures

Distal femur fractures commonly occur in geriatric patients and have two conflicting considerations—early weight bearing is desired to allow for more predictable patient mobilization, but this must be balanced against the risk of fixation failure due to poor bone quality. There is always a race between fixation failure and healing. When considering geriatric patients, one also needs to consider the detrimental effect of limiting weight bearing. Early weight bearing as tolerated should be considered for all geriatric distal femur fractures. To improve fixation in osteopenic patients, flexible fixation using long plates with bicortical nonlocking diaphyseal screw fixation using traditional internal fixator principles is recommended. If the plate contour causes malreduction when the plate is compressed against the bone, the plate may be manually contoured to fit the patient or locking screws can be used to fix the plate to the bone even though it may not be compressed against it—i.e., locking internal fixator concept (▶ Fig. 6.1). Titanium implants are less rigid than stainless steel, and the increased flexibility of titanium plates in distal femur fractures is thought to lead to improved fracture healing. There is a greater risk of catastrophic failure with the use of stiff stainless steel locking plates in distal femur fractures. Finally, surgeons should consider protecting the entire femur with the implant due to increased risk of peri-implant fractures in the future (▶ Fig. 6.1). If the entire femur is not protected with the plate, the last proximal diaphyseal screw should be a unicortical locking screw to make a transition stress zone to minimize stress concentration at the proximal end of the implant.

6.6.2 Open Fractures

Open fractures lead to bone loss primarily in the metadiaphyseal region. This creates increased implant stress that could lead to early implant failure if using a single plate. If the bone loss is more than a centimeter, the surgeon should consider utilizing a temporary antibiotic-impregnated spacer with planned delayed bone grafting. Consider using a second medial plate, a medullary (or cortical substitution) plate, or an intramedullary nail (IMN) if the articular component of the fracture is relatively simple, due to the expected prolonged healing time of the metaphyseal segment in an open injury.

6.6.3 Chondral Damage or Loss

Chondral damage or loss is an unsolved problem for the majority of periarticular fractures in patients that are not arthroplasty candidates. Current strategies are to create a fibrous cartilage substitute for damaged articular cartilage by debriding the damaged area and performing microfracture with or without biological

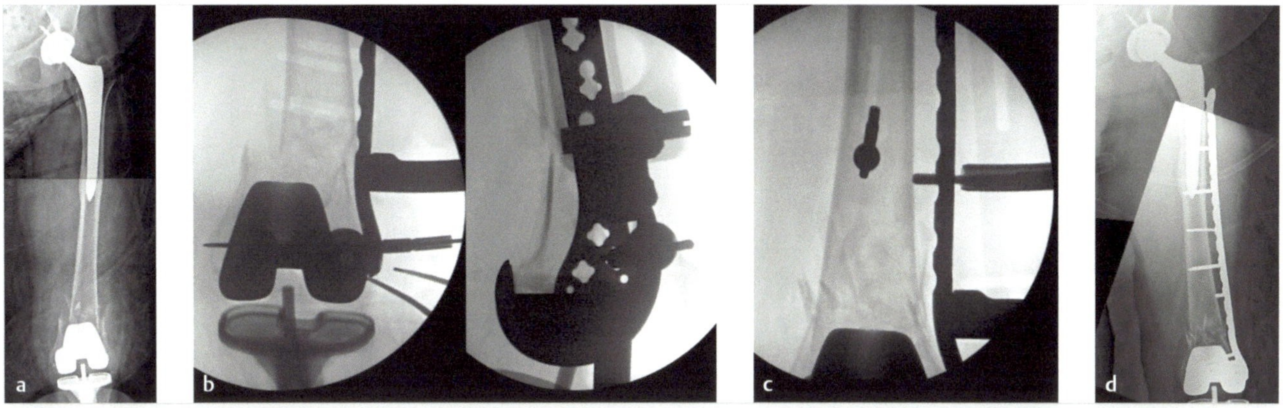

Fig. 6.1 **(a)** Anteroposterior (AP) femur radiograph of an interprosthetic distal femur fracture with initial valgus displacement of the fracture that dictates the fracture to be plated laterally for the plate to have a buttress function for the articular block. **(b)** Intraoperative AP and lateral fluoroscopic views with the 95-degree-axis wire placed through the plate and parallel to the articular surface (left panel). Despite this, the articular block was medialized with initial lateral plate application creating a "golf club" deformity. The plate was repositioned more anteriorly on the lateral view (right panel), but the articular block was still medialized due to plate contour. A periprosthetic locking screw was used (c) to push against the articular block to aide with coronal plane reduction and the locking plate was not compressed to bone. **(d)** The plate functions as a bridging "internal fixator."

stimulation (i.e., platelet-rich plasma). Delayed osteochondral allograft (OCA) may be an option for both damaged cartilage and areas of complete cartilage loss, as long as the bony defect is not significant. If there is more than a centimeter of subchondral bone loss, then the procedure becomes similar to an oncological grafting procedure with prolonged bone incorporation time and increased risk of late failure.

6.7 Special Instructions, Position, and Anesthesia

- A standard radiolucent operating room table should be used, including a diving board–type table, or completely radiolucent table.
- General or spinal anesthetic may be used based on anesthetist, surgeon, and patient preference. Peripheral nerve blocks may be beneficial for postoperative pain control, but affect the patient's ability to mobilize for the first 24 hours after surgery, and may require use of a knee brace locked in extension to minimize risk of falling prior to recovery from the nerve block.
- Positioning:
  - Supine positioning is probably most commonly used due to ease of positioning, lack of special equipment needed, and the ability to address other injuries without having to change patient positioning. Besides ease of positioning, it is easier to visualize and reduce the entire articular surface, reduce the coronal and sagittal planes of the metadiaphyseal component, and assess the alignment profile both lower extremities clinically and radiographically in the supine position.
    - Place a nonsterile bump under the ipsilateral buttock to neutralize hip external rotation, and secure the uninjured extremities and torso.
    - To improve fluoroscopic visualization proximally on the lateral view and to better assess reduction, it is beneficial to prep both lower extremities into the surgical field. This allows the surgeon to flex the nonoperative hip and knee to improve visualization on the cross table lateral view of the operative proximal femur.
  - Lateral positioning is mostly beneficial for the exposure of the extra-articular components of the fracture, and laterally based implant positioning. It, however, precludes the ability to utilize a medially-based plate. During the lateral femur exposure, gravity assists with posterior soft tissue retraction. This is particularly helpful if an extensile lateral exposure to the femur is planned.
    - Utilize a beanbag to secure the torso and pelvis. It is more difficult to fluoroscopically visualize everything on the lateral view due to the opposite lower extremity.
    - Caution: Coronal plane and rotational reduction can be more difficult to judge in the lateral position. The tendency is to malreduce the femur into valgus and external rotation.

6.8 Tips, Pearls, and Lessons Learned

6.8.1 Preoperative Plan

- Mentally creating a preoperative plan is helpful, but committing it to paper or a digital record is even better. Full-length femur and knee orthogonal radiographs are required. A computed tomography (CT) scan should be obtained to evaluate articular involvement (▶ Fig. 6.2). It is critical to make sure there is no coronal plane (Hoffa) fracture. Missing these will lead to a poor outcome. The goal of the preoperative planning exercise is to make the procedure go as efficiently and effectively as possible. To paraphrase Jeff Mast, it is better to make a mistake that can be thrown in the trash or deleted, rather than committing a mistake on a patient. The plan should include perioperative care (i.e., antibiotics, postoperative weight-bearing status, etc.), operative table, patient position, reduction instruments, implants, intraoperative reduction and fixation steps, and closure.

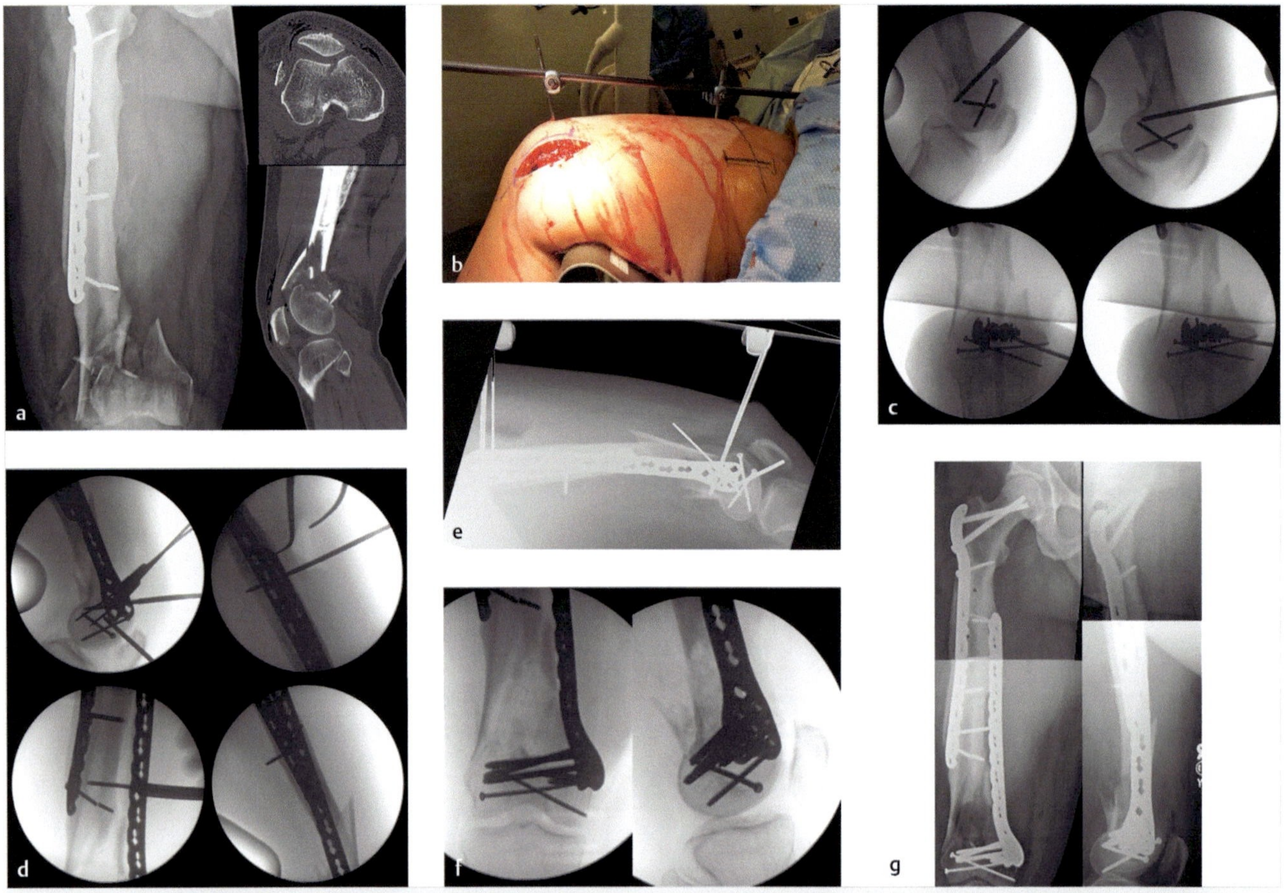

Fig. 6.2 (a) Anteroposterior (AP) femur radiograph (left panel) and computed tomography (CT) scans (right panel) of an AO/OTA 33-C2 type 2 Gustilo-Anderson open distal femur fracture with initial varus displacement. Because of the deformity, the plate should be placed medially to function as a buttress plate. In this case, medial plating avoids having to remove the pre-existing lateral proximal femoral plate. The axial CT scan (upper right) reveals the articular involvement on the axial series. The sagittal reconstruction view (lower right) shows no coronal plane (Hoffa) fracture. (b) An "all femur" external fixator is applied to restore length and provide sagittal plane reduction. (c) Fluoroscopic views showing sequential steps in fracture reduction. Lateral view showing distal Schanz pin in the articular block (upper left). The articular block is rotated and translated to correct the extension deformity and connected to the proximal pin (upper right). AP fluoroscopic views showing a media-to-lateral Schanz pin is placed in the articular block to correct coronal plane alignment (lower panels). (d) Lateral fluoroscopic views showing the anterior placement of the plate distally (upper left) and the plate centered proximally on the diaphysis (upper right). AP fluoroscopic view showing a cortical screw used to reduce the bone to the plate to affect the coronal plane reduction (lower left). However, the screw caused too much anterior translation on the lateral fluoroscopic view (lower right). (e) This was verified on the intraoperative lateral plain femur radiograph. (f) Final intraoperative AP and lateral fluoroscopic views after reduction revised, and fixation complete. (g) Postoperative AP and lateral radiographs.

- When plating a distal femur fracture, evaluate the initial injury radiographs to determine what direction in the coronal plane the articular segment displaced, and determine whether to plate laterally or medially in order to effectively buttress the fracture. If the fracture displaces into valgus, I plate laterally (▶ Fig. 6.1). However, if the main fracture displacement is varus or if the medial aspect of the fracture exits proximally, I will plate medially (▶ Fig. 6.2).

6.8.2 Surgical Exposures

- Direct lateral with modification.
- TARPO.
- Swashbuckler.
- Medial/subvastus.

6.8.3 Common Reduction Instruments

Reduction instruments are critical to a successful surgery and the surgeon should plan for every clamp they need. Common instruments are:

- Large and small pointed reduction forceps, including modified clamps with one straight tine.
- Periarticular reduction forceps.
- Pelvic reduction forceps.
- Collinear reduction clamp (DePuy Synthes, West Chester, PA).
- "All femur" external fixator—5-mm Schanz pins, two external fixator clamps, and one rod.
- 2.0-mm Kirschner wires for joystick reduction of condylar fragments, or individual fracture fragments.

6.8.4 Reduction Aids that Facilitate the Reduction

- Radiolucent triangles.
- Bumps.
- Skeletal traction.

6.8.5 Implants

- Stainless steel or titanium 4.5-mm precontoured periarticular locking distal femur plate, 3.5-mm nonlocking or locking plates.
- Long 2.7-mm and 3.5-mm cortical screws (similar metal to the intended plate or IMN) for articular fixation.
- Retrograde IMN with multiple distal fixation options.

6.8.6 Reduction Tips

Articular Reduction

Do not use skeletal traction during the articular reduction. Longitudinal traction increases the tension on the collateral ligaments and makes reducing the condylar fragments more difficult.

Metadiaphyseal Reduction Evaluation

To improve fluoroscopic visualization proximally on the lateral view and gauge overall clinical length and alignment, it is beneficial to prep both lower extremities into the surgical field. This allows the nonoperative hip and knee to be flexed over the sterile c-arm receiver cover to improve visualization of the proximal femur. Both lower extremities can be clinically compared for overall length and alignment, as well as hip and knee range of motion. A Bovie cord or alignment rod (including any long/straight guide rod) can be used to determine the mechanical axis in the coronal plane by placing it at the center of the femoral head and ankle fluoroscopically. The mechanical axis is determined by where the alignment tool passes across the articular surface of the knee. Unless there is pre-existing deformity, the line should pass just medial to the lateral tibial spine. It is important to make sure that the knee is fully extended, and if the Bovie cord is used, it should be kept taught from the hip to knee, to avoid miscalculation of the mechanical axis. The rotational profile of the femur can be determined fluoroscopically and is dependent on an intact opposite femur as a template. To utilize the "lesser trochanteric sign," an anteroposterior (AP) fluoroscopic view of the uninjured knee with the patella-pointed straight anterior is obtained, and then an AP image of the lesser trochanter either intraoperative or prior to prepping and draping, and serves as the template. The same views are taken of the operative femur. Appropriate reduction is achieved when the operative lesser trochanteric profile matches the uninjured side. Alternatively or supplementary, a true lateral fluoroscopic view can be taken of the uninjured knee, and an axial lateral view of the ipsilateral femoral neck can be used to determine the patient's existing femoral version by determining the angular difference needed on the c-arm arc to obtain each view. The same views can be performed on the operative femur to match femoral torsion.

6.8.7 Fixation Tips

- Intercondylar lag or position screws can be placed in predictable areas anteriorly and posteriorly along the condyles to minimize the risk of compromising plate fixation options (▶ Fig. 6.3). Most periarticular laterally based locking plates have a plate foot print template that can be placed along the lateral femoral condyle to help determine where intercondylar screws can be placed that avoid screws being placed through the plate.
- When using a laterally-based plate, plate positioning is critical to avoid malreduction. The condyles project posterior to the femoral diaphysis. If the plate is placed posteriorly and the shaft of the plate is used to pull the bone to the plate, it can create medialization of the condyles relative to the shaft known as the "golf club" deformity (▶ Fig. 6.1). This shifts the mechanical axis medially and leads to an increased varus stress of the knee. To minimize this risk, the plate should be placed as anterior as possible distally. Different plates have different rotational profiles and this can contribute to how the plate is positioned and fixed. If care is not taken, the condyles can be rotated during fixation of the fracture. A sagittal plane and rotational plane deformity can be induced or there is an increased risk of postoperative plate pull-off if

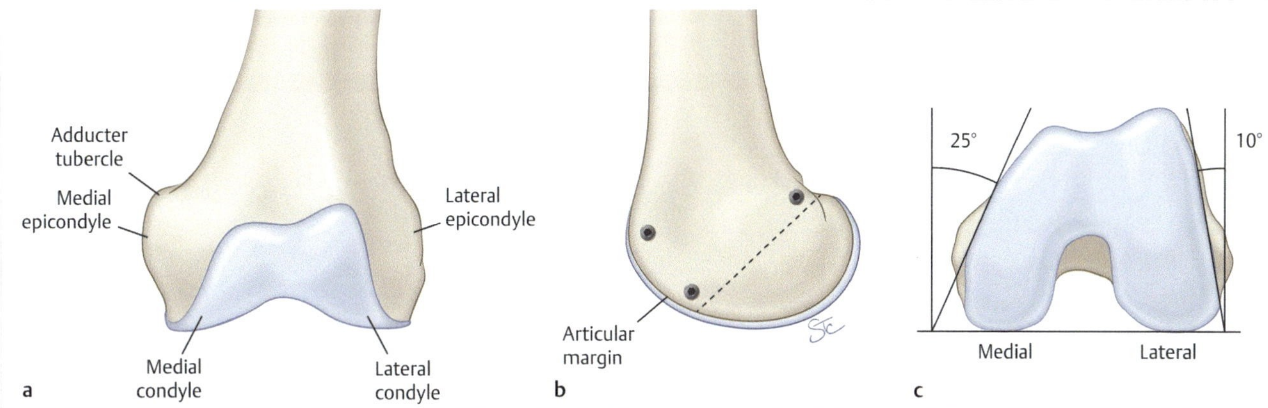

Fig. 6.3 **(a)** Normal anatomy of the distal femur in the coronal plane, **(b)** lateral distal femur showing the normal position of lag screws for the articular fracture fixation, and **(c)** axial view showing the normal angles of the femoral condyles in order to avoid overpenetration of implants.

the plate is not centered proximally. The proximal position of the plate can be verified by either making a large enough incision proximally to clinically visualize or palpate the plate position on the bone, or using lateral fluoroscopy and the percutaneous aiming guide that is incorporated into most systems to reference where the plate will be centered (▶ Fig. 6.2).

6.9 Difficulties Encountered

- The most common malreduction deformity to overcome is extension of the articular segment. However, in bicondylar fractures, the surgeon also has to address the extension deformity of each condyle due to the collateral ligament attachment. The collateral ligament also causes external rotation of each condyle.
- The last difficulty that is encountered with bicondylar fractures is the intercondylar notch reduction. Overcompression of the intercondylar notch causes trochlear stenosis and patellar maltracking. This most commonly occurs when there is anterior intercondylar notch comminution and a single anteriorly-based reduction forceps or lag screws are used. If there is anterior comminution, overcompression with a clamp should be avoided and position screws, rather than lag screws, should be used. If a single anteriorly-based clamp is used, there is also a risk of gapping the intercondylar notch posteriorly. Using a proximal anteriorly-based clamp and a more distal and posterior clamp placed in line with the epicondylar axis decreases the chance of gapping posteriorly (▶ Fig. 6.4).

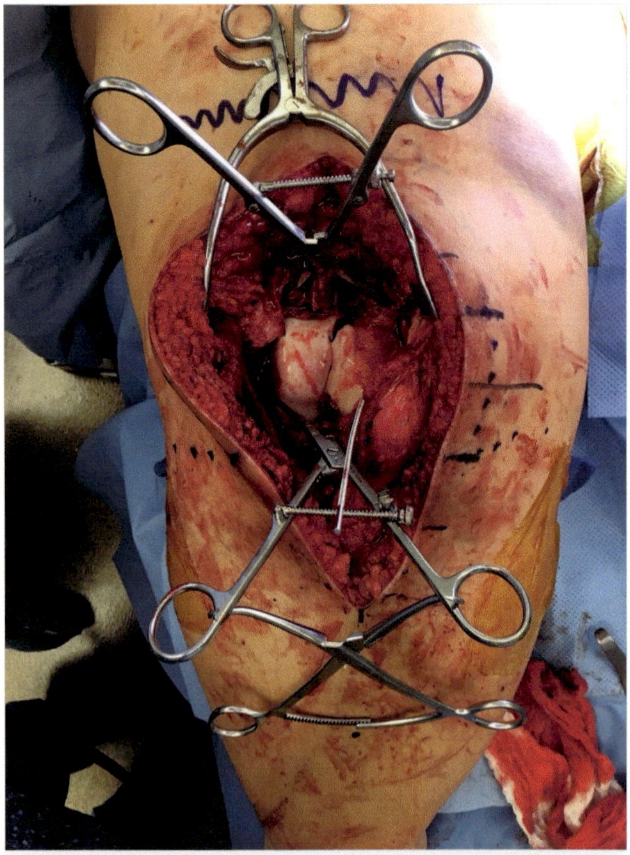

Fig. 6.4 Intraoperative clinical photo showing articular reduction with one large pointed reduction forceps placed proximally, and one placed along the epicondylar axis to reduce the intercondylar articular fracture. The patient had articular cartilage loss proximally.

6.10 Key Procedural Steps

6.10.1 Choosing the Correct Surgical Exposure

Direct Lateral

Indications

- Planning on using a laterally-based implant.
- Lateral Hoffa fracture.
- The initial fracture displacement is valgus:
  - Planning on using buttress/antiglide plating.
- Familiarity with exposure.

Variations

Standard lateral approach with parapatellar arthrotomy.

TARPO (Transarticular Retrograde Percutaneous Osteosynthesis)

Indications

- Intra-articular comminution involving both femoral condyles, particularly if there are two coronal plane fractures, and lateral plating.
- Planning on open reduction of the articular fracture component and medullary nailing.

Description (▶ Fig. 6.5)

- Standard anterior midline incision large enough to gain access to the entire articular surface—3- to 4-cm proximal to the patella and to the tibial tubercle level distally.
- Lateral or medial parapatellar arthrotomy allows for subluxation and retraction of the patella to visualize the entire articular surface—patellofemoral joint and medial and lateral femoral condyles (▶ Fig. 6.6).
- If lateral plating is performed, the plate is passed submuscularly in a retrograde fashion. Using an aiming arm may place too much tension on the lateral skin flap if the patient has a large body habitus.

Swashbuckler Approach

Indications

Same as the TARPO.

Description

A standard midline incision is utilized as discussed in the TARPO section. However, the lateral parapatellar arthrotomy is carried proximal and the quadriceps is split just lateral to the tendon.

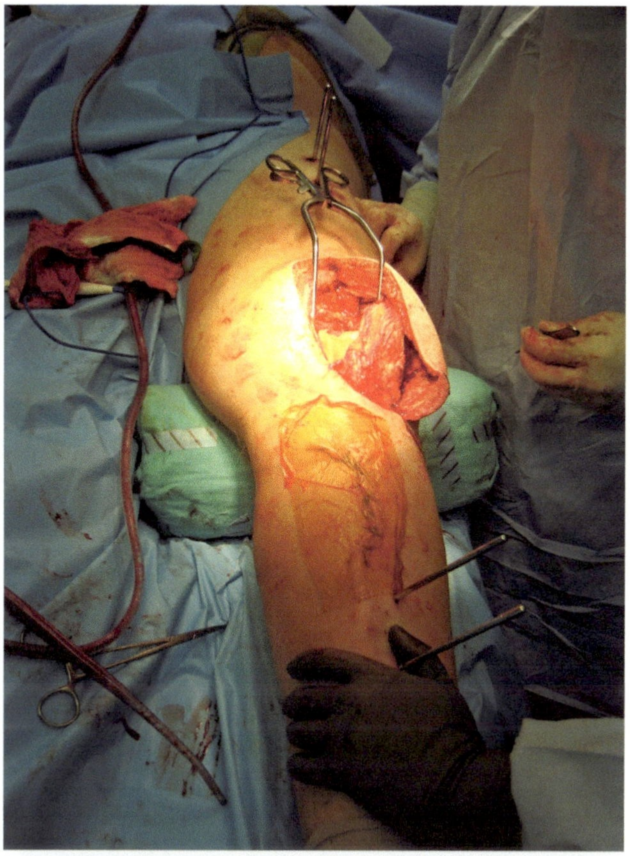

Fig. 6.5 Intraoperative clinical photo showing the transarticular retrograde percutaneous osteosynthesis approach (TARPO) with a medial parapatellar arthrotomy.

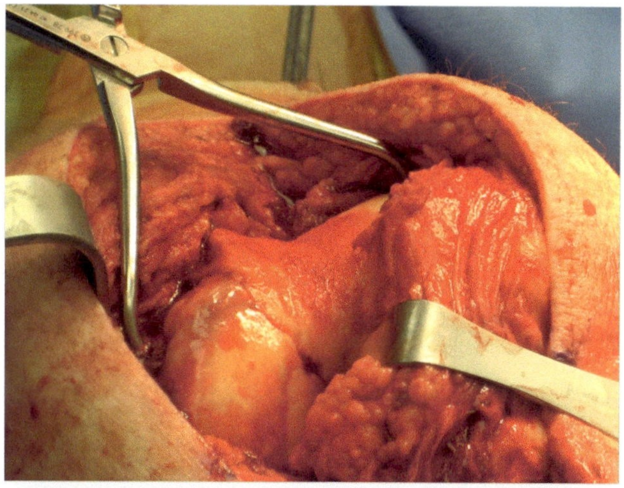

Fig. 6.6 Intraoperative clinical photo showing the articular visualization and reduction afforded with the transarticular retrograde percutaneous osteosynthesis approach (TARPO) with a medial parapatellar arthrotomy.

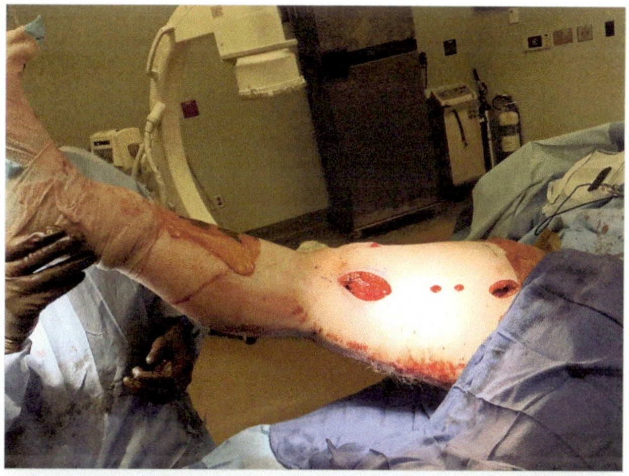

Fig. 6.7 Intraoperative clinical photo showing the medial subvastus approach for medial plating.

Medial Approach—Subvastus

Indications

- Medial Hoffa fracture.
- Medial condylar involvement.
- Initial varus fracture displacement.
  - Planning to use buttress/antiglide plating techniques.

Description (▶ Fig. 6.7)

The vastus medialis is usually palpable just at the proximal margin of the medial femoral condyle. A longitudinal incision is made as proximally as needed for reduction of the fracture including the metaphysis. The superficial femoral artery is posterior to the medial septum and is even more posterior with flexion of the knee. An incision is made proximally where the proximal aspect of the plate will be. This can be determined fluoroscopically by placing the plate over the skin with the distal aspect of the plate in the intended position. A longitudinal incision is made and the superficial interval between the rectus femoris and sartorius is utilized. The vastus medialis is retracted posteriorly which protects the femoral vessels. The descending branch of the lateral femoral circumflex vessel lies over the vastus intermedius and needs to be isolated and protected if plating above the distal 60% of the total femur length. When dissection is within 8 cm of the lesser trochanter, caution must be used to identify and protect the vessels and may require a larger incision for safe dissection. Using careful blunt soft tissue dissection technique, screws that need to be placed between the proximal and distal aspects of the plate can be placed percutaneously.

6.10.2 Articular Reduction and Fixation

- Each femoral condyle is externally rotated and extended due to the collateral ligament attachment. Avoid traction on the limb to minimize the ligamentotaxis. Insert 2.0-mm K-wires into each condyle—one from anterior to posterior along the trochlear ridge, and one more can be added from lateral to medial for the lateral femoral condyle, or medial to lateral for the medial femoral condyle to gain two points of fixation that allows for manipulation of the condyle.
- If a coronal plane fracture is present, it should be reduced first. Usually, a large, pointed, reduction forceps is placed

distally at the peripheral margin of the articular cartilage and proximally along the trochlear ridge to control rotation and compress the fracture.
  - Fixation: Multiple provisional Kirschner wires are inserted from anterior to posterior to control length and rotation while avoiding definitive fixation pathways. Once the provisional reduction and fixation is complete, you can place two definitive anterior to posterior lag screws (3.5-, 4.0-, or 4.5-mm screws) along the trochlear ridge that are countersunk below the articular cartilage, and avoid articular penetration distally/posteriorly. Two screws are used to help control any rotational displacement, and provide symmetric compression for the fracture. It is critical to place these screws in a way to avoid blocking other definitive screw pathways placed from medial to lateral.
- Intercondylar reduction:
  - Use the 2.0-mm K-wires previously placed to independently manipulate and reduce each condylar fragment. Use a large, pointed, reduction forceps (Weber) anteriorly at the level of the trochlea, and another one placed more distally and posteriorly at the level of the epicondylar axis to minimize malreduction (▶ Fig. 6.4). If you only place a reduction forceps anteriorly at the level of the trochlea, there is a risk that you will overcompress the anterior cortex and gap the notch posteriorly. At least two definitive lag or position screws (if comminution is present) are placed transversely and out of the way of definitive plate or IMN fixation pathways. Most plating systems have a template of the distal femur plate footprint that can be used to ensure safe placement of these screws.

6.10.3 Metadiaphyseal Reduction

Coronal and Sagittal Plane Reduction and Length Restoration

It is challenging due to the deforming muscular and ligamentous forces encountered, the limited view that fluoroscopy provides, and fracture comminution that is often present. If there is a simple fracture pattern and the soft tissue envelope allows, a biologically friendly direct reduction is utilized. However, if there is fracture comminution or soft tissue concern, multiple reduction aids and techniques may be used to correct each plane of deformity.

The Metadiaphyseal Deforming Forces

- Length—shortening of fracture is caused by the pull of the adductors, hamstrings, and quadriceps.
- Sagittal plane—extension deformity is caused by the gastrocnemius and hamstring muscles.
- Coronal plane—varus deformity is caused by the adductor muscles.

Techniques for Sagittal Plane and Length Reduction

Although manual or skeletal traction may be helpful, I prefer an "all-femur" external fixator (▶ Fig. 6.2). This allows for correction and maintenance of both the sagittal plane alignment and length. Once the reduction is obtained, and the external fixator clamps are tightened, the reduction is maintained. Sterile bumps or triangles can help supplement and fine tune the reduction. A universal distractor (DePuy Synthes, West Chester, PA) can be used instead of two external fixator clamps and a single rod, but, for me, the weight of the distractor makes it more challenging to maintain the position of the limb.

Pin Placement (All-femur External Fixator ▶ Fig. 6.2)

- Use a 5-mm Schanz pin placed from anterior to posterior in the distal metaphyseal component using fluoroscopy.
- The second pin is placed in the diaphysis from anterior to posterior outside of the zone of comminution.

Techniques for Coronal Plane Reduction

Plate: Author's Preference

When plates are used that have a 95-degree fixed axis hole (▶ Fig. 6.1) or a fixed-angle device that has a known angle distally (i.e., Angled Blade Plate), the device can be used to correct the coronal plane deformity. Once the fixed angle component is placed parallel to the knee joint line, a screw or threaded reduction device can be placed in the diaphysis to restore the lateral distal femoral angle and translation of the femoral shaft on the articular surface (▶ Fig. 6.1). Due to plate contour and patient anatomy mismatch, sometimes this still can overreduce the articular block (▶ Fig. 6.1). The option is to either remove the plate and modify the plate contour, or allow the plate to sit off the bone. A locking screw can be used as a push device to modify the reduction.

Schanz Pin

Placing a Schanz pin into the reconstructed articular segment from medial to lateral allows you to reduce the coronal plane deformity (▶ Fig. 6.2).

Periarticular Reduction Forceps

Either a large pointed or periarticular reduction forceps can be used to reduce the coronal plane deformity and can regain length.

6.10.4 Fixation Strategy

Steps

Articular Fixation

- Type of screws:
  - 3.5-mm, 4.0-mm, or 4.5-mm cortical or cannulated screws.
- Placement:
  - Coronal plane fracture.
  - Intercondylar split.

Plate Fixation vs. IMN for Definitive Fixation

- Plate fixation is advantageous for bicondylar distal femur fractures because the implant can be used to affect reduction and there are more points of fixation in the articular segment.

- However, I will consider using an IMN after articular fixation in older patients with osteoporosis or poor bone quality. I would also consider an IMN in the setting of metaphyseal comminution or bone loss.
- The plate function determines the steps. Usually, the plate is used to affect the coronal plane reduction as previously described. The plate is provisionally fixed proximally and distally—using the 95-degree axis hole for alignment and at least one more wire into the distal segment for rotational control, and one placed proximally through the aiming arm at the most proximal hole to maintain fracture length. If the all-femur external fixator does not control the sagittal plane reduction, another wire can be added through the aiming arm near the metaphyseal fracture component in the proximal segment to increase sagittal plane stability. A cortical screw or threaded reduction device is placed in the proximal segment near the fracture to affect the coronal plane reduction. Once the desired reduction is achieved, the sagittal plane reduction is verified fluoroscopically. Since the plate is positioned anterolaterally on the femur, the sagittal plane reduction can be affected when the bone is pulled toward the plate during the coronal plane reduction (▶ Fig. 6.2). Once the reduction is acceptable, locking screws are placed distally and diaphyseal cortical screws are placed proximally. For both plate fixation and IMN fixation distally, the angle of the medial condyle should be considered when determining screw/bolt length to avoid overpenetration and symptomatic hardware (▶ Fig. 6.3). If there is concern for overpenetration, a merchant view can identify overpenetration of the medial femoral condyle. Locking screws are only used proximally when the coronal plane reduction continues to be effected by placing cortical screws.

6.10.5 Closure

Standard layer closure is performed with absorbable suture deep and nylon skin closure.

6.11 Bailout, Rescue, Salvage Procedures

The most common reasons for difficulty during the procedure are articular comminution and metadiaphyseal reduction. Smaller cortical screws used as lag or position screws, K-wire fixation, or bioabsorbable pins can be used to address the comminuted articular fragments. If there is difficulty in obtaining an appropriate metadiaphyseal reduction, especially in the setting of bone loss, a medial and lateral plate can be applied in a biologically friendly manner. Alternatively, a cortical substitution or medullary plate can be used to affect the medial metaphyseal reduction. This is also a time where I would consider using a retrograde IMN if the articular block is large enough for fixation with the nail in addition to the separate articular fixation. In the elderly with poor bone quality and significant articular comminution or bone loss, a distal femur replacement TKA may be considered.

6.12 Pitfalls

The most common pitfalls are malreduction in the sagittal plane and malpositioning the laterally-based plate too posterior causing medialization of the articular block. If the plate is not centered proximally, poorly placed screws are guaranteed and increase the chance of plate pull-off proximally. Finally, overreduction of the anterior articular surface can occur when there is intercondylar comminution. Throughout this chapter, I attempted to guide the reader to minimize the risk of encountering these pitfalls.

7 Distal Femur Fracture in the Coronal Plane—Hoffa Fracture

Robinson Esteves Pires, Richard S. Yoon, and Frank A. Liporace

7.1 Description

Several surgical approaches and treatment methods are currently described for coronal plane fractures of the distal femur. This chapter aims to outline these treatment methods and the author's preference according to the fracture pattern.

7.2 Key Principles

Distal femur fractures in the coronal plane could be overlooked in the set of multifragmentary injuries. Computed tomography is mandatory to identify the three-dimensional location of the main fracture planes, allowing for a precise preoperative planning. The key factors determining the prognosis and treatment methods are the soft tissue envelope, bone density, the fractured fragment's size, association with sagittal plane fractures, and the degree of comminution.

7.3 Expectations

Posterolateral fractures of the distal femur in the coronal plane can be fixed from anterior to posterior with screws or from posterior to anterior using both screws and buttress plates. Biomechanically, posterior to anterior fixation is more stable than anterior to posterior fixation. However, in associated sagittal plane fractures requiring anterior approach, anterior to posterior screw fixation should suffice. Our treatment preference for coronal posterolateral fractures of the distal femur is the posterolateral buttress plate. Headless screws can be used to fix small osteochondral fragments. For posteromedial fractures, we usually perform posteromedial approach alongside with a posteromedial buttress plate. If necessary, lag screws can be used to complement the fixation.

7.4 Indications

Coronal plane fractures of the distal femur are associated with articular incongruence and knee instability. Therefore, the standard treatment involves anatomical reduction and stable fixation. Conservative treatment may be considered for incomplete fractures or in patients with severe comorbidities that contraindicates fracture fixation.

7.5 Contraindications

- Presence of soft tissue infection or osteomyelitis.
- Clinical comorbidities associated with a surgical risk that outweighs the benefits of surgery.
- Severe vascular insufficiency in the same extremity.

7.6 Special Considerations

Preoperative planning is essential to prevent complications in coronal plane fractures of the distal femur. Radiographs in anteroposterior and lateral views usually show the fracture. In cases of severe articular or metaphyseal comminution, radiographs with gentle traction can be useful for better understanding of the fracture pattern. However, computed tomography is mandatory for the fracture morphology understanding and correct preoperative planning.

7.7 Special Instructions, Positioning, and Anesthesia

The procedure is performed under general anesthesia. Usually, the patient is placed on a radiolucent table in prone or lateral position. For double Hoffa fractures, the prone position is the choice. We apply a pad under the thigh, ensuring that both thighs are not at the same level. The goal is to facilitate fluoroscopic imaging of the distal femur on lateral projections. Lateral positioning with the knee in full extension is an alternative for posterolateral fractures in the coronal plane. Alternatively, supine positioning can be the choice if an anterior surgical approach is required. The medial Hoffa fracture can be addressed with the patient supine with a pad under the contralateral buttock. This facilitates the posteromedial approach. A tourniquet is left on the most proximal aspect of the thigh, but it is not routinely used.

7.8 Tips, Pearls, and Lessons Learned

Fracture pattern determines the surgical approach. For coronal plane fractures, posterolateral or posteromedial approaches are usually the choice. However, in complex fractures combining sagittal and coronal planes, extended anterolateral or anteromedial approach may be required. We use the modified Letenneur classification as a guideline for decision making in cases of fractures of the lateral femoral condyle (▶ Fig. 7.1).

7.8.1 Posterolateral Approach

For Letenneur type I, a posterolateral approach with buttress plating is our treatment choice. If a type I variant (comminution or articular depression) is present, the osteotomy of the Gerdy tubercle facilitates the exposure of the central depressed or comminuted fragment. An anterolateral approach combining anterior to posterior lag screws with a horizontal plate is an alternative treatment option. Double approach, combining posterolateral and anterolateral fixation, is another possibility to address the Hoffa fragment with a posterolateral buttressing plate and the central fragments with headless screws.

For Letenneur type II, plate fixation is almost impossible, since the size of the fractured condyle is too small, representing an osteochondral fragment. Posterior to anterior fixation with headless screws is our preferred treatment method. For Letenneur type III, we usually perform an anterolateral parapatellar approach and fix the fracture using anterior to posterior lag screws, complemented with a horizontal belt plate.

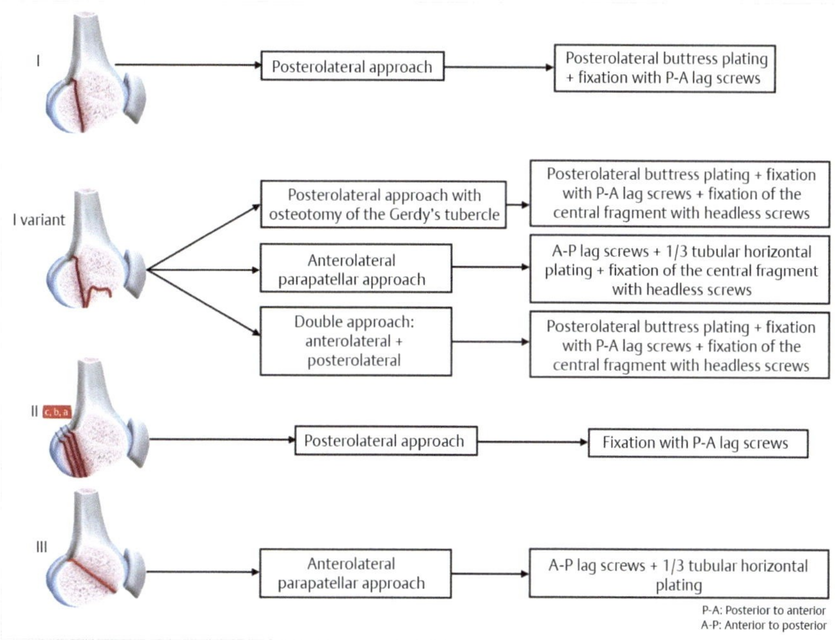

Fig. 7.1 Treatment algorithm based on the modified Letenneur classification for lateral Hoffa fractures.

The posterolateral approach is used for coronal plane fractures of the lateral condyle. A 10-cm longitudinal incision is performed in line with the biceps tendon. Careful subcutaneous dissection is recommended due to the risk of iatrogenic peroneal nerve palsy. The peroneal nerve is identified medially to the biceps tendon. A number 2 Penrose drain or Surg-I-Loop is used to mobilize and protect the nerve. Deep dissection is performed between the biceps tendon and the iliotibial band (▶ Fig. 7.2).

The fracture is reduced with the knee in full extension. Provisional fixation is performed with K-wires, and images are taken in anteroposterior and lateral views. The 3.5-mm locking compression plate (LCP) or the one-third tubular plate is contoured to buttress the posterolateral fracture of the lateral condyle. If an intermediary articular fragment is present (Letenneur type I variant), the standard posterolateral approach may be insufficient to promote adequate exposure of the fracture. In this situation, our preference is the Gerdy tubercle osteotomy and fixation of the intermediary fragment with headless screws. The Gerdy tubercle is then fixed using a 3.5-mm cortical screw with a washer (▶ Fig. 7.3).

In Letenneur types IIa, IIb, and IIc, our preference is the posterolateral approach between the biceps tendon and the peroneal nerve.

Using this approach, one can easily address small fragment fractures of the lateral condyle using headless screws from posterior to anterior. Alternatively, the lateral condyle can be addressed medially to the peroneal nerve, medially retracting the lateral caput of the gastrocnemius muscle to protect the popliteal vessels. We discourage using anterior to posterior fixation in Letenneur type II fractures due to the small fragment size which impedes screw threads from completely bypassing the fracture line, therefore precluding fracture compression.

7.8.2 Anterolateral Approach

An anterolateral approach is our preference to reduce and fix Letenneur type III fractures and our alternative treatment strategy for Letenneur type I variant. The anterolateral approach starts on the lateral edge of the patellar tendon, crosses the lateral retinaculum, and finishes on the metaphyseal area of the distal femur. The patella is moved medially, and the fracture is reduced using bone clamps. Provisional fixation is performed using K-wires.

Letenneur type III fractures generally present horizontal fracture line and a major fragment that can be safely fixed using lag screws from anterior to posterior. To increase construct stability, we recommend using an additional horizontal belt plate (▶ Fig. 7.4).

7.8.3 Medial Approaches

Coronal plane fractures of the medial condyle are less frequent and present morphologic differences in comparison with lateral patterns. Medial Hoffa fractures generally present a more horizontal fracture line. A sagittal fracture mapping showed that fracture lines are concentrated in the middle third of the lateral condyle but are less concentrated in the medial condyle. Comminution is more concentrated in the weight-bearing zone in the lateral condyle, whereas it is more spread in the medial condyle.

We developed a simple comprehensive classification system and a treatment algorithm for medial Hoffa fractures based on the fragment size and presence of fracture comminution (▶ Fig. 7.5).

The great benefit of this fragment-specific fixation strategy over previously described protocols for medial coronal plane distal femur fractures is the choice of surgical approach and ideal fixation strategy according to the fracture pattern. Simple fracture patterns with no comminution (types I and II) can be safely and effectively managed with a posteromedial subvastus approach. When a distal extension is necessary, the posteromedial fragment can be approached in the interval between the gracilis and the medial caput of the gastrocnemius muscle (▶ Fig. 7.6).

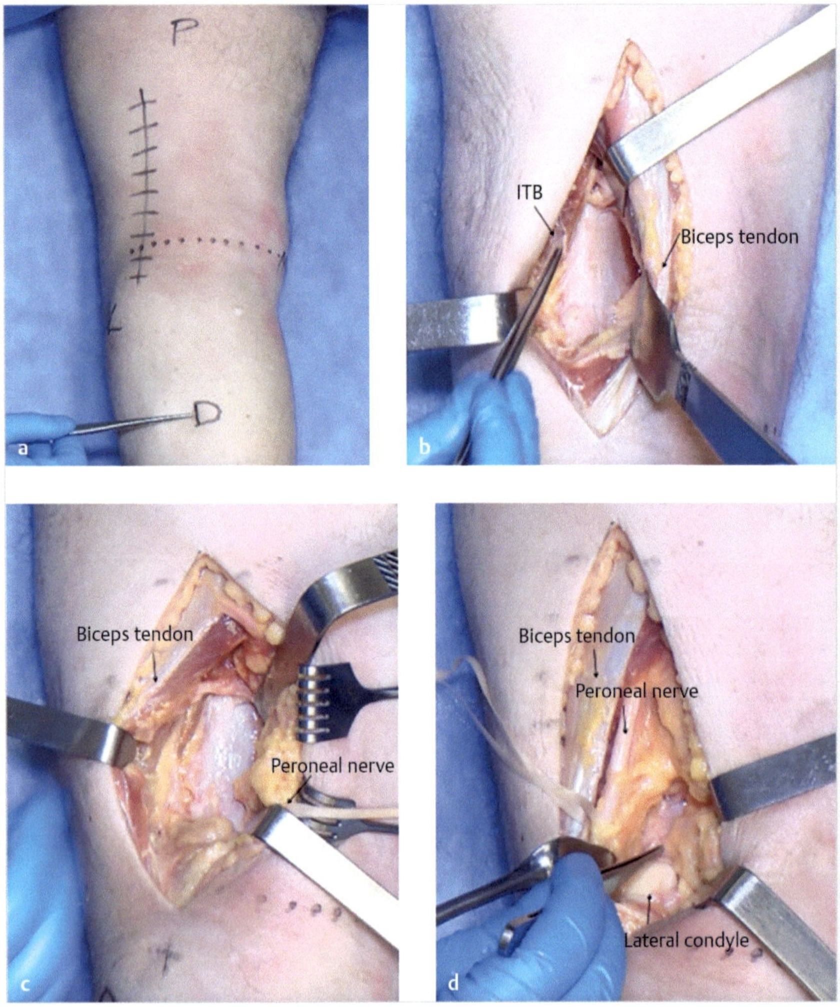

Fig. 7.2 (a) Posterior view of the knee. Longitudinal approach to the distal femur. P: Proximal; D: Distal; L: Lateral; M: Medial. **(b)** Lateral window between the iliotibial band (ITB) and the biceps. **(c)** Posterior view of the knee. Interval between the biceps tendon and the peroneal nerve. **(d)** Alternatively, the lateral condyle can be addressed medially to the peroneal nerve, carefully retracting the lateral caput of the gastrocnemius muscle.

Comminuted patterns (types Ic and IIc) involving both the anterior and posterior zones of the medial femoral condyle require a medial extensile subvastus approach with the two-window fixation technique. Using this approach, two capsulotomies are possible, anteriorly and posteriorly to the medial collateral ligament depending on fracture pattern, location, and degree of comminution. Fragment-specific fixation is performed with multiple screws (2.0, 2.4, or 2.7 mm, depending on the fragment size) in different directions to achieve proper fixation. A buttress LCP or one-third tubular plate is used to fix the Hoffa fragment.

In some fracture patterns with severe comminution, an anteromedial parapatellar arthrotomy and fixation with anterior to posterior lag screws, combined with a horizontal plate may be a helpful and simpler treatment alternative. If an additional fixation with larger footprint is required, the unconventional use of a calcaneal plate or an upside down proximal humeral locking plate plays a strategic role for fracture containment. Precontoured proximal humerus plate turned upside down can offer great fit and an abundance of a locking screw cluster with an ideal trajectory and fixation.

However, although hypothesizing that these plates are interesting alternatives for comminuted fracture patterns, there are no biomechanical studies validating this hypothesis. Osteochondral graft also may be a helpful treatment option.

7.9 Difficulties Encountered

As the Hoffa fracture is usually reduced with the knee in full extension, performing the surgery with an anterolateral approach in supine position is sometimes challenging, since the Hoffa fragment is better visualized with the knee in flexion. Furthermore, placing hardware, plates, and screws from posterior to anterior is very challenging when an anterolateral approach is selected.

Comminuted fractures with central articular depression are challenging and usually require additional Gerdy tubercle osteotomy when doing the posterolateral approach.

The popliteal tendon can be entrapped between the fragments of Letenneur type II fractures, therefore making fracture reduction difficult.

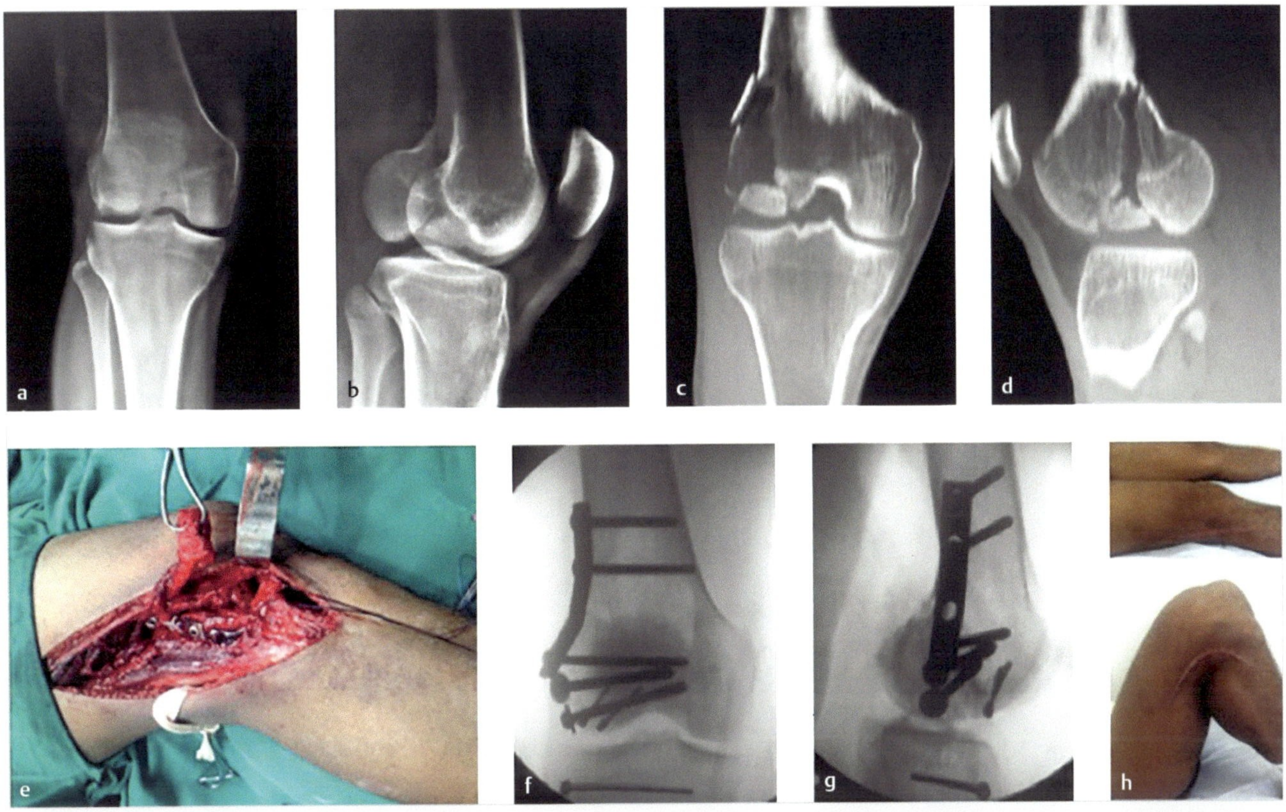

Fig. 7.3 (a,b) Radiographs in anteroposterior and lateral views showing the Letenneur type 1 variant. **(c,d)** Computed tomography (CT) scan in coronal and sagittal cuts showing the central fragment. **(e)** Perioperative image showing the Gerdy osteotomy and the fracture fixation using an antigliding plate and Herbert screws for the central fragment. **(f,g)** Postoperative images in anteroposterior and lateral views showing fracture fixation. **(h)** Clinical images after surgical wound healing showing full range of motion of the fractured knee.

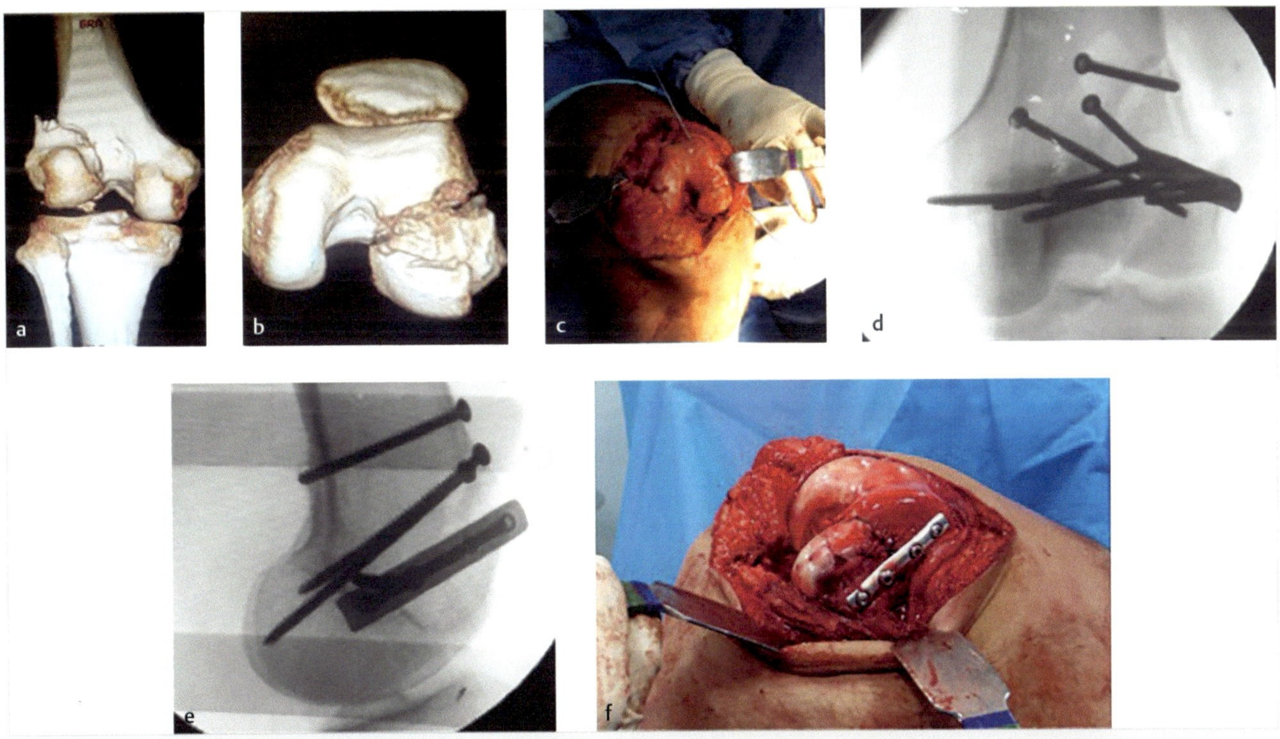

Fig. 7.4 (a,b) Computed tomography (CT) scan in 3D showing the type 1 variant with central comminution. **(c)** Perioperative image of the anterolateral approach showing the fracture reduction and provisional fixation with K-wires. **(d,e)** Postoperative images in anteroposterior and lateral views showing fracture fixation with anterior to posterior screws, complemented with a horizontal belt plate. **(f)** Intraoperative image revealing an horizontal belt plate securing the femoral condyle (Courtesy: Dr. Vincenzo Giordano).

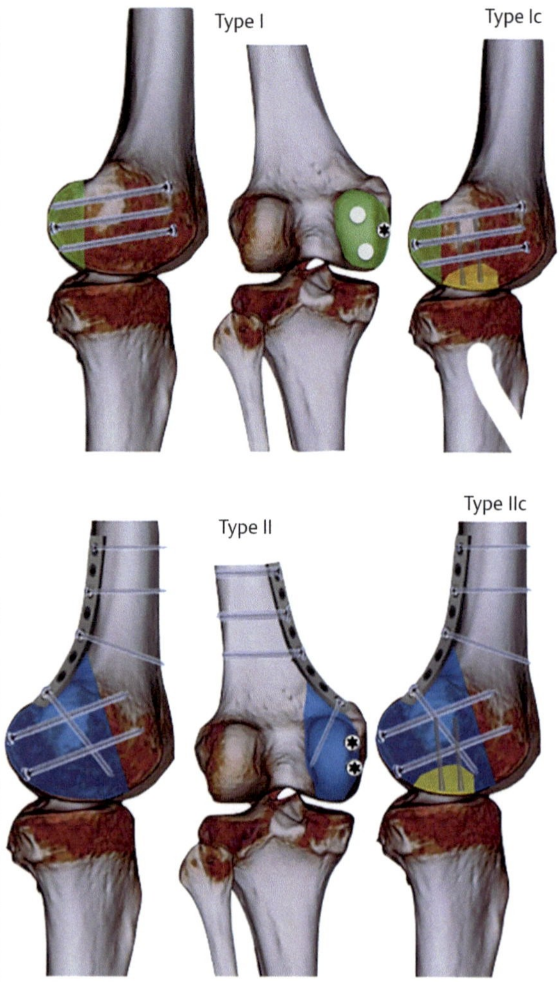

Fracture type	Approach	Fixation strategy
I	Posteromedial fragment can be approached in the interval between the gracilis and the medial caput of the gastrocnemius muscles (alternatively, posteromedial fragment can be approached with the medial extensile subvastus approach	Lag screws to fix the hoffa fragment
Ic	Medial extensile subvastus approach	Lag screws to fix the hoffa fragment + fragment-specific fixation of comminuted fragments with headless or countersunk cortical screws
II	Posteromedial subvastus approach between the vastus medialis and the semimembranosus muscles. If necessary, medial hoffa fragment can be approached in the interval between the gracilis and the medial caput of the gastrocnemius muscles	Posteromedial plate fixation + lag screws
IIc	Medial extensile subvastus approach	Lag screws + fragment-specific fixation of comminuted fragments with headless or countersunk cortical screws

Fig. 7.5 Illustration showing fixation methods according to our classification system. Type I: Osteochondral Hoffa fragment. Ic: Type I with associated comminution (regardless of comminution location). II: Fracture line runs through the metaphyseal area of the posterior cortex of the distal femur. IIc: Type II with associated comminution (regardless of comminution location). Observe the orientation of the lag screws, perpendicular to the fracture line. Observe the projection of the screws placed from anterior to posterior in the posterior view of the knee (*black stars*) for type I fixation. Source: Medial Hoffa fracture: description of a novel classification system and rationale for treatment based on fragment-specific fixation strategy. (Reproduced from Pires RE, Bidolegui F, Pereira S, et. al. Medial Hoffa Fracture: Description of a Novel Classification System and Rationale for Treatment Based on Fragment-Specific Fixation Strategy. Z Orthop Unfall. December 2020.)

7.10 Key Procedural Steps

Preoperative planning, correct fracture classification, and patient positioning, as well as adequate bone clamps, may help diminish problems when fixing coronal plane fractures of the distal femur.

The correct approach and exposure is the key for success. We usually fix Hoffa fractures from posterior to anterior. However, the anterolateral approach can be helpful for comminuted fracture patterns, especially when the fixation from anterior to posterior using lag screws is complemented with the horizontal belt plate to enhance construct stability.

7.11 Bailout, Rescue, and Salvage Procedures

Nonunion and malunions of Hoffa fractures are either a result of overlooked injuries or insufficient fixation. They are extremely symptomatic, leading to a painful joint accompanied by limited range of motion and axis deformity. Preoperative planning with CT scan is mandatory. Prototyping the CT scan can be a helpful procedure to better understand the fracture, therefore facilitating the approach choice, reduction maneuvers, and fixation strategies. ▶ Fig. 7.7 and ▶ Fig. 7.8 show the salvage procedure of a

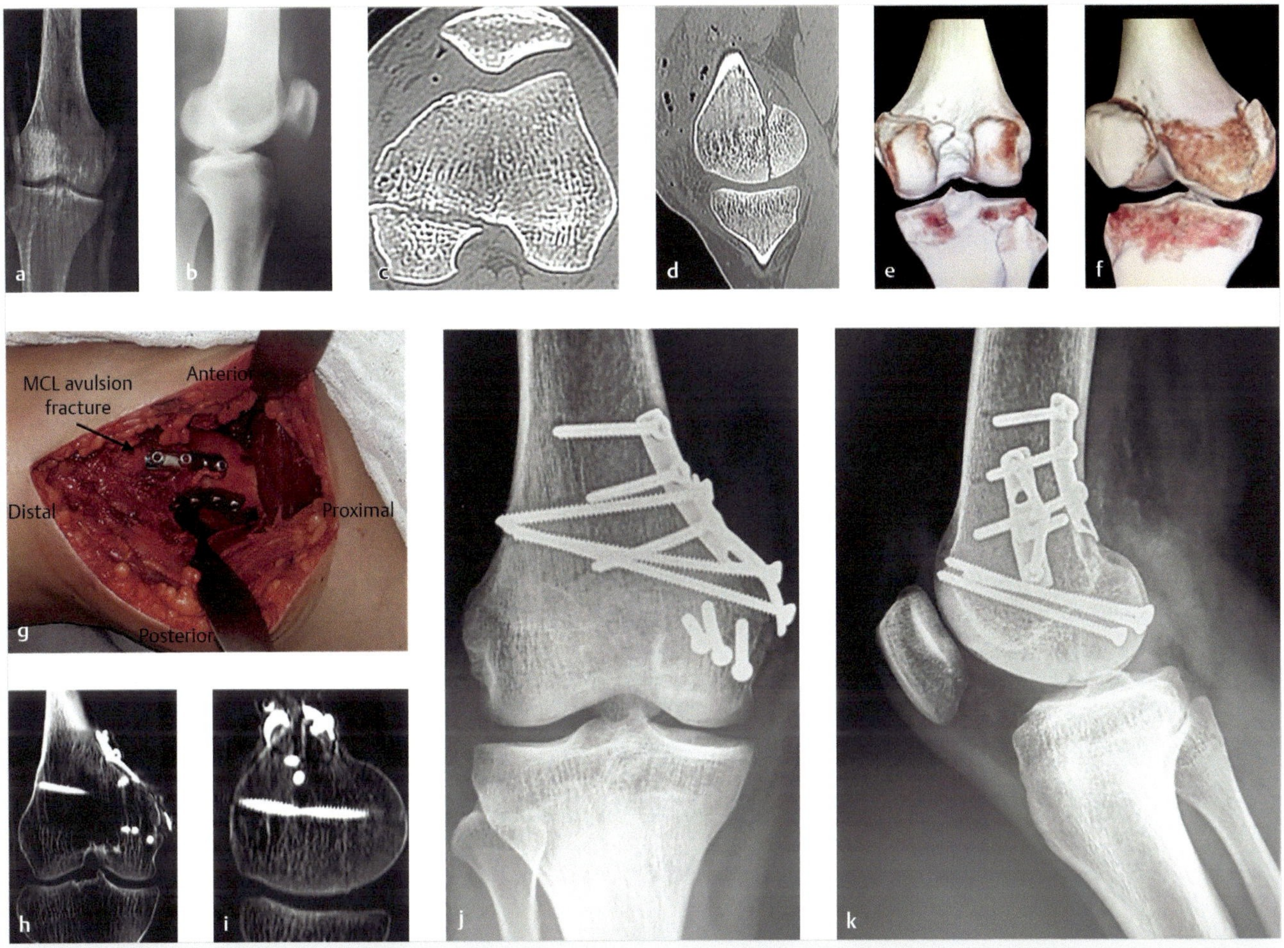

Fig. 7.6 **(a,b)** Radiographs in anteroposterior and lateral projections demonstrating a type II medial Hoffa fracture. **(c,d)** Computed tomography in axial and sagittal cuts depicting the coronal plane fracture of the medial condyle. **(e,f)** Computed tomography with 3D reconstruction highlighting fracture morphology and topography reaching the metaphyseal area of the posterior cortex of the distal femur (type II). Observe that there is a medial collateral ligament (MCL) avulsion fracture. **(g)** Posteromedial subvastus approach between the vastus medialis and the semimembranosus with the patient supine, with a pad under the contralateral buttock. Lag screws from posterior to anterior were placed through the interval between the gracilis and the medial caput of the gastrocnemius muscle. **(h,i)** Computed tomography in coronal and sagittal cuts exhibiting anatomic fracture healing. **(j,k)** Anteroposterior and lateral radiographs exhibiting fracture healing after one year follow-up. The MCL bony avulsion was fixed with an additional plate.

Hoffa fracture malunion after 6 months of surgery. The patient presented knee pain, severe valgus deformity, and important range of motion limitation.

7.12 Pitfalls

The lateral Hoffa fracture internal fixation is challenging with the patient supine, since the reduction is achieved with the knee in full extension, and implants sometimes have to be applied posteriorly to the condyle. We recommend performing lateral Hoffa fracture fixation with the patient in prone or lateral position. Medial Hoffa fractures can be efficiently addressed with the patient supine with a contralateral under gluteal pad.

Letenneur type II fractures present small articular fragments, and the interfragmentary compression is almost impossible from anterior to posterior, since the screw threads do not bypass the fracture line.

Letenneur type I variant (central comminution or depression) is almost impossible to address from posterior approach, unless we carry out a Gerdy tubercle osteotomy or a double approach (anterolateral and posterolateral).

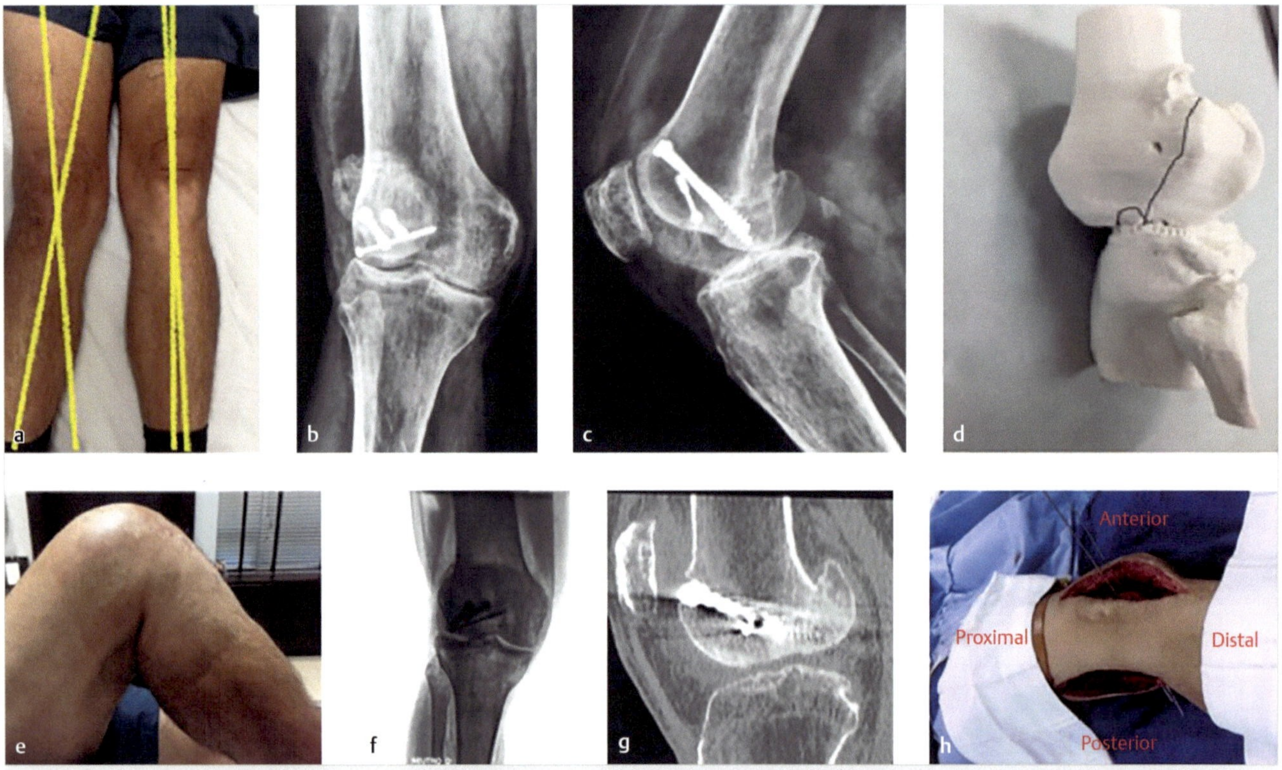

Fig. 7.7 **(a)** Preoperative image showing the clinical aspect of a male patient (55-year-old), presenting significant valgus deformity. **(b,c)** Oblique and lateral radiographic projections depicting a Hoffa fracture malunion. **(d)** 3D prototype reproducing the malunion site. **(e)** Clinical aspect of the knee exhibiting flexion limitation. **(f)** Computed tomography (CT) scan in sagittal view exhibiting the Hoffa fracture malunion. **(g)** Radiograph in anteroposterior view exhibiting the valgus deformity. **(h)** With the patient in lateral decubitus, a double approach was performed (anterolateral and posterolateral). This exposure was needed for the osteotomy and correction of the valgus deformity.

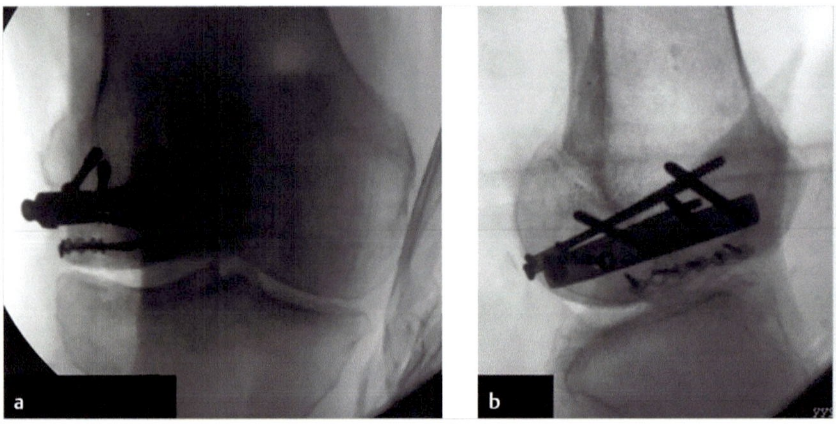

Fig. 7.8 **(a,b)** Postoperative images in anteroposterior and lateral views showing the osteotomy at the malunion site and fixation using posterior to anterior lag screws complemented with a horizontal belt plate. An intra-articular osteotomy was performed to address the depressed central fragment. We fixed the osteotomy with a minifragment plate.

8 Distal Femur Periprosthetic Fracture—Internal Fixation with Plate

Sven Märdian and Michael Schuetz

8.1 Description

This chapter addresses surgical fixation of the distal femur periprosthetic fractures using locking plates.

8.2 Key Principles

Various fixation methods have been described to stabilize periprosthetic fractures of the distal femur. Locking plate systems revolutionized internal fixation techniques, and to date these systems are regarded as the gold standard. Different plating systems are available on the market, with varying philosophies regarding peri-implant fixation options (▶ Fig. 8.1). Although modern fixation techniques tend to be minimally invasive—so-called "biological plating"—stable fixation, restoration of the axis, rotation, and length are of utmost importance for good outcomes and long-term survivorship of the prosthesis (▶ Fig. 8.2). In comminuted distal femur fractures, it is critical to buttress the medial column of the femur. The reconstruction of the medial column may be carried out with either strut grafts or with a plate. The double plating, consisting of lateral and medial plates, has excellent biomechanics properties. Distal femur comminuted fractures are typically seen in the elderly. The authors' preferred method for comminuted distal femur periprosthetic fractures is double plating, as strut bone grafts in this age group are unlikely to be incorporated during the process of bone healing.

8.3 Expectations

In simple fracture types, closed reduction and percutaneous plating using aiming devices provide an excellent and soft tissue-sparing procedure to sufficiently stabilize the femur (▶ Fig. 8.3). Our strategy for long spiral fracture patterns is to apply traction and correct rotation. The reduction is maintained with percutaneous forceps during the plating procedure (▶ Fig. 8.3). In simple fracture patterns, additional lag screws represent a different option to improve stability. Although this seems contradictory to established philosophies, clinical data support the superiority of lag screws in combination with locking plates over stand-alone bridging plate constructs—only in simple fracture types. It has to be emphasized that simple fractures need anatomic reduction. Otherwise, the risk for implant failure or nonunion is increased. Selected cases require open

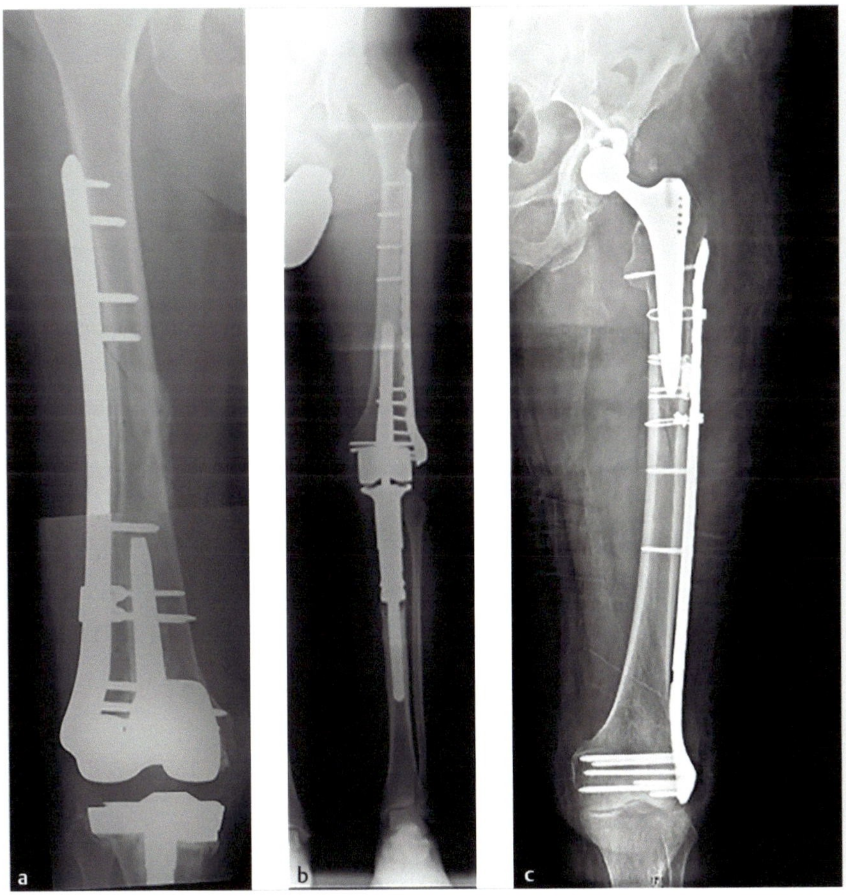

Fig. 8.1 To date, different fixation philosophies for periprosthetic fracture fixation are available. The "L.A.P." (locking attachment plate, Synthes, Umkirch) represents an additional plate **(a)** that is applied to the main implant. Up to four 3.5-mm locking screws can be placed around the intramedullary implant. It has to be taken into account that this plate offers monoaxial screws only. Therefore, it might be difficult to bypass the intramedullary prosthetic stem. Modern plating systems offer the option for polyaxial screw placement (**b**, VA-LCP condyle, Synthes, Umkirch). If the medullary canal is wide enough, bicortical screw anchorage may be achieved around the prosthesis. Recently, a new plating system has been introduced (**c**, aap Implantate AG, Berlin). It offers the option to add "wings" to the main implant. These wings are adjustable to the anatomy of the femur and offer two polyaxial screw option per wing. The fixation philosophy is similar to the L.A.P. but enables the surgeon to achieve the fixation in a variable angle set.

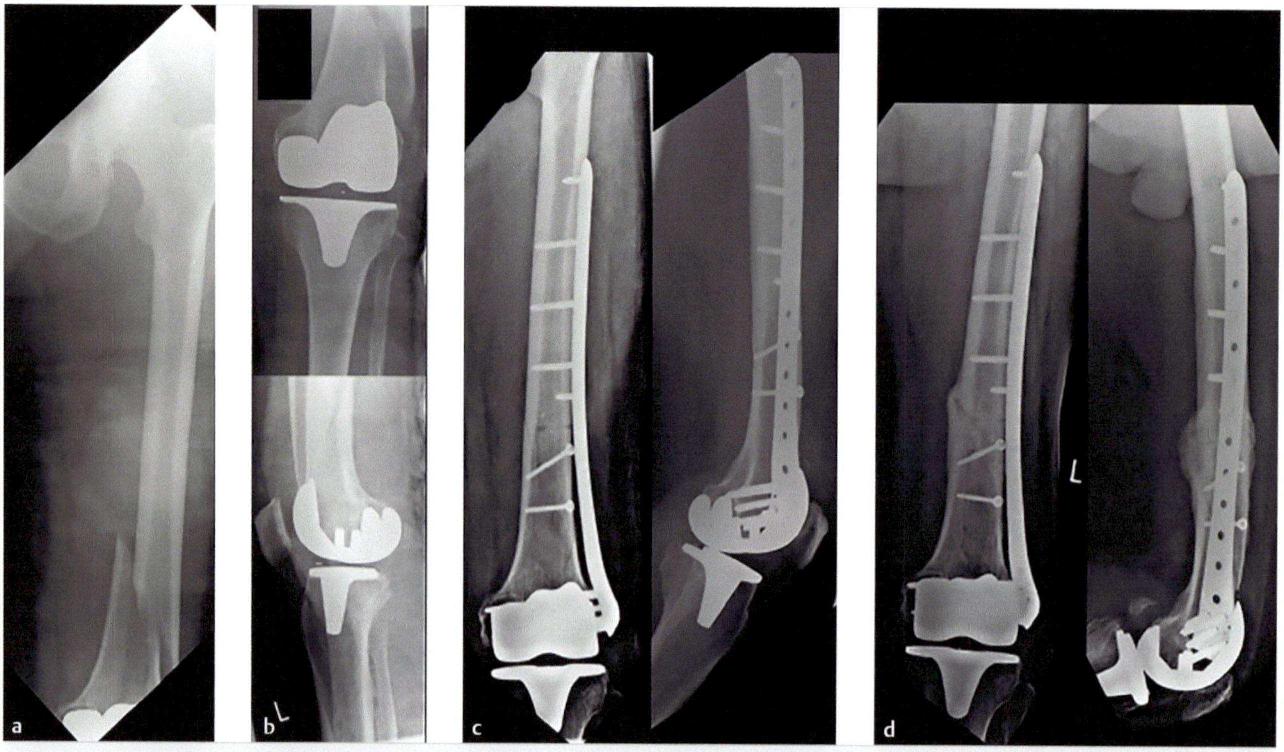

Fig. 8.2 A 77-year-old male suffered a periprosthetic distal femur fracture (**a**, type V.3 C acc. Unified Classification System). He underwent surgery with a locking plate system (**b**, L.I.S.S., Synthes, Umkirch). Immediate postoperative X-ray revealed anatomic reduction (**c**). In addition to the locking plate, percutaneous interfragmentary lag screws were used. Six months postoperatively uneventful healing could be documented (**d**).

reduction to achieve an adequate quality of reduction. In those cases, the lateral subvastus approach grants good fracture exposure allowing for direct plate fixation. By doing so, we can achieve an anatomic reduction in most cases.

8.4 Indications

Surgical fixation of a distal femur periprosthetic fracture is indicated when.

- The fracture is displaced.
- There is enough distal femur bone stock for a stable internal fixation.
- The replacement components are stable.

A relative indication for internal fixation is a nondisplaced fracture in patients with limited mobility.

8.5 Contraindications

- The distal fragment that does not allow for stable screw fixation.
- Loose prosthesis.
- Evidence of infection.
- Significant clinical comorbidities that contraindicate surgery.

8.6 Special Considerations

We obtain plain radiographs of the femur at the patient's admission, including the hip and knee joints on the anteroposterior and lateral incidences. Our decision-making algorithm takes into consideration the following factors.

- Patient's age.
- Patient's overall health status and comorbidities.
- Fracture classification: morphology, location.
- The amount of bone available for a distal femur fixation.
- Bone quality.
- Dedicated history of the knee before the injury: if any mechanical symptoms, pain, or infection had been present before the fracture.
- Prosthesis design: if a cruciate-retaining, a posterior stabilizing, or a revision system.

If the distal femur epiphyseal segment is too short, or if the fracture seems to compromise the stability of the femoral component, we order a computed tomography to determine whether a plate fixation is feasible. High-resolution CT scans with modern software algorithms reduce metal artifacts, improving the interface bone/implant visualization.

8.7 Special Instructions, Position, and Anesthesia

- We place the patient supine on a radiolucent table.
- General anesthesia is our preference.
- The entire femur should be accessible by fluoroscopy.
- If there is no doubt about the stability of the TKA, we prefer a traction table allowing for better control of the femoral length and fracture reduction.

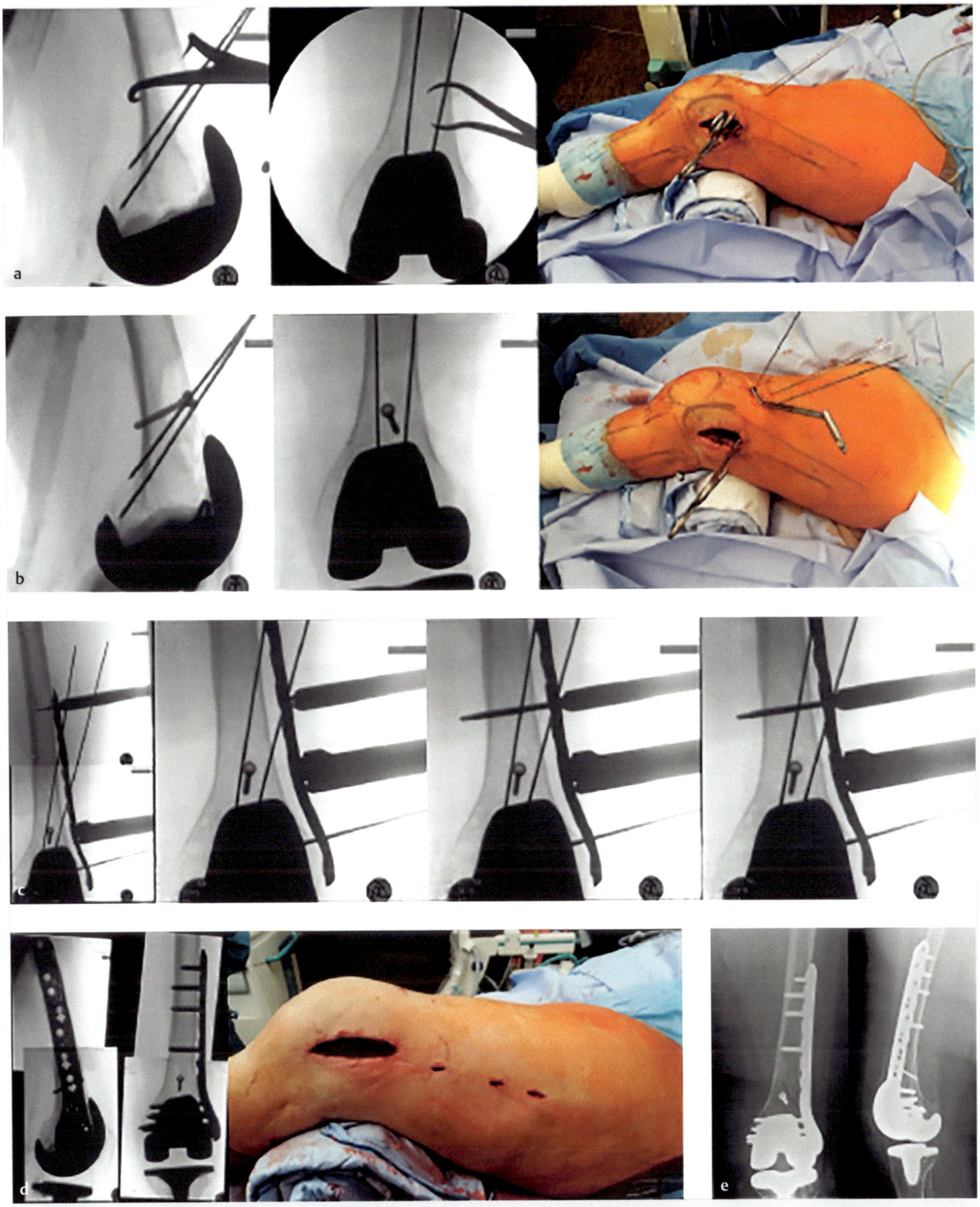

Fig. 8.3 This patient suffered a distal periprosthetic fracture of the femur (type V.3 C acc. Unified Classification System). Closed reduction with a percutaneous applied reduction forceps, and K-wires were inserted **(a)** before introduction of a percutaneous lag screw **(b)**. We used a locking plate with polyaxial screw placement (VA-LCP condyle, Synthes, Umkirch). The axis is finally restored using the reduction tool **(c)** that should be inserted via the aiming device. All screws are applied through the aiming device avoiding additional soft tissues stripping **(d)**. **(e)** Shows a good result 4 weeks postoperative.

- The lower limb is prepped and sterile draped from the midthird of the leg up to the iliac crest.

8.8 Tips, Pearls, and Lessons Learned

- In general, the surgical procedure starts with a standard lateral subvastus approach. If the femoral component is loose, a conversion to a medial parapatellar approach is the option. The skin bridge between the two approaches should be wide enough (at least 8 cm), preventing soft tissue complications.
- The knee should be kept in slight flexion with a pad underneath to counteract the traction forces of the gastrocnemius muscle on the distal fragment facilitating the reduction.
- A preoperative computed tomography (CT) scan determines if bicortical periprosthetic screw placement is possible. If an existing stem prevents the use of bicortical screws to the distal femur, supplemental fixation with locking attachment plates could be an option. Those small plates are connected to the lateral distal femur plates and screw insertion around the femoral stem is allowed.
- In simple fracture cases, the reduction is achieved with traction, correction of the torsion, and percutaneous reduction forceps. By doing so, we achieve an anatomic reduction. Since the reduction forceps prevent the plate from being pushed in, we insert Kirschner wires replacing the forceps. We prefer to insert the wires from anterior to posterior and/or from medial. Sometimes it might be helpful to use cerclages/cables to achieve a sound reduction. We prefer cable cerclages because one can actively reduce the fracture using the clamping device of the cable wire system. The surgeon has to decide whether to use it as a temporary reduction tool or not. If left in place, we place the cable's lock outside of the site where the plate should sit. Furthermore, the use of multiple cerclages/cables is questionable since there is an ongoing debate about the impact of cerclages/cables on the bony blood supply.
- In comminuted fractures, our preference is for relative stability using bridge plates. In these cases, reduction of length, axis, and torsion is the goal. Sometimes it is helpful to apply an anteriorly based external fixator to maintain reduction during the plating procedure. Another suitable method is to insert the plate, fix it to the distal fragment (a perfect plate position is crucial in this case), and then use the plate–distal fragment complex as a reduction aid. Once the fracture is reduced and the plate is centered to the distal fragment, we fix the plate proximally with a threaded Kirschner wire. The wire must be inserted through the drill guide stabilizing the external aiming device. The next step is to insert the reduction tool (*whirlybird*), reducing the proximal fragment to the plate. Once the final reduction is confirmed via fluoroscopy, we complete the insertion of screws through the plate. In most cases of comminuted fractures, we tend to insert a second medial plate.
- What to do if the femoral component is loose?
  It is imperative to answer the following questions preoperatively:
  - What is the design and brand of the knee replacement system already implanted?
  - Is it possible to swap just the femoral component by a revision type, or do we have to perform a complete knee replacement revision?
- Before taking the patient to the operating room, a multidisciplinary approach should be carried out to optimize clinical conditions and foresee all clinical and surgical needs. Special attention is given to the availability of internal fixation and knee revision replacement instruments.

8.9 Difficulties Encountered

Closed reduction may be challenging. If this is the case, a formal open procedure should be performed but respecting the biology of the fracture site. The handling of the soft tissues is of utmost importance following the principles of biological fixation.

The vascular anatomy of the femur should be well known. Special attention is requested when placing a plate to the medial aspect of the femur or inserting bicortical screws from lateral to medial in the subtrochanteric area, or applying cerclage cables around the femur. The surgeon should be prepared in case an unexpected vascular injury happens.

After fixing the fracture with a lateral plate, the knee joint should be stressed in valgus and varus under anesthesia and fluoroscopic control. In case there is residual instability, additional fixation to the medial femoral column should be implemented.

8.10 Key Procedural Steps

We perform a 10-cm incision on the lateral distal aspect of the thigh starting 1 to 2 cm distal to the lateral femoral condyle. The subcutaneous and the iliotibial band are opened in line with the skin. The vastus lateralis muscle is identified and elevated from the posterior septum. We pay attention to the perforator vessels that reach the vastus lateralis from posterior. These vessels have to be coagulated or, in some circumstances, ligated. Following reduction as described above, we apply a plate into the subvastus muscle space.

We position the plate at the distal femur segment with fluoroscopic control in multiple projections. Once we approve its positioning, we apply a provisional threaded wire to hold the plate in place. Our goal is to have the wire parallel to a line tangent to the distal femoral condyles. The lateral fluoroscopic projection is critical in this regard, avoiding hyperextension of the distal femur epiphysis and equivocal distal plate placement. The plate should never be seen below the Blumensaat's line. We use fluoroscopy to confirm that proper placement of the plate is obtained proximally on the femur. Once we approve the position of the plate, we fix it provisionally with a threaded Kirschner wire. At this point, the plate is secured by two Kirschner wires and connected to an external aiming device. Sometimes, a small direct open incision to the lateral aspect of the femur allows for more reliable placement of the plate on the proximal segment of the bone.

Following this, a reduction tool is helpful to reduce the plate to the bone and restore alignment (▶ Fig. 8.3c). It is essential to ensure alignment not only on the anteroposterior but also on the lateral projection of the fluoroscopy. Sometimes having the plate juxtaposed to the lateral aspect of the bone may generate valgus or varus deformity at the fracture site, as precontoured plates do not necessarily fit each patient's anatomy. The surgeon should confirm that pulling the bone against the plate is not generating deformity. Sometimes we leave a space between the plate and the bone, respecting the most anatomical reduction. At the end of the procedure, we detach the aiming device and obtain new fluoroscopic views confirming the fracture reduction's accuracy and the position of the hardware. The wounds are closed following three layers: iliotibial band, subcuticular, and skin.

In distal femur fractures with implants around the hip, long locking plate constructs are favorable as they ensure no stress risers result (▶ Fig. 8.4). However, special considerations have to be made before surgery, reassuring that plate fixation is possible in the case of a femoral stem in the proximal aspect of the femoral canal. New generation implants may overcome this limitation (e.g., L.A.P.—locking attachment plate, Synthes, Umkirch) or polyaxial screw placement. Both options offer the possibility to place bicortical screws around the stem.

In complex fractures or cases in which a significant instability remains following lateral plating, we suggest adding a medial locking plate. To date, no anatomic precontoured plate is available for the medial femur. Alternatively, we have adopted an off-label technique, using an upside-down tibia L.I.S.S. plate (DePuy Synthes). The shape of the plate allows its placement on the anterior medial aspect of the distal femur. This plate position enables the surgeon to safely apply percutaneous screws with the aiming device at the distal third of the femur. When longer plates are necessary, we suggest bending a 4.5-mm L.C.P. to place it anteriorly at the femur's proximal end, avoiding vascular damage.

8.11 Bailout, Rescue, and Salvage Procedures

The literature shows that internal fixation reconstruction of distal femur periprosthetic fractures is accompanied by high failure rates. A revision internal fixation may be considered depending on the patient's general status and the bone stock (▶ Fig. 8.5). However, revision arthroplasty must be considered in cases of multiple failures and insufficient bone stock or other clinical conditions, even if this implies a partial or total femoral replacement (▶ Fig. 8.5). In cases where inadequate stabilization of the distal fragment is seen intraoperatively, revision arthroplasty should be performed instantly. As mentioned above, the decision-making process, whether internal fixation or revision arthroplasty is necessary, should be accomplished before surgery. Therefore, we leave instruments available and obtain appropriate surgical consent. In doubtful cases, when the preoperative screening cannot detect the compromise of the distal femoral component, a small lateral skin incision

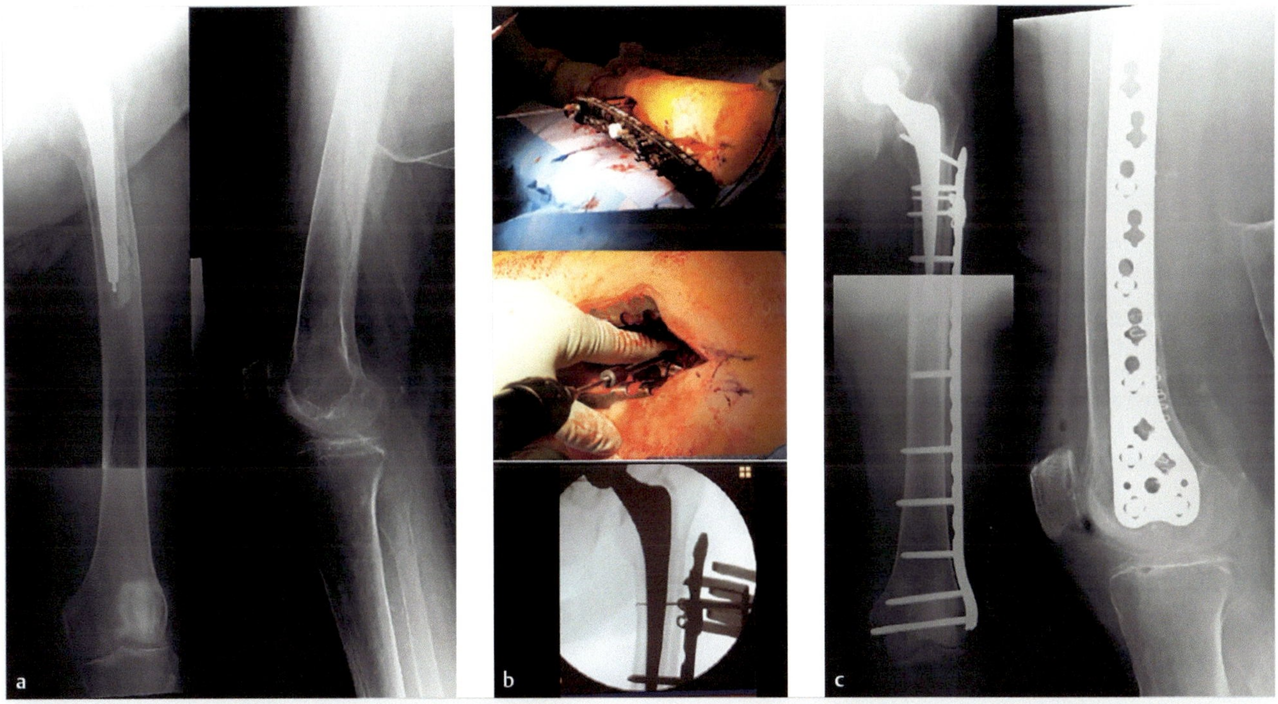

Fig. 8.4 A 101-year-old female sustained a periprosthetic femur fracture (type IV.3 C acc. Unified Classification System, (**a**). Surgery was performed with closed reduction and locking plate fixation (**b**) using the VA-LCP condyle (polyaxial locking plate system, Synthes, Umkirch) with additional L.A.P. (locking attachment plate, Synthes, Umkirch) to bypass the hip stem proximally. In addition, bicortical screw anchorage could be achieved around the hip stem, leading to superior stability compared to monocortical screw anchorage near the stem. Fracture healing was uneventful with a neutral alignment (**c**).

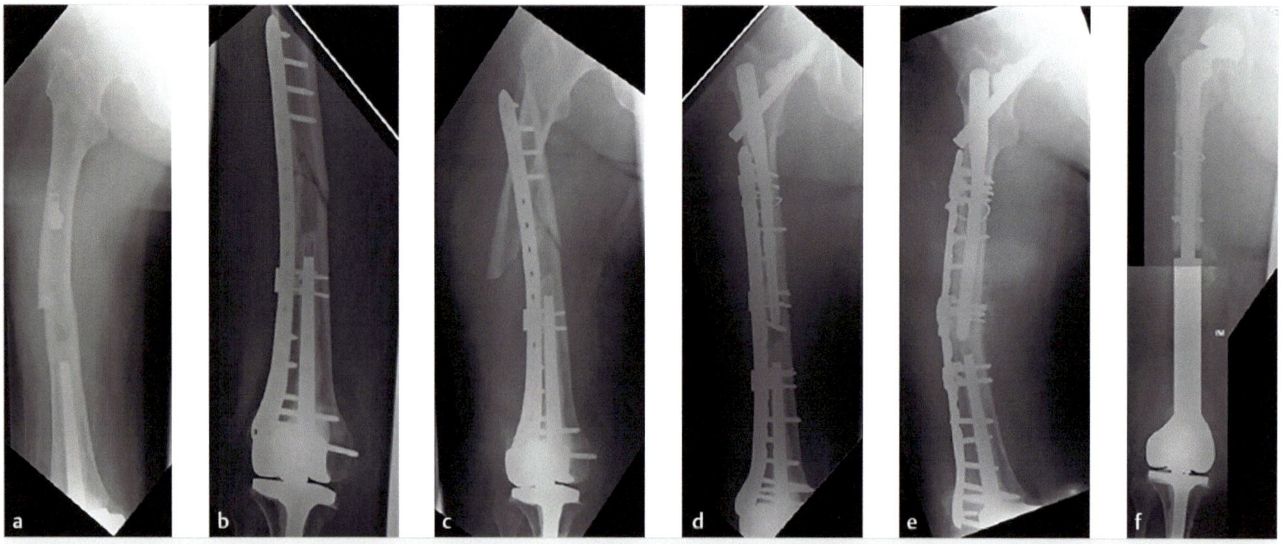

Fig. 8.5 A 98-year-old female sustained a periprosthetic femur fracture (type V.3 C acc. Unified Classification System, (**a**) Emergency surgery was performed with closed reduction and locking plate fixation (**b**) using the L.I.S.S. (less invasive stabilization system, Synthes, Umkirch) with additional L.A.P. (locking attachment plate, Synthes, Umkirch). During the postoperative course, the patient fell again and suffered a peri-implant fracture proximal to the plate but involving the implant bed (**c**). We revised the internal fixation, now bridging the proximal fracture with an intramedullary nail (PFN-alpha, Synthes, Umkirch) in association with a plate (VA-LCP condyle, Synthes, Umkirch). We used bicortical screw fixation around the prosthetic stem (**d**) which was reinforced with the application of the L.A.P. and cerclage wires (**e**). However, this construct failed again (**e**). Salvage procedure was performed by implanting a distal femur replacement connected to an endoprosthesis of the hip (**f**).

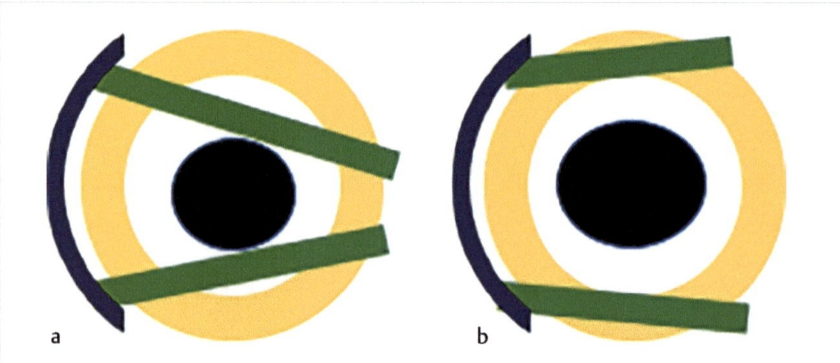

Fig. 8.6 Schematic axial view (*yellow*: femoral shaft) of a locking attachment plate (*blue*) around an intramedullary stem (*black*). (**a**) bicortical screw placement around the stem. Biomechanical data underscore the superiority of this fixation method. (**b**) transcortical screw placement. Although this fixation method also offers enhanced biomechanical stability, there is an increased risk for catastrophic failures with loss of sufficient bone stock for further reconstructions.

to check for the stability of the femoral component might be helpful. Revision T.K.A. with a lateral approach is possible (performed in tumor cases). However, the mobilization of the extensor mechanism needs a comprehensive surgical procedure, which we prefer to avoid.

8.12 Pitfalls

- Not being prepared for an eventual revision knee replacement.
- Transcortical screw placement (screws that are very superficially placed in the cortical) may lead to structural damage to the femur and eventually lead to mechanical failure of the construct (▸ Fig. 8.6).
- Not recognizing instability associated with medial cortex comminution is related to mechanical failure of lateral locking femur plates.
- Short and stiff constructs are related to early mechanical failure. Therefore, a sufficient working length of the plate has to be chosen.
- If a total hip replacement stem is located in the femoral canal, the distal femur plate should overlap the stem, avoiding stress rises at the tip of the femoral stem.

9 Retrograde Nailing of Distal Femur Periprosthetic Fractures

Matthew Stillwagon and George Hanson

9.1 Description

This chapter addresses the management of periprosthetic supracondylar femur fractures with a retrograde femoral nail.

9.2 Key Principles

The goal of surgical treatment of the geriatric patient with a periprosthetic distal femur fracture is to perform timely operative fixation to allow for early mobilization, to obtain fracture union, and to maintain a functional total knee arthroplasty. However, presence of the distal femoral component complicates the procedure tremendously because its dimensions can make it difficult to insert the nail, cause damage to the nail and/or femoral and tibial implants, and make it difficult to obtain an anatomic starting point with resulting malreduction (▶ Fig. 9.1). Cruciate-retaining knees must be flexed 70 degrees to avoid damage to the polyethylene liner; posterior-stabilized knees require 80 degrees or more of flexion, and medial pivot designs also require even greater flexion (80 degrees for cruciate-retaining and 120 degrees for posterior-stabilized). Therefore, the surgeon must be aware of whether the intended implants are compatible and have plans to deal with any of these situations, which may include using an alternative method of fixation.

The use of a retrograde intramedullary nail for a periprosthetic distal femur fracture has both biological and biomechanical advantages. The approach is minimally invasive and can be done using the prior midline surgical incision. Mechanically, the introduction of the retrograde nail in the medullary axis of the femur moves the weight-bearing axis of the fixation construct medially, so that it is aligned with the anatomical axis of the femur. The device is load-sharing, and can be used to span the length of the femur as long as proximal femoral hardware or deformity of the medullary canal is not present.

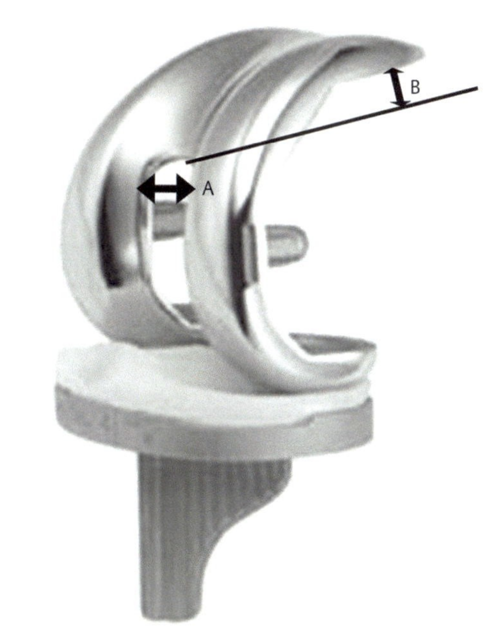

Fig. 9.1 Photograph of total knee components with pertinent measurements to determine suitability for retrograde femoral nailing. The width of the intercondylar box (line A) limits the diameter of the nail. Note that the relevant nail dimension is the distal part of the nail, which for smaller diameter nails can be larger than the labeled nail size. Line B is the distance between the underside of the anterior femoral flange and the top of the intercondylar box. The greater this distance is, the more the retrograde nail will be moved posteriorly, with increased likelihood of femoral hyperextension or anterior translation of the distal femur.

9.3 Expectations

Retrograde nailing of distal femoral periprosthetic fractures is a widely accepted surgical treatment with a high rate of success. When retrograde nailing is utilized for appropriate distal femoral periprosthetic fractures, patient outcomes and fracture healing are similar to distal femoral locking plates, with the advantage of a load sharing device with increased biomechanical resistance to varus and valgus loading. However, retrograde nailing can be technically challenging or impossible due to the design of the total knee implants. The dimensions of a posterior cruciate sacrificing implant or closed-box femoral component can prevent the insertion of the retrograde nail (▶ Fig. 9.1). Diligent preoperative planning and critical evaluation of preoperative radiographs and CT scan are essential to determine the type and stability of existing femoral component. In cruciate-retaining implant designs or open-box femoral components, the typical anatomic starting point for the nail is forced posterior by the anterior flange of the femoral component. One of the most commonly encountered complications is hyperextension deformity of the distal fracture segment due to the posterior to anterior trajectory of the trajectory of the guidewire (▶ Fig. 9.2a–d). Significant malreduction or translation of the distal femur may increase the risk for development of nonunion. Blocking, or Poller screws, is a useful technical trick to avoid malreduction while inserting the nail (▶ Fig. 9.3a–f) Alternatively, a Schanz pin can be inserted into the distal femoral condyle and be used to apply a flexion moment to the distal femur that can assist with reduction (▶ Fig. 9.4a–c). Even with correctly positioned blocking screws, there may be some mild residual hyperextension deformity, which is typically well tolerated, thanks to compensatory motion of the knee joint.

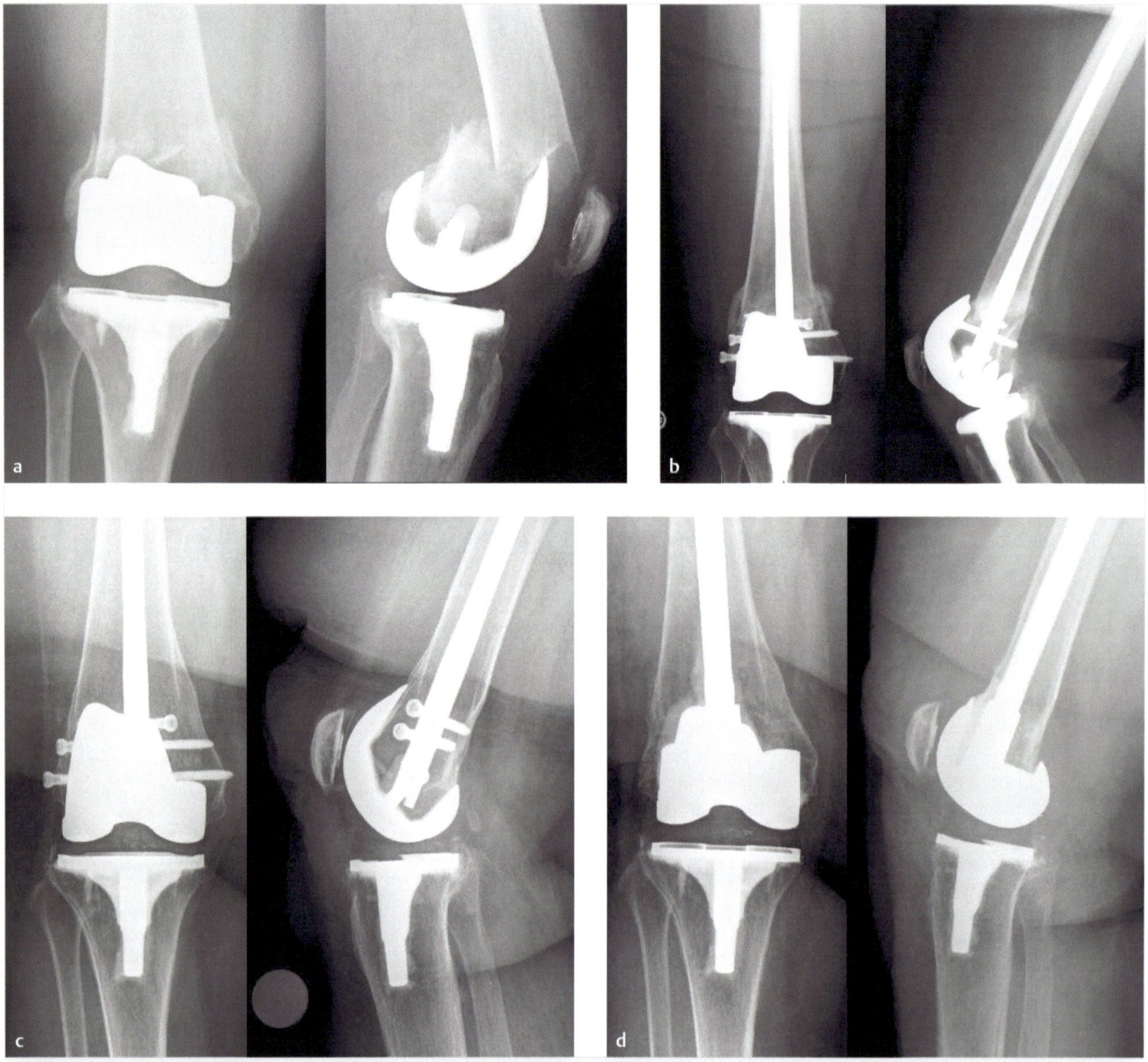

Fig. 9.2 Example of hyperextension deformity after retrograde nailing of a periprosthetic fracture. **(a)** Anteroposterior (AP) and lateral knee radiographs showing a primarily transverse fracture of the distal femur at the level of the femoral component anterior flange. There is no evidence of knee component loosening. **(b)** Radiographs taken about 3 months postoperatively, showing some extension of the distal femur and the femoral component of the total knee. Note that four interlocking screws were used for distal femoral fixation. **(c)** Radiographs taken 12 years postoperatively. The patient had 15 degrees of hyperextension of the knee and could no longer tolerate her altered gait and sense of knee instability. **(d)** Radiographs taken after patient underwent revision of her femoral component, with correction of the deformity done by redoing the distal femoral cuts so that the revision component could be placed in normal sagittal alignment.

9.4 Indications

Supracondylar femur fractures with adequate distal bone stock, no intra-articular or peri-implant fracture extension, and stable implants are amenable to retrograde femoral nailing. Radiographs and computed tomography (CT) scans are useful preoperative tools to evaluate for adequate distal bone stock and stability of the implant. The surgeon must also critically evaluate the total knee implant design, specifically the femoral component, to ensure that it can accept an appropriate sized nail through the open box.

9.5 Contraindications

Fractures with very distal extension may not be amenable to retrograde nailing because of the inability to obtain stable fixation with the distal locking bolts. In addition, posterior cruciate substituting or closed-box femoral components are typically unable to accept a femoral nail due to the dimensions of the femoral component. Also, if the total knee implant appears loose or malpositioned, alternative fixation strategies should be considered such as a revision total knee arthroplasty or distal femoral replacement. Care must be taken when retrograde

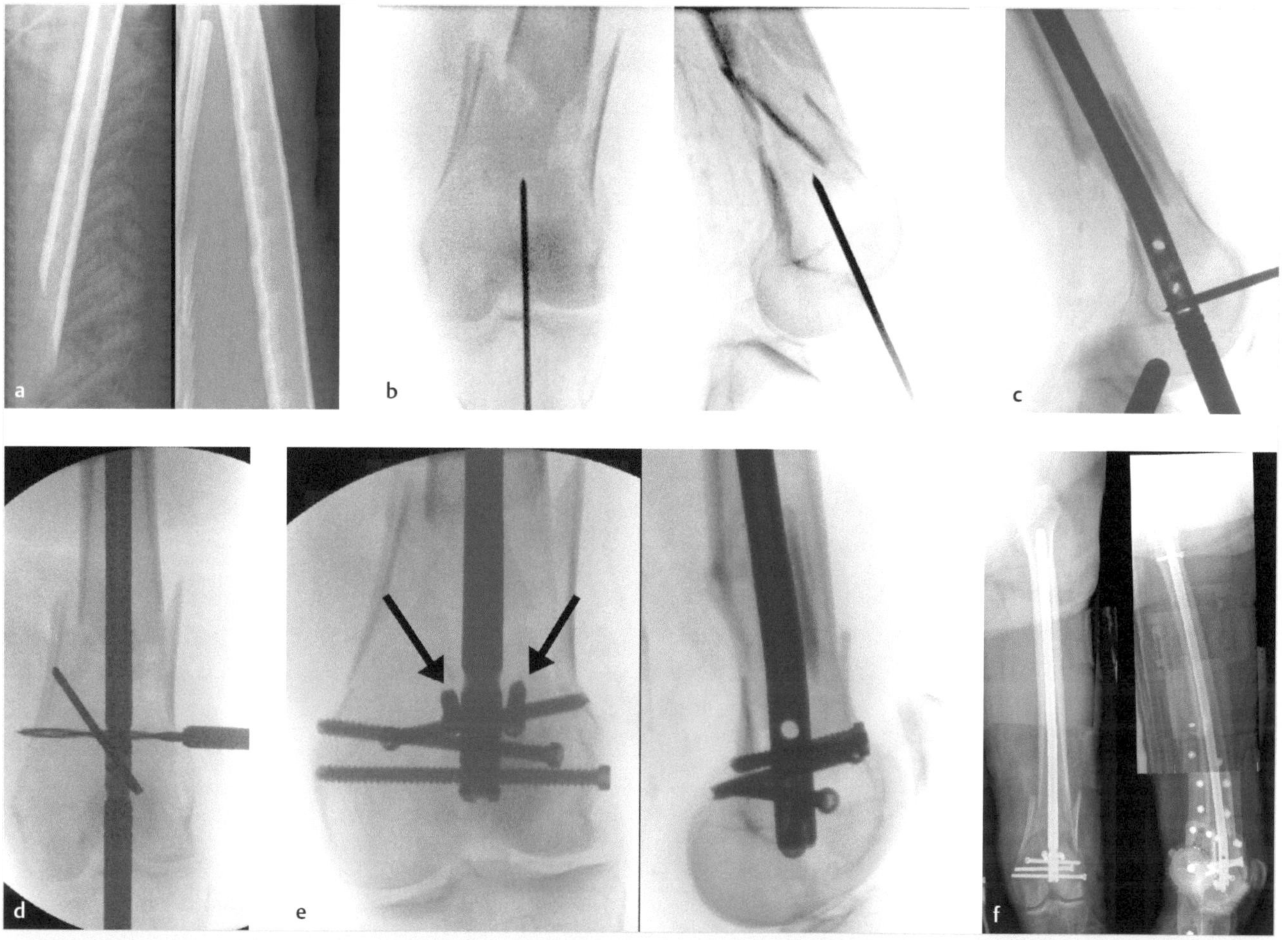

Fig. 9.3 Example of the use of blocking screws to assist with maintaining reduction during retrograde nailing of a distal femur fracture. **(a)** Anteroposterior (AP) and lateral knee radiographs showing a comminuted distal femoral shaft fracture **(b)** Intraoperative fluoroscopic images showing provisional fracture reduction by traction and insertion of a guide-pin into the distal femoral segment. There appears to be some hyperextension of the distal femur. **(c)** A large Steinmann pin has been placed medial to the nail and is used to flex the distal femur. Note the improved sagittal alignment. **(d)** AP fluoroscopic image showing a drill used for insertion of a distal interlocking screw. **(e)** AP and lateral intraoperative fluoroscopic views showing the retrograde nail inserted with three distal interlocking screws and two blocking screws (*black arrows*). **(f)** AP and lateral views of the entire femur demonstrating the entire fixation construct.

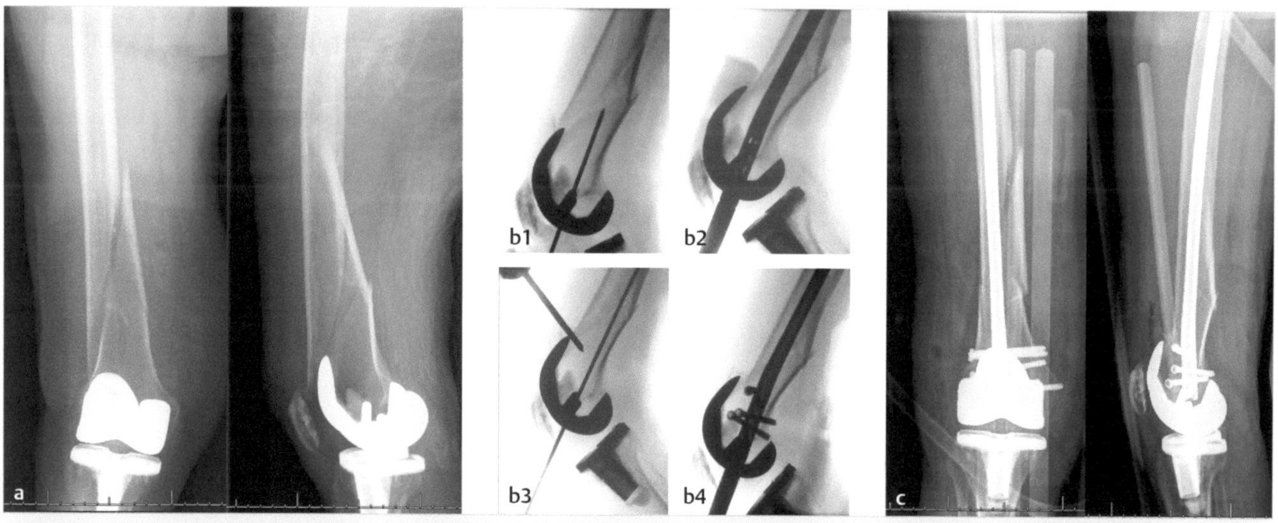

Fig. 9.4 Example of the use of a Steinmann pin for intraoperative correction of alignment and a lateral–medial blocking screw to maintain reduction. **(a)** Anteroposterior (AP) and lateral radiographs of a long oblique periprosthetic distal femur fracture above a well-fixed total knee. **(b1)** Lateral intraoperative fluoroscopic view of initial reduction and passing of guidewire. **(b2)** As the nail is inserted, an extension malreduction becomes evident. **(b3)** The nail was removed, and the deformity corrected with a large Steinmann pin inserted from anterior–posterior in the distal femur while the guide rod for the nail is inserted. **(b4)** Finally, a lateral–medial blocking screw was placed in the femoral shaft to prevent the retrograde nail from moving anteriorly and causing a translational deformity. **(c)** Postoperative radiographs revealing a good alignment at the fracture site.

nailing an interprosthetic femur fracture due to concern for stress riser between the total hip femoral stem and proximal tip of the retrograde nail. In this scenario, a long distal femoral locking plate, overlapping the total hip stem, is often preferred.

9.6 Special Considerations

The typical patient with a periprosthetic distal femur fracture is frail, with morbidity and mortality that are similar to the geriatric hip fracture population. Therefore, multidisciplinary preoperative evaluation and medical optimization prior to surgery is important.

9.7 Special Instructions, Positioning, and Anesthesia

The patient is placed supine on a flat radiolucent table, with the injured side near the edge of the table and the upper extremities perpendicular to the table. General or spinal anesthesia is used depending on the medical needs of the patient. A large rolled towel, blanket (or equivalent), is placed under the ipsilateral buttock to prevent the injured leg from externally rotating. A radiolucent triangle can be used to hold the knee in a partially flexed position, relaxing the gastrocnemius muscles and lessening recurvatum deformity. Preparation and draping of the surgical site should be done from the anterior iliac crest to the ankle. The image intensifier is positioned on the opposite side from the injury.

9.8 Tips, Pearls, and Lessons Learned

- Try to obtain a prefracture history regarding the function of the knee arthroplasty in order to gain clues that might prompt for consideration of loosening or infection.
- Detailed imaging is needed for preoperative planning, including full-length femur films and specific knee views (anteroposterior [AP], patellar skyline, and lateral). Images should be carefully reviewed for evidence of radiolucencies adjacent to the implant that may represent loosening of the total knee components. Finally, computed tomography with 2D and 3D reconstruction is very useful in understanding the fracture pattern.
- When treating a periprosthetic fracture with this technique, specific identification of the total knee arthroplasty implant and ascertainment of its dimensions of the intercondylar notch is critical to ensure that a nail will fit the component (as well as to be prepared to proceed with revision arthroplasty if that may be part of the plan). Important dimensions are the distance between the posterior condyles, and the relationship of the most distal portion of the anterior flange with the top of the intercondylar box (▸ Fig. 9.1). This is best determined by confirming implant dimensions on compatibility reference charts found within published literature or if implants are unknown by measuring on CT scan on reformatted coronal and sagittal axes. The former influences the width of the nail that can be used; the latter can influence the angle and location of the starting point.

9.9 Difficulties Encountered

Hyperextension of the distal femur caused by the deforming force of the gastrocnemius muscles can result in recurvatum deformity (▸ Fig. 9.2, ▸ Fig. 9.3, ▸ Fig. 9.4). This is mitigated by proper choice of starting point in a native distal femur, but in a periprosthetic fracture the anterior flange of the femoral component typically forces the starting point posteriorly. Retrograde Steinmann pins can be placed in cross fashion to help maintain provisional reduction. Blocking screws can be an aid to reduction (▸ Fig. 9.3), as can use of other reduction aids such as clamps and Schanz pins (▸ Fig. 9.4). When placed in the distal femoral segment, blocking screws are typically inserted in an anterior–posterior position direction to bracket the nail and prevent varus or valgus collapse (▸ Fig. 9.3). When trying to prevent hyperextension deformity, blocking screws are most often helpful when placed from lateral to medial and anterior to the nail (▸ Fig. 9.4). This can prevent the nail from moving anteriorly in the femur and causing malreduction or loss of reduction.

9.10 Key Procedural Steps

- Using fluoroscopy, place a bump beneath the distal thigh and obtain traction images. The surgeon will understand what additional reduction steps are needed.
- Make a midline incision. If unsure, a small 1-cm incision can be made to confirm the starting point of the nail within the open notch.
- Flex the knee at least 70 degrees (80 degrees or more is needed if a posterior-stabilized insert is present). Take images to assess reduction with the knee in flexion. If acceptable, place a guide-pin into the distal femoral segment, aligned with the anatomic axis of the distal femur in both AP and lateral images.
- If malreduction is present, redo the reduction or use an anterior–posterior Schanz or Steinmann pin to flex the distal femur.
- Once acceptable reduction is achieved, ream the distal femur over the guide-pin with the opening reamer.
- Pass a ball-tipped guidewire across the fracture and into the intact proximal femur so that the tip is proximal to the lesser trochanter.
- Measure the length of the desired nail using the manufacturer's technique.
- Assess the reduction; beware of hyperextension of the distal femur and/or translation in either coronal or sagittal planes. The placement of blocking screws is a useful technical trick to correct persistent coronal or sagittal malalignment (▸ Fig. 9.3 and ▸ Fig. 9.4).
- Choose a nail with the desired diameter and length and insert it over the guidewire.
- Insert interlocking screws.
- Perform a standard, layered wound closure.

9.11 Bailout, Rescue, and Salvage Procedures

Malreduction, inability to insert the nail due to implant design, unstable total knee implants, or very distal fractures are all technical challenges with retrograde nailing periprosthetic femur fractures. Hyperextension deformity caused by posterior starting point can be corrected by using a blocking screw positioned anterior to the nail in the distal fracture segment (▶ Fig. 9.3). It should be noted that even with correctly positioned blocking screws, there may be some mild residual recurvatum deformity, which is typically well tolerated, thanks to compensatory motion of the knee joint. Very distal fractures should have enough bone stock to allow for fixation with two interlocking screws, at a minimum. However, three or even four interlocking screws may be desired in osteoporotic bone (▶ Fig. 9.4). Distal fixation can be further augmented with anterior to posterior metaphyseal blocking screws (▶ Fig. 9.3), which improves nail fit in the distal metaphysis and provide additional resistance to varus and valgus load. A blocking screw placed just anterior to the nail in the lateral-medial plane in the distal femoral shaft can also prevent anterior migration of the nail and prevent loss of reduction (▶ Fig. 9.4). If the total knee implant is unexpectedly found to be loose intraoperatively, a revision total knee arthroplasty or distal femoral replacement must be considered. Fractures that are very distal, making it difficult to obtain adequate fixation with the nail interlocking bolts can be supplemented by a locking plate, or nail-plate fixation. Dual implant, or nail-plate, fixation should be strongly considered in very distal femur fractures, severely osteoporotic bone, and fractures with significant medial comminution.

9.12 Pitfalls

Always be aware of the potential for chronic infection and implant loosening through careful history, radiographic imaging, and additional workup when treating a periprosthetic fracture. Distal supracondylar periprosthetic fractures should be scrutinized, and confirmed with CT scan if needed, for fracture lines that extend below the level of the distal interlocking screws.

10 Nail-Plate Combination and Double Plating for Complex Distal Femur Fractures (Native or Periprosthetic)

Robinson Esteves Pires and Vincenzo Giordano

10.1 Description

This chapter addresses the management of complex distal femur fractures (native bone or periprosthetic) by the combined use of a retrograde femoral nail and lateral locking plate, as well as the double-plating technique. Both surgical procedures are rapidly gaining favor because they provide stable and balanced fixation, allowing early knee mobilization and in particular situations early weight-bearing.

10.2 Key Principles

The goal of surgical treatment of the complex distal femur fracture is to perform timely operative fixation to reduce overall mortality rate and allow for early mobilization. Surgical treatment more than two days after injury is associated with increased patient mortality after native bone and periprosthetic distal femur fractures in the elderly population. However, especially in this population, the combination of osteopenia and fracture comminution that defines these injuries, combined with the frailty of the typical patient, often means that weight-bearing must be delayed whenever a standard locking plate or retrograde intramedullary nail is used alone. When both techniques are combined (nail-plate combination) or the double-plating technique is applied, a more balanced and load-sharing fixation construct is achieved so that patients can be mobilized immediately after treatment with decreased morbidity and complications.

The biomechanical rationale of a combined nail-plate is that the introduction of the retrograde nail in the medullary axis of the femur moves the weight-bearing axis of the fixation construct medially, so that it is aligned with the anatomical axis of the femur, yet with the added mechanical stability provided by the lateral plate. Although not always possible, either or both implants can span the entire length of the femur, further increasing mechanical stability while also reducing stress-risers that may contribute to a later peri-implant fracture. Although most distal femur fractures can be safely and effectively addressed with just a single lateral locking plate, particular cases require a more stable and balanced construct. The double-plating technique is also a helpful treatment alternative in those situations, especially when there is a severe comminution or reduced bone stock of the medial distal femur metadiaphyseal area. In these situations, there is a relatively high-risk of persistent instability, mainly on the coronal plane; therefore, the use of a medial plate potentially facilitates reduction and improves rigidity in a very short distal segment, thus reducing complication rates compared to traditional single implant constructs.

10.3 Expectations

Reported nonunion rates using nail-plate combination or double plating to repair native bone or periprosthetic distal femur fractures are very low and better than reported for isolated locking plates or retrograde nails. In addition, there is an expected overall lower-mortality rate when these patients are operated on before 48 hours, which is mainly attributed to the benefits of increased fixation, allowing for early postoperative range of motion and up-to-chair activities. Of importance, despite the advantage of immediate weight-bearing, most patients require some assistance with walking and approximately half lose some level of independence. Also, surgical complications and the presence of comorbidities are expected in this patient age population, which can jeopardize the outcome.

10.4 Indications

A nail-plate combination is indicated for periprosthetic fractures of the distal femur with a stable prosthesis (Lewis and Rorabeck type 2), especially in patients with poor bone quality and short metaepiphyseal fragment. Interprosthetic fractures are also a potential indication, depending on whether enough of the intramedullary canal is available for a retrograde nail. Native bone distal femur fractures with severe comminution or bone loss due to high-energy trauma can be effectively addressed with a nail-plate combo or double plating. Periprosthetic distal femur fractures with a stable prosthesis (Lewis and Rorabeck type 2) and a short lateral epiphyseal fragment and medial fracture apex can be safely managed using the double-plating technique. Aseptic nonunions of the distal femur that require a more stable and balanced fixation are also indications for nail-plate combination and double plating.

10.5 Contraindications

Nail-plate combination is contraindicated for periprosthetic distal femoral fractures associated with a closed-box femoral prosthesis component. Soft tissue infection, osteomyelitis, and infected nonunions are also contraindications for both nail-plate combination and double plating. Malunion or abnormal bones with obliterated medullary canal are also contraindications for nail-plate fixation unless a clamshell osteotomy allows for intramedullary nail placement.

10.6 Special Considerations

The typical patient with an osteopenic distal femur fracture is frail, with documented morbidity and mortality rates that are similar to the geriatric hip fracture population. Therefore, appropriate multidisciplinary evaluation and medical optimization prior to surgery is important. A meticulous preoperative planning is mandatory for periprosthetic fractures, carefully evaluating prosthesis stability, design, and dimensions. High-energy distal femur fractures usually occur in polytrauma patients that require total and multidisciplinary care with hierarchy of treatment priorities. When using the double-plating technique, one should be cautious with the possibility of iatrogenic injury of the femoral artery or its perforating rami, especially when a long plate is used. Although the anteromedial surface of the femur is considered a relatively safe zone until the distance of 8 cm from the lesser trochanter, studies using computerized tomographic angiography of the lower limb demonstrated that the medial superior genicular artery presents a posterosuperior to anteroinferior pathway, being therefore an important source of intraoperative bleeding. A helical medial plate is an elegant and safer treatment alternative when using double-plating technique.

10.7 Special Instructions, Positioning, and Anesthesia

Typically, a radiolucent flat table is used to facilitate intraoperative imaging, and the patient is placed supine with the upper extremities perpendicular to the table. General or spinal anesthesia is used depending on the condition of the patient. A bump is placed under the ipsilateral buttock to prevent the injured leg from externally rotating. To facilitate the lateral surgical exposure, the patient can be moved toward the edge of the table. Preparation and draping of the surgical site should be done from the anterior iliac crest to the ankle. A bump and/or radiolucent triangle can be placed under the distal thigh to be used during surgery, especially when a retrograde nail is used. Typically, the image intensifier is positioned on the contralateral side. The contralateral lower limb should be either positioned slightly above or below the segment to be operated to facilitate lateral view of the knee and distal thigh during surgery. If a nail is used, the surgeon may consider positioning the contralateral lower limb in lithotomy position to adequately check both the upper thigh and hip of the operated segment.

10.8 Tips, Pearls, and Lessons Learned

- Periprosthetic distal femur fractures are not typically associated with loosening of the femoral or tibial component, but nevertheless, one should try to obtain a prefracture history regarding the function of the TKA and the sequential control radiographs performed since the index procedure. A history of local pain and gait disturbances can alert for a loose total knee prosthesis component, as well as obvious radiographic risk signs for cement loosening. Periprosthetic infection should be appropriately excluded before proceeding with osteosynthesis. Laboratory findings in the setting of TKA infection are often nonspecific; therefore in suspected cases a knee joint aspiration has been found to be extremely useful in diagnosing joint infection. Culturing should be done for aerobic germs, anaerobic germs, and fungi, with sufficient time allowed for observing their growth. Independently of the clinical and radiological findings, during the surgery, it is strongly recommended to collect at least three to five samples from different locations and preferably before administering prophylactic antibiotics.
- Proper imaging is needed for preoperative planning and should include full-length femur films and dedicated knee radiographs (anteroposterior, patellar skyline, and lateral projections). In case of periprosthetic fractures, prefracture images are helpful in assessing implant stability, and all images should be scrutinized for radiolucencies adjacent to the implant that may be evidence of loosening of the total knee components. Finally, computed tomography with 2D and 3D reconstruction provides more information regarding coronal fracture lines and fracture comminution.
- When treating a periprosthetic fracture with nail-plate combination, specific identification of the implant and ascertainment of its dimensions are important to ensure that a nail will fit the component (as well as to be prepared to proceed with revision arthroplasty if that may be part of the plan).
- The surgeon must choose between one open, midline incision for both retrograde nail insertion and exposure of the lateral surface of the lateral femoral condyle for the lateral plate (which is then inserted submuscularly), and two incisions (distal midline for the retrograde nail and small lateral incision for femoral plating). For periprosthetic fractures, use of the entire prior skin incision and a lateral arthrotomy can provide adequate exposure for fracture reduction and implant insertion. For native bone intra-articular fractures, the anterolateral parapatellar approach (TARPO) is recommended. For extra-articular distal fractures, a dual approach is an option. For the double-plating technique, although the proximal extension of the anterolateral approach provides sufficient exposure for both lateral and medial plating, we usually prefer the dual approach (anterolateral parapatellar and medial subvastus).
- An appropriate lateral plate is one that has a curve that mimics the anatomical radius of curvature of the femur and flares a bit at its proximal end to allow for the plate to sit properly on the greater trochanter. Using a variable-angle locking plate facilitates the positioning of the screws in the normally very short distal fragment.
- Use of a small diameter nail facilitates bicortical screw plate fixation around the nail.
- Precontoured proximal humeral and proximal tibial plates are helpful implants that adequately fit the medial condyle surface. However, either nonlocked or locked small-fragment

straight plates can also be used in the medial distal femur, always trying to touch the lateral plate screws to increase their interdigitation in the distal fragment.
- Helical proximal humeral plates (manufactured or customized) placed upside down, although in an off-label indication, may be an elegant and safer treatment option, since implants especially designed for the medial aspect of the distal femur are still unavailable for most hospitals.
- When there is a severe comminution on the medial metadiaphyseal cortex, the use of intramedullary bone augmentation with a fibular strut graft can be a good option, as performed in other segments, such as the proximal humerus.

10.9 Difficulties Encountered

Hyperextension forces on the distal segment caused by the gastrocnemius muscles acting on the posterior aspect of the distal femur can result in recurvatum deformity. This is mitigated by proper choice of starting point in a native bone distal femur, but in a periprosthetic fracture, the anterior flange of the femoral component may force the starting point to be more posterior than desired. Poller (blocking) screws can be an aid, as well as special clamps and Schanz screws. Retrograde nails with a more curved and distal end shape are also an interesting treatment option to prevent such deformity. Multiple interlocking screws provide a more stable construct. When double-plating, the medial plate can be used as a reduction tool, mainly when there is an incompetent medial wall, allowing the medial plate to act as a buttress during the application of the periarticular clamp.

10.10 Key Procedural Steps

1. For periprosthetic fractures, the previous surgical skin incision is preferred and a lateral arthrotomy is used for the deep exposure. In some cases of a native bone extra-articular distal femur fracture, the surgeon may choose to do a small midline incision for the nail, using a second small lateral incision over the lateral femoral condyle for plate insertion. When using the double-plating technique, our preference is the anterolateral parapatellar approach in combination with a medial subvastus approach.
2. Using fluoroscopy, place a bump beneath the distal thigh and obtain traction images. This will help the surgeon to understand which additional reduction maneuvers are needed.
3. **Nail-plate combination:**
   - Placement of retrograde nail:
     - Place a guide-pin into the distal femoral segment, aligned with the anatomic axis of the distal femur in both anteroposterior and lateral projections. Ream over the guide-pin with the opening reamer using the concept of "ream to fit."
     - Pass a ball-tipped guidewire across the fracture and into the intact proximal femur, beyond the lesser trochanter (unless this isn't possible due to presence of a proximal femoral implant). The ideal position for the upper end of the nail is just below the lesser trochanter in case proximal femoral neck fixation is needed.
     - Measure the length of the desired nail using the manufacturer's technique recommendation.
     - Assess the reduction; beware of hyperextension of the distal femur and/or translation in either coronal or sagittal planes.
     - Choose a small diameter nail of the appropriate length and insert it over the guidewire.
   - Placement of lateral plate:
     - First, choose plate length by overlaying it on the skin under fluoroscopic imaging. Ideally, a long, curved plate will be placed all the way to the lateral aspect of the greater trochanter. Whenever possible, prefer variable angled plates.
     - If needed, contour the plate using a large plate bending press and bending irons. The plate should sit on the anterior aspect of the lateral femoral condyle and on the posterior portion of the greater trochanter, especially if screw placement into the femoral neck and head is planned.
     - The plate is inserted retrograde from the lateral femoral condyle incision. A separate proximal approach to the lateral femur is performed, or at the surgeon's discretion a proximal screw targeting arm can be used for percutaneous screw insertion, when available.
     - The C-arm is positioned in lateral projection until at least one plate hole matches one distal nail hole. Be sure that the plate is well accommodated in the anterolateral surface of the distal femur to prevent soft tissue issues.
     - The plate is provisionally fixed at each end and reduction of the fracture is checked.
   - Linking the nail-plate combination:
     - Using fluoroscopy, place a locking screw through both the plate and the nail. The nail targeting arm facilitates this. Small adjustments in the position of the plate may be necessary.
     - Insert the remaining distal femoral plate locking screws.
     - Insert a nonlocking screw at the proximal end of the plate, fixing both ends of the construct.
     - If possible, consider placing screws into the femoral neck and head to protect the whole femur.
     - Place a limited number of screws into the femoral shaft (▶ Fig. 10.1).
     - Perform a standard, layered wound closure after a thorough hemostasis.
   - Double-plating technique:
     - For periprosthetic fractures of the distal femur with stable prosthesis component (Lewis Rorabeck type 2),

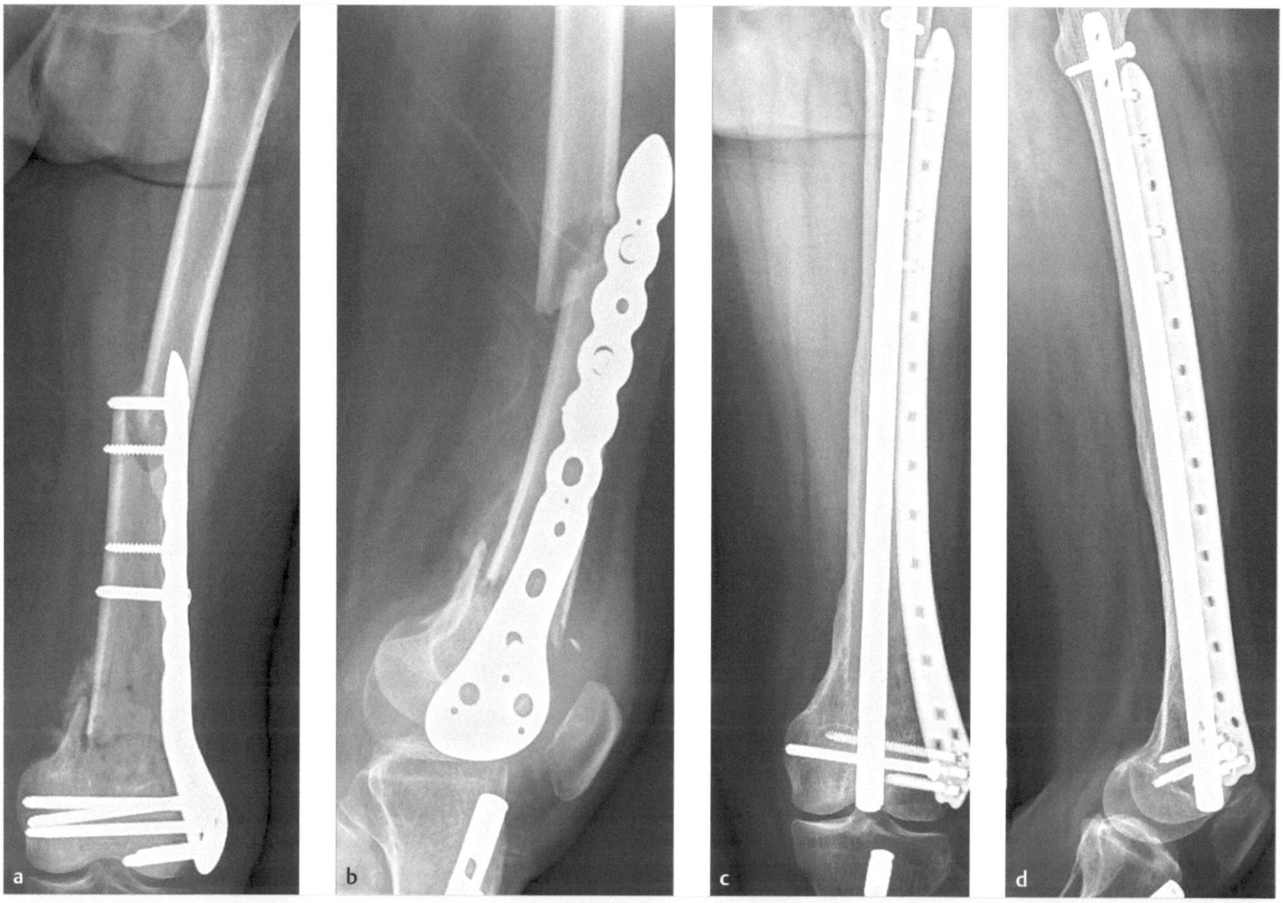

Fig. 10.1 A 37-year-old female patient with kidney failure and osteopenia. The patient sustained a previous distal femur fracture and underwent lateral plate fixation. Observe that the plate is short and incorrectly positioned on the anterior aspect of the distal femur. Due to the stress area on the anterior cortex of the distal femur, the patient presented a peri-implant fracture, proximally to the plate, before complete healing of the distal femur fracture. **(a,b)** Radiographs in anteroposterior and lateral projections depicting the peri-implant femoral fracture. **(c,d)** A nail-plate combination was used for fracture fixation and the fracture healed uneventfully.

short lateral epiphyseal fragment, and medial fracture apex, start the fixation using a medial subvastus approach, reduce the fracture and apply multiple K-wires to maintain the reduction. If a concern about the stability of the prosthesis is present, a mini-open arthrotomy is recommended to evaluate the prosthesis stability prior to fixation.

- After confirmation of adequate reduction, apply a buttressing medial proximal humerus plate (upside down) or another implant as mentioned previously over the medial surface of the distal femur. Lateral proximal tibial plates and 3.5-mm nonlocked or locked plates are helpful implant alternatives.
- Use an anterolateral parapatellar approach for submuscular retrograde plate placement.
- Provisionally fix each end of the lateral plate with K-wires.
- Use multiple screws interdigitated with the medial plate screws to enhance stability.
- Combine cortical and locking screws to proximally fix the plate, providing a balanced and stable construct (▸ Fig. 10.2).
- Perform a standard, layered wound closure after a thorough hemostasis.
- If the distal femur fracture is not the above-mentioned periprosthetic pattern, start the procedure with lateral fixation, followed by the medial fixation, or perform the dual approach simultaneously to reduce the fracture and achieve proper fixation. Fibular strut graft can be used as an augmentation tool.
- Minimally invasive medial plating is also a valuable alternative, especially when using an upside-down helical proximal humerus plate (▸ Fig. 10.3).

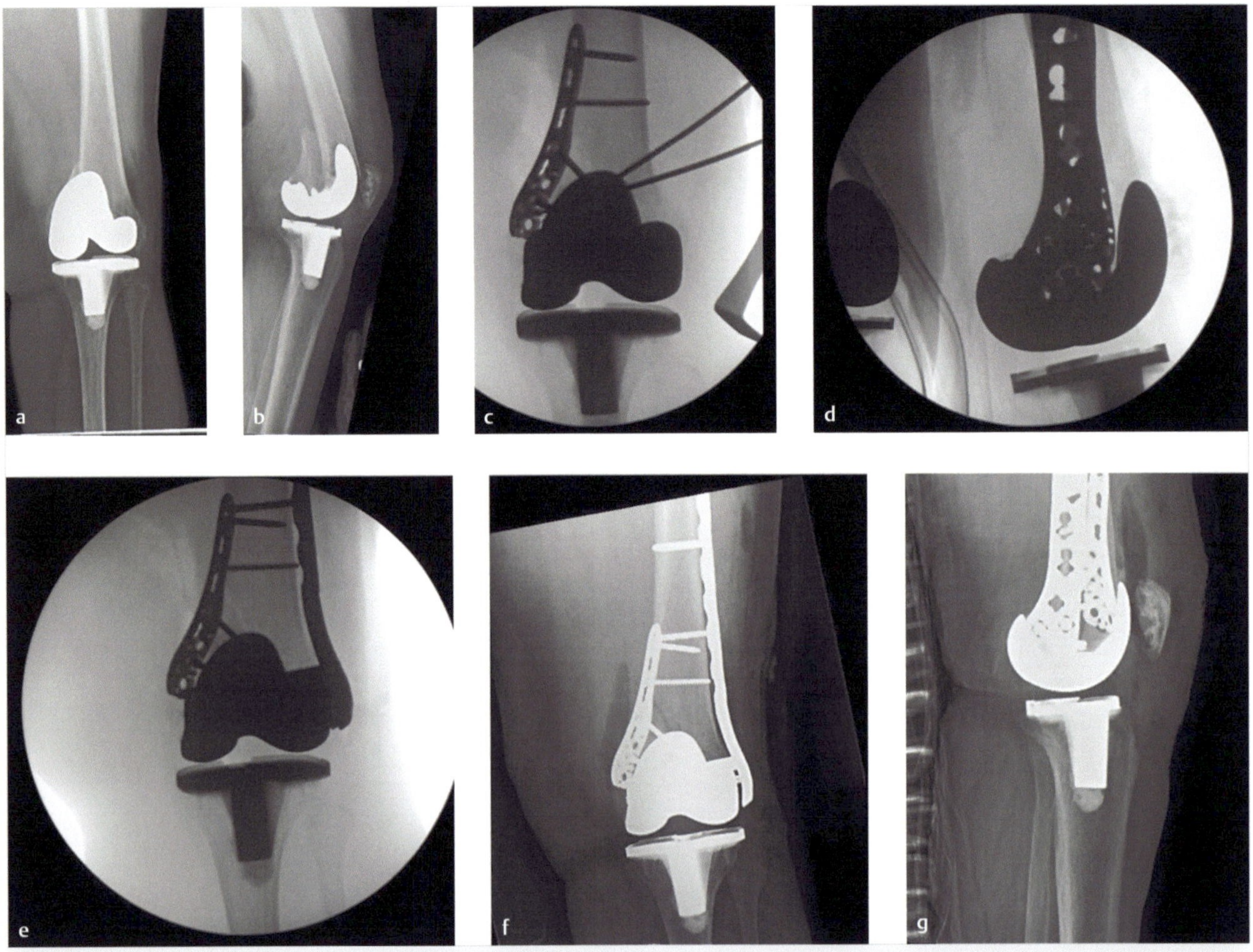

Fig. 10.2 A 67-year-old female patient has a fall at home and presented a Lewis Rorabeck type 2 periprosthetic distal femur fracture. **(a,b)** Radiographs in anteroposterior and lateral projections depicting the periprosthetic distal femur fracture. Observe the short lateral epiphyseal fragment and the medial apex of the fracture. After a miniopen arthrotomy to confirm the prosthesis stability, a medial subvastus approach was performed to reduce and fix the medial apex of the fracture with a proximal humerus plate. K-wires were applied to provisionally maintain the reduction **(c)**. **(d,e)** Fluoroscopy views depicting the fracture reduction and fixation using the double-plating technique. **(f,g)** Radiographs of the left knee in anteroposterior and lateral projections demonstrating fracture healing after achieving a stable and balanced fixation (Courtesy: Prof. Mauricio Kfuri—University of Missouri, USA).

10.11 Bailout, Rescue, and Salvage Procedures

Nail-plate combination and double plating are extremely helpful techniques in the therapeutic arsenal for complex periprosthetic and native bone distal femur fractures. However, both techniques are not exempt of complications. Meticulous preoperative planning is recommended to prevent complications and optimize outcomes. In patients with severe osteopenia, insufficient bone stock, or bone loss, augmentation techniques may contribute to enhance mechanical properties and improve the biological environment for fracture healing (▶ Fig. 10.4). The revision arthroplasty is also a bailout alternative in cases of failed distal femur fracture fixation if a formal contraindication for fixation revision exists.

10.12 Pitfalls

Always be aware of the potential for chronic infection when treating a periprosthetic fracture. Carefully evaluate the patient history and the prosthesis design (dimensions, open or closed box) when dealing with a periprosthetic knee fracture if a retrograde nail is part of the therapeutic plan. Depending on the prosthesis design, the anterior flange of the femoral component

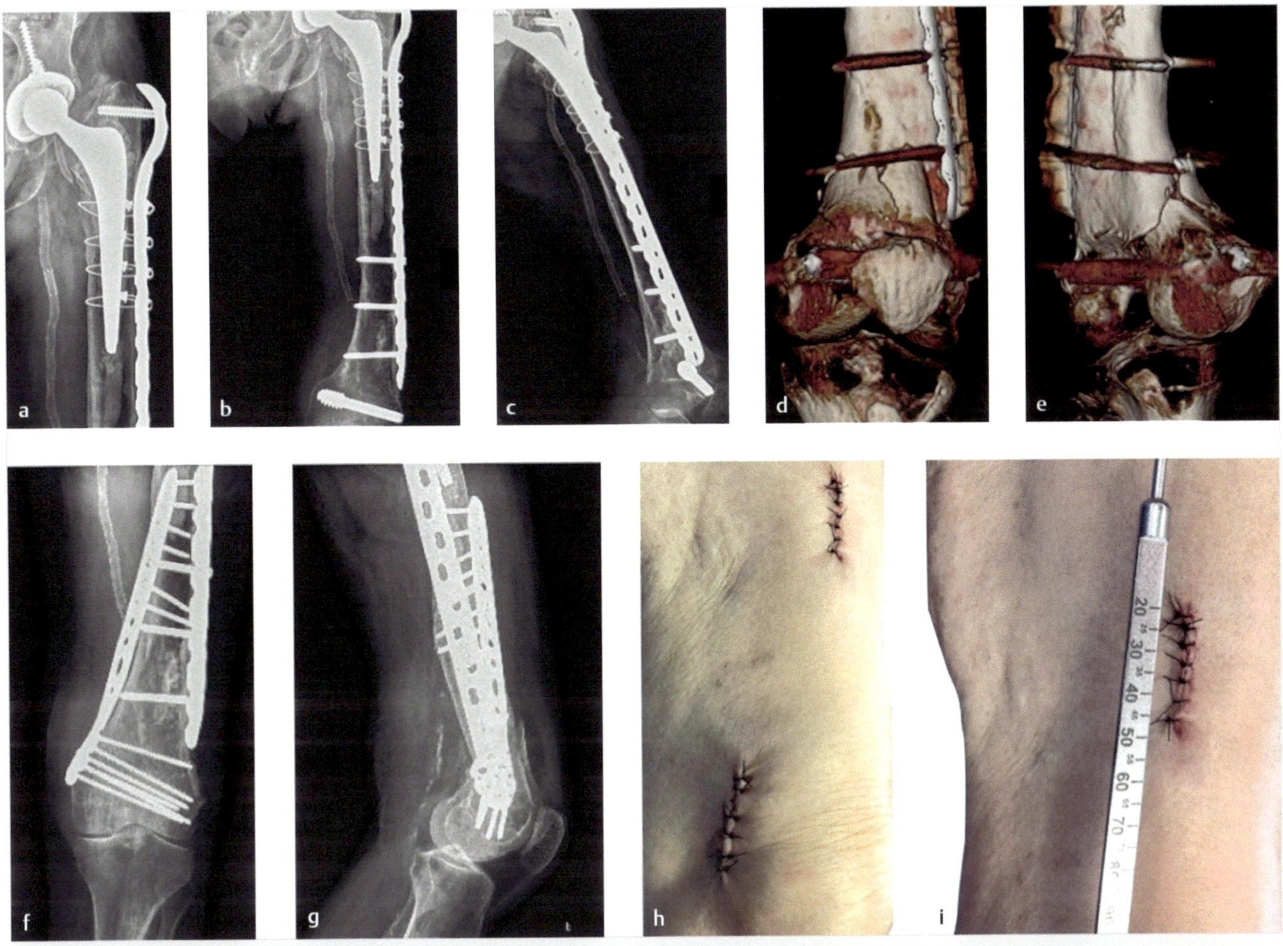

Fig. 10.3 A 92-year-old female patient with severe osteopenia presented a peri-implant distal femur fracture. Note that the patient previously underwent a distal femur fracture (fixed with a Dynamic Condylar Screw—DCS) and a periprosthetic fracture of the femur (Vancouver B1). This fracture was fixed with a long trochanteric plate, leaving the DCS screw in place. After a new low-energy trauma, the patient presented another distal femur fracture in the stress area between both implants. **(a–c)** Radiographs depicting the peri-implant femoral fracture. **(d,e)** Computed tomography with 3D reconstruction demonstrating the distal femur fracture and the poor bone quality. Due to the critical clinical scenario, with multiple comorbidities and chronic use of anticoagulants, a major procedure was contraindicated. Thus, an exception treatment was performed, using a precontoured helical proximal humerus plate. **(f,g)** Observe the fracture fixation and the plate pathway avoiding the "dangerous zone" of the femoral artery. **(h,i)** Skin incisions in the medial (distal) and anterior (proximal) aspects of the thigh, with 2.5 cm length.

forces the starting point to be more posterior than desired, leading to recurvatum deformity. Poller (blocking) screws and nails with a curved end may prevent such deformity (▶ Fig. 10.5). Removing the jig immediately after retrograde nail introduction is also an option to allow for a more anterior nail positioning. Create a stable construct, avoiding excess stiffness when using a nail-plate combination. The closed-box concept of the nail-plate combination needs balanced fixation. Combine standard cortical and locking screws to proximally fix the lateral plate. If possible, protect the whole femur to prevent further peri-implant fractures. Although the distance of 8 cm below the lesser trochanter is considered a relatively safe zone on the anteromedial aspect of the femur, be extremely careful to avoid distal perforating rami and medial superior genicular artery iatrogenic injuries. Considering periprosthetic knee fractures fixation, the surgeon must be aware about the possibility of intraoperative detection of prosthesis instability, therefore requiring prosthesis revision.

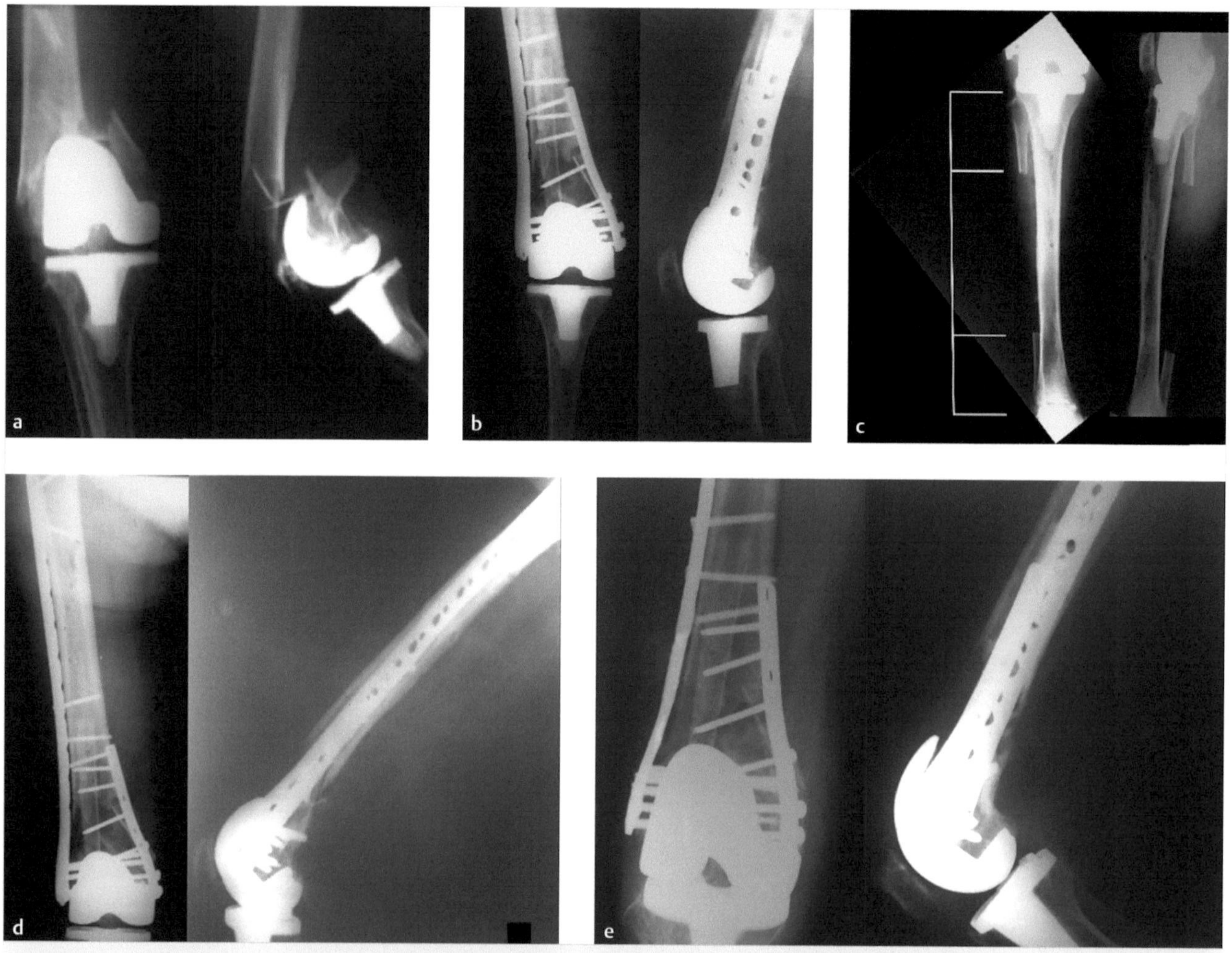

Fig. 10.4 This patient is an 86-year-old woman who suffered a minor fall at home and presented with a right comminuted distal femur fracture around a stable total knee arthroplasty. **(a)** Knee radiographs in anteroposterior and lateral projections depicting the complex distal femur periprosthetic fracture (Lewis Rorabeck type 2). Note the severe comminution in the metaphyseal area, including the medial wall of the distal femur. **(b)** Postoperative radiographs depicting satisfactory fracture reduction and a stable construct consisting of double-plating technique augmented by a nonvascularized fibular strut autograft. **(c)** Observe the resected portion of the fibula. **(d,e)** Final follow-up radiographs demonstrating that the fracture healed uneventfully.

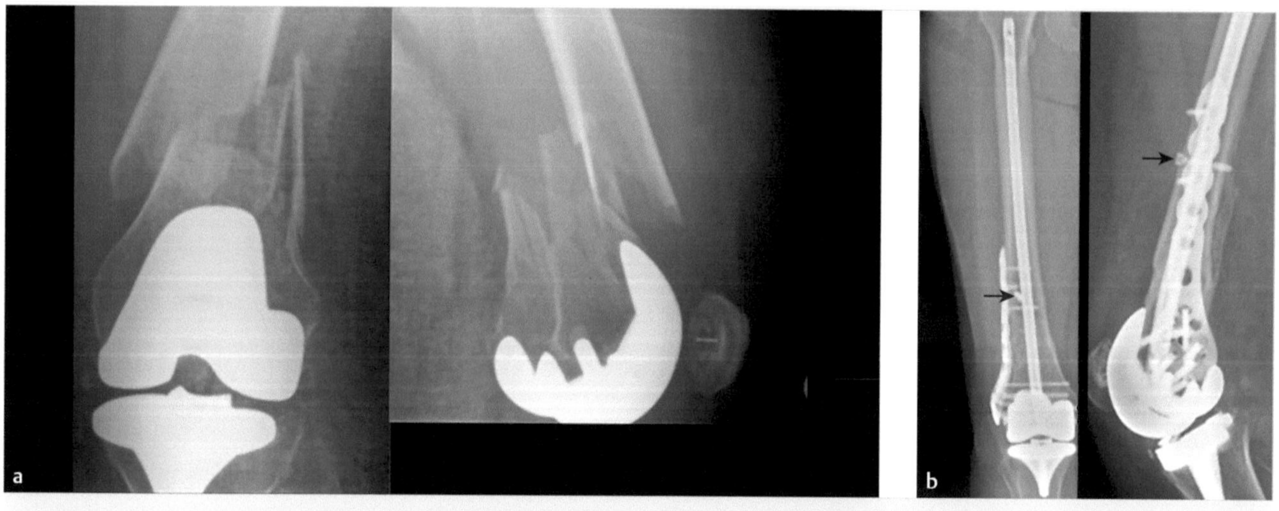

Fig. 10.5 Example of the use of a Poller (blocking) screw to assist in the reduction of a comminuted distal femoral periprosthetic fracture. **(a)**: Injury radiographs demonstrating a displaced, comminuted distal femoral fracture just proximal to a well-fixed total knee replacement. **(b)**: Postoperative radiographs showing a nail-plate combination with anatomic reduction. The Poller (blocking) screw is identified by the *black arrowheads*. The Poller screw keeps the nail centered in the canal and creates a more biomechanically stable construct.

11 Distal Femur Periprosthetic Fracture: ORIF and Revision Arthroplasty

Idemar Monteiro da Palma and Rodrigo Satamini Pires e Albuquerque

11.1 Description

This procedure addresses the revision of a total knee replacement in cases of distal femoral periprosthetic fractures with a loose total knee replacement component.

11.2 Key Principles

Distal femur periprosthetic fractures are associated with significant morbidity and are a challenging complication to be dealt with after a total knee replacement (▶ Fig. 11.1a). Decision making regarding the best therapeutic option for a given patient is based on his/her characteristics (age, comorbidities, bone density), fracture classification (morphology, location), and history of the existing knee replacement (design, time since implantation, symptoms/complications preceding the fracture). The outcomes of fracture fixation have improved significantly with the advent of new fixation devices (locking plates and retrograde intramedullary nails). Nevertheless, in some cases, successful internal fixation is not feasible due to the characteristics of the injury (for example, a short epiphyseal segment and a loose femoral component), necessitating consideration of revision knee replacement as the best therapeutic option.

It is essential to know the specific history of the existing knee replacement: the time elapsed since implantation, the presence of any symptoms or complications preceding the fracture, its manufacturer, design and review of all radiographs before the fracture occurred, if available.

In simple injury patterns, the fracture and the loose femoral component may be addressed using a femoral revision component with a long stem. Alternatively, in the absence of significant bone loss but with proximal fracture extension to the femoral shaft, the use of internal fixation and a femoral revision component with a long stem allows for the preservation of bone stock and augmented fixation at the level of the fracture site.

A distal femoral replacement (DFR) arthroplasty is indicated in the presence of significant bone loss, poor bone quality, and fracture extension to the femoral shaft.

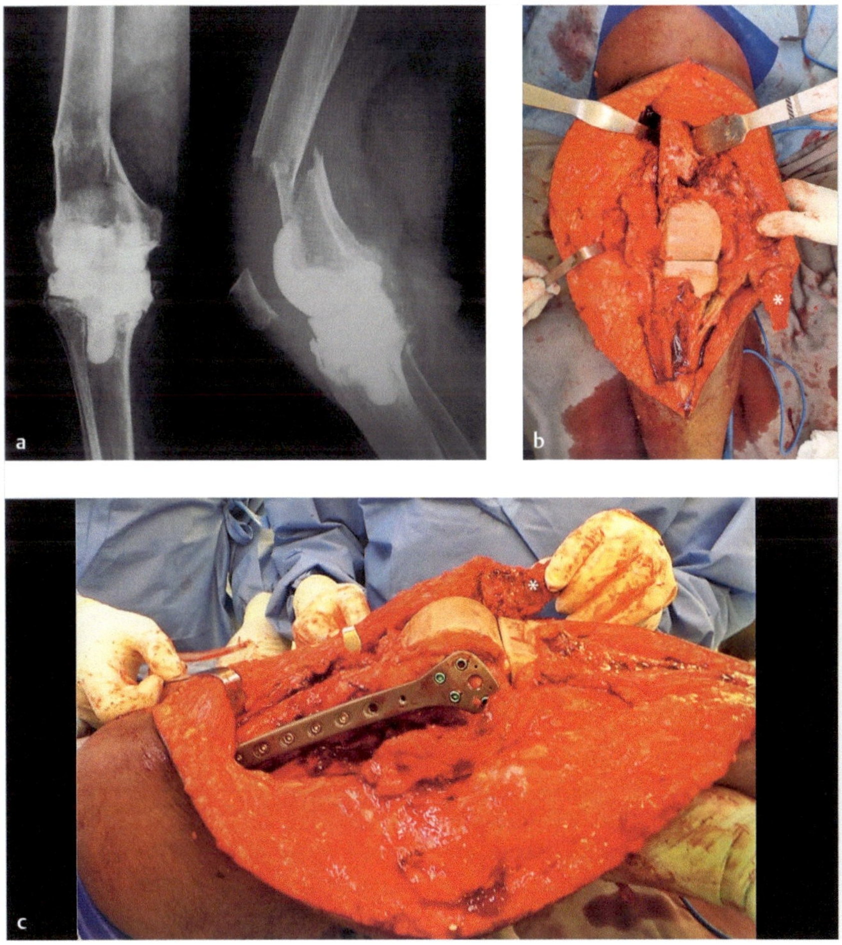

Fig. 11.1 Periprosthetic distal femur fracture. **(a)** Radiographs of the knee depicting a metaphyseal distal femur in association with a mobile knee antibiotic-loaded cement spacer implanted 2 years before the fracture. **(b)** Extensile approach including a tibial tubercle osteotomy with excellent and complete exposure of the fracure site as well as of the joint. The tibial tubercle is elevated from its original location (*). **(c)** Observe that the fracture was fixed with the cement spacer in place.

11.3 Expectations

Revision arthroplasty after distal femur periprosthetic fractures may occur as a primary procedure (when there is a loose femoral component) or as a secondary procedure (in those cases with a failed internal fixation).

Revision to a DFR allows for early total weight-bearing and is not associated with complications typically associated with internal fixation (nonunion or malunion). Difficulties in this group are related to torsional and/or axial malalignment (patellofemoral instability).

The use of femoral revision components and stems augmented by plates also allows for early weight-bearing.

Management of the extensor mechanism during surgical exposure of the knee is challenging in these cases and may require particular techniques, such as a quadriceps snip or a tibial tubercle osteotomy, if joint exposure is difficult. (▶ Fig. 11.1b)

11.4 Indications

Lewis and Rorabeck categorized distal femur periprosthetic fractures into three groups. Type I are nondisplaced fractures. Type II are displaced fractures. Type III are fractures, displaced or not, associated with a loose femoral component.

A revision knee replacement is indicated for Type III distal femur periprosthetic fractures. Another indication is the surgical treatment of a recalcitrant distal femur periprosthetic nonunion.

11.5 Contraindications

The contraindications for a revision total knee replacement are:

- Active infection.
- Presence of comorbidities severe enough such that risks outweigh the benefits of the procedure.

11.6 Special Considerations

A detailed preoperative history and physical exam are of utmost importance. Identification of prior surgical scars is critical in deciding where to place the new surgical incision. By and large, one should avoid making narrow skin bridges and whenever possible, incorporate previous scars into the new incision.

The brand and the design of the existing knee replacement should be determined. If the tibial component is stable, a femoral revision component may be implanted without revising the tibial one, but only if the components are compatible with one another.

If joint infection is a possibility, the authors proceed with a staged treatment. In the first stage, an antibiotic spacer is placed after articular debridement of the joint and removal of the femoral component. Then, once the infection has been controlled, definitive knee revision is carried out.

The authors recommend use of extensile surgical approaches, including appropriate mobilization of the extensor mechanism, granting appropriate exposure of the knee. A proper surgical approach is decisive to ensure thorough debridement and optimal access to the distal femur (▶ Fig. 11.1 b and c).

11.7 Special Instructions, Positioning, and Anesthesia

The procedure is performed under general anesthesia or regional peripheral nerve block. The patient is placed supine on a radiolucent table. The ipsilateral arm placed on top of the chest, supported by foam or blankets. The goal is to leave the ipsilateral arm comfortable without stretching the shoulder and brachial plexus during the case. Some of these procedures take several hours, and keeping the shoulder abducted for a long period of time may be detrimental, especially in the elderly population. The involved lower limb is prepped and sterile-draped from the foot up to the iliac crest. A sterile tourniquet is left in place but it will be inflated only in case of acute and significant bleeding. Leg holders should be available to support the knee in varying degrees of flexion during the operation. We like to have the two lower limbs at different levels to facilitate imaging, either by lowering the noninvolved leg or elevating the operated one. Proper positioning of the lower limbs is necessary for the adequate use of fluoroscopy, if needed during the surgery.

11.8 Tips, Pearls, and Lessons Learned

- Preoperative computed tomography is of paramount importance, providing information about the fracture pattern and the interface between the bone and the femoral component of the knee replacement.
- A complete examination of the contralateral leg determines the length of the lower limb and range of hip rotation. Knowing the parameters associated with the nonoperated lower extremity aids in reconstructing the injured leg.
- Preoperative planning determines the surgical strategy. A Lewis Rorabeck III fracture requires a revision of the femoral component of the knee replacement.
- An extensible approach should be utilized in most cases to optimize exposure, including either a quadriceps snip or a tibial tubercle osteotomy (▶ Fig. 11.1 b and c).
- Attempt to preserve as much bone as possible, securing the distal segment with an anatomic distal femur locking plate. We plan the placement of screws to not interfere with the insertion of a femoral component stem (▶ Fig. 11.2a).
- Stabilize the distal femur segment prior to revising the knee replacement. To avoid conflict between the distal femoral component and the plate, reconstruct the metaphyseal femoral fracture with unicortical screws.

11.9 Difficulties Encountered

Preoperative images may fail to demonstrate loosening of the femoral component, so the surgeon should be prepared if this is found out to be the case during surgery.

Existing scars around the knee may compromise the ideal surgical approach to the knee. Any skin bridges between prior incisions and a new incision should be at least four-finger breadths wide. In case multiple scars are present, the most lateral one should be preferred.

Previous patella baja and a stiff knee pose difficulties for adequate exposure of the distal femur. In those cases, extensible approaches, including quadriceps snip or a tibial tubercle osteotomy might be necessary (▶ Fig. 11.1 b,c).

The determination of the length and rotation of the distal femur component may be challenging with comminuted injuries. In those cases, a radiograph of the contralateral femur is of assistance as a template.

Active infection imposes a need for staged treatment. The surgeon should be prepared to use provisional knee spacers until a definitive surgery may be carried out. In exceptional cases, when complete resection of the distal femur was performed, the use of a spanning knee external fixator in association with a cement spacer provided reasonable stability to the lower limb.

Advanced osteoporosis is a risky condition for applying plate and screws, even if the implants are angle stable. Variable angle locking plates help allow screw insertion with varying directions.

11.10 Key Procedural Steps

- Surgical Incision and Exposure. Most of these patients have a surgical scar located on the anterior aspect of the knee. If the goal is to add a medial plate, extension of the existing incision proximally with a medial subvastus approach is possible. If a plate is to be implanted laterally, two separate incisions may be considered, one for the distal femur component revision (parapatellar medial) and another one for the plate placement (minimally invasive direct lateral incision, with percutaneous submuscular plate application to the shaft). If the plan is to perform an extended exposure of the distal femur, an anterolateral incision to the knee is extended to the lateral aspect of the thigh. A tibial tubercle osteotomy or a quadriceps snip is usually needed for adequate exposure. The extensor mechanism is retracted medially or elevated proximally in order to enhance visualization. The entire distal femur is exposed, offering great exposure for a total knee revision augmented by a lateral plate (▶ Fig. 11.1 b,c).
- Fracture Exposure and Reduction. The perforator vessels come from the posterior septum and should be identified and ligated. The vastus lateralis is carefully elevated, and the lateral corridor of the femur is exposed. One may preserve the vascular supply to the bone by keeping the periosteum intact. The fracture is reduced by gentle manipulation of the fragments, sometimes using joysticks (Schanz or Steinmann pins).
- Fracture Fixation. We fix the metaphyseal and diaphyseal components of the fracture with a lateral locking plate. Fluoroscopy in multiple projections may be used to confirm proper fracture alignment and adequate hardware positioning. On the lateral radiographic projection of the knee, plate and screws should not sit below Blumensaat's line which in our experience is extremelly difficult to be seen due to the presence of hardware. (▶ Fig. 11.3a–c).
- Removal of Femoral Prosthesis. Once the fracture is stabilized, we carefully remove the femoral component of the prosthesis, using flexible osteotomes, oscillating saw with short and narrow blades and Gigli's saw, aiming to preserve as much bone tissue as possible (▶ Fig. 11.2a). If the tibial component is stable, only the femoral component may be revised, but in the author's experience this is a most rare event. A complete knee replacement revision is done if the tibial component is not stable or if it shows to be incompatible with the femoral revision component available (▶ Fig. 11.2 b,c). If there is a suspicion of infection, we may leave the internal fixation with a plate and implant an antibiotic spacer into the joint. This method attempts to preserve bone stock by performing a staged total knee revision replacement once the infection is under control.
- Wound Closure. The closure of the extensor mechanism is of paramount importance. We use absorbable sutures to repair the quadriceps snip, but many others prefer nonabsorbable ones. Our preference is to use 3.5-mm cortical screws for the fixation of the tibial tubercle osteotomy. The screws should not be driven completely parallel to each other but rather in

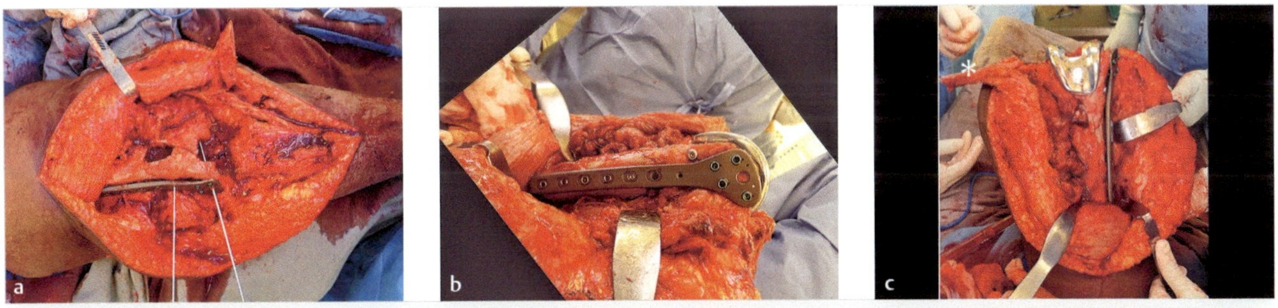

Fig. 11.2 Intraoperative pictures. **(a)** Removal of the cement spacer. Observe the tibial tubercle osteotomy. The plate is secured to the metaphyseal area with locking screws. The Kirschner wires demonstrate the correlation between the end of the plate and the intercondylar notch. **(b,c)** Perspectives of the knee revealing the relationship between the distal femoral plate and the definitive femoral component of the revision knee replacement. Note a long lag screw over the superior margin of the plate.

differing directions in order to strengthen fixation. The tibial tubercle osteotomy should be at least 8 cm long, 1 cm thick and 1.5 to 2 cm wide (▶ Fig. 11.3b,c).

11.11 Bailout, Rescue, and Salvage Procedures

Some fracture patterns may benefit from the use of cerclage wires or cables.

Variable angle locking plates allow the insertion of bicortical screws, skipping the distal femoral stem.

Unicortical screws should be considered in the distal portion of the plate, avoiding conflict with the femoral component. The authors believe that a long femoral stem combined with a locking plate and unicortical screws provide a means of stable fixation for these difficult fractures without interfering with each other (▶ Fig. 11.3c).

A sterile tourniquet is an alternative for significant and unexpected bleeding. Eventually, sterile Doppler and an angiogram are required to rule out vascular injury alongside the fracture repair.

Persistent infection or recalcitrant symptomatic distal femur nonunion is eventually managed with an above-the-knee amputation.

11.12 Pitfalls

Insufficient exposure of the distal femur prevents proper implantation of the revision component and/or a plate construct.

Metaphyseal bone defects should, whenever possible, be augmented with bone graft, providing a healthier biological enviroment for bone healing (▶ Fig. 11.3a).

The tibial component should also be revised if a more constrained joint replacement system is indicated. Residual instability will lead to poorer outcomes.

The fixation of the tibial tubercle osteotomy should be carefully planned to avoid the occurence of fracture or fixation loosening.

The knee should be tested under anesthesia for stability throughout the complete range of motion before closure of the soft tissue layers. Articular instability is a major cause for failure after these technically demanding procedures. Due adjustments (e.g., polyethylene exchange, realigment of components, gaps balancing, bone recuts, et cetera) have to be performed before the final components are positioned and cemented in place. At the end of the day, we expect to be able to provide our patients with a stable, well-aligned, functional, and painfree joint that allows full weightbearing improving their quallity of life (▶ Fig. 11.4a–d).

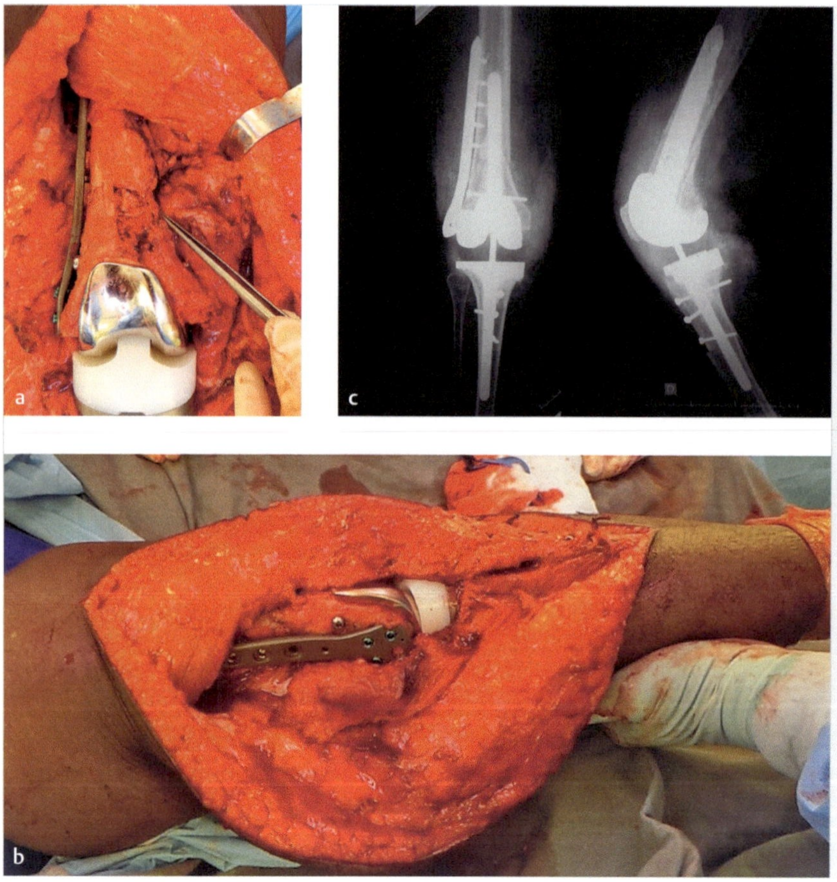

Fig. 11.3 Intraoperative images and postoperative radiographs. **(a)** AP view of the distal femur showing the relationship between the plate and the femoral component. Observe the bone grafting on the medial aspect of the distal femur; **(b)** lateral view of the knee. Aspect of the wound after reattachment of the tibial tubercle with screws. **(c)** Postoperative radiographs depicting a long femoral stem and a lateral locking plate bypassing the fracture area.

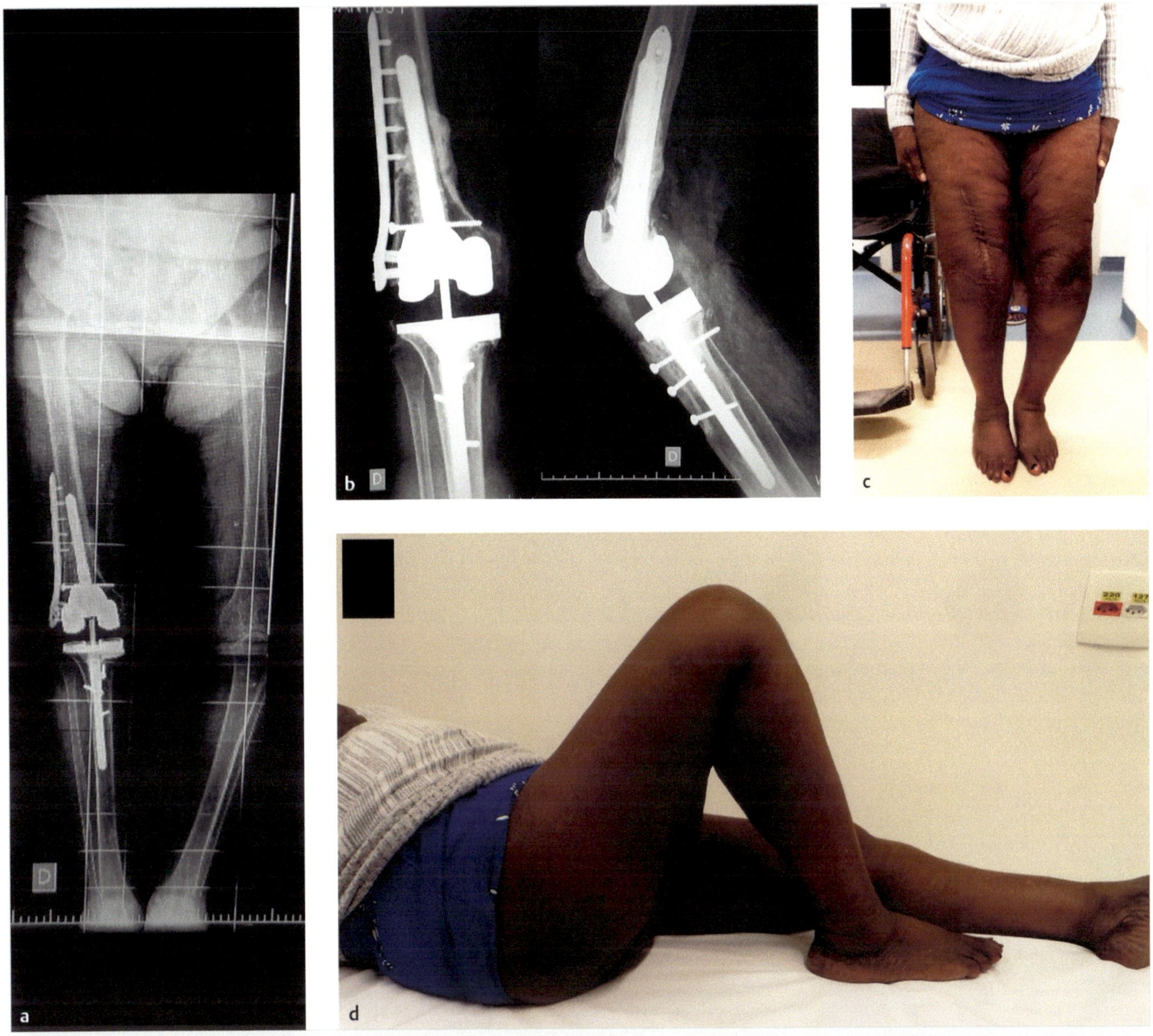

Fig. 11.4 Postoperative follow-up. **(a)** Long leg standing radiograph demonstrating neutral alignment of the operated limb; **(b)** radiographs revealing progressive healing of the distal femur fracture with no signs of hardware failure; **(c)** Full weightbearing on a stable lower limb; **(d)** Range of motion: 0 - 0 - 110.

12 Patellar Fracture—Simple Transverse Pattern

Suthorn Bavonratanavech and Chatchanin Mayurasakorn

12.1 Description

Patella fractures constitute up to 1 to 2% of all fractures, with 70 to 90% of them having a transverse fracture pattern. Because of its anterior subcutaneous location and anatomical attachments, the patella is prone to injury from direct or indirect mechanisms. Most patellar fractures are caused by a combination of direct and indirect forces. Direct injury, such as a dashboard injury or a fall on the anterior knee, often results in a comminuted stellate fracture pattern. When a direct injury occurs, the extensor mechanism may remain intact but significant chondral injury may occur. The indirect mechanism results from exaggerated distraction force on the extensor mechanism which overcomes the tensile strength of the patella. This indirect force usually results in a simple transverse fracture extending to the adjacent medial and lateral retinacular tears, causing fracture displacement and disruption of extensor mechanism.

Associated injuries have been reportedly found in 26 to 44% of patellar fractures, most frequently ipsilateral distal femur or proximal tibia fractures. High-energy mechanism and open fractures are predictors for associated injuries.

12.2 Key Principles

The patella is the largest sesamoid bone in the body. It plays an important biomechanical role for knee function by increasing the moment arm of the extensor mechanism by 30%. The proximal three-fourths of the patella is covered with thick articular cartilage which can be 1 cm or greater in a normal patella. Henceforth, patella fracture could result in discontinuity of extensor mechanism and potential patellofemoral joint incongruity. Failure to restore the articular surface contour results in posttraumatic arthritis. Despite the relatively uncommon incidence of this fracture, careful assessment is essential for planning an effective treatment strategy.

Patellar fractures are usually classified in terms of displacement. Displaced patellar fractures are defined by separation of fragments by more than 3 mm or articular incongruity of more than 2 mm. Descriptive classification may be further categorized according to fracture geometry which could represent the mechanism of injury (▶ Fig. 12.1). The Orthopaedic Trauma Association (OTA) classification is based on articular involvement and number of fracture fragments; however, the clinical utility of this system remains uncertain. This chapter focuses on the simple transverse pattern.

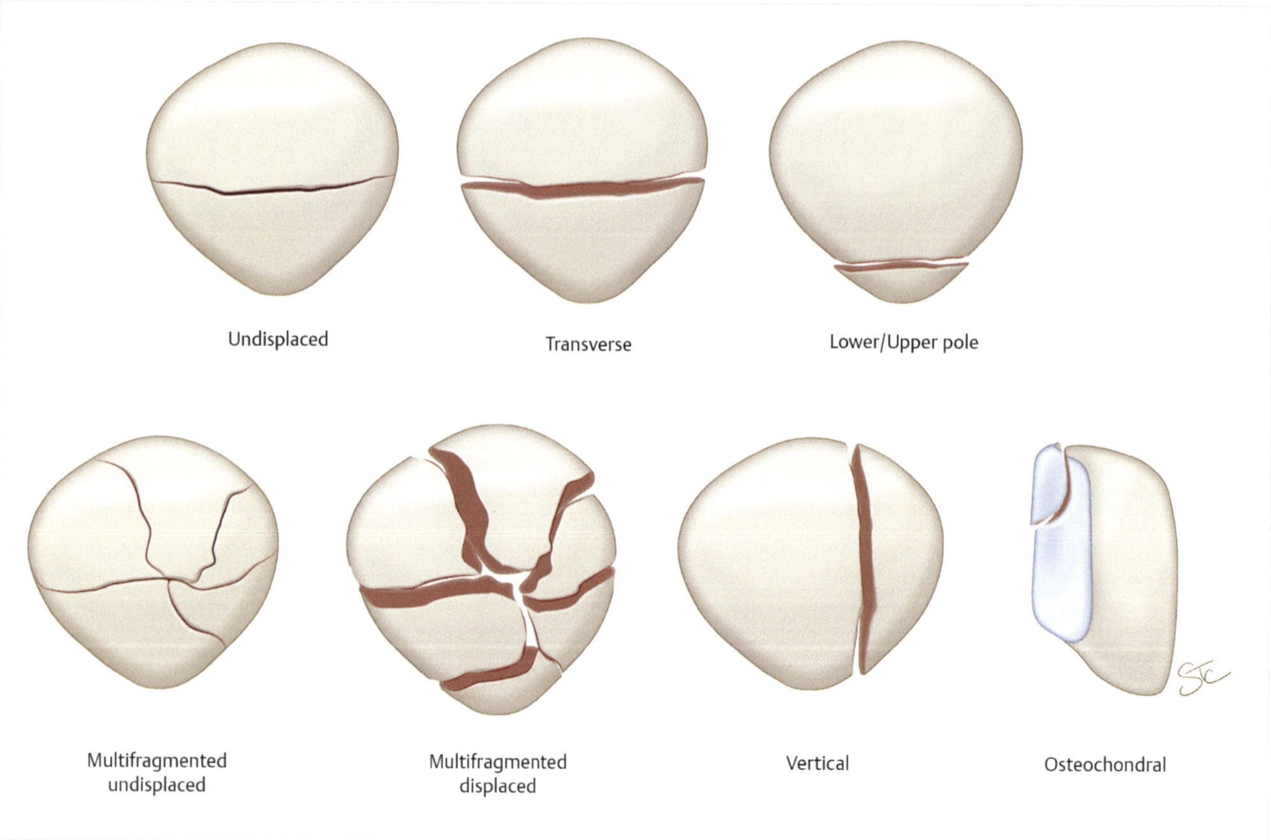

Fig. 12.1 Descriptive classification of patellar fractures.

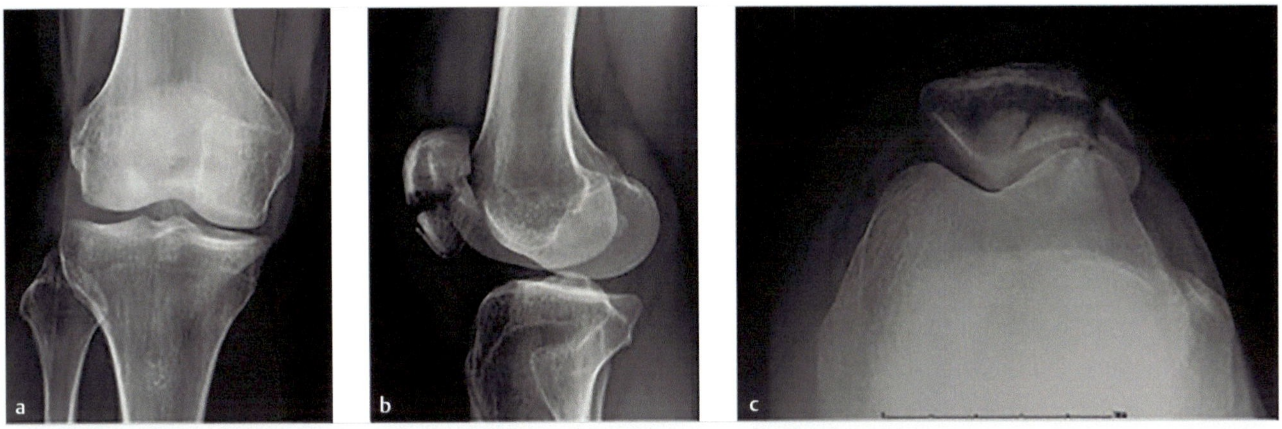

Fig. 12.2 (a,b) Anteroposterior (AP) and lateral views of transverse patella fracture. In AP view, evaluation of fracture may be difficult due to its superimposition with the femoral condyles. Transverse fracture is best seen in lateral view. **(c)** Vertical fracture is demonstrated in Merchant's view.

Initial evaluation of a patient with knee injury includes detailed history and physical examination. Mechanism of injury helps the surgeon to anticipate possible fracture pattern and extent of the injury. Anterior knee pain, swelling, and limited range of knee motion are commonly associated with patellar fractures. Inability to extend the knee usually indicates disruption of extensor mechanism.

When there is a suspicion of open fracture, the saline loading test can be used with caution. Several publications report that using a standard saline volume of 60 mL is inadequate to diagnose traumatic arthrotomies of the knee (36–46% of sensitivity). Arthroscopy-based studies demonstrated that saline volumes of 155 to 194 mL are required to achieve 95% sensitivity. The surgeon should be aware that small arthrotomy wounds can give a false negative result. Addition of methylene blue did not improve the diagnostic value of the saline load test.

Plain radiographs in anteroposterior (AP) and lateral views (▸ Fig. 12.2a,b) are typically sufficient to diagnose most of patella fractures. The Axial or Merchant's view (▸ Fig. 12.2c) is a useful addition in suspicion of vertical fracture, osteochondral defects, and for assessment of articular incongruity. CT scan is rarely necessary for evaluation of an isolated patellar fracture. However, in distal pole patellar fractures it has been demonstrated that the addition of a CT scan may modify the AO/OTA classification and alter treatment plans. The distal pole fracture is often unappreciated when using plain radiographs alone. Magnetic resonance imaging (MRI) can be used to help determine osteochondral fragments and associated ligamentous or extensor mechanism injuries.

12.3 Expectations

Regardless of the fracture morphology and degree of displacement, the goal of treatment remains restoration of the extensor mechanism and maintenance of articular surface congruity to allow early motion. Failure to minimize the articular incongruity could result in posttraumatic arthritis.

12.4 Indications and Contraindications

12.4.1 Nonoperative Treatment

Indications for nonoperative treatment are < 2 mm articular incongruity, < 3 mm displacement with an intact extensor mechanism. Relative indications include severe medical comorbidities or severe osteopenia. In a minimally displaced transverse fracture with active knee extension, the retinaculum is intact and these patients can be managed conservatively.

Treatment protocol consists of immobilization in long cylindrical cast or locked knee brace in extension for 4 to 6 weeks with weight bearing as tolerated. Once the pain subsides, straight leg raise and isometric quadriceps exercises are initiated to minimize quadriceps atrophy. When there is evidence of callus formation, begin gradually increasing range of motion exercises to prevent intra-articular adhesions.

12.4.2 Operative Treatment

Our operative indications are as follows: > 2 mm of articular incongruity; > 3 mm of displacement; compromised extensor mechanism with loss of active extension; osteochondral fractures with intra-articular loose bodies; and open fracture. For simple transverse fractures, the preferred current surgical option is open reduction and internal fixation (ORIF) with tension band fixation. The tension band concept is to convert the distractive tensile force of the extensor mechanism into compressive force across the fracture interface. A modified tension band wiring involves two parallel Kirschner wires and a stainless-steel figure-of-eight wire loop.

12.5 Special Considerations

Modification of implants have been substantially proposed in an effort to reduce complications while maintaining fixation strength. Those modifications include use of interfragmentary

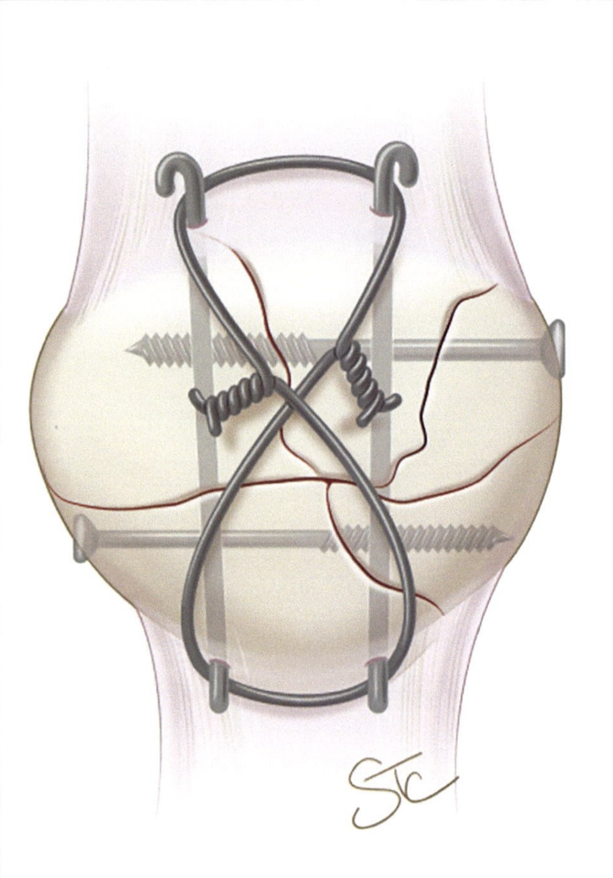

Fig. 12.3 Comminuted fracture can be fixed with lag screw creating simple fracture, which is amenable for tension band fixation.

lag screws, nonmetallic implants, different wiring techniques such as cerclage wiring, Lotke loop, and Magnusson wiring.

In the authors' practice, we have been using tension band fixation with two interfragmentary lag screws in combination with a vertically oriented figure-of-eight FiberWire loop (▸ Fig. 12.3). This combination offers comparable fixation strength to allow early motion and a satisfactory union rate. The nonmetallic figure-of-eight loop has a low-profile resulting in less hardware complication and no secondary surgery is needed for implant removal.

Partial patellectomy is rarely indicated in simple transverse fractures. Total patellectomy alters knee biomechanics, reducing quadriceps strength > 49%. These procedures should be reserved as salvage procedures in case of severe comminution, failed internal fixation, and patellar osteomyelitis.

12.6 Special Instructions, Position, and Anesthesia

The patient is usually placed supine on the operating table. A small bump can be placed beneath the hip to align the limb in neutral rotation. Another small bump is prepared in the sterile operative field to provide knee flexion. A nonsterile tourniquet is an optional addition and may be inflated only in the event of uncontrolled bleeding. The inflated tourniquet may trap the quadriceps muscle proximally, complicating the reduction process of the patella.

12.7 Tips, Pearls, and Lessons Learned

- In order to use tension band fixation, the posterior articular cortex cannot be comminuted as it must provide sufficient fracture interface to allow compression.
- To achieve adequate tension band fixation, the figure-of-eight loop needs to be tightened with the knee in extension.
- The placement of figure-of-eight loop should be as close to the bone as possible, as the tension band became more stable while turning over adjacent bone surface.

12.8 Difficulties Encountered

When operative treatment is planned, it is essential to meticulously evaluate the fracture pattern in order to formulate a stepwise approach for reduction and internal fixation. Frequently, the fracture consists of some comminution or more than two main fragments which might not be visualized on the preoperative radiographs. If needed, minor fragments can be fixed to the main fragment to simplify the fracture to a pattern that is amenable to tension band fixation (▸ Fig. 12.3). Some useful instruments such as cannulated screws and pointed reduction clamps should be anticipated with thorough preoperative planning.

12.9 Key Procedural Steps

The author's preferred method is modified tension band fixation by using two 4.0-mm cannulated screws and braided polyester figure-of-eight loop (▸ Fig. 12.4).

- A midline/lateral parapatellar longitudinal incision is made through the skin and prepatellar bursa. This is usually made with the knee in slight flexion.
- Usually, there is subcutaneous hematoma and contused soft tissue anteriorly to the patella. Avoid unnecessary soft tissue removal or undermining. In the case of an open fracture, the debridement of contaminated soft tissue is essential.
- Once the fracture is exposed, the fracture edges are cleaned just for determining the reduction. At this step, the surgeon may encounter comminuted fragments which may be overlooked from the preoperative radiographs. Minute fragments which do not contribute to the stability should be removed. Major fragments can be fixed together to create a simple fracture pattern. Options include lag screws, cannulated lag screws, or transosseous suture.
- The medial and lateral retinaculum are assessed.
- The joint is thoroughly irrigated to remove debris.
- **Interfragmentary fixation with 4.0-mm cannulated screw**: One 1.6- or 2.0-mm double-tipped K-wire is used for temporary fixation and serves as a guide for subsequent cannulated screw guidewire. The K-wire is inserted in the midline from the fracture site into the proximal fragment in retrograde fashion, to ensure the most optimal position and direction of the K-wire. The K-wire should lie approximately 5 mm from the anterior surface of patella.

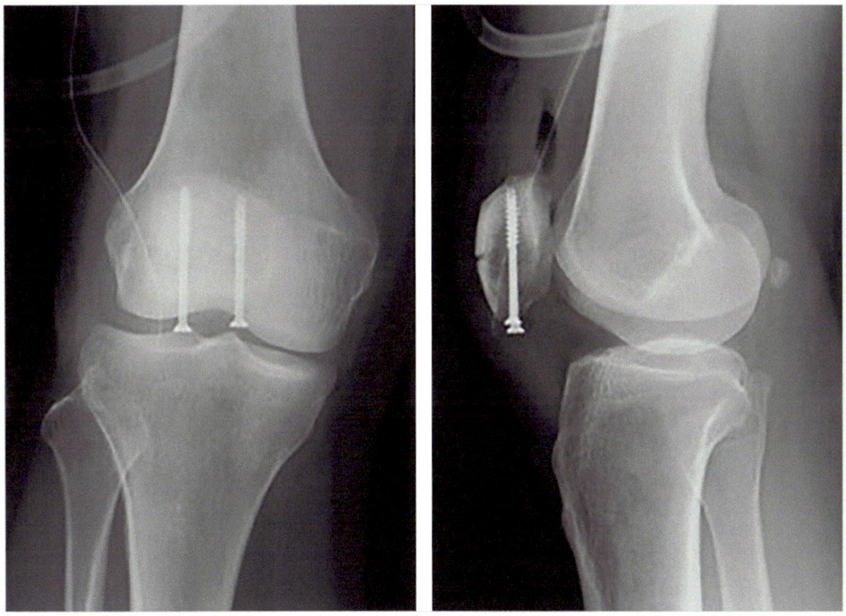

Fig. 12.4 Authors' preferred method of fixation: Cannulated screws in combination with braided polyester figure-of-eight loop.

- The fracture is directly reduced to obtain articular reduction and maintained with pointed reduction clamps. Careful assessment of the articular reduction has to be done by direct palpation through the defect of the retinaculum. Extension of the arthrotomy or retinacular tear may be necessary.
- The midline K-wire is then advanced across the fracture to the distal fragment.
- Two parallel guidewire fixation: Guidewires for 4.0-mm cannulated screws are usually 1.0- to 1.2 mm in diameter. Location for these guidewires will spread from the midline K-wire to the right and left, separating patella into thirds. The guidewires are inserted from the proximal to distal fragment with the direction parallel to the midline K-wire in both AP and lateral planes.
- The length of each guidewire is measured. Drilling for cannulated screws is performed.
- Two 4.0-mm cannulated screws are inserted through the guidewires in regular fashion. We prefer the partially threaded screw to achieve interfragmentary compression. The screw head needs to be countersunk slightly to minimize hardware complications. (▶ Fig. 12.5).
- **Alternate option for interfragmentary fixation with traditional two parallel K-wires:**
  - Usually, 1.6- to 2.0-mm K-wires are used for interfragmentary fixation. We recommend K-wire fixation in retrograde fashion to ensure the optimal position of the K-wires. The K-wires are made double-tipped by cutting the blunt end of the wires.
  - The first K-wire is driven from the fracture site proximally, ensuring the correct position of the K-wire. The second K-wire is placed in similar manner, parallel to the first K-wire
  - The fracture is directly reduced. Then the two K-wires are advanced into the distal fragment.
- Making a figure-of-eight loop: We have used #5 FiberWire (Arthrex, Naples, FL), a braided polyester cable for a figure-of-eight loop. The material is passed underneath the quadriceps and patellar tendons and cross anterior to the patella forming a figure-of-eight loop. The cable is then tightened and tied with five to seven surgical knots on the superolateral surface of the patella. The knot is then buried in the soft tissue.

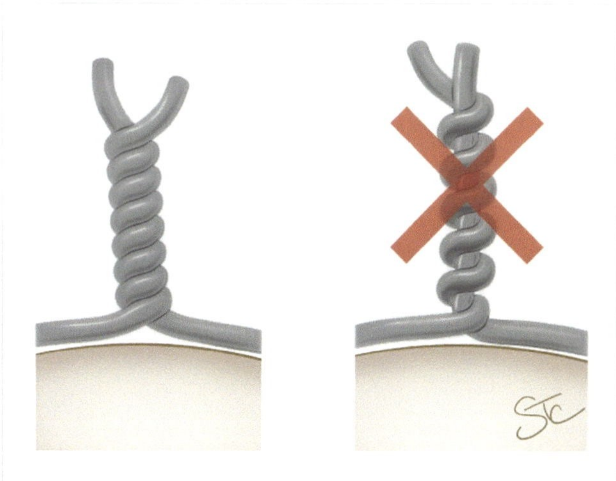

Fig. 12.5 Knot tightening, as emphasized by AO, the twist should be equally turned on each other limb.

12.10 Bailout, Rescue, and Salvage Procedures

In case of severely comminuted fractures, cerclage wiring is a useful option provided that it holds fracture reduction and maintains the extensor mechanism.

12.11 Pitfalls

12.11.1 Indication for Treatment Issue

Intact extensor mechanism does not exclude the articular incongruity which may require surgical treatment.

12.11.2 Technical Consideration

Malreduction

Articular congruity and quality of reduction can be directly assessed intraoperatively. Relying on fluoroscopy is not sufficient for the assessment of articular reduction.

Intra-articular Implant Penetration

Screw or K-wire penetration can be prevented by drilling through the fracture site before reduction.

K-wire Migration

In case the K-wire is used for interfragmentary fixation, proximal wire migration can occur. This complication can be prevented by bending the K-wire into a loop.

Wire Breakage

If stainless-steel wire is chosen for the figure-of-eight loop, overtightening may cause excessive strain on the wire and lead to premature wire breakage.

Wound Dehiscence

Avoid creating subcutaneous flaps.

Hardware Prominence or Symptomatic Hardware

Metallic implants have been associated with symptomatic hardware. Wire twisting can be made at the superior aspect and buried in the deep soft tissue which can reduce this complication. Otherwise, consider using nonmetallic implants such as braided polyester.

13 Patellar Fractures—Comminuted Pattern

Mauricio Kfuri, Juan Manuel Concha, and Igor A. Escalante Elguezabal

13.1 Description

This procedure addresses surgical fixation of multifragmentary fractures of the patella using an anterior mesh plate.

13.2 Key Principles

The morphology of the fracture is related to the energy of the trauma, direction of the blow, and bone density. Comminuted patellar fractures result from a high-energy mechanism of trauma. The main goals in managing comminuted patellar fractures are to restore the integrity of the extensor mechanism of the knee and to pursue an anatomical reduction of the articular surface, when possible. In some of these injuries the extensor mechanism may be intact, despite the fragmentation of the bone. The soft tissues envelope status determines the timing of surgical intervention (▶ Fig. 13.1).

Simple transverse patellar fractures are adequately addressed with the tension band principle described by the Arbeitsgemeinschaft für Osteosynthesefragen (AO) group. The tension band principle requires circumferential contact between the two main poles of the patella, which must be achieved through anatomical reduction. The tension band principle allows for early motion of the knee. Once the patient bends the knee, the tension forces existing on the anterior surface of the patella will be converted into compression forces at the fracture site. However, this principle is not applicable in cases of severe comminution, where circumferential bone contact is not achievable, increasing the risk of a postsurgical mechanical failure. The use of a dorsal patella neutralization mesh plate is an alternative in cases of comminuted patellar fractures. It restores the continuity of the anterior patellar cortex, neutralizing shearing forces along with the knee range of motion.

13.3 Expectations

Tension band wire constructs are associated with high failure rates in the management of comminuted patellar fractures. In recent years, plate fixation became the standard method for comminuted patellar fractures. In most cases, patients complain of anterior knee pain/discomfort associated with the presence of hardware on the anterior aspect of the knee. All patients undergoing a patellar fixation should be advised that, most likely, they will need a second procedure for hardware removal. In cases of severe comminution, the anatomical reduction of the articular surface may not be feasible. The surgeon should disclose this information to the patient at the beginning of the treatment. Posttraumatic arthritis and patellofemoral pain are potential outcomes associated with articular surface incongruency. Bone healing is expected in the majority of cases in less than 3 months.

13.4 Indications

The classic indications for internal fixation of patellar fractures are:

- Compromise of the integrity of the knee extensor mechanism.
- Articular step off equal or superior to 2 mm.
- Open injuries.

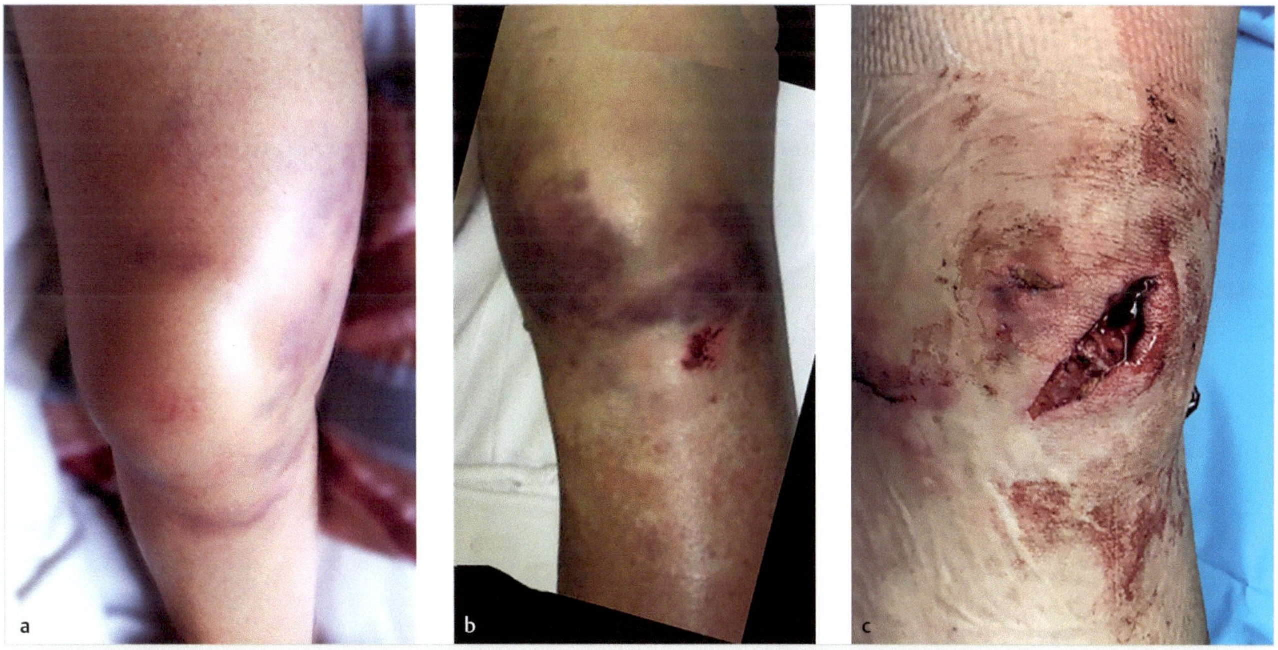

Fig. 13.1 Soft tissues envelope in cases of patellar fractures. **(a)** Bruised and swollen knee, with intact skin; **(b)** bruising, swelling, and abrasion; **(c)** open fracture.

- Association with an ipsilateral femur or tibial fractures, allowing for the early motion of the limb.

13.5 Contraindications

The contraindications for internal fixation of patellar fractures are:

- Current infection.
- Soft tissue damage to the prepatellar skin (severe contusion, swelling, abrasion) or loss (in which case internal fixation should be only carried out along with a coverage procedure).
- Nondisplaced fractures with an intact knee extensor mechanism.
- Patients that may not benefit from a surgical procedure due to other comorbidities (i.e., paraplegia, nonambulatory patients, severe osteopenia).

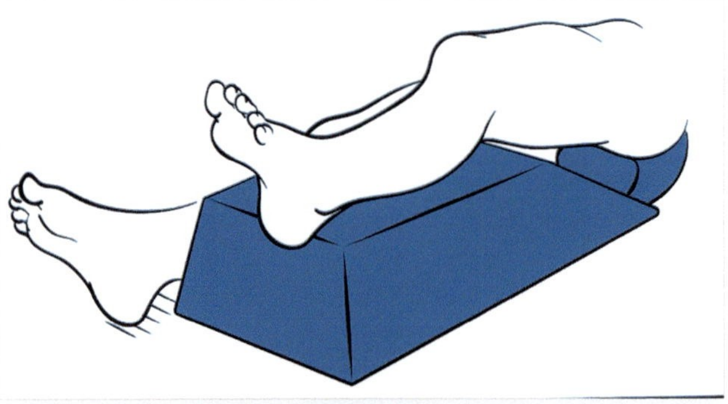

Fig. 13.2 Patient positioning in the operating room. A small foam/gel bump is placed under the ipsilateral buttock, maintaining the leg in neutral rotation, with the patella facing the ceiling. A foam ramp is placed under the leg. The injured leg will sit higher than the opposite limb. This allows for optimal fluoroscopic control in multiple projections (anteroposterior [AP], lateral, medial facet tangent, lateral facet tangent).

13.6 Special Considerations

The patella is the most prominent sesamoid bone in the musculoskeletal system. A thin layer of soft tissues covers the patella, which also has a sizeable articular surface covered by cartilage. A majority of these fractures are closed but often are associated with injury to the overlying soft tissues (massive swelling, skin abrasions) that must be considered when planning surgery. The physical exam at admission is of critical importance, although it may be compromised by pain. Sometimes, it is possible to palpate a gap between the patella's superior and inferior poles, confirming the diastasis between the fracture fragments. The best way to test the knee extensor mechanism is by having the patient sit up and ask the patient to raise his/her leg from 90 degrees of flexion to 0 degrees of extension. This test cannot be performed by individuals with a complete tear of the extensor mechanism. The radiographic evaluation of the knee should include the anteroposterior, lateral, and axial projections of the joint. The computed tomography is very helpful to determine the characteristics of the fracture and the best strategies to address it. The soft tissue envelope on the anterior aspect of the knee is thin and easily compromised by injury. In case of significant swelling, blisters, or loss of continuity of this envelope, the internal fixation should be postponed until safe coverage is assured. The most crucial goal of the surgical treatment is restoring the continuity of the extensor mechanism. The patient should be advised that an anatomical reconstruction of the patellofemoral joint may not be possible, either because some fragments were lost in open fractures or are too small for internal fixation.

13.7 Special Instructions, Positioning, and Anesthesia

The patient is positioned supine and induced under general anesthesia or spinal block. A tourniquet is left on the proximal aspect of the thigh, but in most cases, it is not inflated. The lower limb is placed over a foam ramp. A small, folded blanket or a gel pad is placed under the patient's ipsilateral buttock to keep the leg in neutral rotation (▸ Fig. 13.2). Elevation of the injured limb during surgery allows for intraoperative fluoroscopic control in multiple projections. It is essential to consider that the lateral fluoroscopic incidence does not reflect each of the patella's facets. It is necessary to obtain oblique views of the patellofemoral joint to evaluate the fracture reduction separately at the medial and lateral facets. An accurate lateral view of the patella is obtained when the beam is perpendicular to the long axis of the bone. The limb's internal and external rotation will respectively position the X-rays parallel to the medial and lateral facets. A lateral radiograph of the contralateral knee set with 30 degrees of flexion provides a good template for the surgeon regarding the intact patella's morphology and height. Individuals with a previous history of patellofemoral instability may pose an additional challenge to the surgeon. In those cases, the repair of the patella and the extensor mechanism will not necessarily be associated with a stable patellofemoral joint. A detailed preoperative history provides a better understanding of the patient's pretraumatic activity levels and ruling out preexistent knee disorders.

13.8 Tips, Pearls, and Lessons Learned

- Patella fractures may be associated with other injuries to the knee, femur, and acetabulum, and the treating surgeon should examine the images of these areas.
- Longitudinal extensible surgical incisions should be used. Full-thickness skin flaps should be obtained. Do not undermine the layer in between the subcuticular and the superficialis fascia.
- Preserve small osteochondral fragments when cleaning the fracture hematoma.
- Try to convert a multifragmentary pole to a larger bone block fixed by either lag screws or provisional Kirschner wires.
- Once the two main poles are identified, the goal is to connect them with temporary 1.25-mm Kirschner wires.
- With the main fragments in place confirm the reduction of the articular surface with a lateral longitudinal arthrotomy.

- Suture the soft tissues of the ruptured extensor mechanism with a number 1 or number 2 nonabsorbable suture.
- Besides sutures applied to the transversely oriented tear of the extensor mechanism, consider using a circumferential suture on the rim of the patella, containing the perimeter of this bone.
- Mold and apply a low-profile anterior locking mesh plate to the patella.
- Consider biplanar fixation of the patella, with unicortical screws inserted from anterior to posterior and bicortical screws inserted longitudinally from inferior to superior.
- Utilize fluoroscopy during the entire procedure certifying that fracture reduction and hardware placement are satisfactory.
- Confirm that the construct is stable along with the entire range of motion of the knee, obtaining fluoroscopic lateral views of the patellofemoral joint with the knee set at 0, 30, 60, 90, and 120 degrees of flexion.
- If the construct does not seem to be completely stable in cases of severe comminution, consider adding a safety cerclage. The cerclage may be performed with metal wires or nonresorbable tapes. The cerclage is passed through the fibers of the quadriceps and the tibial tubercle. The cerclage is tied without excessive tension and with the knee flexion of 90 degrees avoiding patella baja.
- If the inferior pole is comminuted and not entirely captured by the edge of the plate, consider Krakow sutures to the patellar tendon and transosseous sutures tied at the level of the superior pole of the patella.

13.9 Difficulties Encountered

Capturing the patella's comminuted inferior pole is challenging, even while using a low-profile anterior mesh plate. The patellar tendon covering the inferior pole makes it difficult to wrap the plate around the tip of the patella. Obtaining a normal patella height is not easy in the presence of comminution or loss of patellar fragments. Reducing and fixing small osteochondral fragments, as well as managing peeled off pieces of cartilage, is sometimes not feasible.

13.10 Key Procedural Steps

- A longitudinal incision is placed on the anterior aspect of the knee. It should expose the attachment of the quadriceps tendon and the anterior tibial tubercle. The skin should not be undermined. A full-thickness flap should be elevated, including the superficialis fascia located under the subcuticular tissue.
- The fracture is quickly exposed, and the extent of the damage to the extensor mechanism is assessed. It is essential to evaluate the fracture pattern and the extent of the soft tissue injury into the medial and lateral knee retinacula.
- The initial goal is to convert a multifragmentary fracture into two main blocks, corresponding to the superior and inferior poles. The fragments are carefully manipulated, reduced, and provisionally fixed with small 1.25-mm Kirschner wires. In selected cases, nonresorbable sutures were used to group small pieces. The provisional Kirschner wires are applied as a raft into the subchondral bone. Larger fragments may be fixed with 2.7- or 2.4-mm lag screws.
- Once we obtain two main patellar bone blocks, we set them provisionally with two longitudinal Kirschner wires, inserted from the superior to the inferior pole or vice versa. Fluoroscopy in multiple projections (AP, Lateral, Medial Facet Tangent, and Lateral Facet Tangent) is used to confirm that a satisfactory alignment has been obtained.
- A lateral longitudinal parapatellar arthrotomy is eventually performed to assess the articular surface.
- Once the multifragmentary fracture is provisionally stabilized, the next step is to repair the extensor mechanism's soft tissues. We use nonresorbable sutures to sew the medial and lateral retinacula and the fibers of the extensor mechanism located on the anterior aspect of the patella. We also place a circumferential nonresorbable suture around the patella, aiming to contain its peripheral rim.
- Once the patella is reduced and contained, we apply a low-profile molded locking mesh plate to the anterior aspect of the bone. The plate captures the bone as a cage, allowing for the insertion of bicortical screws in the longitudinal axis of the patella and unicortical locking screws from anterior to posterior. Fluoroscopy in multiple projections (lateral, tangent medial facet, and tangent lateral facet) is used to confirm satisfactory fracture reduction and proper hardware placement.
- At the end of the fixation, we range the knee from 0 degrees of extension up to 120 degrees of flexion. Lateral fluoroscopy of the knee is used to assess proper patellar height and assure that the bone-implant construct is stable along with the entire knee range of motion.
- Irrigate the wound with saline solution copiously at the end of the procedure.
- The lateral arthrotomy is repaired at this time with resorbable sutures. The superficialis fascia is closed with resorbable sutures, with the knee at 45 degrees of flexion. The closure of the subcuticular and skin must be done without tension, with the knee in flexion. Suturing the soft tissues anterior to the knee with the joint flexion of at least 45 degrees facilitates early motion in the postoperative set.
- Final radiographs should be obtained in the postoperative setting (▶ Fig. 13.3).

13.11 Bailout, Rescue, and Salvage Procedures

Some fracture patterns present significant comminution with small osteochondral fragments. If some pieces are too small to be fixed and are not attached to soft tissues, we remove them. A partial patellectomy is a consideration in those cases. The goals associated with partial patellectomy are the restoration of an intact and stable knee extensor mechanism. The shortening of the patella with resultant loss of patellar height may have implications on knee flexion. Besides the incongruence of the patellofemoral joint, it is difficult determining the proper patella height. The patient should not leave the operating room without a complete assessment of the patellofemoral stability along with the entire knee range of motion. We recommend supplementing the repair in cases of severe osteoporosis,

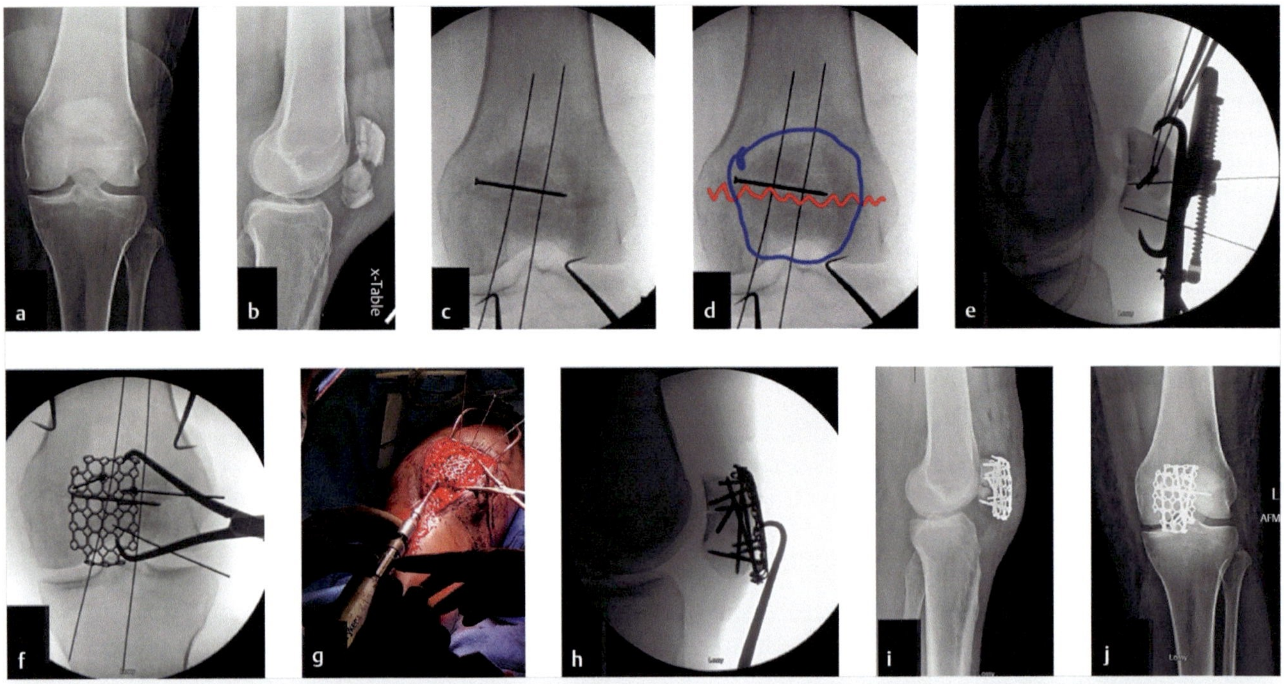

Fig. 13.3 Internal fixation of a comminuted patellar fracture using plate and screws. **(a,b)** Anteroposterior and lateral knee radiographs depicting a comminuted patellar fracture; **(c)** the initial strategy consists in grouping the principal fragments of the fracture with interfragmentary screws and provisional Kirschner wires; **(d)** once the fracture is reduced, nonresorbable suture repairs are applied not only to restore the continuity of the fibers of the extensor mechanism but also to contain the rim of the patella; **(e,f)** a point reduction clamp compresses the two main patellar poles and a low-profile mesh locking plate is applied on the anterior aspect of the bone. Kirschner wires secure the plate in place and push the plate onto the anterior cortex of the patella; **(g)** an essential step is to ensure the insertion of longitudinal screws from the inferior pole to the superior pole, or vice versa. A biplanar fixation has excellent biomechanical properties if compared with a construct with only unicortical anteroposterior screws; **(h)** a bone hook is placed into one of the plate holes. This allows tilting the patella internally and externally at the time of the fluoroscopy. We obtain accurate lateral and oblique views tangent to the patella's medial or lateral facet. **(i,j)** Lateral and anteroposterior postoperative radiographic incidences.

comminution, or revision of failed fixations. We have added a nonresorbable tape passed through the fibers of the quadriceps tendon and the tibia tubercle level, configuring a circumferential cerclage. We apply this construct with the knee flexed at 30 degrees. The cerclage should not be tightened with tension; otherwise, it may cause patella baja. The knee should be ranged again after applying the cerclage, confirming no interference with the patellar height and the stability of the extensor mechanism's repair. The cerclage system acts as a seat belt, holding the superior pole of the patella and avoiding that quadriceps forces may pull the entire repair apart. In cases where the hardware placed on the anterior aspect of the knee is too proud, patients may have pain mobilizing the joint. In those cases, the hardware may be removed after 6 to 9 months, provided image studies confirm that the fracture is healed. If radiographs cannot offer certainty about bone healing, computed tomography should be ordered. Impending soft tissue conditions may lead to hardware exposure, knee stiffness, and sometimes infection. If the soft tissues are compromised, a medial gastrocnemius rotational flap is an excellent alternative providing a robust coverage and blood supply to the patella.

13.12 Pitfalls

Comminuted fractures of the inferior pole of the patella are challenging. If the comminuted inferior pole is not captured by the plate construct, the repair of the extensor mechanism will fail. The failure mode will simulate an avulsion of the patellar tendon. Osteoporotic fractures may require extra soft tissue reinforcements. Those are injuries where one may not rely just on hardware fixation. A tourniquet should be avoided in the management of patellar fractures. A tourniquet applied to the upper portion of the thigh may limit the excursion of the superior pole of the patella, making the fracture reduction harder.

14 Patellar Tendon Repair with Ipsilateral Semitendinosus Autograft Augmentation

Vishal S. Desai and Michael J. Stuart

14.1 Description

This procedure describes a method of primary patellar tendon repair with bidirectional fixation using both transosseous tunnels and suture anchor fixation combined with an ipsilateral hamstring autograft inserted into a distal patellar pole socket.

14.2 Key Principles

The mechanism for a patellar tendon rupture typically involves a forced contraction of the quadriceps against a resisted knee during flexion. Tendon failure usually occurs at the distal patellar pole in patients younger than age 40. Failure to address this injury acutely can lead to tendon retraction and scarring which ultimately compromises the functional result. Early repair provides the highest probability of restoring full knee range of motion, extension strength, and return to preinjury activities. The postoperative rehabilitation program can also influence success of the procedure since prolonged immobilization can lead to knee stiffness.

14.3 Expectations

Outcomes will vary depending on tendon quality, surgical precision, patient comorbidities, the timing of surgery, and rehabilitation compliance. Intraoperative findings and knee examination after repair dictate the postoperative protocol. The patient will need to wear a rehabilitation brace locked in full extension, bear partial weight using crutches and perform active flexion/passive flexion range-of-motion exercises during the first 6 weeks after surgery. Patients are then allowed full-active range of motion and begin progressive resistance strength training (▶ Fig. 14.1 and ▶ Fig. 14.2).

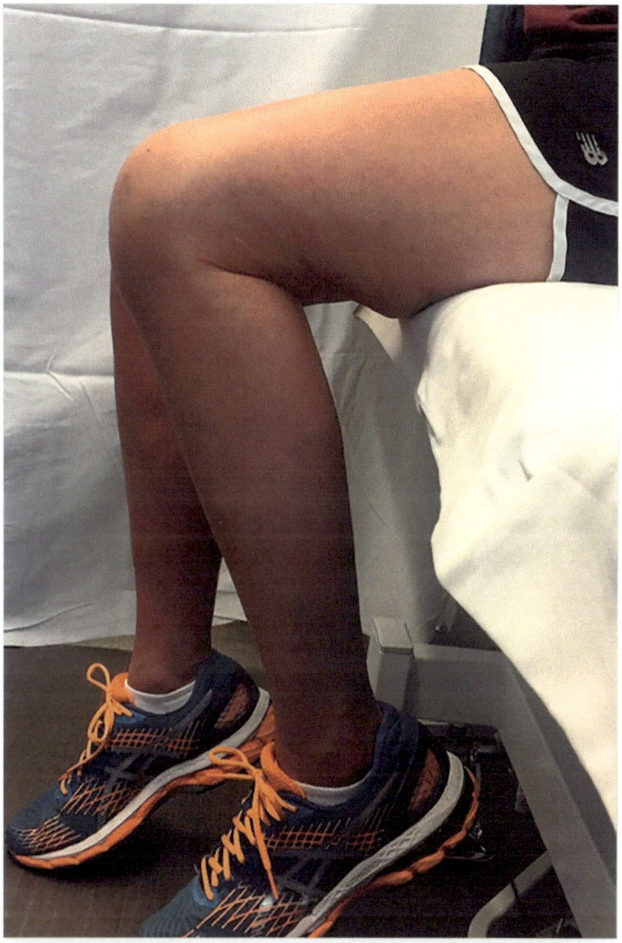

Fig. 14.1 Patient demonstrating 110 degrees of left knee flexion at 3 months after patellar tendon repair with semitendinosus autograft augmentation.

14.4 Indications

The primary indication for this procedure is acute repair of a completed patellar tendon rupture in patients with poor tissue quality due to any of the following predisposing factors: chronic tendinopathy, distal patellar enthesophyte, systemic steroid therapy, fluoroquinolone use, and selected medical conditions, such as renal failure, diabetes, hyperparathyroidism, and rheumatologic diseases. Additional indications include patients with a prior failed patellar tendon repair, chronic patellar tendon rupture, and previously failed tendon debridement for chronic infrapatellar tendinopathy.

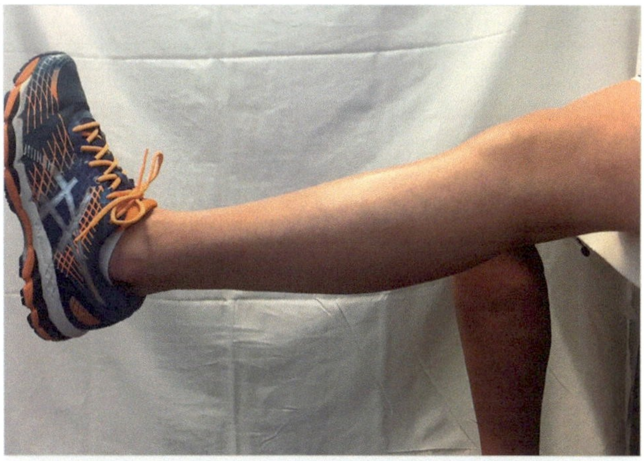

Fig. 14.2 Patient demonstrating full active left knee extension at 3 months after patellar tendon repair with semitendinosus autograft augmentation.

14.5 Contraindications

An open or contaminated wound or active infection is an absolute contraindication. Deficient patellar bone and poor native tendon quality may necessitate tendon reconstruction with Achilles tendon allograft.

14.6 Special Considerations

The following equipment is required to perform the described technique: tendon stripper, No. 2 nonabsorbable sutures (× 2), 2.5-mm drill (× 2), spade tip pin, 5- or 6-mm reamer, TightRope RT with a button and suture anchors (× 2).

14.7 Special Instructions, Position, and Anesthesia

General or spinal anesthesia is administered. The patient is placed in a supine position and a pneumatic tourniquet is placed on the proximal thigh. Extremity exsanguination and tourniquet inflation are performed only if necessary. After completion of the procedure, the soft tissues are injected with a mixture of ropivicaine, ketorolac, saline, and epinephrine. The subcutaneous tissue along the margins of the incision is injected with 0.25% ropivicaine without epinephrine. Sterile gauze, soft roll, an elastic sock, and a rehabilitation brace locked in full extension are applied. The procedure is performed in the outpatient setting.

14.8 Tips, Pearls, and Lessons Learned

The spade tip pin starting point should be in the central location on the distal patellar pole with the exit point at the midpoint of the proximal patellar pole. A freehand technique or a standard anterior cruciate ligament (ACL) tibial guide can be used to ensure proper pin position and to avoid intra-articular or anterior cortex penetration. Parallel longitudinal drill holes are placed 1-cm medial and lateral to the central hole. The smallest diameter drill possible is used to allow later insertion of a Hewson suture passer. The reamer size for the distal pole socket is determined by measuring the diameter of the double semitendinosus graft. The socket is drilled to a maximum depth of 10 mm. After advancing the tightrope through the central tunnel, direct visualization of the flipped TightRope button on the proximal pole of the patella is encouraged to ensure proper positioning. The suture anchors are placed between the central socket and the medial/lateral drill holes. The tendon sutures are pulled proximally and the graft is pulled distally until the tendon is approximated to the distal patellar poll and patellar height is restored. Comparison to the contralateral knee using a lateral fluoroscopic view is helpful in order to avoid patellar tendon overreduction (patella infera). After the procedure is complete, the construct should be tested during surgery by slowly flexing the knee to ensure graft purchase was successful and to guide postoperative rehabilitation.

14.9 Difficulties Encountered

The guide pin and drill bits need to be inserted in a parallel fashion and should exit through the proximal patellar pole. Perforation of the anterior cortex of the patella may increase the risk of fracture.

14.10 Key Procedural Steps

- The patient is positioned and the knee is prepped.
- A 10- to 15-cm anteromedial incision is made from the proximal patellar pole to the tibial tubercle. The paratenon is preserved for a layered closure.
- The patellar tendon is exposed and nonviable tissue is debrided.
- Medial and lateral nonabsorbable, locking whipstitches are placed in the remnant of the proximal patellar tendon.
- The semitendinosus graft is harvested in the standard fashion and passed through the loop of the TightRope device. The diameter of the double graft is measured with a sizing cylinder.
- The distal patellar pole is prepared by removing enthesophytes to create a smooth surface of healthy, bleeding bone.
- The spade-tipped guide pin is placed from the center of the distal pole to the center of the proximal pole. Two parallel 2.5-mm drills are then inserted from distal to proximal located 10 mm lateral and medial to the central pin (▸ Fig. 14.3).
- Two suture anchors are inserted adjacent to the drill bits ensuring a minimum 5-mm osseous bridge (▸ Fig. 14.3).
- A 5- or 6-mm-diameter cannulated reamer equal to the doubled semitendinosus tendon is placed over the spade tip pin to create a 10-mm deep socket in the distal pole.
- The medial and lateral drill bits are removed and the most medial and lateral whipstitch sutures are passed proximally through the transosseous tunnels. Similarly, the central sutures are passed with the TightRope Fixation device through the central tunnel.
- The TightRope button is visualized through a small incision in the quadriceps tendon, flipped and engaged onto the proximal pole of the patella. The semitendinosus graft is reduced into the distal pole socket (▸ Fig. 14.4). The patellar tendon sutures are then tied over the proximal patellar pole restoring the patellar height (▸ Fig. 14.5). The anchor sutures

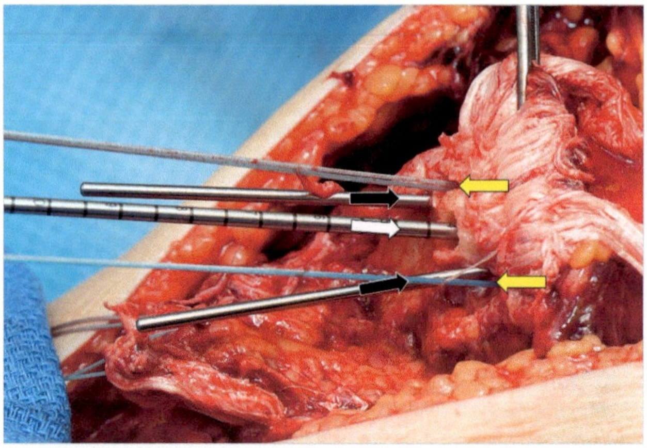

Fig. 14.3 Distal patellar pole preparation for transosseous suture fixation and semitendinosus autograft augmentation: a central spade-tipped pin (*white arrow*), two parallel drill bits (*black arrows*), and two suture anchors (*yellow arrows*).

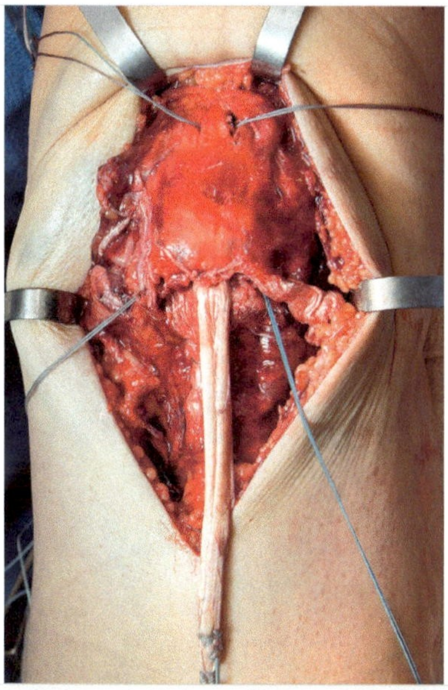

Fig. 14.4 Semitendinosus autograft being advanced into the patellar socket. The doubled semitendinosus tendon is bottomed out within the 10-mm patellar socket.

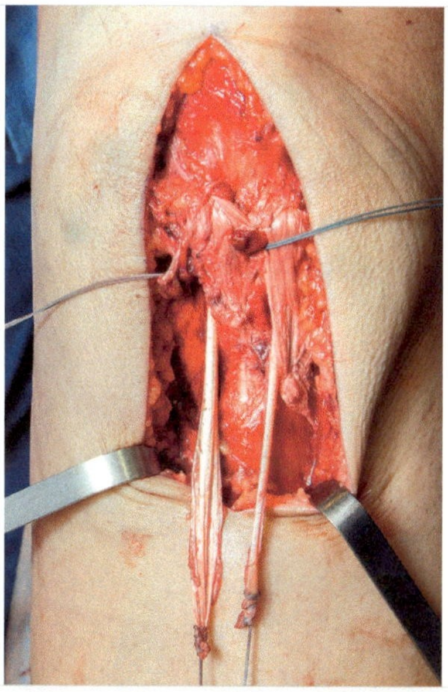

Fig. 14.5 The remaining native patellar tendon is approximated to the distal pole with the transosseous sutures. The autograft is tensioned distally, then sutured to the native patellar tendon at the tibial tubercle.

are tied to the native proximal patellar tendon. The free ends of the semitendinosus graft are tunneled beneath the patellar tendon, tensioned and sutured in place to the distal, native tendon. The remaining graft is flipped proximally and sutured to the proximal, native tendon producing a quadruple augmentation (▶ Fig. 14.6).

- Following closure of the medial and lateral retinacula, paratenon, subcutaneous tissue and skin, the knee is placed in a rehabilitation brace locked in full extension.

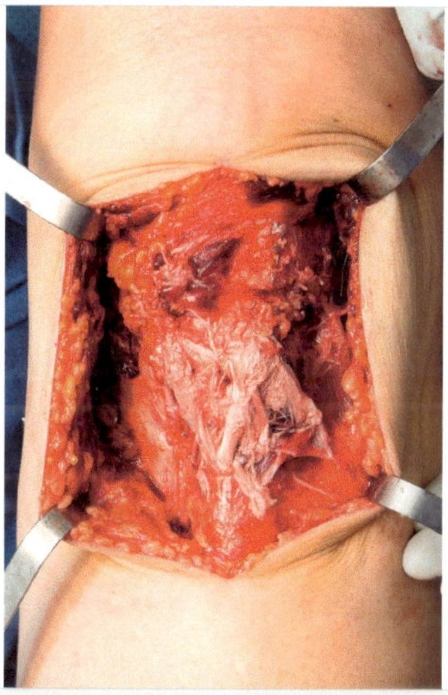

Fig. 14.6 The autograft is folded proximally and then incorporated into the native tendon and distal patellar pole to create a four-stranded construct.

14.11 Bailout, Rescue, Salvage Procedures

Repair with augmentation may not be possible if there is inadequate remaining native patellar tendon. This is an indication for an Achilles tendon allograft reconstruction with insertion of the calcaneal bone block into a tibial tubercle trough and fixation of the graft to the distal patellar pole with both transosseous sutures and suture anchors.

14.12 Pitfalls

There are several considerations to be aware of when executing this technique. It is critical that an adequate distance is maintained between the three transosseous tunnels on the distal pole of the patella in order to avoid tunnel convergence and inability to utilize the suture anchors. Be cautious not to overreduce the patellar tendon with the initial transosseous sutures and cause patellar baja. Finally, the TightRope may have the tendency to flip within the quadriceps tendon. The construct may feel secure at first, but has the potential to subside and lead to gap formation. Visualization of the button through a split in the quadriceps tendon will prevent this problem.

15 Quadriceps Tendon Rupture

Fabricio Fogagnolo and Mauricio Kfuri

15.1 Description

We describe the repair of acute quadriceps tendon ruptures with transosseous repair, and describe our preferred technique for augmented repair in the setting of chronic quadriceps tears.

15.2 Key Principles

Quadriceps tendon ruptures are not as frequent as injuries compromising either the patellar ligament or the patella. The typical patient is a middle-aged male, older than 40 years, with a minor traumatic event rupturing a degenerated tendon. The acute quadriceps tear typically follows a violent eccentric contraction of the quadriceps muscle in sports or home accidents. Males are affected eight times more frequently than females. Usually, the disruption occurs at the proximal pole of the patella or in an area very close to it (within 2 or 3 cm) and involves all three layers of the quadriceps tendon. The patient experiences partial or complete loss of active knee extension following the injury. A defect or gap may be palpated in the suprapatellar region, but this sign may be difficult to observe in obese patients. Lateral projection radiographs of the knee show patella baja or patella ptosis associated with a complete tendon tear. In cases of partial tears, radiographs may not depict noticeable changes, which can mislead the attending physician. Unfortunately, quadriceps tendon ruptures are sometimes unrecognized in the emergency room setting. Ultrasonographic examination is an excellent imaging diagnostic tool, and recent studies have shown sensitivity, specificity, and accuracy above 90%. Magnetic resonance imaging (MRI) should be ordered only in high-energy trauma cases due to the possible association with other overlooked knee injuries. Bilateral lesions occur in 10% of patients. A late diagnosis is frequent as the extensor lag is sometimes attributed to pain following trauma. Ruptures of the quadriceps tendon require early surgical repair in order to restore active knee extension. Partial ruptures may cause extreme weakness and extensor lag if conservatively treated. In acute cases, the goal is to accomplish a robust direct repair of the injury. Neglected or chronic tears require additional augmentation of the repair with soft tissue grafts.

15.3 Expectations

Quadriceps tendon ruptures have a successful recovery with a good prognosis in more than 90% of patients if diagnosed and treated quickly. When a sound repair is carried out promptly, patients regain active full extension and recover an excellent functional level, although some atrophy and loss of flexion may be observed. Fifty percent of patients will have a decreased level of sports performance. Neglected ruptures and excessive surgical delay are associated with a worse prognosis due to muscle retraction and further tendon degeneration. Re-ruptures occur in about 10% of cases and are associated with worse outcomes. High complication rates and poor outcomes are reported on patients who sustained partial or complete quadriceps tendon rupture following total knee arthroplasties.

15.4 Indications

The vast majority of quadriceps tendon ruptures require early surgical intervention. Any complete rupture or partial rupture with weak knee extension with an extension lag should be operated on.

15.5 Contraindications

Small partial tears, severe medical comorbidities, or nonambulatory patients are situations in which conservative treatment is appropriate.

15.6 Special Considerations

Medical comorbidities or other predisposing factors (such as previous tendinopathy or tendinosis) are commonly associated with quadriceps tendon tears and the patient should be carefully investigated. Pathologies such as rheumatoid arthritis, gout, systemic lupus erythematosus, diabetes mellitus, and uremic patients with secondary hyperparathyroidism are related to tendon degeneration. Medications have also been implicated, particularly corticosteroids, anabolic steroids, and antibiotics (fluoroquinolones). Quadriceps disruptions after total knee arthroplasties and quadriceps tendon harvesting for ligament reconstruction procedures are reported and should also be considered for a tendon repair. Once the injury is repaired, the postoperative rehabilitation regimen is of utmost importance. A short period of 4 to 6 weeks with knee immobilization in a brace locked in full extension is recommended. During this period, patients may bear weight as tolerated, provided they have a knee brace locked in extension and are using crutches for balance. Patients are also encouraged to perform isometric quadriceps exercises, avoiding excessive muscle atrophy. Active knee extension and full unprotected weight-bearing is avoided until 6 weeks postoperatively. The knee immobilizer is removed during physiotherapy sessions, and progressive active knee flexion is introduced. We aim to reach the maximum range of motion by the 12- to 16-week mark. Resistive strengthening exercises are initiated after 12 weeks and return to sports should occur only after six months. One may expect poor results in these cases. Partial tears with preserved knee function without any extension lag may be conservatively treated. Partial weight-bearing and knee immobilization for 6 weeks, followed by cautious rehabilitation, is the general rule.

15.7 Special Instructions, Positioning, and Anesthesia

Patients are positioned in the supine position on the operating table. A tourniquet is placed on the proximal aspect of the thigh in the case marked bleeding is associated with the procedure, which is rare. We avoid using a tourniquet as it may restrict mobilization of the proximal end of the quadriceps tendon, contributing to an increased gap at the injury site and increased tension on the repair. Complete muscle relaxation has paramount importance during tendon repair, and this information should be provided to the anesthesiologist. Contrary to patellar tendon ruptures, radiolucent table and image intensification are not mandatory because there is no risk of altering the patellar height if too much tension is applied when tying sutures.

15.8 Tips, Pearls, and Lessons Learned

- Quadriceps tear should be ruled out in the face of suprapatellar pain and lag of active knee extension.
- Once the tear is diagnosed, risk factors should be identified—comorbidities, steroid use.
- Ultrasonographic examination is associated with high sensitivity. MRI should be ordered in doubtful cases or after high-energy trauma.
- The surgical repair should be done within the first 2 weeks of the injury if the patient is clinically stable.
- Very strong nonabsorbable braided sutures in locked fashion (Krackow or similar) are the standard procedure after tendon debridement.
- Lesions at the osteotendinous junction require bone decortication before tunnel drilling and suture passing.
- Biological augmentation is recommended in chronic, neglected ruptures or with midsubstance tears of degenerated tendons. The same applies to patients with predisposing factors.
- Careful rehabilitation and knee brace in extension on the first 4 to 6 weeks should be emphasized. Slight knee range of motion under supervision only.

15.9 Difficulties Encountered

Chronic tears and patients with highly degenerated tendons are tough to manage sometimes because it is hard to fix the quadriceps tendon to the patella securely. Patellar tendon ruptures, for instance, allow us to use two bone extremities to anchor or protect our sutures, namely the patella and tibia tuberosity. When dealing with quadriceps tendon injuries, the quadriceps site of repair should be strong enough to overcome massive traction forces when knee range of motion is started during rehabilitation.

15.10 Key Procedural Steps

15.10.1 Preparation

The first steps of the procedure are similar in acute and chronic cases. We examine the knee under anesthesia in all cases. Any associated ligament injury is recorded and considered for repair or reconstruction.

15.10.2 Incision and Exposure

A midline longitudinal incision is made, centered on the patella and measuring 12 to 15 cm in length. It is essential to extend the incision at least 5 cm proximal to the superior pole of the patella. Full-thickness skin flaps are developed to expose the site of injury adequately. Besides the quadriceps tendon, the medial and the lateral retinaculum are generally compromised and are thoroughly examined. The associated hematoma is evacuated, and the surgical wound is irrigated with saline. Frayed and necrotic tissues are debrided, thus leaving healthy tissue for healing. The quadriceps tendon and muscle are carefully mobilized from any surrounding scars or adhesions.

15.10.3 Tendon Repair

Acute Repairs

In acute ruptures occurring at the osteotendinous junction, transosseous heavy nonabsorbable sutures passed through three longitudinal transpatellar tunnels and tied over the distal pole of the patella are a standard nonexpensive and straightforward method of the tendon to bone repair (▶ Fig. 15.1). Long-term studies confirm excellent healing and remodeling following direct repair using transpatellar drilling sutures. However, while some authors report similar repair strength, others have shown better resistance with suture anchors at the proximal pole of the patella in cadaveric experiments. One of the possible advantages of transosseous sutures is the possibility of adjusting the suture tension at the docking site of the quadriceps tendon on the patella, maximizing surface area contact and optimizing healing. The other possible advantage is that the pull-out forces are not concentrated in one spot (anchor) but dissipated across the entire length of the patella.

Acute Ruptures at the Osteotendinous Junction

The superior pole of the patella is decorticated to promote healing. The quadriceps tendon is debrided, and sutures are performed with two No. 5 nonabsorbable sutures. Krackow stitches are used along the edges of the tendon to 4 to 5 cm proximal of the tear, then coming back again to the tear site, leaving four ends of sutures exiting the quadriceps tendon at the defect, right within the area, which will be reattached to the proximal pole of the patella. The free four suture strands from the proximal tendon are passed through the three 2.0-mm bone longitudinal patellar tunnels using a suture passer with the two central strands passing through the central tunnel. The four free ends of sutures are retrieved through the bone tunnels and tied to each other over the distal pole of the patella. The knee is maintained in full extension while the sutures are tied. We test the repair by flexing the knee and confirming that

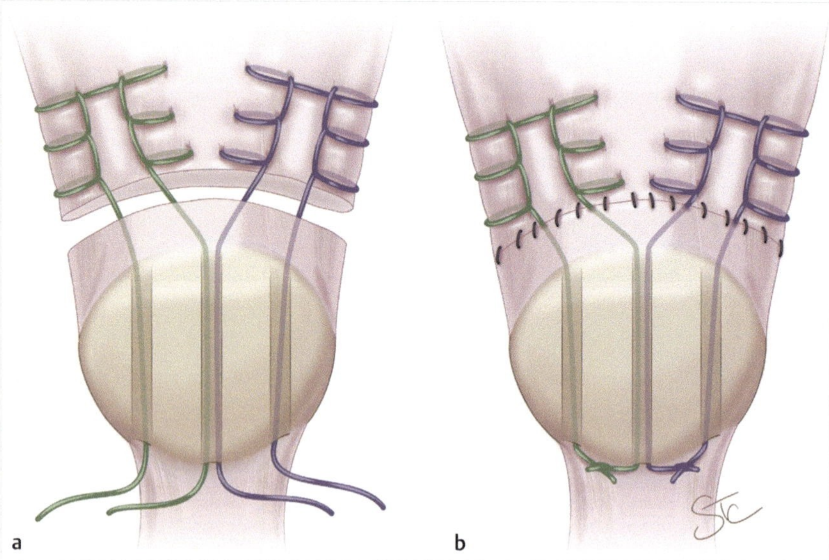

Fig. 15.1 Acute transosseous repair. **(a)** Nonresorbable sutures are applied to the quadriceps tendon. On the lateral side of the quadriceps tendon, a suture is placed in the tendon using locking Krackow technique, advancing in a retrograde manner to 4 cm above the level of the tear. Then, the suture is turned down toward the area of the tear. Two free arms of the suture are left at the end of the quadriceps tendon (*green*). The same procedure is performed on the medial side of the tendon (*blue*). Three longitudinal tunnels are drilled in the patella using a 2.5-mm drill bit. The sutures are passed through the tunnels, with the middle strand of each suture placed in the middle tunnel. **(b)** The sutures are tied under tension at the level of the inferior pole of the patella. The quadriceps tendon and the retinacula are also sewed using nonresorbable sutures (running locking suture).

the quadriceps tendon is stable in place along the entire range of motion.

Acute Ruptures at the Midsubstance

If the rupture is located in the midsubstance of the tendon, direct repair using Krackow stitches or a similar locked technique on both sides is the method of choice. The surgeon should carefully examine tissue ends at the site of the rupture to perform an adequate debridement of local tissue and judge the need for grafting or biological augmentation. We also believe that applying two sets of Krakow sutures to the proximal aspect of the tendon and sending those through patellar tunnels would reinforce the direct repair performed at the midsubstance level.

Chronic Ruptures

In chronic cases, significant gaps may result from muscle retraction of the proximal part of the ruptured tendon. These gaps may also be a consequence of surgical debridement of degenerated areas. We avoid excessive traction on the tissues while closing the defect. A proximal release of the quadriceps muscle group from the scar tissue is performed, mobilizing its distal end. In chronic tears, lengthening or grafting procedures are our preferred methods of reconstruction. Transosseous repair is performed similarly as previously described for acute injuries at the osteotendinous junction. Hamstring grafts are the most commonly used grafts to bypass the defect or to enhance repair strength as biological augmentation. The semitendinosus tendon usually provides adequate length to be passed through a transverse bone tunnel at the patella's proximal pole, and then the two free tendon ends are passed through the quadriceps tendon several times. Sutures connecting graft and quadriceps tendon reinforce the augmentation.

Another very reliable technique is to reinforce the repair with the anterior tibialis tendon if allograft is available. This is a long graft that measures more than 20 cm in length. We usually fold the graft at its half. The resulting loop diameter is measured. The loop has two free arms. Each arm will measure at least 10 cm in length. Under fluoroscopy, we insert a guidewire into the superior pole of the patella and then a loop of the prepared graft is docked to a hole performed from the central third of the superior pole of the patella toward the inferior pole. A cannulated reamer is applied to drill a socket, whose diameter matches the diameter of the allograft loop. The loop should contain a suspensory fixation, which will be passed through the patella from proximal to distal. The loop portion of the graft is driven into the socket in the superior pole of the patella. The two arms of the graft are then passed through the fibers of the quadriceps tendon proximally up to 4 cm above the level of the injury. Then, we turn each arm of the graft distally in the direction of the patella. The ends of each arm are then docked to suture anchors placed on the medial and lateral aspects of the superior pole of the patella (▶ Fig. 15.2).

15.11 Bailout, Rescue, and Salvage Procedures

Significant defects should be bypassed by biological tissues, such as hamstrings, allografts, fascia lata, or quadriceps turndown flaps as described by Codivilla. The Codivilla technique is an alternative method where an inverted-V flap from the proximal quadriceps tendon is turned down to approximate and close the defect. The lower margin of the inverted-V should be 1 to 2 cm proximal to the rupture, and the apex is folded distally and sutured in place. The open proximal portion of the inverted-V is sutured longitudinally. Full extensor mechanism

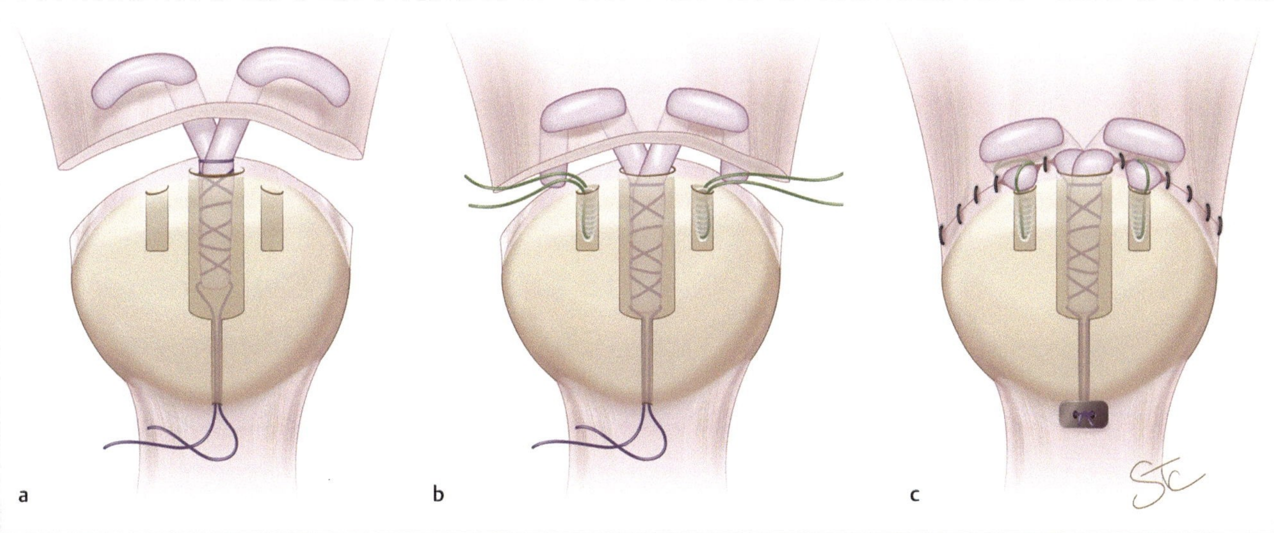

Fig. 15.2 Augmented repair of the quadriceps tendon. **(a)** Drawing showing a graft docked into a central patellar socket. The graft is folded, and the loop has sutures and a suspensory device which are passed with a suture passer toward the inferior pole of the patella. The two free arms of the loop are then passed into each one of the halves of the quadriceps tendon. Each arm is passed from distal to proximal, and then a 90-degree turn is made toward the periphery of the tendon. Two suture anchors are inserted; one on each side of the central socket. The socket has a diameter of 8 to 10 mm and a depth of 20 mm. The anchors are 3 to 4 mm in diameter. The distance between each anchor and the socket is 10 mm. **(b)** Each arm is passed distally toward the area of the tear. It is important to mention that the graft is not only passed throughout the fibers of the quadriceps tendon, but also sutured to it with nonabsorbable stitches. The anchors have stitches which will be passed through the graft and through the quadriceps tendon. **(c)** The grafts are tied to the anchors. A nonresorbable running suture closes the quadriceps tear.

allografts may be used in exceptional cases, such as failed repairs, poor quality autografts for biological augmentation, chronic ruptures with diastasis and degenerated tendon margins or traumatic cases with severe loss of tendinous tissue.

Some recent papers describe the use of synthetic mesh augmentation. Mobilization of quadriceps tendons and muscles may be difficult in old cases due to severe scarring tissue at the suprapatellar region and muscle contractures.

15.12 Pitfalls

- Missed diagnosis leading to late surgeries with severe adhesions and scaring tissues.
- Failure to recognize associated intra-articular knee injuries.
- Inappropriate repair technique with weak sutures or few passes through the tendon edges.
- Failure to decorticate proximal pole of the patella or bad technique deploying bony anchors.
- Weak anchors.
- Anchor fixation in frail bone.
- Transpatellar tunnel drilling too deep or too superficial.
- Inappropriate or aggressive rehabilitation too early during postoperative rehabilitation.

16 Knee Dislocation—Acute Management

John D. Adams Jr

16.1 Description

The acute management of a knee dislocation is vital to patient outcomes and avoidance of devastating long-term complications. This chapter will focus on diagnosis, physical exam, and external fixation.

16.2 Key Principles

Successful acute treatment of a knee dislocation relies on a high index of suspicion in any patient with knee pain following a high-energy traumatic injury. Many patients (60–80%) present with their dislocation reduced on initial radiographs. A careful ligamentous knee exam allows identification of patients with multiligament injuries if other ipsilateral injuries (fractures) do not prevent a good exam. If the knee is dislocated on presentation, emergent reduction should be performed. Once the diagnosis of a knee dislocation has been established, careful physical examination with identification of vascular or neurologic injury is paramount in the acute management. The knee should remain reduced until definitive surgical management is performed. A static external fixator is used in the setting of vascular compromise, open dislocations, and severely unstable knees that do not remain reduced in external braces.

16.3 Expectations

Acute management should help avoid the devastating complications associated with a dysvascular limb, infection, and compartment syndrome. In patients with a vascular injury, emergent revascularization should be performed. Placement of an external fixator prior to vascular repair stabilizes the knee, preventing recurrent vascular compromise. Patients with an open dislocation should receive antibiotics and early surgical irrigation and debridement. Serial exams help identify patients who develop compartment syndrome which is treated with emergent four compartment fasciotomies.

16.4 Indications for External Fixation

Indications for acute placement of an external fixator.

- Vascular injury.
- Open knee dislocations that require soft tissue management.
- Severely unstable knees in which reduction is not maintained in an external brace.

Relative indications for the use of an external fixator are discussed in "Special Considerations.

16.5 Contraindications to External Fixation

While not specifically contraindicated, the routine use of external fixation for knee dislocations is not recommended. After reduction, most knees will stay reduced in a knee immobilizer or a well-fit knee brace. Unless the indications described earlier are met, the use of an external fixator should be questioned.

16.6 Special Considerations

16.6.1 Intimal Tears Resulting in Vascular Occlusion

The traumatic injury to the vasculature that occurs after a knee dislocation can result in perfusion loss in more than one way. In addition to complete transection of the popliteal artery, the dislocation can cause intimal tears within the popliteal artery. These small intimal tears can occlude on a delayed basis, resulting in loss of perfusion to the distal extremity. In this setting, the loss of vascular supply to the leg does not occur abruptly but can occur many hours later. As a result, ruling out an initial vascular injury does not obviate the need for serial vascular exams of the patient for at least 48 hours after the initial assessment.

16.6.2 External Fixation in the Polytrauma and/or Obese Patient

Knee dislocations frequently occur in trauma patients. External fixation can be considered in patients with multiple injuries. The fixator may allow for easier nursing care in the intensive care unit (ICU) and mobilization of the polytrauma patient. In addition, obese patients pose significant challenges in regards to the fit of external braces and should be considered for external fixation.

16.7 Special Instructions, Position, and Anesthesia

16.7.1 Reduction

Emergent reduction should be performed in patients who present with the knee dislocated. After reduction, a knee immobilizer should be applied. Postreduction radiographs should confirm reduction. Occasionally, an irreducible dislocation may present which requires open reduction in the operating room. A good vascular exam pre- and postreduction should be documented.

16.7.2 Vascular Exam

The diagnosis of a vascular injury relies primarily on physical exam. The routine use of angiography is not recommended. A vascular injury can be successfully ruled out with symmetric distal pulses and an Ankle Brachial Index (ABI) greater than 0.9. Asymmetric dorsalis pedis and/or posterior tibial pulses raise concern for vascular injury. An ABI less than 0.9 is indicative of vascular injury and a vascular surgeon should be urgently consulted.

16.7.3 Serial Examinations

Serial examinations, focusing on vascular status and signs of compartment syndrome, should be performed for at least 48 hours, as intimal tears can occlude hours after injury.

16.7.4 External Fixation

When placing an external fixator, the patient is usually positioned supine on a radiolucent operating table. General anesthesia with paralysis is recommended.

16.8 Tips, Pearls, and Lessons Learned

16.8.1 External Fixation—Pin Placement

In cases where an external fixator is indicated, a simple uniplanar construct can be applied (▶ Fig. 16.1). Predrilling for the half pins should be done to avoid thermal necrosis. The diameter of the pin should not be greater than a third of the diameter of the bone. Two bicortical pins, usually either 5 mm or 6 mm in diameter, are placed in the lateral or anterior aspect of the femur. Two bicortical 5-mm tibial pins are placed in the anteromedial tibia. The pins should be placed well away from the knee joint, outside the zone of injury, and should not compromise eventual reconstruction tunnels.

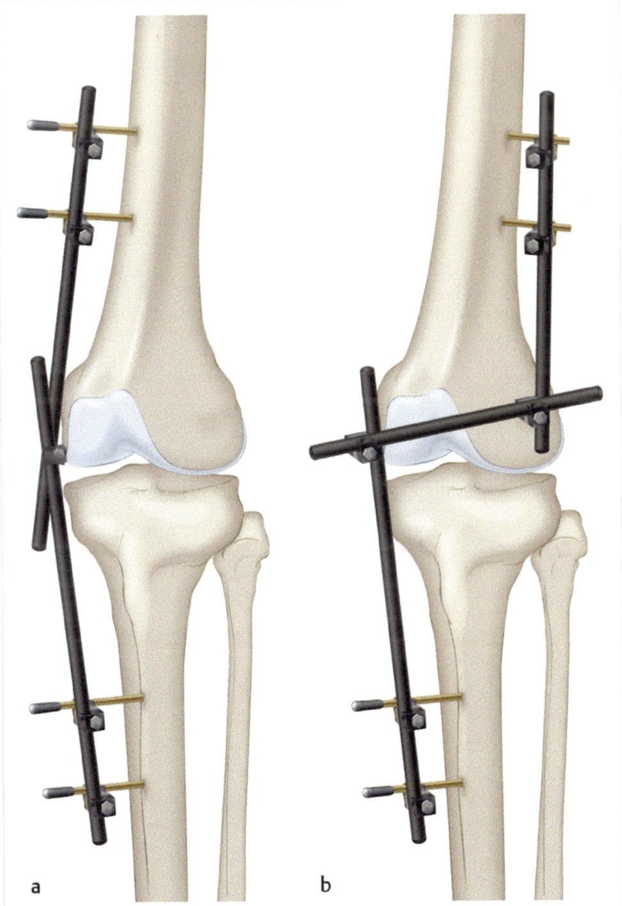

Fig. 16.1 (a) Four examples of configurations for external fixation of a knee dislocation. Anterior-based frame with pins in the anterior femur and tibia, (b) lateral-based frame with lateral pins in the femur and anterior pins in the tibia.

16.8.2 External Fixation for Open Dislocations

In cases of severe soft tissue injury after an open dislocation, the position of the fixator bars and clamps should be carefully planned to allow for easy access and soft tissue management.

16.8.3 Tips

- Assure that reduction of the knee has been maintained prior to discharge. A radiograph of the knee once the patient has mobilized should be performed prior to discharge.
- Because of the risk of late occlusion of the vasculature, admission with serial examinations should be performed for 48 hours.
- Compartment syndrome can develop after a knee dislocation. Especially if pulses are absent prior to reduction, but return after reduction, the provider should maintain a high index of suspicion for the development of compartment syndrome.
- If vascular repair is needed, the external fixator should be applied prior to revascularization if possible. If the vascular repair is performed prior to the application of an external fixator, the placement of the fixator, with subsequent reduction, can potentially disrupt the repair.

16.9 Difficulties Encountered

A knee dislocation which presents reduced in a polytrauma patient who is obtunded can be quite challenging to accurately diagnose. A thorough ligamentous exam of the knee should be performed in all of these patients. A knee effusion in the setting of normal radiographs is a clue there may be an undiagnosed multiligamentous injury.

16.10 Key Procedural Steps

16.10.1 External Fixation

The placement of the external fixator half pins should be done with the definitive surgery in mind. The pins should be placed outside the zone of injury and should not compromise eventual repair or reconstruction options. Once the position of pins has been decided, a small stab incision is made in the skin. The triple drill sleeve with the trocar is then advanced down to the bone. All pins are predrilled to avoid thermal necrosis and potentially stripping the near cortex. The trocar is then removed and the appropriately sized drill is inserted. Palpating the medial and lateral edges of the femur allows an understanding of the femoral bony anatomy and ensures bicortical pin placement. Once predrilled, the half pins are inserted. Blunt tip pins are preferred. Fluoroscopic imaging allows orthogonal views of the pins to assure bicortical placement. To assure adequate purchase of the pins in the far cortex, three to four full turns of the pin should be done once the pin engages the far cortex. Once the half pins are placed into the femur and tibia, the bars and clamps are applied and tightened with the knee reduced. Reduction is confirmed by fluoroscopy. In general, the knee is placed in 20 to 30 degrees of flexion. The bars should be close to the skin, but should not touch the skin. Two fingerbreadths of clearance are usually sufficient. After tightening the construct, the stability of the knee is evaluated by exam and fluoroscopy. Final tightening of the clamps should be done with wrenches, as the torque produced using the lever arm of the wrench is much higher than a T-handle type device.

16.11 Bailout, Rescue, Salvage Procedures

Fortunately, the placement of an external fixator is a relatively simple procedure; however, problems occasionally occur, which are usually associated with the placement of the half pins. The most important step to avoid problems with the pins is carefully planning their position in the femur and tibia. If a unicortical path occurs during predrilling, another position 2 to 3 cm away should be chosen. Occasionally, the far cortex can be broken when inserting a half pin. This usually occurs if the trajectory of the pin is not the same as the one drilled. Self-drilling pins are especially prone to creating their own path and can increase this occurrence. Therefore, blunt tip pins are recommended.

If stability of the knee cannot be obtained with a standard anterior-based uniplanar external fixator, there are several strategies to increase stability. Double stacking external fixation bars (▶ Fig. 16.2) can provide increased stability. In severely unstable knees, especially in the coronal plane, special external fixation constructs can be considered. Lateral femoral pins can provide the force vector needed to maintain reduction. Adding a third pin, off-axis from the two initial femoral pins, can allow for multiplanar constructs and increased stability (▶ Fig. 16.3).

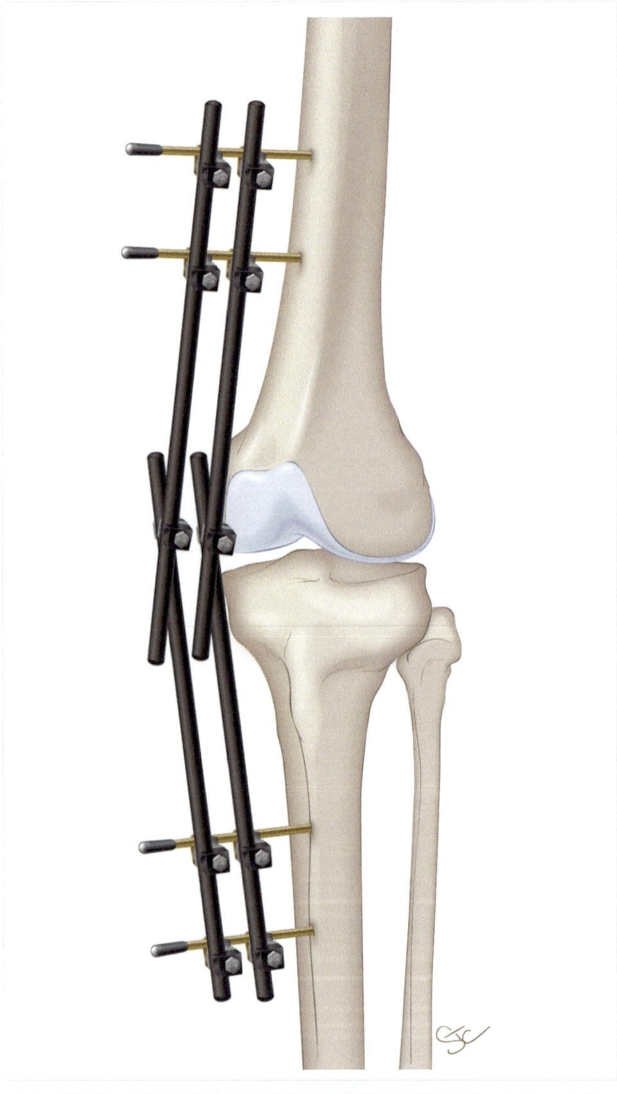

Fig. 16.2 Double-stacked anterior frame.

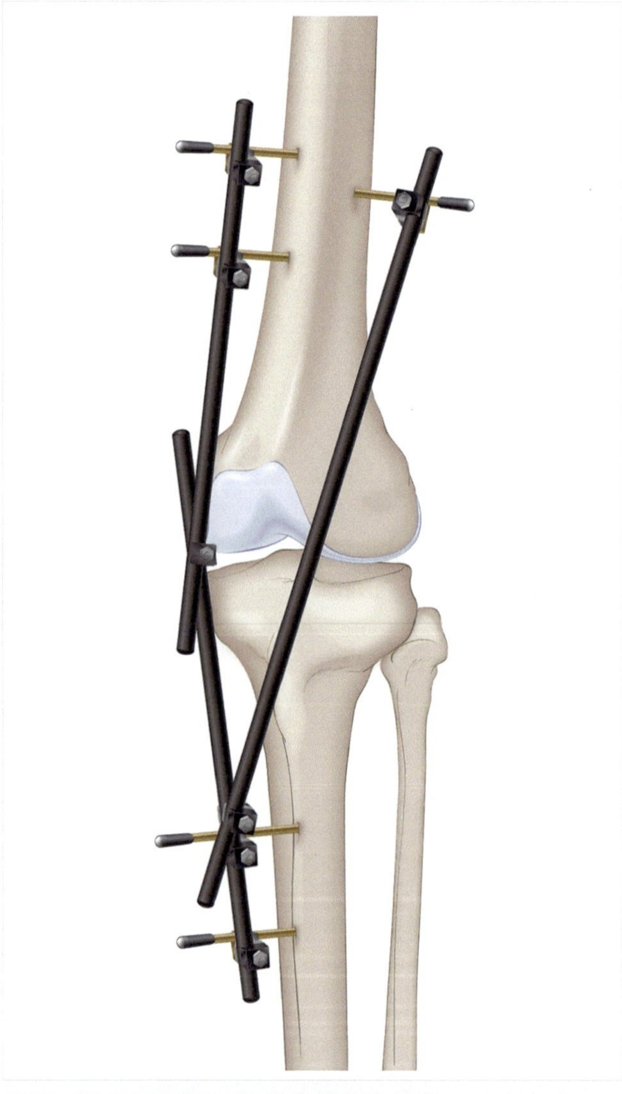

Fig. 16.3 A multiplane frame.

The morbidly obese patient can create significant challenges in providing stability using an external fixator. This is primarily due to the distance between the bone and the bars due to the patient's body habitus. Although rarely needed, cross pinning the knee, with buried large Steinman pins, is an option to maintain reduction. If cross pinning is done, an external fixator should still be used to protect the pins and prevent pin breakage.

16.12 Pitfalls

There are a few scenarios in which pitfalls occur in the acute management of a knee dislocation.

- A lack of suspicion and inadequate physical examination can lead to a missed or delayed diagnosis. This can lead to delayed treatment or a chronic dislocation, which can be disastrous.
- A missed vascular injury can be devastating and may lead to amputation. If the patient does not have symmetric distal pulses and an ABI 0.9 or greater, emergent vascular surgery consultation should be done in an effort to restore blood flow to the distal extremity. Revascularization should occur in less than 8 hours after injury.
- Discharging the patient without serial examinations for at least 24 hours (48 hours is recommended) can lead to a delayed diagnosis of vascular thrombosis and/or compartment syndrome.

17 Correction of a Periarticular Knee Deformity with External Fixation

J. Spence Reid

17.1 Description

This chapter describes the use of modern ring fixation with software-assisted hexapod technology for the correction of complex periarticular deformities of the knee. This procedure offers the advantages of very precise correction of all components of the deformity simultaneously. The ability to provide complete deformity correction and appropriate lengthening makes this approach the current method of choice in these situations and offsets the patient inconvenience and discomfort inherent in ring fixation.

17.2 Key Principles

The hallmark of the clinical problem is one of malalignment in any plane that results in a mechanical axis deviation across the knee. Sometimes, often a result of trauma, there is a combination of intra-articular as well as extra-articular deformity that requires correction in both regions.

In addition to appropriate patient selection, a complete analysis of the deformity in all planes is essential to correct all aspects of the deformity and at the correct location. Placement of a stable hexapod frame with atraumatic technique of pin-and-wire insertion, as well as an atraumatic corticotomy technique, is crucial to successful outcome.

17.3 Expectations

The treatment of a complex deformity about the knee with a software-assisted hexapod frame is a very reliable procedure as long as the technical aspects of preoperative planning and frame placement are well managed. This is a stressful procedure for the patient and family, in that daily frame adjustment and pin care are usually the responsibility of the patient. It is not unusual for an unplanned procedure to be needed during the course of treatment to manage a pin problem or other unforeseen problem. However, major complications are rare. It is difficult to precisely predict when frame removal will occur since the biologic response of the patient plays such a key role. Despite these difficulties, this procedure can provide a dramatic solution to an often complex and debilitating problem and may delay or eliminate the need for joint arthroplasty.

17.4 Indications

Indications for treatment include any deformity that interferes with function, alters the natural history of the knee in a negative way over time, or is unacceptable cosmetically for the patient. The ideal deformity for this technique is a multiplanar periarticular deformity with or without limb shortening. Younger patients may present with functional issues or unacceptable cosmesis. Older patients with long-standing deformity may present with recent onset of knee pain in conjunction with radiographic arthritis. This group may occasionally be referred from arthroplasty surgeons for consideration of deformity correction prior to, or in conjunction with knee arthroplasty.

17.5 Contraindications

- Psychological intolerance to the presence of the fixator.
- Inability to make daily adjustments (patient or caretaker).
- Inability to return for follow-up appointments (social support).
- Inability to care for the external device or unsafe home environment.
- Severe soft tissue issues (obesity) precluding the placement of pins or wires.
- Systemic issues such as poorly controlled diabetes mellitus (DM) which will increase the pin infection rate.

17.6 Special Considerations

Because of the burden on the patient, external fixation techniques usually are reserved for complex deformity in multiple planes—particularly associated with shortening of the limb.

In selected situations, it is possible to remove the hexapod frame before complete regenerate consolidation and place a plate or an IM nail. This conversion carries the risk of increased infection rate. If all pin sites are free of any signs of deep infection, conversion can be done in one stage. Otherwise, a 2- to 3-week pin-free internal may be needed with the caveat that there may be a risk of loss of correction/length during the interval. In a single-stage conversion, oral antibiotics are started 5 days prior to the planned procedure and continued until all pin sites are dry. In the case shown in ▶ Fig. 17.1, an intramedullary (IM) nail was placed at 16 weeks postcorrection in a single stage using a femoral distractor to maintain reduction during nailing (▶ Fig. 17.1b, c).

17.7 Special Instructions, Position, and Anesthesia

17.7.1 Preoperative Evaluation

The preoperative evaluation of a periarticular knee deformity prior to treatment with a hexapod ring fixator is more complicated than treatment with an osteotomy and internal fixation. There are three distinct aspects to the preoperative phase of care as discussed next.

Radiographic and Clinical Evaluation

We prefer to begin with a standing weight-bearing radiograph in which the pelvis, knees, and ankles are visible (both sides)

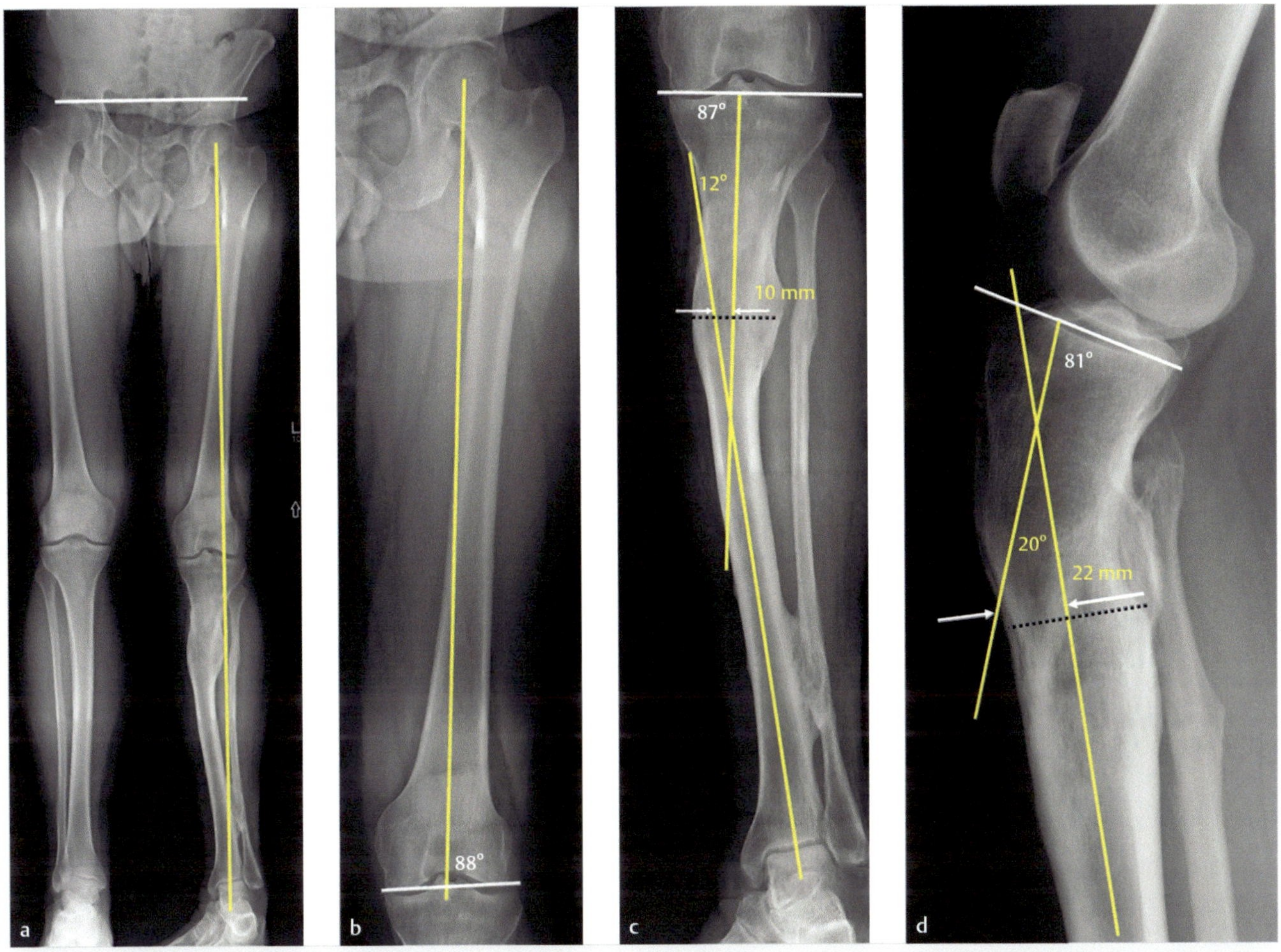

Fig. 17.1 Deformity analysis: 32-year-old male following trauma. **(a)** A standing weight-bearing alignment radiograph is obtained with the patellas centered over the femoral condyle. The mechanical axis is determined by extending a line from the center of the ankle to the center of the femoral head. There is a lateral mechanical axis deviation at the knee and shortening of the left leg (20 mm). **(b)** The mechanical of the femur is normal –but a computed tomography (CT) analysis revealed a 15-degree external rotation deformity that was corrected by transverse osteotomy (intramedullary saw) and IM nail. **(c)** Analysis of the anteroposterior (AP) tibia radiograph shows valgus, internal rotation, and medial translation. The black dotted line is the proposed corticotomy site (see ▶ Table 17.1). **(d)** Analysis of the lateral radiograph shows apex anterior angulation and posterior translation. The black dotted line is the proposed corticotomy site (see ▶ Table 17.1).

(▶ Fig. 17.1a). This is typically done with digital merging of three radiographs centered on the hips, the knees, and the ankles to minimize parallax error. If a leg length discrepancy is present, the short leg should be elevated on blocks so that the analysis can be performed with the pelvis level. Finally, a true anteroposterior (AP) orientation of the involved knee should be achieved in which the patella is centered over the distal femur. This is very important and can dramatically affect any apparent deformity measurement. The first step in analysis is to determine the overall mechanical axis by drawing a line from the center of the femoral head through the center of the ankle joint. A mechanical axis deviation is present if the line deviates significantly from the centerline of the knee (▶ Fig. 17.1a). A separate analysis of the tibia and the femur is then performed to determine the magnitude and location of the deformity on each segment and how it contributes to the overall deformity. ▶ Fig. 17.1b shows a normal femur mechanical axis (88 degrees), indicating that the mechanical axis deviation is a result of the tibial deformity. In deformities close to the knee joint, the normal joint line axis is typically used (87 degrees) (▶ Fig. 17.1c). An analysis in the sagittal plane is then performed. The measured values in the deformed limb can be compared to published norms, or compared to the contralateral leg if it is normal. Finally, if significant rotational malalignment is suspected or detected, a CT scan with imaging through both femoral necks, distal femur, proximal and distal tibia is performed. This allows precise determination of rotational differences and yields a value that can be used in a hexapod software program. The goal of the radiographic deformity analysis is to determine if the deformity requires correction in the femur, or tibia or both, and the complete description of the deformity. ▶ Fig. 17.1c, d shows the deformity analysis for this

Table 17.1 Deformity parameters (see ▸ Fig. 17.1c and d)

	Angulation	Translation
Anteroposterior	12-degree valgus	10 mm medial
Lateral	20-degree apex anterior	22 mm posterior
Axial	15-degree internal rotation	20 mm short

posttraumatic deformity in a 32-year-old man, and the findings are summarized in ▸ Table 17.1. In addition to the radiographic evaluation, clinical examination of the hips, knees, and ankles and gait observation are mandatory to document range of motion (ROM), joint laxity, contractures, and verify rotational differences.

Metabolic Evaluation

A metabolic work-up is often indicated and will vary with age and medical condition of the patient. In young patients, a serum vitamin D level (25 OH vitamin D total) is very useful. It is well established that vitamin D deficiency is common in the population, and if significant (< 30 ng/mL), it may adversely affect new bone formation via the regenerate, and delay consolidation. We routinely administer 2,000 to 5,000 IU of vitamin D3 daily to our patients during treatment or until their serum levels are > 40 ng/mL.

Patient Education

Should include allowing the patient to handle an external frame similar to the one that they will have applied, as well as make frame adjustments (patient, spouse, caretaker). The expectations for frame hygiene, pin care, pain management, physical therapy, and return visits should all be clear prior to surgery.

17.7.2 Positioning

The patient is positioned with bumps into true anteroposterior (AP) position on the table.

17.7.3 Anesthesia

General or spinal/regional anesthesia may be performed depending on both the surgeon's and anesthesiologist's assessment of the particular case, with consideration of the anticipated length of the procedure, any medical comorbidities, and the wishes of the patient.

17.7.4 Postoperative Deformity Correction

The exact details of the software correction are beyond the scope of this chapter. In most adult cases, the delay prior to initiation of correction in the tibia is 7 to 10 days and the rate of lengthening is 0.75 mm/d in the tibia, and 1.0 mm/d in the femur. For the case shown in ▸ Fig. 17.1, a prescription with a 10-day latency was planned with 35-day period of correction. It should be remembered that this is a dynamic correction with the patient as an active participant. Patients are seen in the outpatient clinic with radiographs at least every week or two during the active phase of the correction. When the treatment is complete, it is very important to obtain a new standing weight-bearing long-leg alignment radiograph like the one used for planning and watch the patient ambulate. The new mechanical axis, length, and clinical rotation should be confirmed as the bone will often be undercorrected compared to the frame. Sagittal plane correction should be confirmed as well (▸ Fig. 17.5b, d and ▸ Fig. 17.6a). Often, one additional correction prescription is required in a complex deformity prior to satisfactory alignment. When the patient and surgeon are satisfied with the correction, the hexapod struts can be removed and replaced with four threaded rods as this will simplify the frame and increase stability.

17.8 Tips, Pearls, and Lessons Learned

- It is extremely important that two surgical aims be accomplished during frame application. The first is frame stability, and the second is atraumatic pin-and-wire application. Attention to these two details will maximize patient comfort, promote weight bearing during correction, ensure accurate movement of the bone segments via the hexapod, and minimize complications.
- A Gigli saw technique is useful in the proximal tibia as it allows very precise control of the location of the corticotomy. A multiple drill hole/osteotome technique is equally effective.
- Preplacing a suture along the path of the corticotomy prior to the placement of any pins/wires simplifies this step significantly.
- Placing the knee in about 30 degrees of flexion using a small bump under the distal femur relaxes the posterior structures, facilitating safe osteotomy.
- Postoperative care: It is very useful to generate the patient treatment prescription via the hexapod software while the patient is still in the hospital. This allows additional radiographs to be obtained or an immediate strut change prior to discharge. It is also extremely helpful for the patient to see the prescription and be observed performing a strut adjustment. Patients are encouraged to undergo weight bearing as tolerated. Physical therapy as an outpatient to monitor knee and ankle ROM and encourage weight bearing is essential.

17.9 Difficulties Encountered

In a periarticular knee correction, maintenance of knee terminal extension is critical as the posterior structures will tighten and drive a flexion contracture. Splintage of the knee in terminal extension at night is important. Pin care is via daily saline cleaning and all pins are wrapped with gauze and slight pressure applied via a skin clip to minimize pin/skin motion. Patients are allowed to shower when incisions are dry. Antibiotics in the postop period are reserved for pin tract infections.

17.10 Key Procedural Steps

- Identify location of corticotomy (distal to tubercle) and place suture subperiosteally around tibia (Gigli saw osteotomy) (▶ Fig. 17.3a, b).
- Perform fibular osteotomy—close wound.
- Begin the frame application by placing a 1.8-mm smooth wire parallel to the knee joint at the proposed level of the proximal ring. This reference wire is parallel to the AP plane and approximately 2.5 cm from the knee joint.
- Use 5/8 ring proximally to maximize knee ROM. Slight rotation of the proximal ring may optimize knee flexion (▶ Fig. 17.2a).
- Identify strut locations on proximal ring to avoid conflict with fixation elements.
- Stable fixation of proximal ring (two wires and two half pins minimal). An anterior-to-posterior half pin is then placed from the center of the master tab to a location about 1.5 centimeters proximal to the proposed corticotomy site. This first half pin should be placed in such a way as to render the proximal ring "orthogonal" to the proximal segment on both AP and lateral views (▶ Fig. 17.2b). An additional 1.8-mm wire is then placed in a posterolateral-to-anteromedial direction on the distal surface of the ring at about a 30-degree angle to the reference wire. This pin is started at the anterior border of the fibula and it is generally proximal enough to not be a concern with respect to the peroneal nerve. The final fixation for the proximal ring is anteromedial-to-posterolateral 6-mm half pin about 10 mm proximal to the AP half pin (▶ Fig. 17.2c).
- Confirm orthogonal relationship of proximal ring to proximal segment.
- Six-mm-diameter hydroxyapatite (HA)-coated stainless steel pins are preferred in the adult.

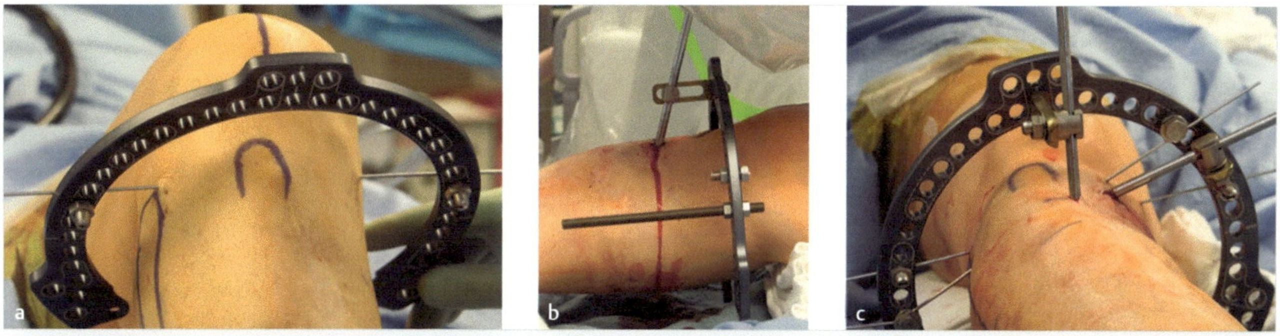

Fig. 17.2 Alignment of proximal ring. **(a)** A reference wire is placed parallel to the knee joint and a partial ring is mounted and rotated to maximize knee flexion. **(b)** An A-P half pin is then placed with the proximal ring orthogonal to the proximal segment. **(c)** Proximal fixation is completed with an additional wire and additional half pin.

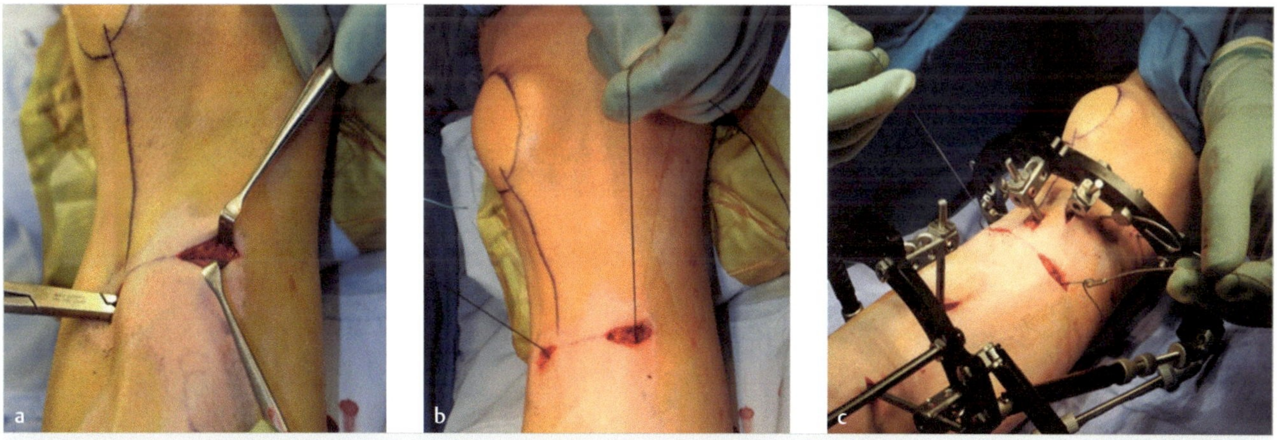

Fig. 17.3 Preplacement of corticotomy suture. **(a)** If a Gigli saw technique is planned, it is helpful to pass a suture at the site of the corticotomy prior to placement of the proximal ring. Two transverse incisions are made, and a vascular clamp is passed from posteromedial to anterolateral. **(b)** A suture is then passed and left in place until frame application is complete. **(c)** At the time of the corticotomy, a Gigli saw is tied to the suture and passed across the back of the tibia.

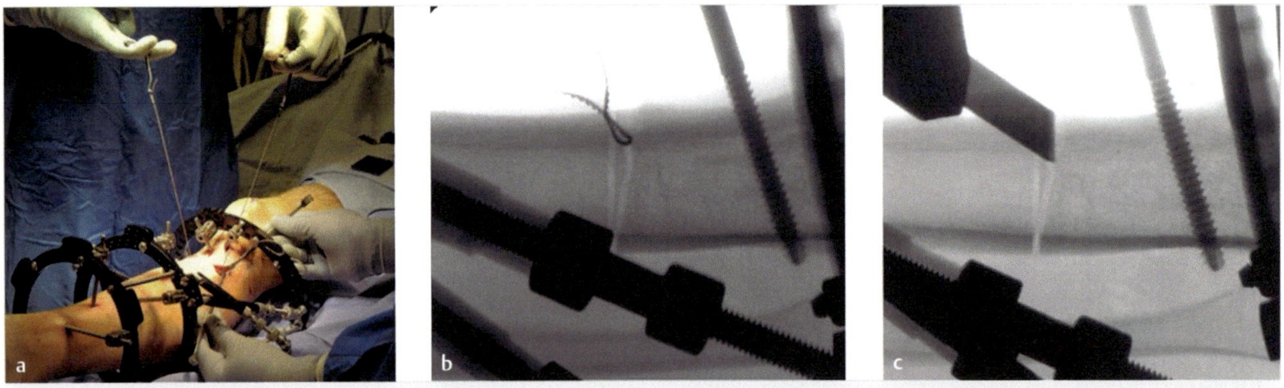

Fig. 17.4 Completion of the corticotomy. **(a, b)** The two anterior hexapod struts are disconnected, and the Gigli saw is gently advanced up to (but not through) the anteromedial face of the tibia. **(c)** The anterior corticotomy is then completed with a narrow osteotome, introduced from the anterolateral incision, with care taken to avoid injury to the skin.

- If significant lengthening is planned (> 2–3 cm), a 4.5-mm cannulated screw can be placed across the tib/fib joint to prevent fibular migration.
- Stable fixation of distal ring (three divergent half pins—minimal). In the clinical case shown, a three-ring frame with two distal rings was chosen for increased stability. A single distal ring with widely spaced pins will offer similar stability. The distal ring or ring block should be slid over the leg into position. It is helpful to keep in mind that the farther apart the two rings that attach the hexapod struts, the fewer strut changes are needed. In general, this distal ring block can be fixed with two half pins off each ring about 60 degrees divergent (anteromedial face and medial to lateral).
- If significant lengthening is planned, a 4.5-mm cannulated screw or a tensioned 1.8-mm wire should be placed across the distal ankle syndesmosis to protect it.
- The hexapod struts are then applied and labeled and the type and length of each strut is recorded. If a significant valgus deformity is being corrected, consideration should be given to a proximal peroneal nerve decompression.
- Record strut settings. The anterior two hexapod struts are then detached from the proximal ring to provide space.
- The corticotomy is then performed by tying the Gigli saw to the preplaced suture and passing it across the back of the tibia (▶ Fig. 17.3c). In the clinical case shown, the planned osteotomy is in the metaphysis just distal to the tibial tubercle. Two small transverse (1.5 cm) incisions are carried down to and through the periosteum. The first is at the level of the medial posterior cortex of the tibia and the second is over the anterior compartment just lateral to the crest of the tibia (▶ Fig. 17.3). A small periosteal elevator is passed via the medial incision and across the back of the tibia in a subperiosteal fashion. The periosteal elevator is then passed in a subperiosteal fashion along the anterolateral face of the tibia. A large, curved, vascular clamp holding the braided suture is then passed from the medial incision to the lateral incision. The tip of the clamp is located laterally, and a #2 suture is grasped with a hemostat as the vascular clamp is opened and removed. At this point, the suture is gently tied over the front of the tibia. If there is any concern that the suture has been placed around a vessel, the suture can be pulled anteriorly as pulses are palpated or confirmed distally via a Doppler examination (▶ Fig. 17.3c).
- The Gigli saw is then carefully used to cut the tibia up to (but not through) the anteromedial face (▶ Fig. 17.4a, b). The Gigli saw is then divided and withdrawn. The corticotomy is then completed under lateral c-arm imaging with a sharp osteotome (▶ Fig. 17.4c). A complete corticotomy should be confirmed.
- The incisions are closed and the two anterior struts reattached and placed at their precorticotomy length.
- Obtain images for mounting parameters.
- Prior to leaving the operating room, it is very important to make sure all pins and wires have been released from soft tissue tension. A dressing that provides mild pressure against the skin to prevent skin/pin motion is useful.
- It is helpful if all radiographs needed for the hexapod software (deformity and mounting parameters) are obtained in the operating room under surgeon control.

17.11 Bailout, Rescue, Salvage Procedures

Several problems can develop during treatment.

- **Poor regenerate bone formation during correction:** This may be a result of a damaging corticotomy or "too rapid" correction of the deformity. This can usually be first identified at about the 5- to 6-week mark after surgery as a lack of bone formation in the developing gap. The first step in treatment is to slow down the distraction rate to 0.5 or 0.25 mm/d and continue to monitor.
- **Loss of knee terminal extension or ankle equinus:** This is often a problem when significant lengthening (> 4 cm) is associated with deformity correction. Patients need to be educated regarding this problem and taught daily stretching

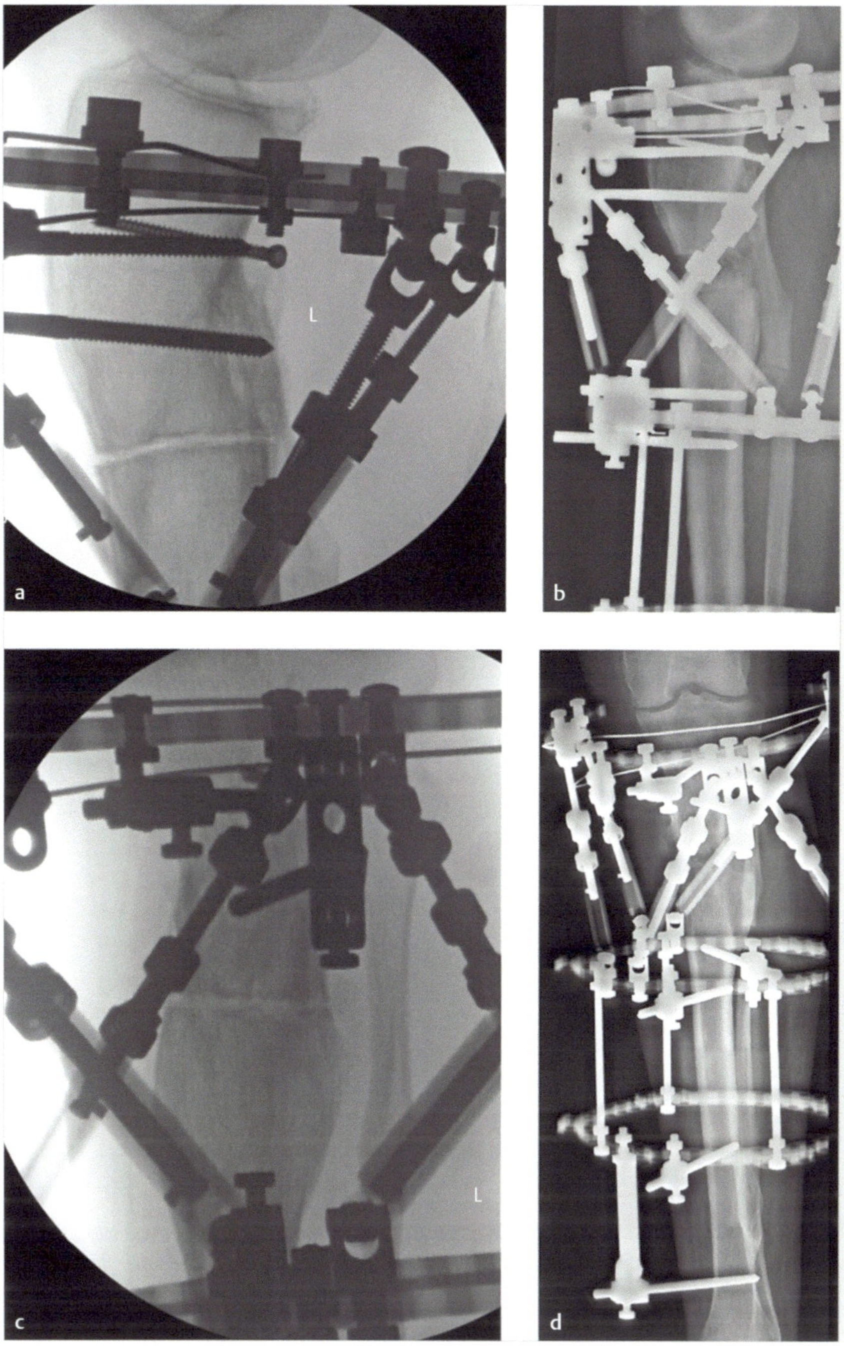

Fig. 17.5 Deformity correction. **(a, b)** Immediate postop lateral image and at completion of correction (40 days postop). **(b, c)** Immediate postop anteroposterior (AP) image and at completion of correction. **(d)** Anteroposterior radiograph of the leg revealing a neutral tibial mechanical axis.

exercises. If refractory, the patient should be referred to physical therapy for stretching and extension splinting.

- **Painful frame/wires:** Frame instability can present as activity-related pain. Wire tension may have been lost or pin loosening may have occurred. A pin or wire may be near a superficial nerve. Pin tract infection can also present with pain. A painful frame should be investigated and revised as needed because the patient will reduce weight bearing secondary to pain and this will hinder bone formation.
- **Frame removal/conversion to internal fixation:** In selected cases, conversion to internal fixation prior to complete regenerate consolidation may be indicated. This can be done in one stage in the absence of a pin tract problem in a healthy patient. However, if a significant pin tract infection is suspected, a staged conversion is probably wise with the first step being frame removal in the operating room and curettage/culturing of the involved pin followed by a course of antibiotics prior to placement of the internal fixation.

17.12 Pitfalls

A power saw **must not be used** in the tibia to create the corticotomy as this will generate heat and result in very poor bone formation during correction.

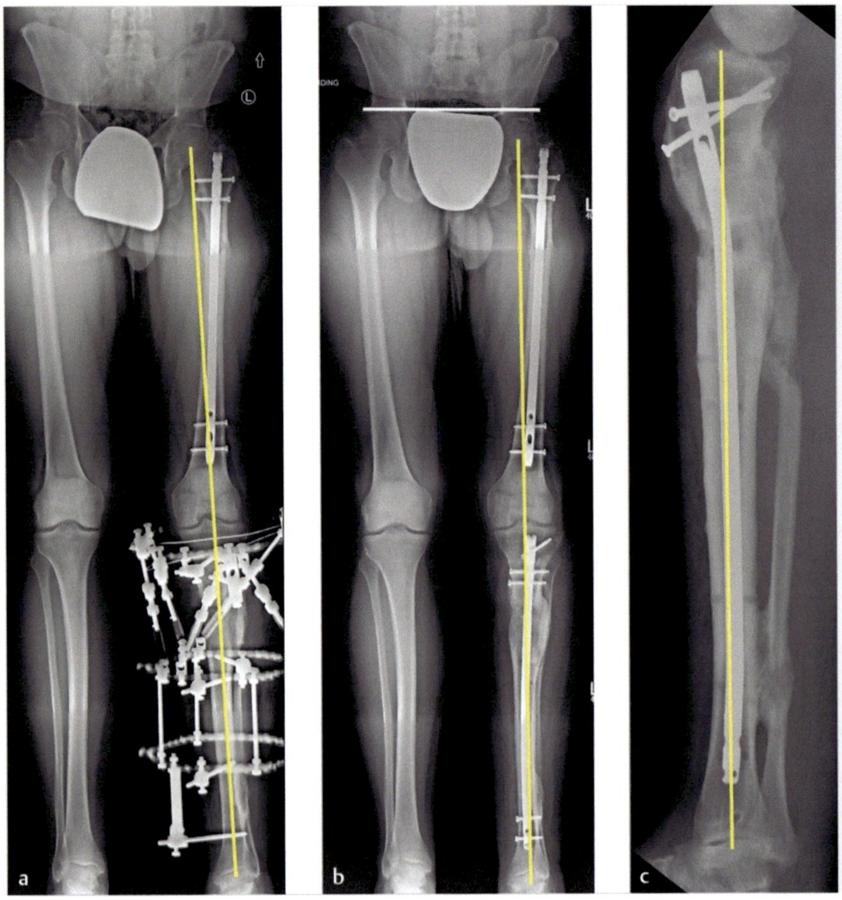

Fig. 17.6 Final deformity correction – conversion to internal fixation. **(a)** A long leg alignment radiograph is obtained at the end of treatment to confirm satisfactory restoration of the mechanical axis. **(b, c)** The patient was free of pin tract problems, so to ease the burden on the patient, conversion to intramedullary nail was performed at 16 weeks with excellent final restoration of alignment and rotation in both planes. The patient experienced some problems with ankle equinus during correction, and was intentionally left 10mm short at the end of treatment.

18 Floating Knee Injuries

Christian Krettek

18.1 Description

This technique addresses combined, ipsilateral fractures of either the diaphyseal, metaphyseal, and/or epiphyseal (intra-articular) regions of both the femur and the tibia, resulting in what has been called a "floating knee".

18.2 Key Principles

Surgical stabilization of both fractures is recommended. Treatment goals are to restore fracture and ligament stability, physiologic alignment (mechanical axis, articular plane), and articular congruency in order to allow early mobilization of the extremity and the patient, and soft tissue cover (▶ Box 18.1). The Blake and McBryde classification is useful for surgical planning, and is based on the presence or absence of an intra-articular fracture (▶ Table 18.1). Type I injuries have extra-articular fractures of both bones. Type IIA injuries represent the combination of a femoral shaft fracture with an intra-articular proximal tibia fracture, while type IIB injuries represent the combination of a tibia shaft fracture with an intra-articular distal femur fracture. In type IIC injuries, both the femoral and tibial levels are represented by an intra-articular fracture.

Box 18.1 Principles of fixation

Principles
Healing has priority over length
Use a radiolucent table
Have tools ready for intraoperative alignment control
The more diaphyseal the fracture, the more a nail might be appropriate
Start with the more simple fracture

Fracture fixation is typically achieved with intramedullary (IM) nails in the diaphysis, plates in the metaphysis, screws in epiphyseal injuries, or external fixation, which may be temporary or definitive, and is usually done in cases with severe associated soft tissue injury, polytrauma, or damage control situations.

18.3 Expectations

Open soft tissue injury, fracture comminution, compartment syndrome, vascular injury, ligamentous and meniscal injury, age, smoking, and injury severity score are predictive for the outcome (fracture healing, malalignment, knee stability and stiffness, and overall function). Better results and fewer complications are observed when both fractures are diaphyseal, compared to when one or even both are intra-articular.

18.4 Indications

Floating knee injuries are best treated operatively. The timing of definitive fracture stabilization must be adapted to the physiological status of the patient. If definitive fixation is not possible, temporary fixation with external fixation should be considered. Patients with compartment syndromes, vascular injuries, and most open fractures require immediate surgery.

18.5 Contraindications

Even patients in extremis usually benefit from fixation. In some rare instances, emergency external fixation can be done even on ICU without any C-arm control.

18.6 Special Considerations

Frequently, these are high-energy injuries, often complicated with open soft tissue and/or vascular injuries, and most often occur in polytrauma patients. Those initially evaluating a floating-knee injury should consider measuring ankle-brachial indices (ABI) to look for clinically occult vascular lesions.

There is not a single ideal method of treating the different fractures in a patient with a floating knee. A first treatment plan for each fracture should be done individually. Then these individual plans need to be adjusted in order to fit the priorities best in an overall master plan (▶ Table 18.1).

18.7 Special Instructions, Positioning, and Anesthesia

Positioning: The use of a flat radiolucent table rather than a fracture table allows simultaneous surgical setup for fixation of both the femoral and the tibial fracture. A pelvic and chest support on the contralateral side allows longitudinal rotation of the OR table lifting the ipsilateral side up. In conjunction with a bolster under the knee, the injured leg is more accessible for lateral fluoroscopic C-arm images (▶ Fig. 18.1).

18.8 Tips, Pearls, and Lessons Learned

18.8.1 Alignment References

Prior to draping, one should obtain anatomic reference information from the contralateral leg regarding femoral (lesser trochanter shape sign) (▶ Fig. 18.2) and tibial torsion (clinical foot position relative to the tibia), and in cases with fracture comminution, about the femoral/tibial length. In addition, the configuration of the femoral condyle (anteroposterior [AP] and lateral images) should be stored in the C-arm memory as a reference for recurvatum alignment (notch sign, Blumensaat angle) (▶ Fig. 18.3).

18.8.2 Type I Injuries

Intramedullary nailing of both fractures is the preferred method of treatment (▶ Fig. 18.4, ▶ Table 18.1). The more distal the femoral shaft fracture is located, the more retrograde nailing should be considered as the best option.

Sequence

Since retrograde femoral nailing requires only little manipulation of the leg, doing the retrograde femoral nail first is recommended. Once the femur is stabilized, the knee and tibia can be more easily manipulated. For example, flexion of the knee is needed for a transligamentous/paraligamentous approach to tibial nailing. Alternatively, the suprapatellar approach allows tibial nailing with the knee in an extended position. A trans- or paraligamentous approach requires 90 degrees of knee flexion and a stabilized femur, either by a nail or a temporary external fixator.

Table 18.1 Classification, main implant choice priority, and fixation sequence

Type	Fracture pattern	Main implant choice priority femur	Main implant choice priority tibia	Fixation sequence	Comment
I	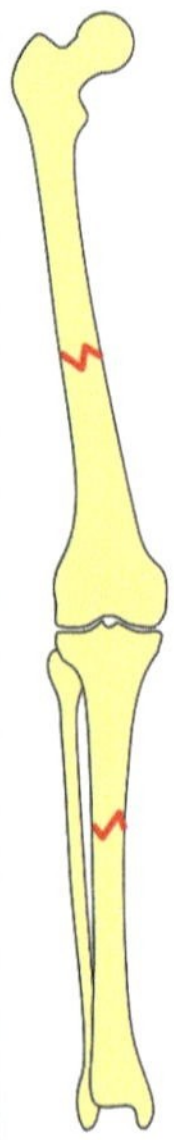	• Nail • Plate • Ex Fix	• Nail • Plate • Ex Fix	• Femur • Tibia	Femur first, then tibia or Femur temporary Ex-Fix, then tibia, then femur definitively
IIa	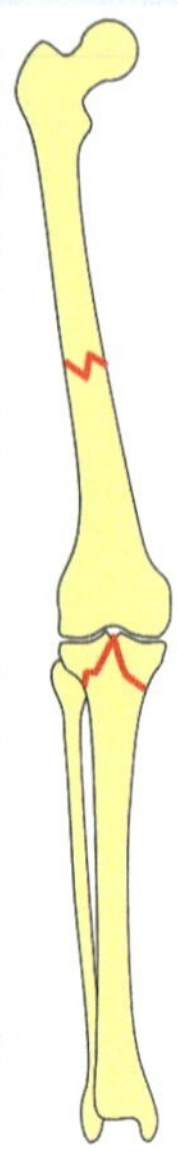	• Nail • Plate • Ex Fix	• Plate • Ex Fix	• Femur • Tibia	Femur first, then tibia Make sure, weight-bearing line is centered to the knee and articular plane is horizontal

Table 18.1 (*Continued*) Classification, main implant choice priority, and fixation sequence

Type	Fracture pattern	Main implant choice priority femur	Main implant choice priority tibia	Fixation sequence	Comment
IIb	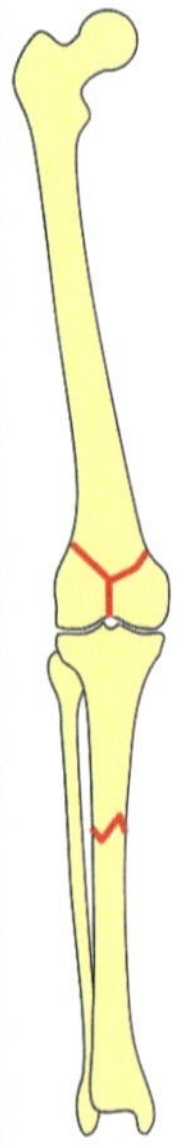	• Plate • Ex Fix	• Nail • Plate • Ex Fix	• Tibia • Femur	Tibia first, then femur make sure, weight-bearing line is centered to the knee and articular plane is horizontal
IIc	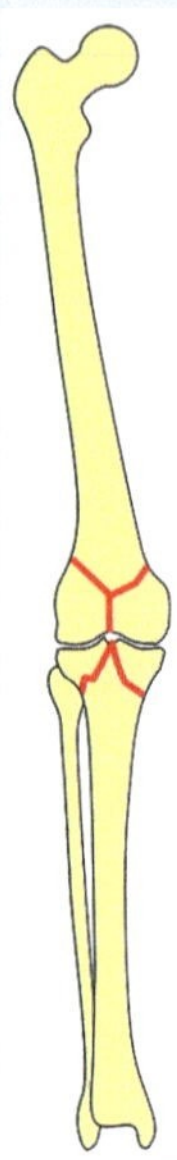	• Plate • Ex Fix	• Plate • Ex Fix	Start with easier fracture	Make sure, weight-bearing line is centered to the knee and articular plane is horizontal

Minimally Invasive Single Portal Approach

Retrograde femoral and antegrade tibial nailing can be done through the same surgical approach (▶ Fig. 18.4). As in all metaphyseal fractures, intramedullary nails get effective mechanical support by supplemental Poller (blocking) screws.

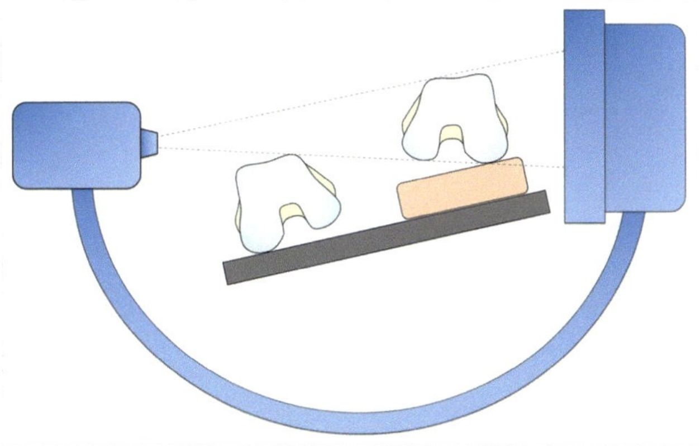

Fig. 18.1 Positioning on the operating table (bump, knee flexion 20–30 degrees, table rotation).

18.8.3 Type IIA and IIB Injuries

Depending on the fracture configuration and location, diaphyseal fractures are usually fixed with nails. The more metaphyseal the extra-articular fracture component gets, the more (locking) plates are preferred. Since the extra-articular fracture is usually (though not always) easier to fix, this is typically where to start. If the intra-articular fracture is easier to fix (e.g., an undisplaced fracture), it is advisable to start with it first.

18.8.4 Type IIC Injuries

These are the most complex and difficult fractures to treat. Again, one should start with the more simple fracture first. The choice for medial or lateral parapatellar approach depends on the fracture configuration(s).

Tibia Tuberosity Osteotomy

If a tibial tuberosity osteotomy is considered to facilitate exposure, make sure the osteotomized bone fragment is not too small (should be a minimum 5 × 1 × 1 cm) in order to get reliable fixation with one-third tubular plate to allow for unrestricted rehabilitation. In certain proximal tibia fractures, the

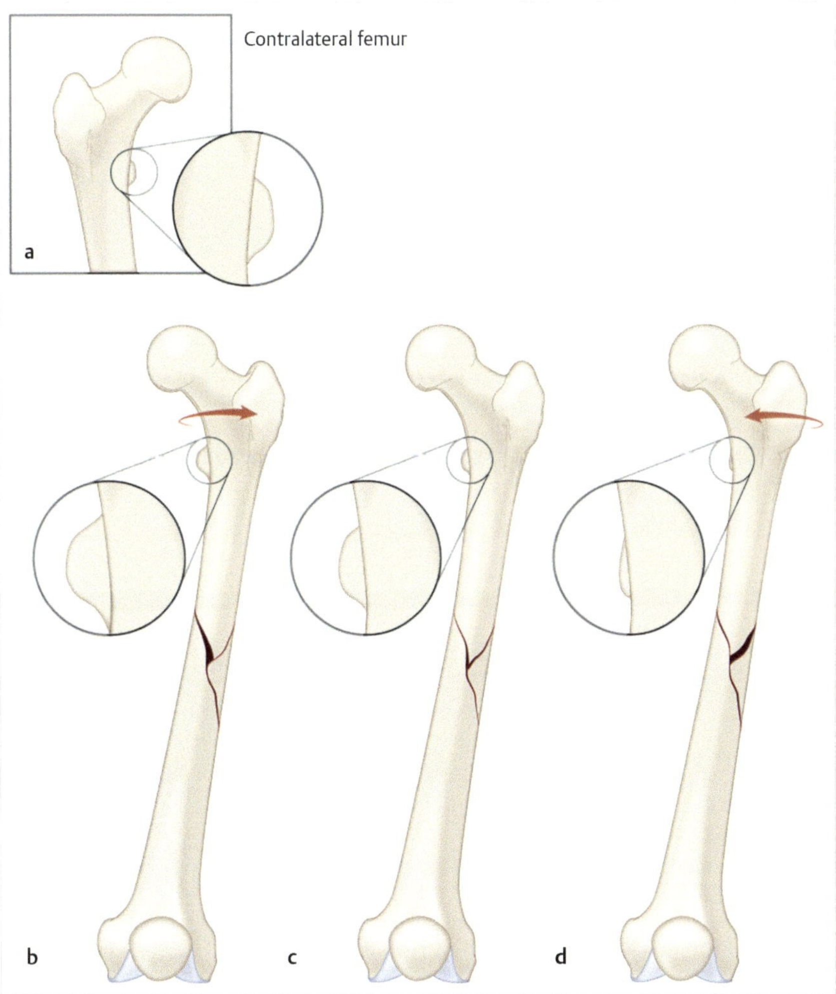

Fig. 18.2 Lesser Trochanter Shape Sign (LTSS): With the patella precisely centered over the distal femur, the shape of the lesser trochanter of the uninjured contralateral femur (**a**, inset upper left) is compared to the profile of the lesser trochanter of the injured femur. **(b)** The shape of the lesser trochanter is more prominent compared to the healthy contralateral side (**a**, inset upper left) indicating an external torsional deformity (*arrow*). **(c)** The lesser trochanter profiles match, indicating correct rotational alignment of the injured femur. **(d)** The shape of the lesser trochanter is less prominent compared to the healthy contralateral side **(b)** indicating an internal torsional deformity (*arrow*).

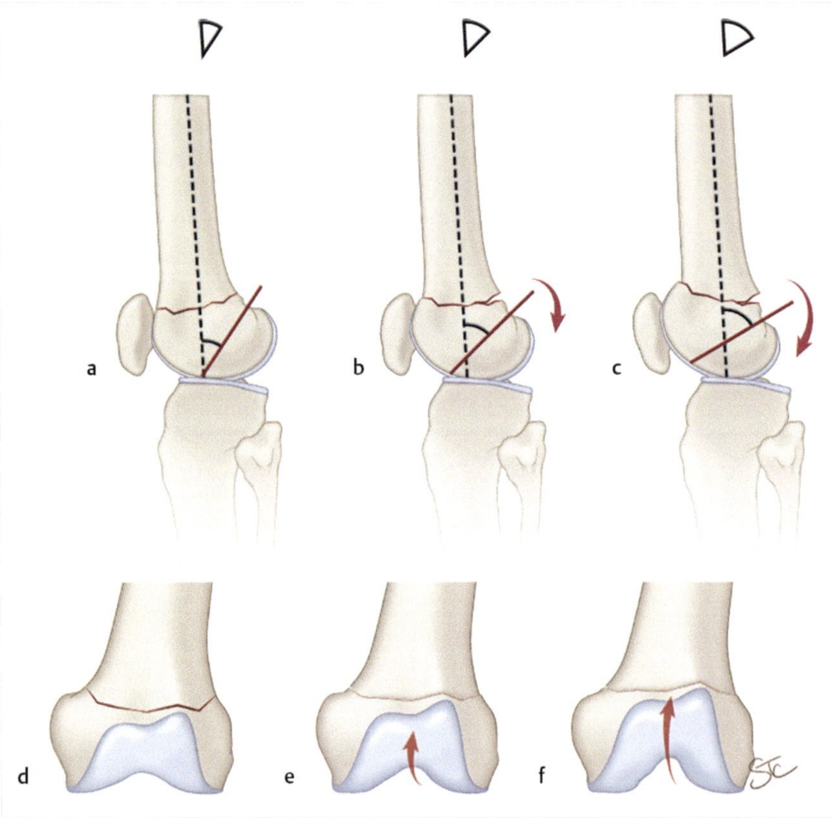

Fig. 18.3 Notch sign and recurvatum malalignment: Schematic drawings demonstrate the depth of the notch of **(a)** in normal positioned distal main fragment block and **(b)** and **(c)** increasing degree of recurvatum deformity. If the distal fragment is short, recurvatum deformity is difficult to recognize in the lateral view **(d–f)**. In this case, the analysis of the Blumensaat line can be a helpful reference.

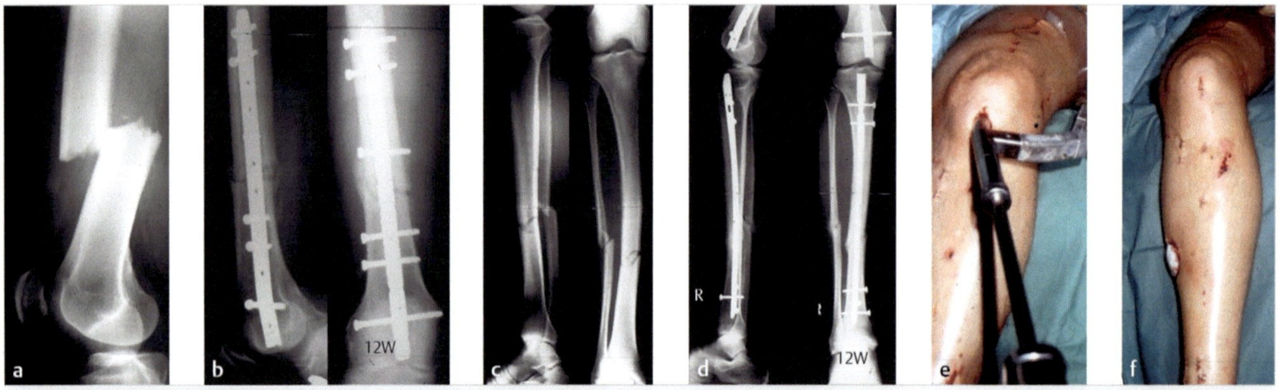

Fig. 18.4 Floating knee type I: Minimally invasive single incision approach. Femoral shaft fracture **(a)** before and **(b)** 12 weeks after retrograde nailing. **(c)** Ipsilateral tibial shaft fracture **(c)** before and **(d)** 12 weeks after retrograde nailing. **(e)** Intraoperatively, with the femoral nail instrumentation still in place, and **(f)** after wound closure. Reproduced from Krettek C, Gosling T. Femur diaphysis. In: Rommens PM, Hessmann, Martin H, ed. Intramedullary nailing: a comprehensive guide. London: Springer; 2015:245–316.

tuberosity fragment is fractured and is a movable and retractable piece, allowing good access to all tibial and femoral compartments.

Temporary Miniplates

When traditional temporary K-wire fixation fails (e.g., oblique fracture lines in cases with associated bone defect), small plates (two-hole one-third tubular plates or minifragment plates from hand set) can help by temporarily supporting the reduction and fixation. This simplifies the fixation of the condylar block to the femoral shaft in case of bone defects and comminution. Miniplates work well as antiglide plates. Since the fixation is not rigid with such plates, this still allows some flexibility for moderate bending and torque (varus/valgus, ante/recurvatum, torsion) for final reduction and fine-tuning of limb alignment, but not for length (▶ Fig. 18.5).

Difficulties Encountered: Difficulties encountered include soft tissue problems, malalignment, problems to achieve a step- and gap-free articular reduction, management of bone defects, instability due to fixation problems or meniscal and ligamentous injuries, postoperative stiffness, pain, and other. The careful selection of correct starting point in retrograde femoral and antegrade tibial nailing is crucial.

Correct alignment means not only that the mechanical axis of the limb is centered in the knee joint, but also that the articular plane of the knee is horizontal in the AP projection. This means that the sum of the lateral distal femoral angle (lDFA) and medial proximal tibial angle (mPTA) not only should be exactly 180 degrees, but also that they stay within the physiologic range. The use of an alignment rod with a radiopaque 90° outrigger element can be extremely helpful in defining the articular plane in cases where there is no other good reference.

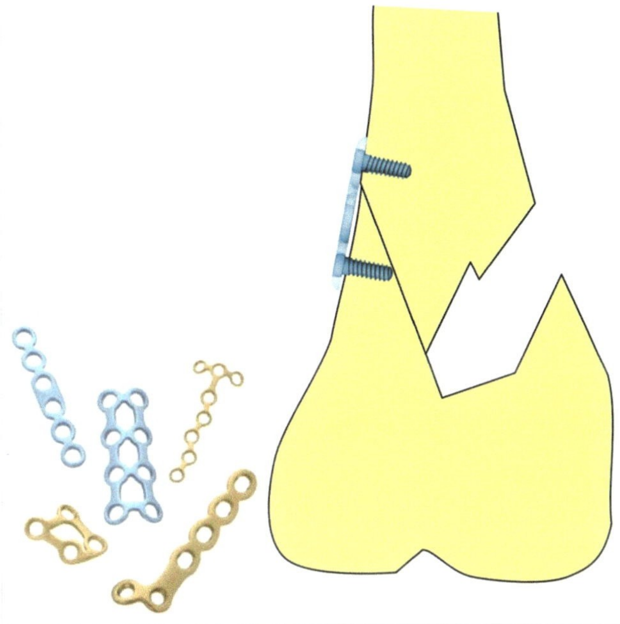

Fig. 18.5 Use of miniplate fixation as temporary stabilizer. Miniplate(s) provide provisional fixation while allowing for minor "alignment fine tuning," except for length. Stainless steel bends/torques better than titanium (less stiff).

18.9 Key Procedural Steps

The key procedural steps in femoral or tibial nailing, in plate and screw fixation, or external fixation of the distal femur or the proximal tibia are the same as the procedures described in the specific sections of the book for the technique of interest.

18.10 Bailout, Rescue, Salvage Procedures

Proper soft tissue management is crucial. Local and free flaps might need to be considered in severe open injuries with soft tissue loss. If soft tissues are compromised, temporary or definitive external fixation has an important role as an alternative to plates or nails. In situations with vascular injuries, limb salvage versus amputation needs to be considered carefully. In the geriatric patient and/or unreconstructable articular or metaphyseal destruction, early arthroplasty might be an option. In addition, if the extensor mechanism is missing or unreconstructable, arthrodesis needs to be considered.

18.11 Pitfalls

Pitfalls include lack of fracture or ligamentous stability, failure to restore physiologic alignment (mechanical axis of the limb or correct articular plane), and articular incongruency. Potential additional problems are prominent hardware, locking screws on the medial femoral condyle, and intra-articular prominence of the distal ends of a retrograde femoral nail (▶ Fig. 18.6).

Ninety-five-degree plate devices for distal femoral fractures usually have targeting devices referring to the lateral femoral cortex and/or knee joint line. If the patient has a diaphyseal bow (sometimes in elderly patients), the use of the reference guide can result in deformity. The use of the cable technique/alignment rod can help to prevent this.

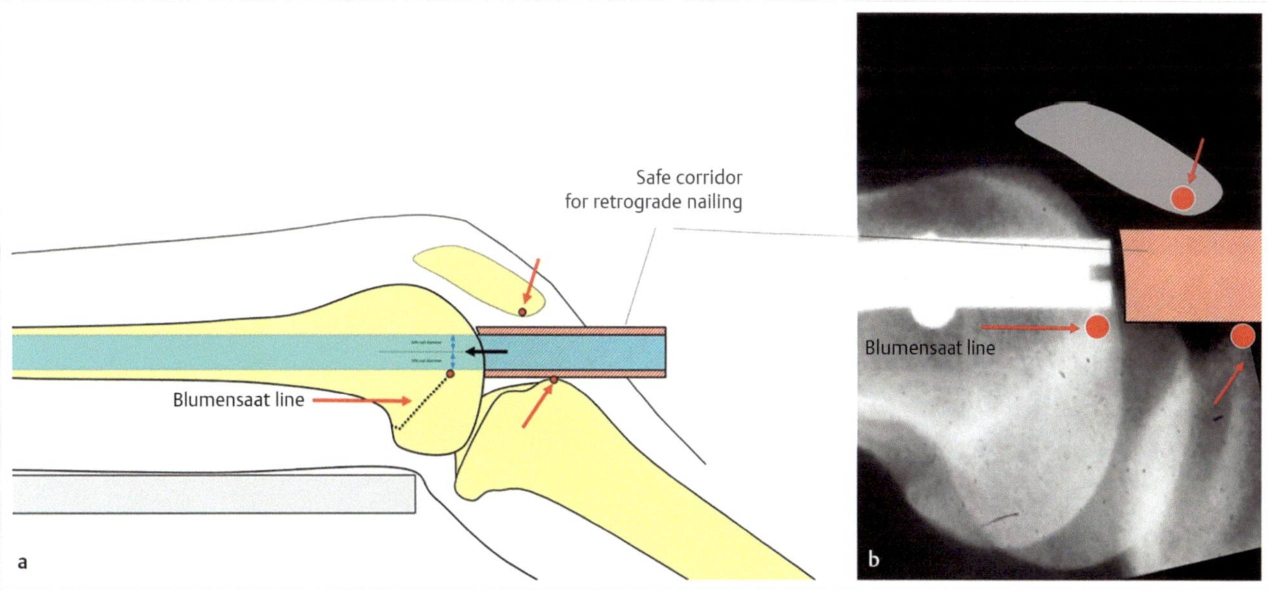

Fig. 18.6 Starting point and landmarks for retrograde femoral nailing. **(a)** Schematic drawing of the knee in 30-degree flexion (*red arrows* represent the three important landmarks for a safe corridor). This allows for avoiding potential obstacles (arrows: tibial tuberosity, patella). The ideal bone starting point (*black arrow*) is anterior to the anterior end of the Blumensaat line + ½ nail diameter (*blue arrows*). **(b)** Lateral radiographs after nail insertion. Correct position relative to the Blumensaat line; however, incorrect incomplete insertion (prominent distal nail end) can cause retropatellar cartilage damage).

19 Open Knee Fractures: The Use of Rotational Flaps

David Volgas

19.1 Description

Open fractures of the distal femur and proximal tibia are dangerous as they imply a great deal of energy dissipation in an anatomical region that has many important neurovascular structures which are at risk for injury (▶ Fig. 19.1). Furthermore, the knee capsule extends over much of the distal femur and proximal tibia, making wounds in this area potential sources of septic joints. Soft tissue coverage in this area is problematic because of the need to maintain range of motion of the knee. The knee is also an area which is prone to wound-healing problems because of the paucity of perforating arteries at the joint level. As a result, open knee injuries may require a durable, vascularized soft tissue flap to replace damaged capsule, cover exposed bone or articular cartilage, and supply a vascular bed for wound healing. The gastrocnemius rotation flap meets these requirements and is the workhorse flap for coverage of wounds around the knee joint. Either the medial or lateral portions of the gastrocnemius may be used; both heads have a dominant vascular pedicle off of the popliteal artery that enters the muscle proximally; each head also has independent innervation.

19.2 Key Principles

Early soft tissue coverage is optimal for satisfactory bone healing without infection. The infection rate is significantly higher when coverage is delayed more than 3 to 5 days. Local rotational flaps can be performed by orthopaedic surgeons without microvascular training and, when done in appropriate patients, these lead to excellent functional and acceptable cosmetic results. Careful assessment of the quality of the muscle in light of local injury must be performed.

19.3 Expectations

A gastrocnemius flap can be expected to have greater than 95% survival in properly selected patients. There will be pain associated with muscle spasm for the first 2 weeks and may be managed with splinting of the ankle and medication. The skin graft will "take" in 3 to 5 days and will completely epithelialize within 2 weeks. During the first 12 months, the muscle will atrophy approximately 50%, resulting in much less bulk. Weight bearing may be initiated as soon as the skin graft has epithelialized, depending on the restrictions imposed by the fracture.

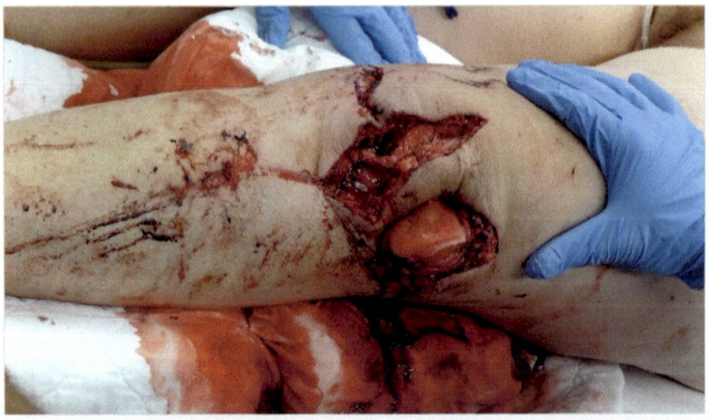

Fig. 19.1 A traumatic wound to the left knee after a motorcycle crash. Note the exposed lateral femoral condyle associated with a posterior knee dislocation, the injury to the patellar tendon, and the loss of articular cartilage on the condyle.

19.4 Indications

A gastrocnemius flap is able to cover wounds involving the proximal third of the tibia, the anterior knee, and the distal femoral condyles. It is limited to the area from the superior aspect of the patella to approximately 4 cm distal to the tibial tubercle, but body habitus and individual variation in the length of the muscle belly may increase the reach of the muscle flap.

19.5 Contraindications

Severely comminuted fractures of the proximal tibia or distal femur may damage the blood supply to the gastrocnemius muscle or may directly lacerate the muscle, making it unusable as a flap (▶ Fig. 19.2).

19.6 Special Considerations

A common scenario is that a lateral hockey-stick incision over the proximal tibia dehisces, requiring coverage. Mobilization of the lateral head of the gastrocnemius is potentially riskier because of the peroneal nerve proximally and the need to bring the muscle belly around the fibula, effectively shortening its

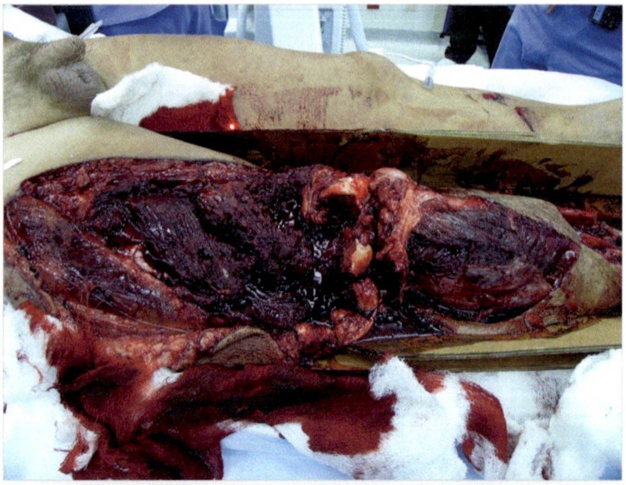

Fig. 19.2 Clinical photograph of a mangled lower extremity. Note the extensive damage to muscle, which renders local muscle transfer not feasible.

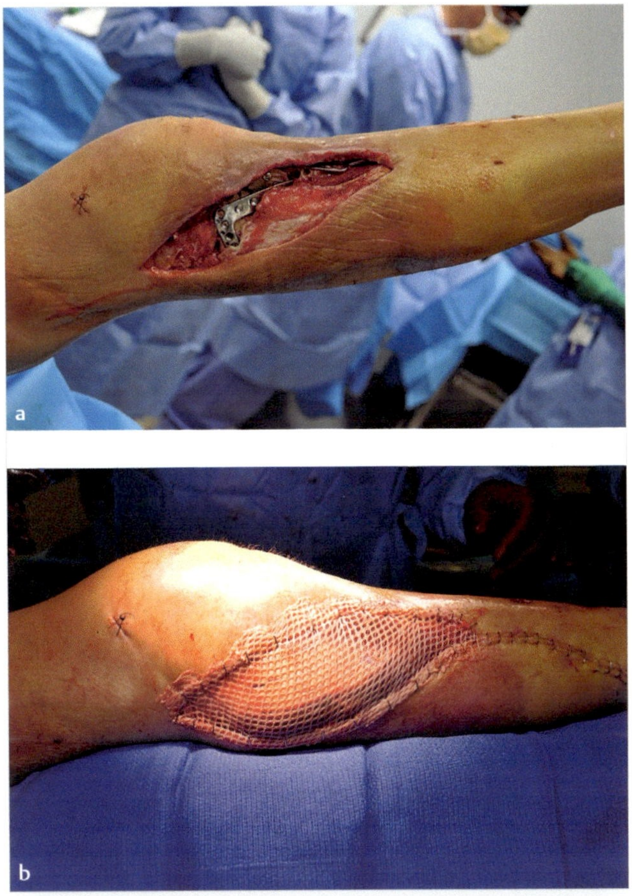

Fig. 19.3 **(a)** Intraoperative photographs of a wound dehiscence of a lateral surgical wound and **(b)** subsequent coverage by a gastrocnemius flap with split-thickness skin graft.

excursion. The lateral gastrocnemius will rarely cover medial to the midline, but is well-suited to coverage of the typical anterolateral surgical wound which dehisces (▶ Fig. 19.3a). There are differences in the surgical techniques between medial and lateral gastrocnemius flaps described below. The normal width of the gastrocnemius muscle flap is 6 to 8 cm proximally and 4 cm distally, so leaving a wound defect of this size is not only acceptable but may be desirable.

19.7 Special Instructions, Position, and Anesthesia

The procedure is done with the patient supine and the affected leg draped free. The gastrocnemius flap will generally require a split-thickness skin graft over the muscle after it is sewn into its new position. Therefore, remember to prep the entire leg up to the hip so that access to the thigh for a skin graft is possible. If a tourniquet is required, consider a sterile tourniquet. Muscle relaxation is not typically required during the procedure.

19.8 Tips, Pearls, and Lessons Learned

- The length and bulk of the gastrocnemius is variable, more so than the soleus.
- When muscles are transected, patients often experience significant spasm. Consider placing them on diazepam for the first 2 to 3 days after surgery.
- Muscle spasm may also be ameliorated by using a splint or knee immobilizer to keep the gastrocnemius stretched out.
- During the initial debridement and irrigation of the traumatic wound, assess and document the viability of the gastrocnemius. Muscle belly lacerations, dark color, and crushing injuries may make the gastrocnemius a poor choice for coverage.
- If required for coverage, both medial and lateral gastrocnemius muscles may be used in a given patient. There will be some loss of plantar flexion, but it will affect primarily jumping activities.

19.9 Difficulties Encountered

Occasionally, the gastrocnemius, especially in muscular males, will be difficult to rotate because of the thickness of the flap. In these cases, it is not possible to thin the flap by taking only half of the muscle. This will compromise blood supply. In elderly patients, the quality of the muscle tissue is more friable and will not stretch as much.

19.10 Key Procedural Steps

- Thorough and aggressive debridement of the traumatic wound.
- Dissection of the hemigastrocnemius from the origin of the muscle to the insertion on the triceps surae. This is described separately for the medial and lateral flaps.

19.10.1 Medial Gastrocnemius Flap

- The tourniquet is inflated.
- A line is drawn approximately 2 cm posterior to the posterior aspect of the tibial shaft beginning about 4 cm proximal to the knee joint to point approximately at the junction between the middle and distal third of the tibia (▶ Fig. 19.4a).
- Identify and protect the saphenous vein.
- Dissect through subcutaneous tissue using scissors. Identify the crural fascia and incise it longitudinally.
- Dorsiflexion of the foot may help the surgeon identify the soleus and gastrocnemius. The plane between gastrocnemius and soleus can be easily identified, especially proximally where the sural nerve lies between the gastrocnemius and soleus muscle bellies. Finger dissection can develop the plane between the gastrocnemius and soleus down to the merging of the gastrocnemius and soleus tendons at the triceps surae.

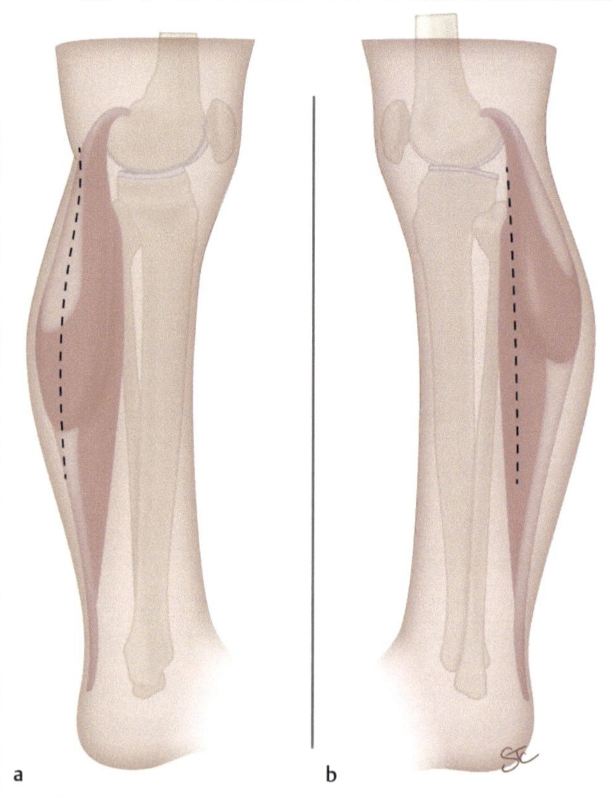

Fig. 19.4 The incision for the gastrocnemius flap is shown for **(a)** medial and **(b)** lateral flaps.

19.10.2 Lateral Gastrocnemius Flap

- The tourniquet is inflated.
- A line is drawn approximately 1 cm posterior to the posterior aspect of the fibular shaft beginning about 4 cm proximal to the knee joint to point approximately at the junction between the middle and distal third of the tibia (▶ Fig. 19.4b).
- Dissect through subcutaneous tissue using scissors. Identify the deep muscular (crural) fascia and incise it longitudinally.
- Identify and protect the common peroneal nerve proximally. It does not need to be mobilized.
- Dorsiflexion of the foot may help the surgeon identify the soleus and gastrocnemius. The plane between gastrocnemius and soleus can be easily identified, especially proximally where the sural nerve lies between the gastrocnemius and soleus muscle bellies. Finger dissection can develop the plane between the gastrocnemius and soleus down to the merging of the gastrocnemius and soleus tendons at the triceps surae.

Mobilization of the Hemigastrocnemius and Transection of the Gastrocnemius Belly Distally

- Identify the raphe between the medial and lateral gastrocnemius. Identification of the sural nerve, which perforates the gastrocnemius in its midline, may help identification of the hemigastrocnemius (▶ Fig. 19.5).
- Beginning proximally, use a finger to develop a plane between the medial and lateral hemigastrocnemius and continue separating the muscle belly down to the triceps surae.

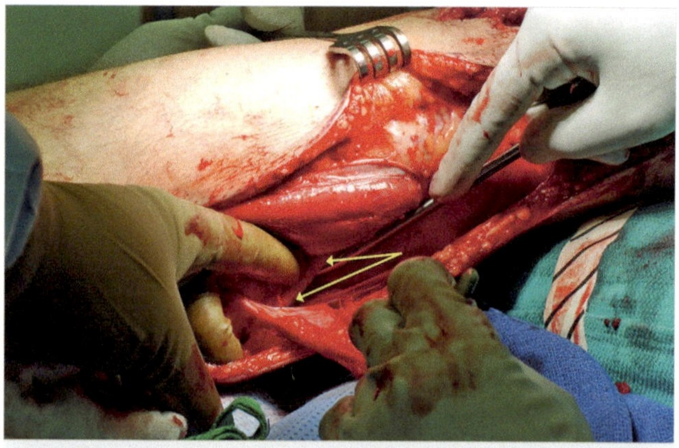

Fig. 19.5 The interval between medial and lateral hemigastrocnemius muscles is easy to identify proximally where the sural nerve (*arrow*) penetrates the gastrocnemius in midline.

- Sharply transect the hemigastrocnemius at the level of the triceps surae, leaving about 1 cm of tendon attached to the hemigastrocnemius. Mobilize the flap proximally as far as the knee joint.

Rotation of the Flap either Subcutaneously or Through a Transverse Incision

- On the lateral side, the muscle must pass around the fibula and superficial to the peroneal nerve. This requires mobilization of the muscle and dissection of the fascia more proximally than is typically the case for a medial gastrocnemius flap.
- The muscle may be tunneled under the subcutaneous tissue between the surgical incision and the wound defect or the surgeon may elect to resect the skin (more commonly) between the incision and the defect (▶ Fig. 19.6).
- The flap is then rotated into the wound defect.
- The flap is then secured distally by undermining the skin where the tendinous portion of the flap will be secured with a bolster. A large nonabsorbable suture is passed through a bolster consisting of cast padding and an occlusive dressing such as Adaptic or Xeroform.
- The suture is then placed through skin approximately 3 to 4 cm distal to the skin defect in line with the long axis of the flap. A Krakow suture through the tendinous portion of the flap is used and then the suture is brought back up through skin and the bolster. The suture is then tied down. There is usually a thick fascia on the deep side of the muscle which may be used to place several small, absorbable sutures to tack down the edges of the flap.

Coverage of the Flap with a Split-Thickness Skin Graft

- A split-thickness skin graft is then harvested from the ipsilateral thigh and placed over the flap.
- It may be secured using staples at the edges.
- A drain is placed in the space where the muscle was removed.

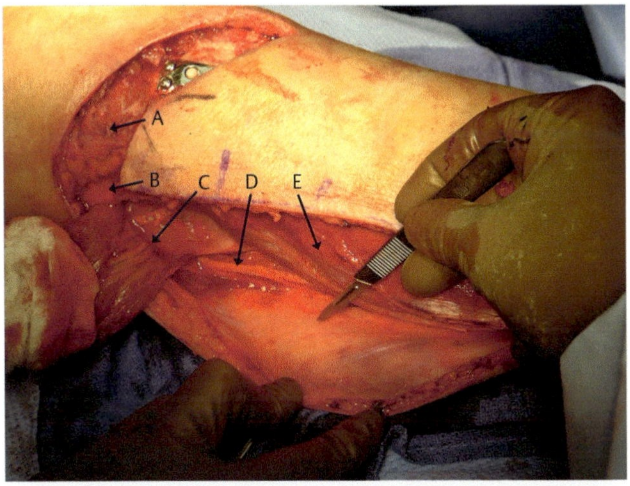

Fig. 19.6 Intraoperative photograph showing **(A)** proximal mobilization of the lateral gastrocnemius muscle and the transverse incision **(B)** connecting the wound defect with the surgical incision to raise the flap. Note the peroneal nerve, **(C)** perforator artery to gastrocnemius muscle, **(D)** sural nerve, and **(E)** soleus muscle.

- The donor site is closed.
- A negative-pressure wound dressing is applied over the skin graft.
- A splint is placed across the ankle to prevent plantar flexion.

19.10.3 Aftercare

- Splint, negative-pressure wound therapy × 3 days.
- Patients will often complain of significant muscle spasm. Diazepam may be given on a scheduled dose during the initial hospitalization, and other antispasmodic medications may be given upon discharge.
- Weight-bearing is limited during the first 3 days and elevation is encouraged. Weight-bearing on discharge is determined by the fracture.

19.11 Bailout, Rescue, Salvage Procedures

The gastrocnemius flap is extremely reliable when patient selection is good (see Contraindications). However, occasionally, there is more muscle damage than is appreciated initially. When this is recognized, the salvage procedure is a free flap.

19.12 Pitfalls

Failure to recognize the extent of injury to the gastrocnemius muscle will result in compromise or loss of the flap. It is possible to dissect the muscle proximally and inadvertently divide the arterial supply to the muscle. Finger dissection is recommended for proximal dissection.

20 Tibial Plateau Revision Surgery

Peter Kloen and Mauricio Kfuri

20.1 Description

Malunion, incongruency, and instability are possible outcomes after tibial plateau fractures. The malunion can be extra-articular, intra-articular, or both. The intra-articular deformities may compromise one or both tibial condyles. We describe a systematic approach to evaluating and addressing cases of malunion of the tibial plateau aiming to preserve and reconstruct the joint. We intend to restore joint stability, congruency, and alignment, therefore postponing whenever possible a joint replacement.

20.2 Key Principles

The history of the injury and its treatment is of critical importance. It is essential to understand patient's complaints (pain, instability, mechanical symptoms of locking), prior level of activity (young/old, active/sedentary), expectations (low vs. high level of activity), body habitus (obesity), comorbidities (diabetes mellitus, tobacco use, venous insufficiency, knee arthritis before the injury). Preoperative images include.

- Radiographs of the knee (anteroposterior [AP], lateral, plateau, and oblique views).
- Computed tomography with 3D reconstruction (very helpful in determining the three-dimensional location of the principal plane of the deformity).
- Long-leg standing radiograph, which is used to assess deformities in the coronal and sagittal planes.

Preoperative planning is a critical step of this procedure. We use software to calculate the mechanical proximal tibial angle (MPTA), the mechanical lateral distal femur angle (mLDFA), the joint line convergence angle (JLCA), and the mechanical femorotibial angle. Printed 3D prototypes are instrumental for preoperative visualization of the deformity and planning of the corrective osteotomy. The joint preservation concept is based on performing an osteotomy that improves the knee joint's overall alignment, stability, congruency, and orientation in all three dimensions (axial, sagittal, and coronal). Once the surgeon determines the osteotomy plan, the ideal surgical approach is chosen. Our experience is that an extensile surgical approach (e.g., Gerdy osteotomy, fibular head osteotomy, lateral femoral epicondyle osteotomy) allows a better exposure of the lateral tibial condyle. The surgical approach provides good exposure to the site of the deformity and the best access for plate fixation. We position the plate parallel to the principal osteotomy plane, where it will withstand shearing forces, provide containment, and restore joint stability.

20.3 Expectations

Osteotomies around the knee aim to improve the biomechanics of the joint. In the case of a posttraumatic deformity, the goal is to restore alignment, stability, and congruency. A stable and aligned joint is suitable for weight-bearing, even when it is not entirely congruent due to cartilage destruction. Osteotomies should be considered in young and active individuals as an alternative to a total joint replacement. Multiple series have shown that if joint stability and alignment are restored, the development of symptomatic knee arthritis is a late occurrence. In the elderly population, especially in osteopenic and arthritic individuals, a joint replacement should be favored, acknowledging that the outcomes of this procedure after a tibial plateau fracture are inferior if compared to a knee arthroplasty performed for the management of a nontraumatic degenerative joint disease.

20.4 Indications

The decision making for a joint preservation procedure after a malunited tibial plateau fracture (fixation) includes one or a combination of the following criteria.

- Biological age (active and young individuals).
- Intra-articular step off > 2 mm.
- Metaphyseal deformity > 5 degrees.
- Joint instability caused by bony pivoting.

20.5 Contraindications

The status of the menisci and the soft tissue around the knee is of great importance. If the patient has no menisci left or has a grossly unstable joint caused by multiligament injury, osteotomies around the tibial plateau may not restore stability. If the joint is aligned but not stable, the reconstruction will fail. The surgery is also contraindicated in the following conditions.

- Active infection.
- Significant knee stiffness.
- Advanced posttraumatic tricompartmental knee arthritis.
- Osteonecrosis.
- Patient's comorbidities and associated risks that would outweigh the benefits of surgery (peripheral vascular disease, morbid obesity, heavy tobacco use, alcoholism, drug addiction).
- Noncompliance with postoperative rehabilitation.

20.6 Special Considerations

Tibial plateau malunion may result from either neglected management or a failed internal fixation (▶ Fig. 20.1). The majority of the cases are indeed related to open internal fixation without satisfactory reduction. The definitive surgical treatment should be staged. The first stage should rule out the presence of low-grade infection and includes hardware removal and a knee exam under anesthesia. Before the first surgical procedure, we obtain a blood sample to determine the baseline inflammatory markers, and we may perform a knee aspiration if a knee effusion is present. At the time of the hardware removal, bone biopsies are also obtained and sent for cultures. If possible, an arthroscopy may be carried out at the time of hardware removal. The purpose of the arthroscopy is to document the status of the soft tissue (cartilage, menisci, and ligaments). A knee exam

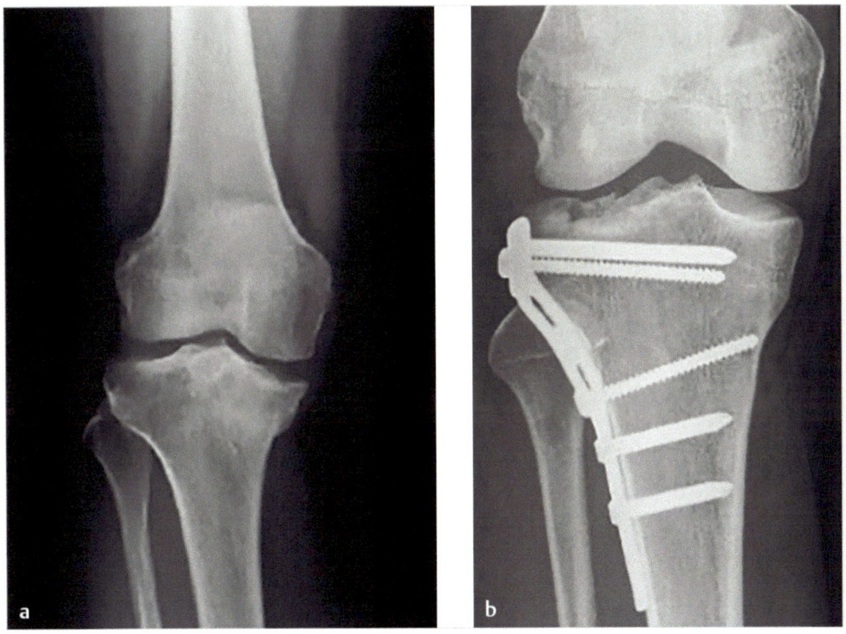

Fig. 20.1 Radiographic presentation of a tibial plateau malunion. **(a)** Anteroposterior knee radiograph revealing a neglected medial tibial plateau fracture; **(b)** Anteroposterior knee radiograph of a failed open reduction and internal fixation of the lateral tibial plateau.

under anesthesia determines the range of motion and stability of the joint. Alternatively, when a knee arthroscopy is not performed concomitant with hardware removal, a postoperative knee magnetic resonance imaging (MRI) may be obtained to determine the extent of associated knee soft tissues compromise. 3D-CT (computed tomography) planning is now standard in our practice. 3D-cutting jigs for this type of osteotomy are becoming more popular, although the articular surface is difficult to see on CT. Currently, we cannot do 3D planning based on MRI images yet, which we think would be more precise.

20.7 Special Instructions, Positioning, and Anesthesia

General anesthesia is favored over peripheral nerve blocks, as we should monitor compartment syndrome and unplanned neurological changes in the postoperative time. We document the neurological exam pre- and postoperatively. Most patients are placed supine on the operative table, but it depends on the surgical approach selected for the case. On some occasions, split-wedge deformities in the coronal plane are better addressed with the patient prone, as the main fracture plane is located on the posterior aspect of the knee. In selected cases where the posterolateral and anterolateral quadrants of the knee should be addressed, the patient was placed on a lateral decubitus.

Access to the posterolateral quadrant of the tibial plateau is possible with the patient in the supine position, provided the surgeon performs either a fibular head osteotomy or a lateral epicondyle osteotomy. The fibular osteotomy grants excellent access to the posterolateral quadrant of the tibial plateau, enabling a posterolateral buttress plate placement. The lateral epicondyle osteotomy also provides visualization of the posterolateral quadrant of the tibial plateau, without the option of buttressing the metaphyseal area, but the epiphyseal space with a horizontal rim plate. Each one of these approaches has pros and cons. The fibular head osteotomy requires dissection of the peroneal nerve and disruption of the proximal tibiofibular joint. The lateral epicondyle osteotomy does not allow buttressing of the posterolateral tibial metaphysis. When operating on the medial tibial plateau, the surgeon stands on the opposite side of the involved leg and the fluoroscopy equipment comes from the same side as the involved leg.

20.8 Tips, Pearls, and Lessons Learned

- The surgeon should be familiar with extensile approaches to the lateral tibial plateau. The chevron osteotomy for the fibular head grants great exposure to the posterolateral corner (▶ Fig. 20.2). The lateral epicondyle osteotomy also comprehensively exposes the lateral tibial plateau, preserving the tibiofibular joint (▶ Fig. 20.3). The osteotomy of the anterolateral tibial plateau rim allows for the exposure of depressed areas of the lateral tibial plateau (▶ Fig. 20.4). A direct medial approach to the tibial plateau grants access to the anteromedial and posteromedial quadrants of the medial tibial condyle (▶ Fig. 20.5).
- A tibial plateau malunion may present as a unicondylar angulation, an epiphyseal widening, a combination of metaphyseal and epiphyseal deformity, a combination of angulation and depression. Some strategies should be considered while dealing with each one of these deformities.
- As a rule of the thumb, unicondylar tibial plateau angulations are represented by a tilt of the tibial condyle. They result from an incomplete reduction of the condyle, and in most cases, the apex of the split wedge is located lower than where it should belong. In those cases, a unicondylar open-wedge tibial osteotomy should restore the joint orientation line (▶ Fig. 20.6).
- The widening of the tibial plateau occurs when fragments are interposed at the fracture site, and the reduction between the

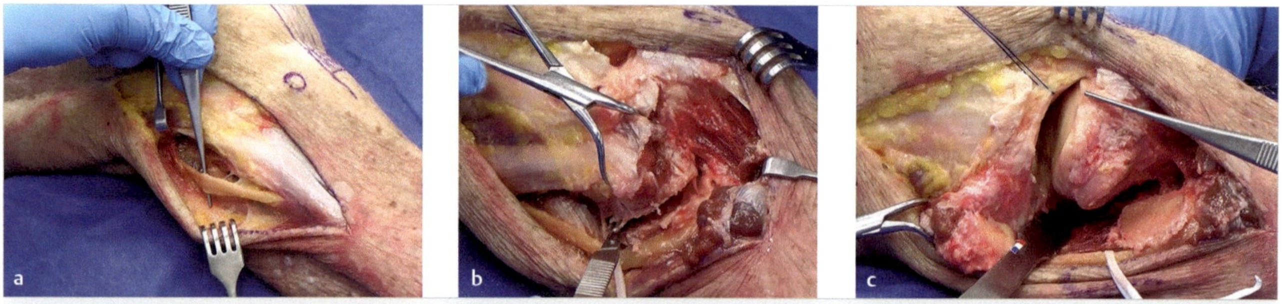

Fig. 20.2 Extensile lateral approach with a fibular head osteotomy. **(a)** Dissection of the peroneal nerve; **(b)** fibular head osteotomy, proximal to the peroneal nerve; **(c)** exposure of the anterolateral and posterolateral quadrants of the tibial plateau obtained with a fibular head osteotomy.

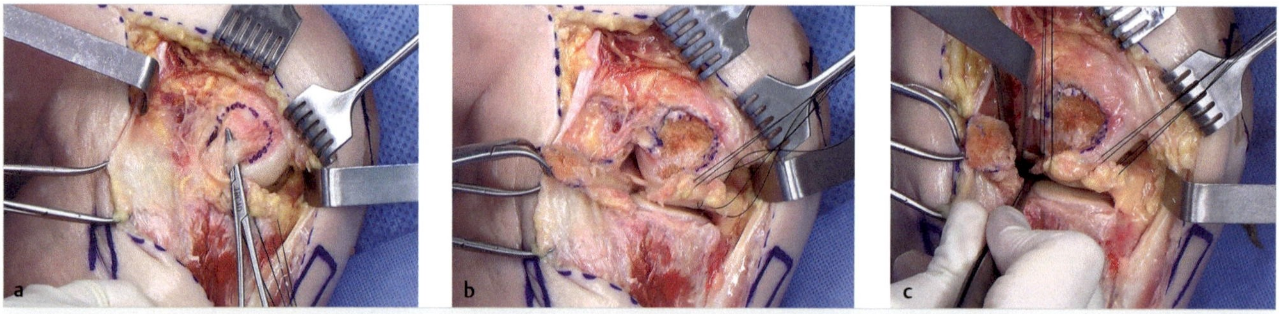

Fig. 20.3 Extensile lateral approach with a lateral epicondyle osteotomy. **(a)** Lateral view of the knee depicting the lateral epicondyle (*blue dotted line*) and the popliteus tendon (elevated by a clamp); **(b)** lateral perspective of the knee after the elevation of the lateral epicondyle with the attachments of the lateral collateral ligament and popliteal tendon. We applied sutures to the tibial meniscal ligament; **(c)** exposure of the anterolateral and posterolateral quadrants of the tibial plateau with a lateral epicondyle osteotomy.

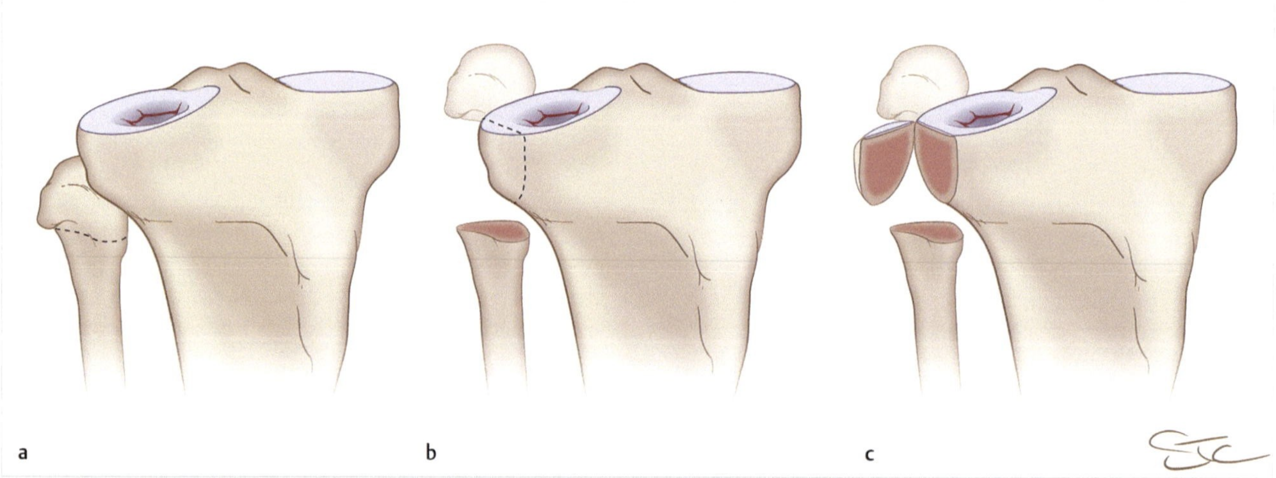

Fig. 20.4 Illustration of a lateral tibial plateau rim osteotomy. **(a)** A fibular head osteotomy is planned; **(b)** after the fibular head osteotomy, one gets access to the tibial plateau rim, but not the area of depression in the lateral tibial plateau; **(c)** an additional osteotomy to the lateral tibial plateau rim grants access to the more central portion of the lateral tibial plateau.

two condyles leaves a gap between them. As a result, an area of fibrous tissue is interposed in between the two tibial condyles. In those cases, the resection of the interposed fibrous tissues, using a closing wedge osteotomy, restores the width of the tibial plateau, the congruency of the articular surface, and the continuity of the tibial plateau rim (▸ Fig. 20.7).

- Impacted areas of the tibial plateau that were not reduced may be accessed when the surgeon performs an osteotomy of the tibial plateau rim, getting access to the impacted area. The area of depression must be mobilized and then elevated to the level of the tibial plateau rim so we may restore the joint surface (▸ Fig. 20.8).

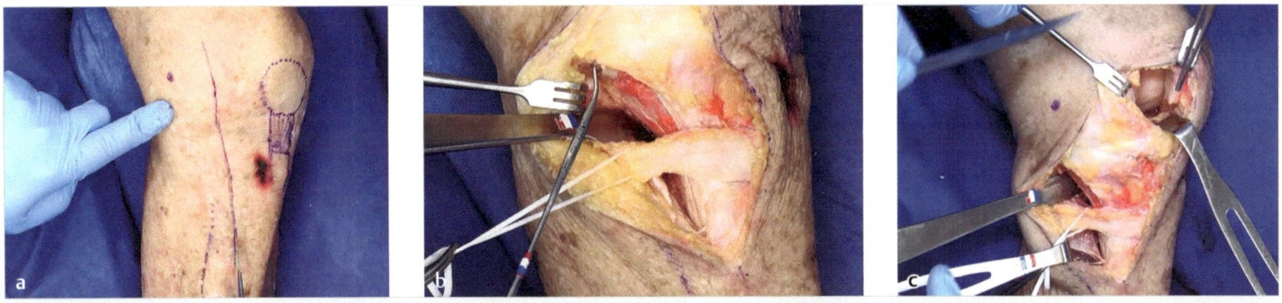

Fig. 20.5 Extended direct medial approach to the knee. (a) The incision is placed at a midline point in between the anterior and posterior tibial crests, extending itself from the medial femoral epicondyle to the proximal tibial shaft. (b) The popliteus muscle is elevated directly from the posterior tibial crest, granting access to the posteromedial quadrant of the tibial plateau. (c) A medial parapatellar arthrotomy exposed the joint from above, and a limited medial submeniscal arthrotomy allows for visualization of the anteromedial quadrant of the tibial plateau. It is imperative to avoid stripping of the medial collateral ligament.

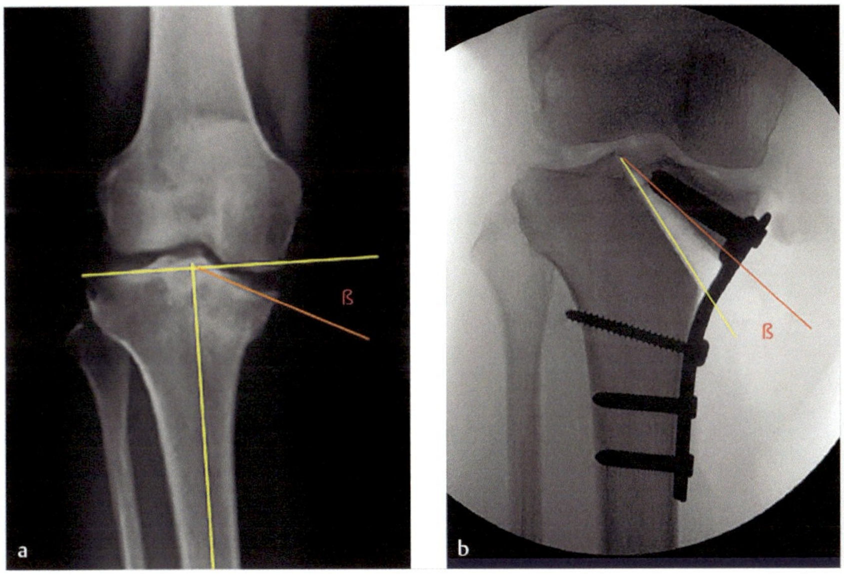

Fig. 20.6 Unicondylar tibial plateau angulation. (a) Radiograph on an anteroposterior projection reveals an inclination of the medial tibial plateau articular surface to the joint orientation line. The angle of inclination is measured as β. (b) Postoperative radiograph revealing an open-wedge unicondylar osteotomy. The angle of the wedge matches the β angle measured preoperatively.

- Bone graft should be available when we perform open-wedged osteotomies or mobilize the initially impacted osteochondral fragments. Tricortical iliac bone autograft is instrumental in supporting subchondral and epiphyseal voids.
- When the articular joint is elevated on the lateral tibial plateau, we use Kirschner wires inserted from lateral to medial, and we retrieve these wires on the medial side. Before retrieving the wires, we support the metaphyseal and epiphyseal bone with a bone graft and a buttress plate.

20.9 Difficulties Encountered

A complex deformity can preclude its treatment with a single-cut osteotomy. Understanding the deformity in preoperative planning is, therefore, a must. 3D-printed models of the injured and the contralateral tibial plateau should be sterilized and available in the surgical field if possible. The scarring around the peroneal nerve poses an additional risk, especially if we plan to perform a fibular osteotomy. External neurolysis of the peroneal nerve is required in these cases. Converting a posttraumatic concavity into the normal convexity of the lateral plateau is challenging. "Overdoing" may create a fracture of the osteotomized fragment.

20.10 Key Procedural Steps

Our discussion will focus on the management of deformities that result in either a condyle inclination or the widening of the articular surface.

20.10.1 Unicondylar Angulation

This may be a result of a malunion of the Schatzker type II (lateral split depression) or Schatzker type IV (medial tibial plateau condyle). Most frequently, this occurs on the lateral tibial condyle and results in valgus alignment of the lower limb. Besides the angulation of the condyle, one may find some degree of articular impaction. We use an extensile anterolateral surgical approach. We release the anterior tibial muscle and the iliotibial band insertion (Gerdy's tubercle osteotomy). We elevate the lateral meniscus through a horizontal submeniscal horizontal

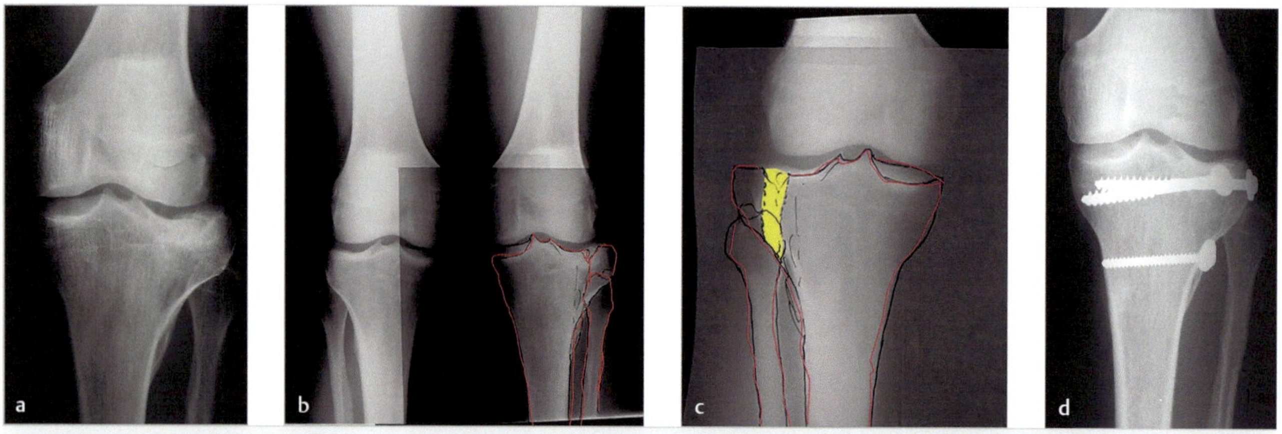

Fig. 20.7 Lateral tibial plateau malunion. **(a)** Radiograph on an anteroposterior projection revealing a healed and widened tibial plateau as a result of conservative management of lateral tibial plateau fracture. **(b)** A paper drawing was performed over the radiograph of the widened left tibial plateau fracture. **(c)** The drawing is then flipped and superimposed over the opposite and nonfracture tibial plateau. The drawing shows how much broader the left tibial plateau is when compared to the normal opposite side. The *yellow area* represents the site of widening, filled by fibrous tissue. **(d)** Postoperative radiograph, after a lateral closing wedge was performed preserving the lateral meniscus and narrowing the width of the tibial plateau. The continuity of the tibial plateau rim is restored, and the joint is now stable and congruent.

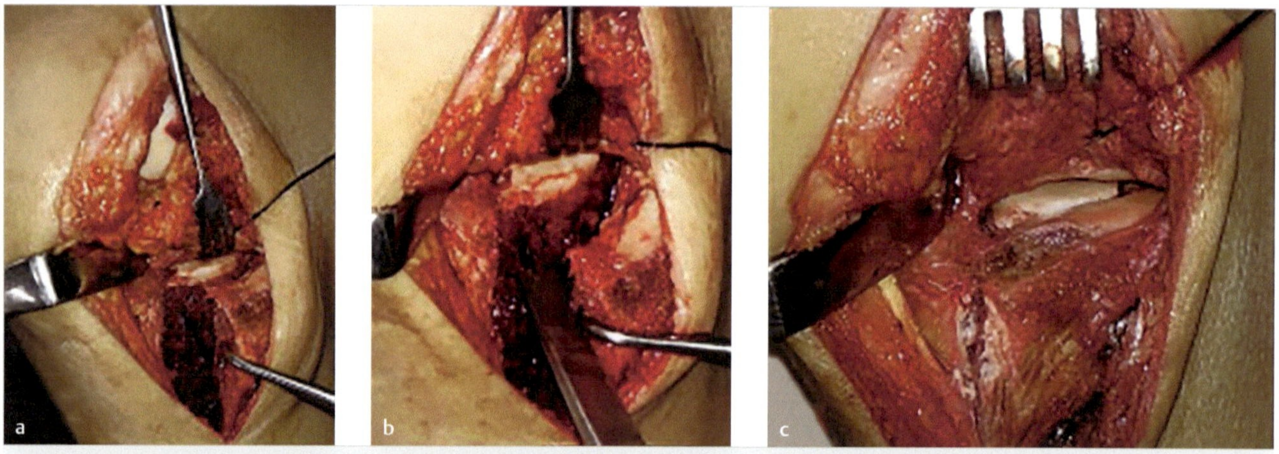

Fig. 20.8 Lateral tibial plateau malunion. **(a)** An osteotomy to the lateral tibial plateau rim is performed, and the area of depression on the anterolateral quadrant of the tibial plateau is identified under the lateral meniscus. **(b)** The osteochondral depressed fragment is then elevated after being osteotomized. **(c)** The articular surface is reduced anatomically, as the depressed fragment is elevated to the level of the lateral rim. The joint will be fixed with lag screws and a buttress plate, restoring the continuity of the rim and the joint's congruity and stability.

arthrotomy. Often, the lateral meniscus is torn; small tears should be debrided to a stable meniscus, whereas larger ones should be sutured. Sutures are placed in the peripheral rim of the meniscus for later reattachment. Placing a large femoral distractor with the knee flexed allows for good visualization. Increased access to the posterolateral quadrant of the tibial plateau is possible via either a fibular head osteotomy or a lateral femoral epicondyle osteotomy. Often the peripheral osseous rim of the plateau is at the correct level, and impaction is seen in the weight-bearing area. We osteotomize the rim cortex with a thin oscillating saw, granting us access to the depressed site. We leave a hinge intact of the osteotomized cortex in the metaphyseal area, maintaining its blood supply and facilitating later reposition and fixation. Multiple small (1.0–1.25 mm) K-wires are placed in the subchondral bone under the plateau to prevent breaking through the subchondral bone and cartilage when performing a unicondylar osteotomy. The osteotomy of the depressed fragment is done with an oscillating thin-bladed saw under saline cooling. The starting point of the osteotomy is 1.5 to 2 cm below the articular surface. A laminar bone spreader or stacked osteotomes will allow gentle elevation of the osteotomized fragment. An essential aspect is to prevent breakage of the cartilaginous hinge opposite the starting point of the osteotomy. Once the osteotomy is completed, the iliac bone graft is harvested. A triangular tricortical graft is taken in one piece. Smaller wedges can then be fashioned from this graft. Use these tricortical wedges of iliac crest graft cut to fit the subchondral void and placed under the osteotomized fragment(s) (▶ Fig. 20.9). Often, more than a few attempts are needed to get the perfect height. A slight 1-mm overcorrection is better than an undercorrection.

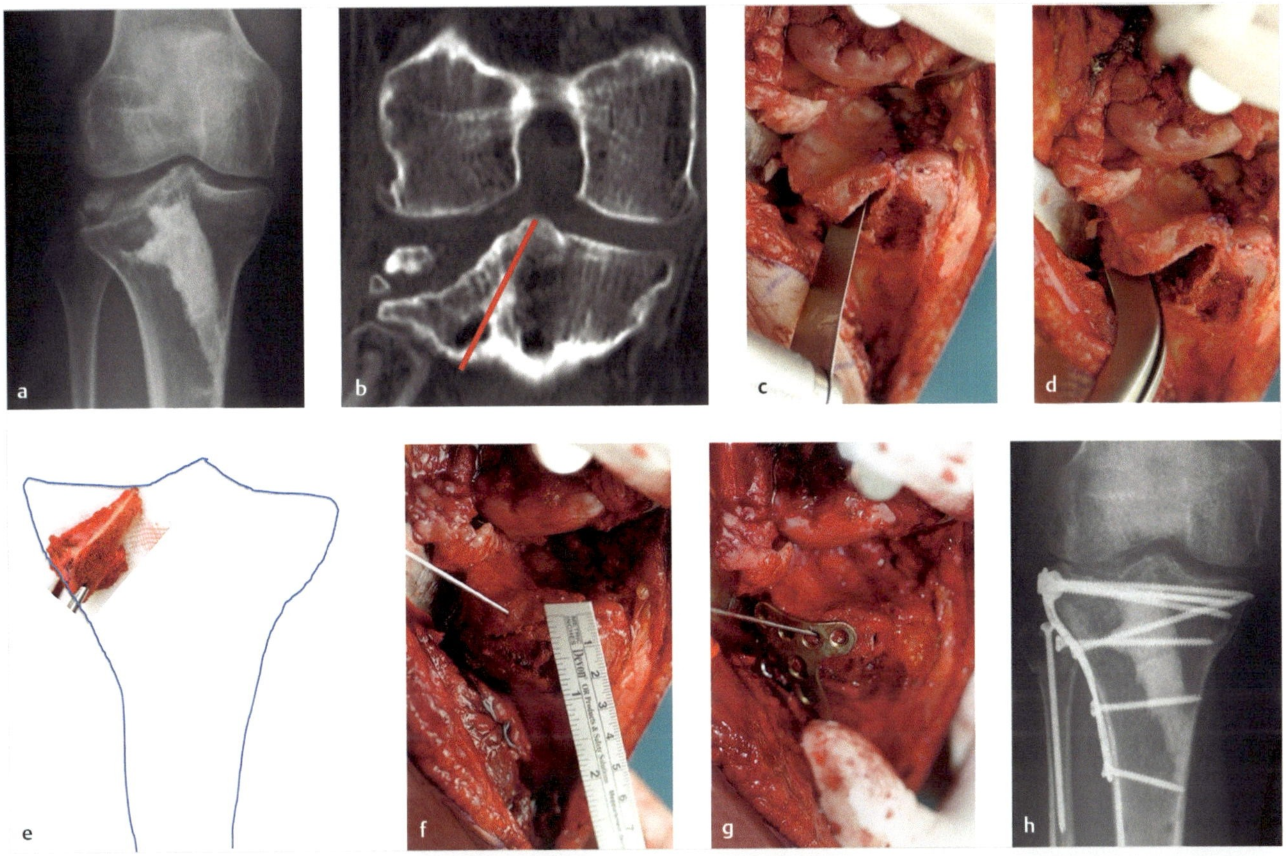

Fig. 20.9 Example of an intra-articular open-wedge osteotomy to address a unicondylar inclination and depression. **(a)** A healthy 56-year-old male was referred after internal fixation of a Schatzker 2 tibia plateau fracture. During the initial internal fixation, the surgeon used a bone graft substitute placed under the depressed area; **(b)** this led to a malunion with poor knee function, pain, and instability. Despite hardware removal at the other hospital, his symptoms did not improve. **(c)** Using an extensile approach including a fibular head osteotomy and a Gerdy's tubercle osteotomy, we did a unicondylar osteotomy of the lateral plateau using an oscillating saw. **(d)** Using a laminar bone spreader the unicondylar fragment was gently elevated. **(e,f)** A tricortical wedge from the iliac crest was cut to size, and placed under the osteotomized condyle. **(g)** Fixation with a small 3.5-mm T-plate. **(h)** At final follow-up all osteotomies had healed. His knee was now well-aligned without a residual bony pivot. Although not perfect, his range of motion was very good with good pain relief.

The cortical fragment is repositioned, and the reconstruction is temporarily fixed with K-wires. Testing the knee in full extension should determine whether the pseudolaxity is corrected. Evaluation of mechanical axis using comparison with the contralateral leg and fluoroscopy is done. A small fragment plate (T-shaped or L-shaped) is positioned on the anterolateral cortex. The sutures in the lateral meniscus are placed through the plate for reattachment. The fibular head osteotomy is fixed with a 1.25-mm cerclage wire or a 3.5-mm screw. If a lateral epicondyle osteotomy is performed, it will be fixed with a 3.5-mm cortical screw and a plastic spiked washer.

20.10.2 Widened Tibial Plateau

This is caused by incomplete reduction during the initial treatment. The axial valgus force during the injury did not only compress and split the lateral plateau leading to a concavity, but it also caused subsequent widening of the plateau. When this comminuted area is not "narrowed" back to its original width, there will be a mismatch with an overhang of the lateral plateau. In these cases, resecting a wedge will reestablish the regular width. Because this wedge is covered by poor-quality cartilage, there is a dual benefit of this resection. For these cases 3D-CT-based planning and the use of patient-specific cutting jigs are helpful (▶ Fig. 20.10).

20.11 Bailout, Rescue, and Salvage Procedures

- Gastrocnemius rotational flaps are limb salvage procedures in case of a compromised soft tissue envelope.
- If a lateral reconstruction has compromised the cortical stability on the medial side, lateral fixation alone may not provide enough stability. In that case, a temporary two-pin external fixation can be placed on the medial side as a buttress. This can be removed in the outpatient clinic after 6 weeks.
- Focal cartilage defects can be filled with locally harvested cartilage from the proximal tibiofibular joint. The cartilage of this joint is often of good quality and is especially easy to access after a chevron fibular head osteotomy.

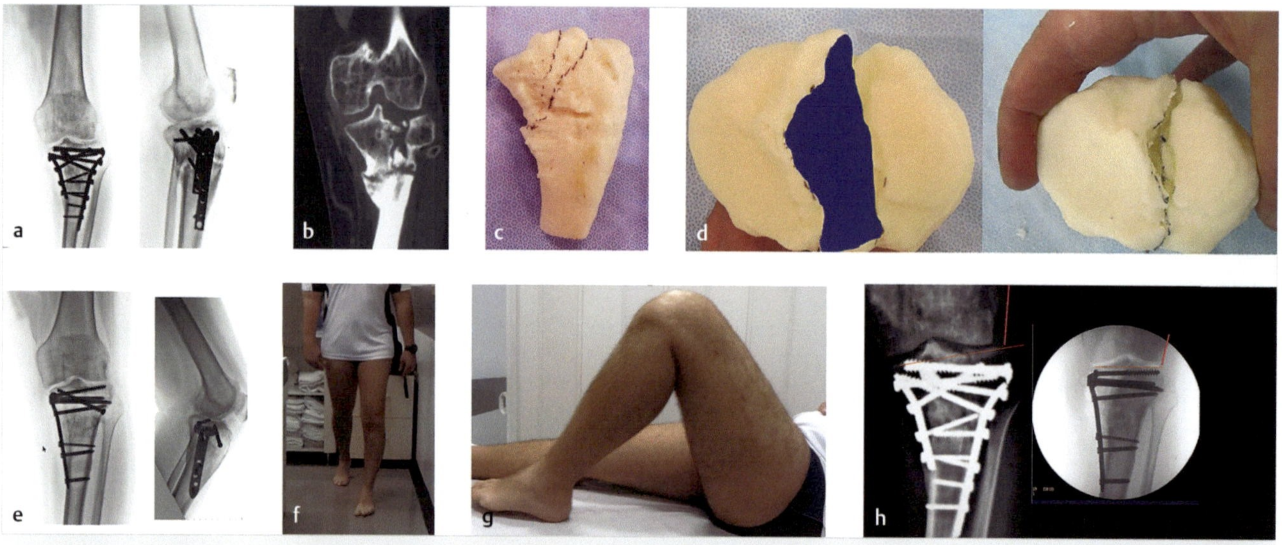

Fig. 20.10 The use of a three-dimensional prototype in preoperative planning of a complex tibial plateau malunion. **(a)** Radiographs of a 24-year-old male who sustained a bicondylar tibial plateau fracture and ended up with a malunion of the proximal tibia. The tibial plateau is wider than expected, the knee is unstable, and there is varus deformity. **(b)** Computed tomography image after removing the hardware reveals widening of the tibial plateau metaphyseal varus deformity. **(c)** A three-dimensional prototype base on computed tomography (CT) images was obtained. The visualization of the prototype allows for the planning of an intra-articular closing wedge osteotomy. **(d)** Axial views of the prototype revealing the area to be resected (*blue*), and the narrowing of the articular surface after a closing wedge osteotomy with a metaphyseal apex was performed in the model. **(e)** Postoperative radiographs revealing a significant improvement in the alignment and congruency of the joint. **(f)** Follow-up at 8 months postoperative. The patient has a stable and pain-free knee. **(g)** Knee range of motion at 8 months postoperative. **(h)** Comparison of radiographs before and after the corrective osteotomy. There is a significant improvement in the knee alignment.

20.12 Pitfalls

After a fibular head osteotomy, there is a significant increase in the varus opening of the joint. This might lead to too much stretching of the peroneal nerve and neuropraxia, mainly if a femoral distractor is used to increase visualization of the knee.

Undercorrection is more common than overcorrection. We test the knee stability with the joint positioned in full extension, confirming that the pseudolaxity (bony pivot) is absent.

One should avoid reconstructive attempts with joint preservation procedures in the presence of extensive damage to the cartilage in the weight-bearing area of the tibial plateau in patients older than 50 years of age.

Acknowledgment

The authors would like to thank Prof. Dr. Cleber Paccolla, MD, who has made significant contributions in the field of posttraumatic osteotomies around the knee and who was the principal surgeon in the case illustrated in ▶ Fig. 20.7.

Section II

Sports Medicine

II

21 Quadriceps Autograft: All-Inside Anterior Cruciate Ligament Reconstruction

Patrick A. Smith, Jordan A. Bley, and Corey Cook

21.1 Description

Multiple graft options exist for anterior cruciate ligament (ACL) reconstruction. This technique description details the utilization of autograft quadriceps tendon tissue for all-inside ACL reconstruction. Quadriceps tendon grafts offer unique benefits for ACL reconstruction such as ease of harvest and predictably large diameter. Compared to patellar tendon BTB (bone-tendon-bone) grafts, the advantages of quadriceps tendon grafts include: low donor site morbidity with less anterior knee pain, less risk of skin sensitivity loss by avoidance of the infrapatellar branch of the saphenous nerve, larger diameter graft if desired, and elimination of risk of patellar fracture if only a soft tissue graft is harvested.

21.2 Key Principles

Quadriceps tendon harvest is done through a small incision with available specialized equipment. Minimally invasive all-inside ACL reconstruction with bone sockets in both the femur and tibia is performed utilizing adjustable length suspensory fixation.

21.3 Expectations

Quadriceps tendon harvest provides reproducible large size graft diameter and good graft length with minimal harvest site morbidity. This option also provides adequate flexibility; a quadriceps graft can be harvested with a bone plug from the patella based on surgeon preference. Finally, harvest also allows for either a partial or full-thickness quadriceps tendon graft.

21.4 Indications

Complete ACL tears are diagnosed following history and clinical examination, especially related to a positive pivot shift, and correlated with diagnostic imaging. Quadriceps tendon grafts utilizing the all-inside technique is an excellent option for both primary and revision ACL reconstruction situations.

21.5 Contraindications

This graft should be avoided if the patient has previously experienced a quadriceps tendon tear or significant quadriceps muscle strain.

21.6 Special Considerations

Athletes participating in kneeling sports like wrestling and volleyball are excellent candidates for a quadriceps tendon graft in order to avoid a direct anterior incision such as with a patellar tendon graft. Furthermore, a quadriceps tendon is the ideal graft for any patient worried about kneeling pain from graft harvest. It can also be used for pediatric growth plate sparing ACL reconstruction.

21.7 Special Instructions, Position, and Anesthesia

The patient is placed in the supine position. General anesthesia is usually utilized. It is helpful to have a leg holding device so the knee can easily be flexed to 100 degrees of flexion to facilitate graft harvest and closure. A tourniquet is not used.

21.8 Tips, Pearls, and Lessons Learned

For exposure of the quadriceps tendon, do not excise the overlying fatty tissue over the tendon as that can lead to a postoperative cosmetic deformity. Simple retraction of this tissue allows for full tendon exposure. Regarding graft harvest, it is generally easier to take a full-thickness graft. Plus, this provides a reproducible larger graft. Furthermore, there are no issues with suprapatellar swelling during surgery with full-thickness grafts, as long as the tendon defect is closed. Graft harvest is best done at 100 degrees of flexion, keeping the quadriceps tendon under tension. Also, closing the quadriceps tendon defect in the same degree of flexion prevents shortening of the residual tendon.

Regarding all-inside ACL reconstruction, a femoral socket can be created with either an outside-in technique using a FlipCutter device (Arthrex, Inc., Naples, FL) or from the anteromedial portal utilizing a low-profile reamer.

21.9 Difficulties Encountered

Minimally invasive graft harvest, as described below and highlighted in the video, has a short learning curve. Instrumentation for all-inside ACL reconstruction with the FlipCutter and use of the suspensory TightRope devices (Arthrex, Inc., Naples, FL) for adjustable loop fixation on the femur and tibia also has a bit of a learning curve. However, both techniques are effective and reproducible. It is important to make sure the suspensory button on the lateral femoral condyle is against bone and deep to the iliotibial band to avoid hardware-related pain.

21.10 Key Procedural Steps

For graft harvest, the knee is flexed to 100 degrees of flexion, and a 3-cm incision is made from the superior pole of the patella proximally. Dissection is done through subcutaneous tissue to expose the quadriceps tendon, again without excision of this normal fatty tissue. It is easy to establish a plane between the tendon and the overlying subcutaneous tissue proximally by passing a sponge with a periosteal elevator for blunt dissection. Either a 10- or 11-mm-wide double knife (Arthrex, Inc., Naples, FL) is used to harvest 70 to 75 mm of tendon proximally (▶ Fig. 21.1). The tendon is then released sharply off the superior pole of the patella with a #10 blade. Again, I prefer a full-thickness graft. Next, a #2 FiberWire suture (Arthrex, Inc., Naples, FL) is passed through the released tendon for traction purposes and threaded through the opening of the Quad Tendon Stripper Cutter (Arthrex, Inc., Naples, FL) (▶ Fig. 21.2a, b). The stripper is passed proximally over the tendon while applying traction on the tendon with the suture at the free end. Squeeze the Stripper Cutter handle to cut the proximal tendon sharply at a length of 70 to 75 mm. It is essential to make sure the Stripper Cutter handle is kept in the "closed" position until ready to cut the tendon proximally. The quadriceps tendon defect is then closed with multiple #1 Vicryl horizontal mattress sutures (Ethicon, Inc., Somerville, NJ), keeping the knee flexed at 100 degrees of flexion. The subcutaneous tissue is closed with 2–0 Monocryl suture (Ethicon, Inc., Somerville, NJ), and the skin with a 2–0 Proline subcuticular suture (Ethicon, Inc., Somerville, NJ).

For graft preparation, suspensory fixation is assembled with a TightRope RT (reverse tensioning) on the femoral side and a TightRope No-Button on the tibial side. This is done, as shown in the video, by suturing FiberTag (Arthrex, Inc., Naples, FL) to each end of the graft with a special #2 FiberWire suture on a needle for a "ripstop" technique, incorporating the TightRope devices in the process. The final diameter and length of the graft are then measured (▶ Fig. 21.3).

I prefer all-inside ACL reconstruction as it is minimally invasive. After appropriate treatment for any associated meniscal tearing and/or articular cartilage damage, I debride a minimal amount of torn native ACL tissue, leaving a good footprint of native tissue for remnant preservation on the femur and especially the tibia, to enhance proprioception regeneration with the ACL tendon graft. I do not routinely perform a notchplasty. For creation of the femoral socket, I prefer isometric graft placement more toward the anteromedial bundle attachment. If done outside-in with a FlipCutter, the 6–9 guide (Arthrex, Inc., Naples, FL) is used through the anterolateral portal (▶ Fig. 21.4), viewing through the anteromedial portal for optimal positioning (▶ Fig. 21.5). A small lateral skin incision is made, and the guide sleeve is passed through the iliotibial band down to bone on the lateral femur. The femoral intraosseous distance can then be measured off the guide sleeve. A FlipCutter of the diameter matching the graft is then drilled as a 3.5-mm straight pin into position on the joint side and the guide sleeve is tapped 7 mm into the lateral femur (▶ Fig. 21.6a). Flipping the FlipCutter, the femoral socket is retrocut from the joint side a few mm deeper than the desired amount of graft in the femoral socket (▶ Fig. 21.6b). Usually, this distance is 22 to 25 mm. If a deeper socket is desired, one can ream all the way back until the metal sleeve is encountered, which will leave a 7-mm intact bone bridge for the button fixation. A #2 FiberStick (Arthrex, Inc., Naples, FL) is then passed through the guide sleeve and retrieved on the joint side to serve as a shuttle suture for the graft. The guide sleeve is then removed.

If drilling through the anteromedial portal, I use either a 6- or 7-mm offset guide (Arthrex, Inc., Naples, FL)—depending on

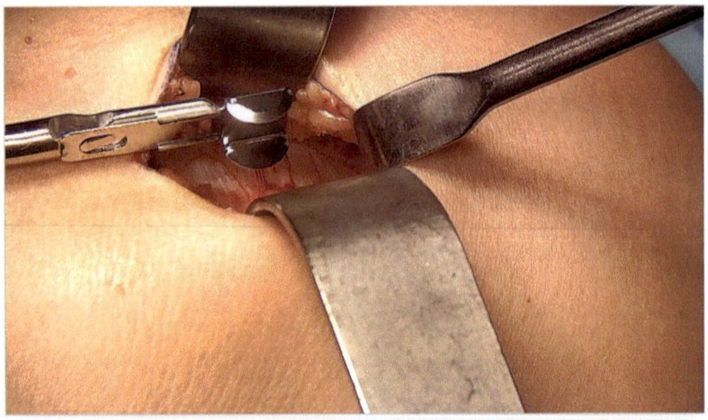

Fig. 21.1 Right knee at 100 degrees of flexion with knee to the left and hip to the right. An 11-mm-wide double knife blade in position to harvest exposed quadriceps tendon graft.

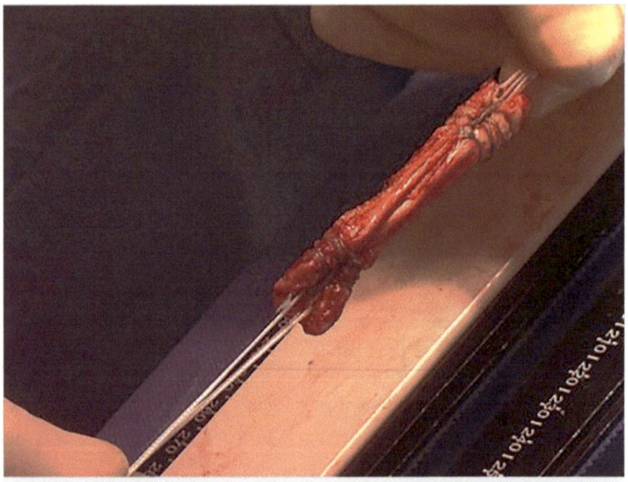

Fig. 21.3 Final prepared quadriceps tendon autograft. TightRope RT (reverse tensioning) secured on femoral side (proximal) and on tibial side (distal) with TightRope No-Button. Both suspensory fixation devices are secured to tendon with Fibertag and #2 FiberWire cerclage sutures.

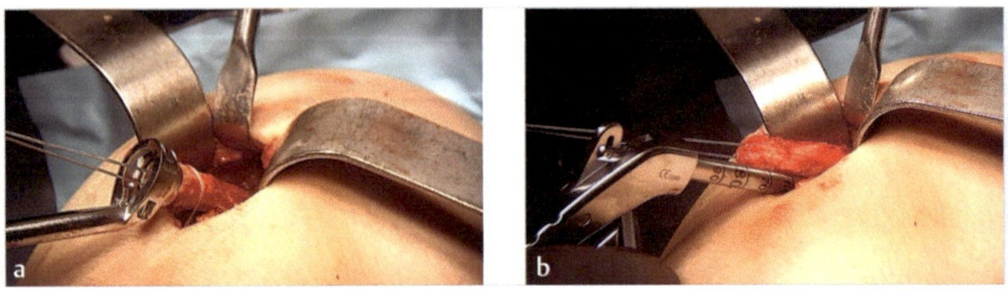

Fig. 21.2 Right knee flexed to 100 degrees. Special quad tendon stripper cutter on left **(a)** passed over quadriceps tendon that has been released off the superior pole of the patella. On the right **(b)** the stripper cutter is passed proximally usually 70 to 75 mm, and then the handle is squeezed to free the graft proximally.

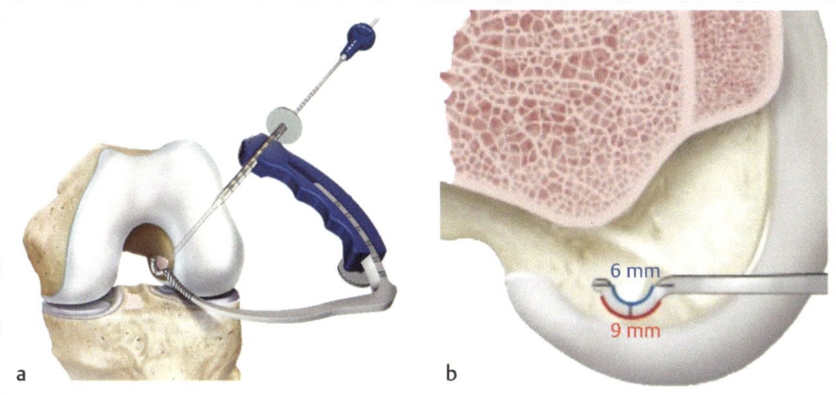

Fig. 21.4 (a) Femoral 6–9 guide in position to create desired femoral socket from outside-in approach. (b) The inner diameter is 6 mm and the outer diameter is 9 mm for ease of orientation of the femoral socket position.

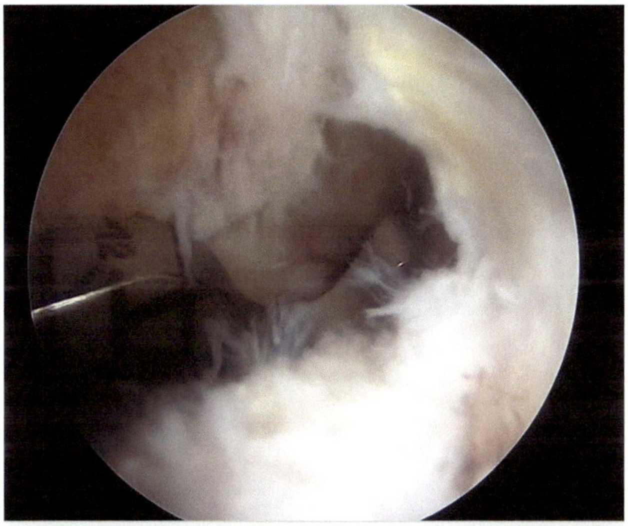

Fig. 21.5 Right knee. Viewing from anteromedial portal. Femoral 6–9 guide in position to create femoral socket.

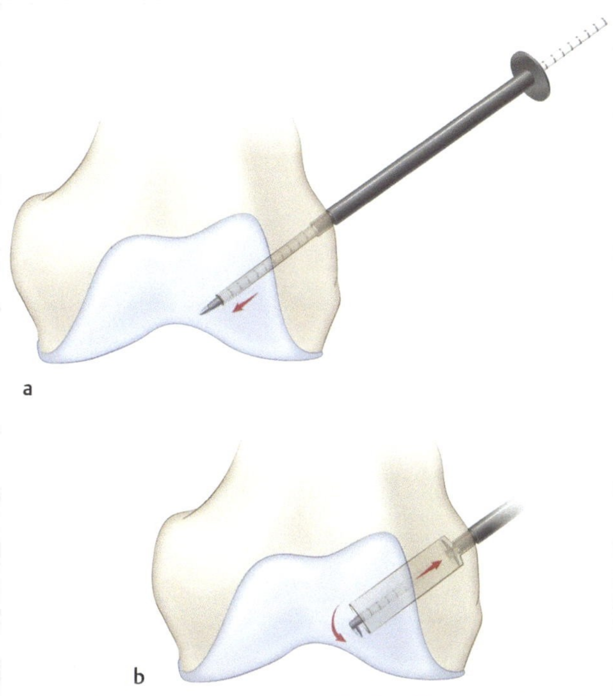

Fig. 21.6 (a) The FlipCutter is drilled from the lateral femoral cortex into the joint, and the guide sleeve is tapped 7 mm into the bone here to provide a bridge of intact bone. (b) Pushing forward on the FlipCutter handle, the pin is "flipped" to now become a reamer to ream back to the guide sleeve preserving the bone bridge for this femoral graft socket.

graft diameter—through the anteromedial portal with the knee flexed to approximately 120 degrees of flexion to create a pilot hole within the anteromedial bundle footprint. I always check this point viewing from the anteromedial portal to be sure I am happy with the position of this pilot hole, which I can easily change if need be. Next, a 3.5-mm special spade tip measuring pin (Arthrex, Inc., Naples, FL) is drilled in to measure the femoral intraosseous distance to facilitate suspensory button flipping later. This pin is drilled out the lateral thigh, and a low-profile reamer (Arthrex, Inc., Naples, FL) (as shown in the video) that matches graft diameter is passed vertically through the anteromedial portal to avoid the medial femoral condyle and reamed for the desired graft depth in the femur (▶ Fig. 21.7). The pin is then used to pass a #2 FiberWire graft shuttle suture here.

All the following surgical steps are well delineated with the surgery video. After creating the femoral socket for all-inside ACL reconstruction, I always measure the intra-articular distance for the graft from the femoral socket to the tibial ACL footprint by using an intra-articular measuring device (Arthrex, Inc., Naples, FL). This measurement added to the femoral socket depth allows me to drill the appropriate tibial socket depth and yet preserves the tibial socket to be all-inside, based on the overall graft length.

For creation of the tibial socket, a FlipCutter matching the graft diameter is used. The tibial guide (Arthrex, Inc., Naples, FL) is placed within the native ACL footprint fibers left at the normal attachment site, also indexing off the anterior horn of the lateral meniscus. With the knee flexed to approximately 80 degrees of flexion, the skin is marked anteromedially, and a short incision is made here and carried through subcutaneous tissue. The periosteum is incised and elevated here so the suspensory fixation button will sit on the bone. Maintaining the guide in position on the joint side, the guide sleeve is passed down to the tibia bone, measuring the intraosseous distance of the tibia, which should be at least 40 mm. The FlipCutter is then drilled as a 3.5-mm straight pin into the joint (▶ Fig. 21.8), and like on the femoral side, the guide sleeve is tapped 7 mm into the tibia.

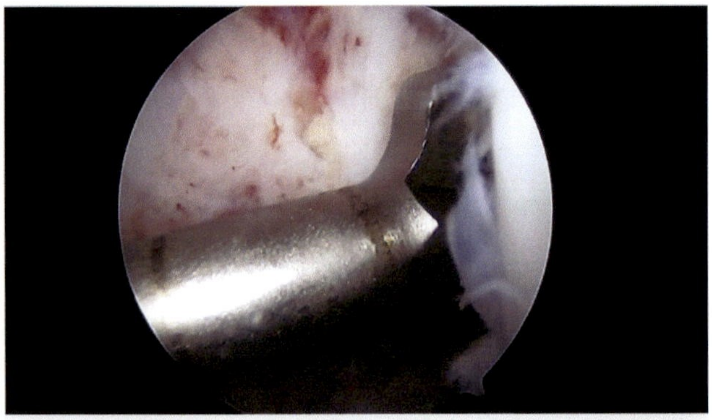

Fig. 21.7 Right knee. Viewing from anterolateral portal. Low-profile reamer in position to create femoral socket from anteromedial portal.

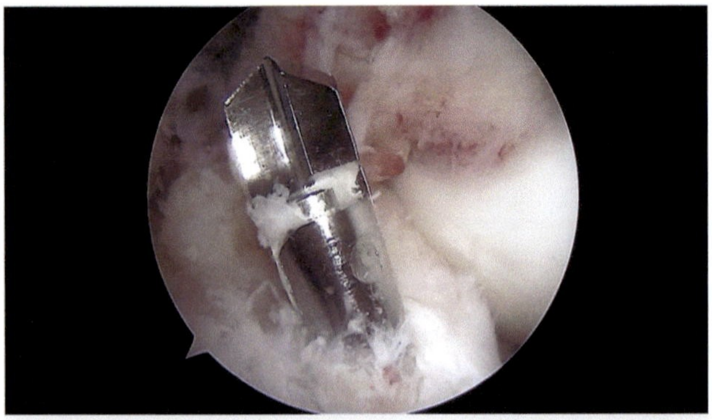

Fig. 21.8 Right knee. Viewing from anterolateral portal. Unflipped FlipCutter drilled in position to retroream tibial socket.

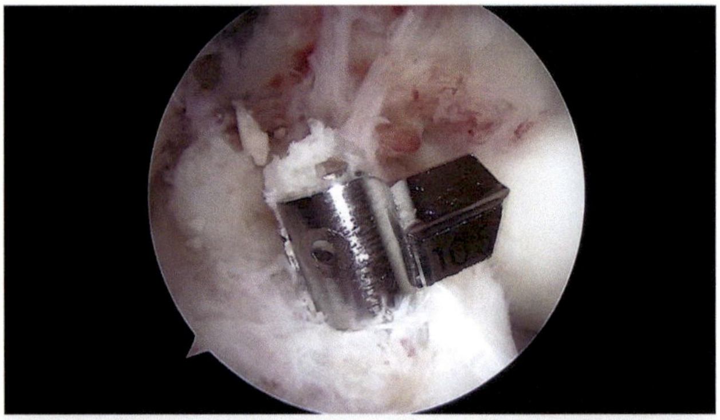

Fig. 21.9 Right knee. Viewing from anterolateral portal. FlipCutter (10.5 mm diameter) flipped for retroreaming of tibial socket.

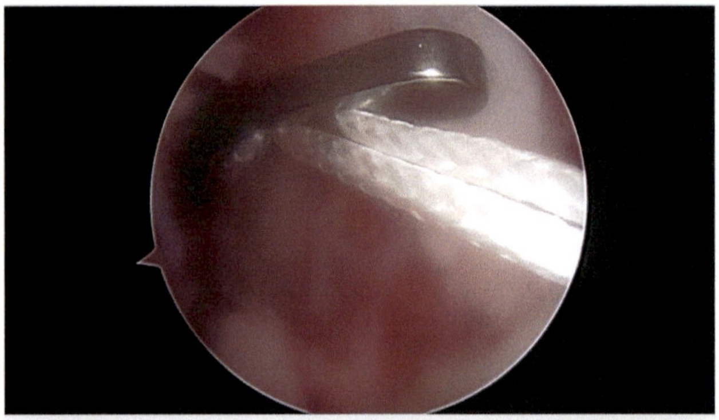

Fig. 21.10 Right knee. Viewing from anterolateral portal. Passage of suspensory tightrope button for femoral graft fixation. White shortening sutures will pull graft into socket.

The FlipCutter on the joint side is then unflipped (▶ Fig. 21.9), and the tibial socket is retroream to the desired depth, always 5 mm longer than the expected graft in the tibial socket to allow for appropriate graft tension. Again, the guide sleeve ensures at least a 7-mm tibial bone bridge. The critical step with any all-inside ACL reconstruction relates to making sure you never "bottom-out" your graft to where it cannot be tensioned, so the total length of the femoral and tibial socket depths and the measured intra-articular distance must be longer than the final graft length. Again, I usually overream the tibia by approximately 5 mm to ensure appropriate graft tensioning.

A "pearl" for graft passage is placement of a PassPort cannula (Arthrex, Inc., Naples, FL) in the anteromedial portal to prevent a soft tissue bridge during graft passage, which can be very frustrating when encountered. I place this with a hemostat through the anteromedial portal after creating the tibial socket. A TigerStick (Arthrex, Inc., Naples, FL) is then passed from the 3.5-mm tibial hole up into the joint and retrieved as a tibial shuttle graft suture through the PassPort cannula.

Graft passage is initiated by retrieving the femoral socket graft shuttle suture through the PassPort cannula in the anteromedial portal. This is then used to shuttle the TightRope RT blue passing suture in the suspensory button, along with the two white shortening strands, out the lateral small skin incision (▶ Fig. 21.10). Before passing the button, I always mark the intraosseous distance that was measured for the femur on the shortening strands from the *trailing* end of the button. In this way, I know when to expect the button to "flip" on the lateral femoral cortex to provide fixation with the shortening strands. In this way, intraoperative X-ray is not needed. Once the button "flips," which also usually can be felt as a "pop," the graft is hoisted up into the joint through the PassPort cannula to the expected depth in the femur by way of alternating pull on the white shortening strands, keeping the strands each at about the same length.

Next, the No-Button TightRope and the tibial end of the graft are passed into the tibial socket. A "pearl" here is to pass a #2 FiberWire suture through the loop of the TightRope as a "luggage tag" suture to shuttle this FiberWire suture into the tibial socket with the graft. In this way, the loop of the TightRope will not shorten prematurely. Then the shortening strands are pulled out the anteromedial tibia through the 3.5-mm drill hole here with the TightRope loop via the "luggage tag" suture, and the graft is pulled into the socket with finger pressure through the TightRope loop. An 8 × 12 mm diameter Attachable Button System (Arthrex, Inc., Naples, FL) is attached to the No-Button TightRope loop on the tibial side, and fixation is done through alternating pull on the two shortening strands. I always fix my grafts holding the foot so the knee is in maximal hyperextension to avoid any chance of overconstraint. At this time, the knee joint is cycled 20 times to eliminate any creep in the system. A major advantage with the use of adjustable loop fixation

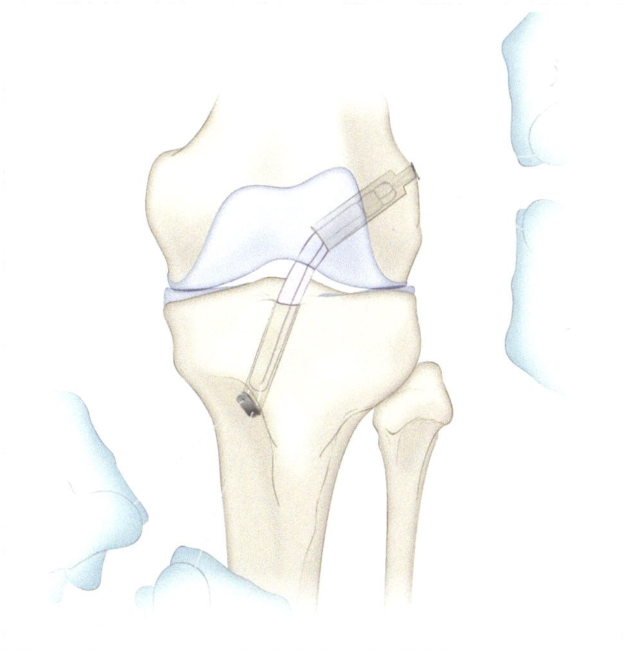

Fig. 21.11 While holding the foot so that the knee is in maximal hypertension, graft fixation is performed by alternating the pulling of the two shortening strands.

is that retensioning of the graft can be done at this point. The femoral TightRope shortening strands are retensioned with the knee hyperextended, followed by retensioning the tibial shortening strands, also with the knee hyperextended to further optimize graft tension (▶ Fig. 21.11). The tibial shortening sutures can then be tied to the button here for additional backup fixation (▶ Fig. 21.12).

21.11 Bailout, Rescue, Salvage Procedures

Probably the one "bailout" situation relates to potential length mismatch of the graft and the socket depths plus the intra-articular distance. If this were to occur, resulting in the graft being too long, the graft could not be tensioned and would be lax. If that situation occurred, the button on the tibial side would have to be removed to free up the graft, so that with a

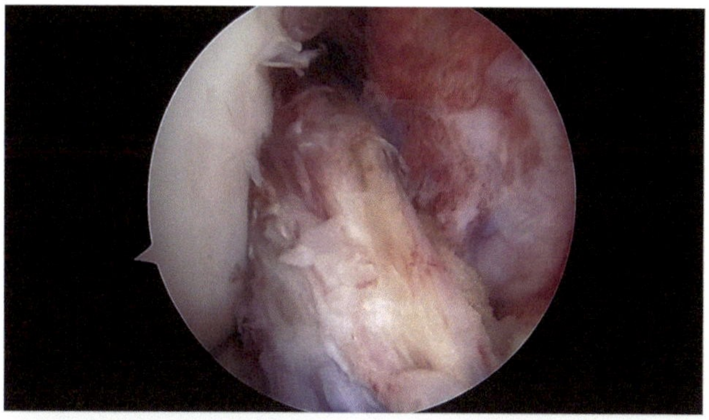

Fig. 21.12 Right knee. Viewing from anterolateral portal. Final quadriceps all-inside tendon autograft.

probe from the anteromedial portal, it could be teased out of the tibial socket. Then, a grasper would be used through the anteromedial portal to pull the end of the tendon graft out this portal to where a suture could be passed through the graft. Next, passing a 3.5-mm pin through the tibial socket into the joint, the tibial socket could be converted into a full tibial tunnel with a reamer, matching the graft diameter. The graft could then be easily passed back into this tibial tunnel and fixated with an interference screw.

21.12 Pitfalls

These have been highlighted above in the procedure description steps. A quick review of the major potential pitfalls.

- Always measure the intraosseous distance of the femur either outside-in with the FlipCutter drill sleeve or inside-out from the anteromedial portal with the special 3.5-mm spade pin. This will greatly facilitate flipping of the femoral TightRope fixation button without the need for intraoperative X-ray.
- Use of the intra-articular measuring device to determine length of the graft across the joint in combination with appropriate socket reaming depth in the femur and tibia will help ensure the ACL graft will never "bottom-out."
- Use the PassPort cannula through the anteromedial portal during graft passage to avoid aggravating soft tissue bridges.
- Place a #2 FiberWire suture through the tibial No-Button TightRope loop to protect this critical loop from premature shortening when pulling the graft into the tibial socket.

22 Anterior Cruciate Ligament Reconstruction: Hamstrings Autograft

John Byron

22.1 Description

Arthroscopic reconstruction with autograft is the gold standard for the treatment of anterior cruciate ligament (ACL) instability. There are a number of graft options available, each with a different set of benefits and liabilities. This chapter will focus on Hamstring autograft ACL reconstruction.

22.2 Key Principles

The ideal graft is the one that is easy to harvest, has similar strength and resistance as the native ACL, a low donor site morbidity, fast integration rate, and that allows early mobility and rehabilitation. Patellar ligament autograft (BTB—bone-tendon-bone) has been, historically, the gold standard; nevertheless, it also has the highest donor site morbidity and incidence of patient complaints. During the last decade, hamstring autograft has become an alternative with comparable results to patellar ligament autograft, lower donor site morbidity, and fewer patient complaints.

22.3 Expectations

Hamstring autografts provide the following biomechanical advantages: higher resistance and rigidity and higher cross-section area, and providing a greater area for incorporation and ligamentization. Hamstring autografts are a safe and efficient alternative for the treatment of ACL rupture and can be performed with a simple and minimally invasive grafting technique. Technical errors related to lack of knowledge of the anatomy may place the reconstruction at risk of failure.

22.4 Indications

Hamstring ACL reconstruction is indicated in active patients with a torn ACL and functional instability in the sagittal plane and/or rotational instability. The decision to reconstruct should be based on the desired activity level of the patient more than on age. Another clear indication is patients who have tried and failed nonoperative therapy and have recurrent episodes of instability. The surgical technique in this chapter is based on individual channels, using medial portal access for the femoral tunnel, seeking an anatomical-functional reconstruction with hamstring tendon autografts with the largest possible diameter, which may require not only quadruple grafts but sextuplets on some occasions, in order to fill between 60 and 80% of the native ACL anatomic footprint.

22.5 Contraindications

Relative contraindications include a prior ipsilateral hamstring ACL reconstruction, a sprinting athlete, and patients with a multiligament injury that includes severe medial corner damage.

22.6 Special Considerations

Patients with exceptionally small hamstring tendons may be better candidates for one of the other graft choices.

22.7 Special Instructions, Position, and Anesthesia

With the patient lying in a supine position, a tourniquet cuff is placed on the thigh, as proximal as possible and is inflated only if required to control bleeding. The leg is then left hanging over the edge of the surgical table, with a roll or sandbag under the tourniquet; a lateral support is placed on the surgical table as fulcrum to perform knee valgus during the examination and the procedures on the medial compartment. In order to examine and perform procedures on the lateral compartment, the limb of the patient is placed in the figure-four position with the heel on the table (▶ Fig. 22.1).

22.8 Tips, Pearls, and Lessons Learned

1. The semitendinosis tendon has an accessory insertion in most patients that goes from the inferior aspect of the tendon down to the tibia. If this accessory insertion is not identified and released when harvest occurs from an anterior incision, it can easily lead to amputation of the tendon with a grossly inadequate length.
2. An alternate transverse incision for tendon harvest can be made posteriorly in the popliteal crease (▶ Fig. 22.2a, b). This decreases the risk of nerve damage and of amputation of the tendon during harvest.

22.9 Difficulties Encountered

Inadequate graft length can occur if the accessory insertion is not identified and released and if the graft is not gently harvested from the muscle with a tendon stripper.

22.10 Key Procedural Steps

22.10.1 Tendon Harvesting

The harvesting of the tendon must be done carefully to avoid saphenous nerve iatrogenic injuries and to obtain tendons of adequate length.

With the knee in the figure-four position, a 4-cm longitudinal incision is made on the skin over the tendons which are

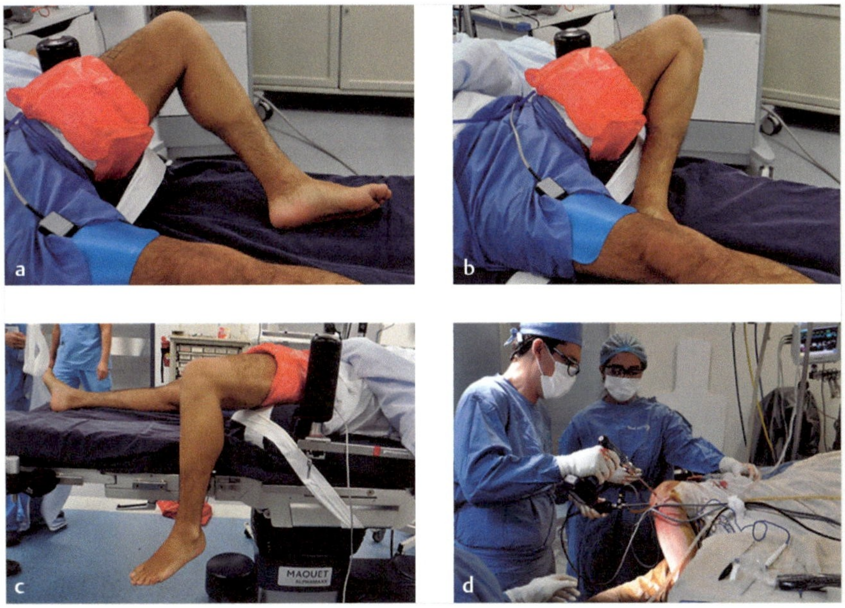

Fig. 22.1 **(a–d)** Patient positioning for hamstring anterior cruciate ligament (ACL) reconstruction.

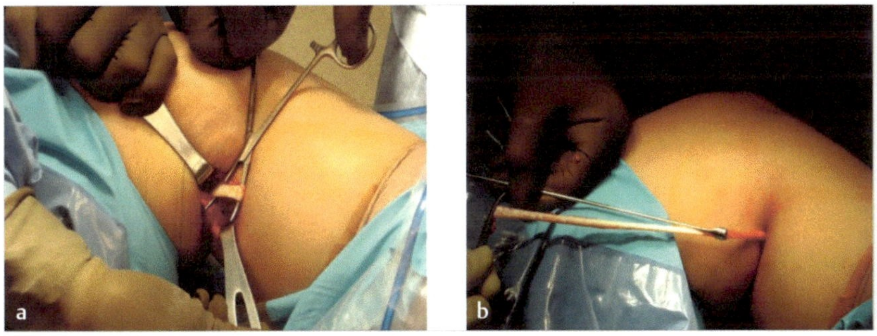

Fig. 22.2 **(a, b)** Alternate posterior harvest from the popliteal crease.

palpated subcutaneously. The incision begins at the height of the anterior tubercle over the medial cortex of the tibia at the union of the anterior third with the medial third of the medial cortex in a distal direction. Blunt dissection of the subcutaneous tissue is done down to the sartorious fascia, the tendon insertion zone is exposed, the most proximal tendon in the proximal edge is palpated and identified (gracilis), and the most anterior edge of the medial collateral ligament (MCL) is also identified. These points of reference are used to incise the sartorious fascia which lies superficial to both tendons; immediately in front of the MCL and proximal to the gracilis tendon. An incision is made down to the periosteum and it is continued distally parallel to the anterior edge of the tibia, forming then an inverted L. The appropriate location is 1.5 cm away from the anterior border being careful not to damage the patellar tendon at the insertion in the anterior tubercle. The length of this vertical part of the incision should be approximately 4 cm to guarantee that both the gracilis and semitendinosus tendon insertions are included. The graft is released from the bone, then the flap is everted, allowing the surgeon to easily identify both tendons deep to the sartorious fascia.

Next both tendons are dissected from the sartorious fascia trying to avoid damaging the fascia so it can be sutured back to its origin. The tendons are separated one at a time from the sartorious fascia starting with the most proximal tendon, the gracilis. The tendon is dissected proximally releasing its vinculum to the gastrocnemius and all of the attachments to the surrounding tissues to avoid the tendon being prematurely amputated when using the tendon stripper. A blunt tendon stripper is preferred to avoid premature amputations of the tendon. The distal end of the tendon is secured with Krakow suture or with a blunt pair of clamps and the tendon stripper is directed proximally toward the ischium, parallel to the tendinous and muscle fibers bypassing the tendon and bringing the stripper deeper to harvest a tendon as long as possible (28–30 cm). The same procedure is repeated with the more distal and thick semitendinosus tendon, which is dissected proximally, releasing every attachment and vinculum; it is essential to look for the accessory attachment to the gastrocnemius muscle to release it. This is the most frequent cause of tendon amputation (▶ Fig. 22.3).

22.10.2 Graft Preparation

The remaining muscle tissue over the tendons is stripped with a blunt dissector from the rest of the tendon graft. The tendon is then folded over itself with the objective of obtaining an 85- to 90-mm-long graft as thick as possible; this is achieved folding the tendons two or three times, in order to have a quadruplet or sextuplet graft. Firm fixation of the graft ends is secured to avoid graft disassembling when introduced into the tibial and femoral tunnels; the distal ends of the graft

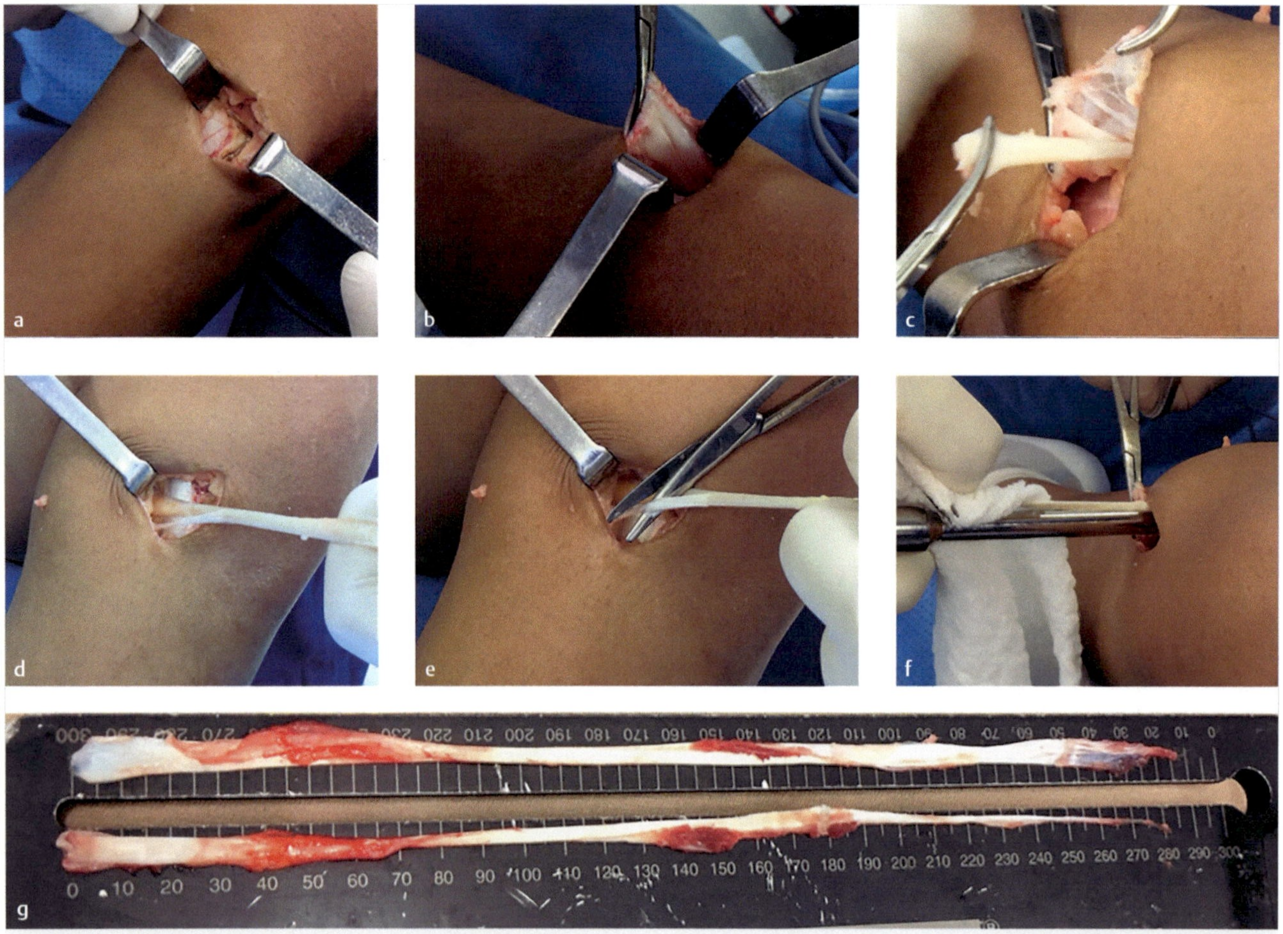

Fig. 22.3 (a–g) Harvest of semitendinosis and gracilis tendons.

are sutured together with Krakow sutures using a #2 suture which also allows the surgeon to obtain additional distal fixation on the tibia using a post and screw. The graft is left in saline solution with antibiotics while the arthroscopy is performed (▶ Fig. 22.4).

22.10.3 Portals

Three portals are generally used.

1. Proximal anterolateral: for notch preparation, located close to the patellar tendon at the level of the distal pole of the patella; the most proximal and central position of this portal allows excellent visualization of the intercondylar zone, the meniscus anterior horn, and the ACL tibial footprint.
2. Proximal anteromedial (that may be replaced by a transpatellar tendon portal): for the general examination, additional procedures, and also becomes the portal for the full visualization of the lateral condyle medial wall, and identifying the anatomical footprint on the ACL on the femur.
3. Accessory distal medial portal: medially located near the medial condyle and immediately proximal to the medial meniscus; this portal is used for the femoral tunnel preparation. Debridement of synovium and fat pad is often necessary to allow clear visualization when the knee is flexed 120 degrees (▶ Fig. 22.5).

22.10.4 Femoral Tunnel Preparation

With the arthroscope through the anteromedial portal, the ACL femoral footprint is visible. In chronic ACL lesions, the footprint is sometimes not as well defined because of fibrosis, sinovitis, and bone remodeling. The remaining ACL stump is easily visualized and can be marked with the electrocautery to identify the center of the anatomical footprint. When the injury is chronic, frequently no stump is found, and it is necessary to find the femoral footprint site with bone anatomic reference points. The intercondylar ridge is located, which is the anterior limit of the anatomical footprint and the bifurcated ridge that divides the anteromedial bundle from the posterolateral bundle corresponding to the center of the femoral footprint, as described by Freddie Fu.

If the ridges are not clearly demarcated, the Watanabe method may be used, which has been recently promoted by Spalding; it includes locating and marking the most proximal and distal margins from the articular cartilage on the condyle-lateral medial wall; in the middle of this area is the center of the femoral footprint. Through the accessory distal medial portal an AWL is introduced (a microfracture AWL is useful) and a pinhole is marked at the center of the ACL footprint. Depending on the tunnel diameter, the AWL is moved anteriorly or posteriorly to ensure that the posterior and proximal walls are spared,

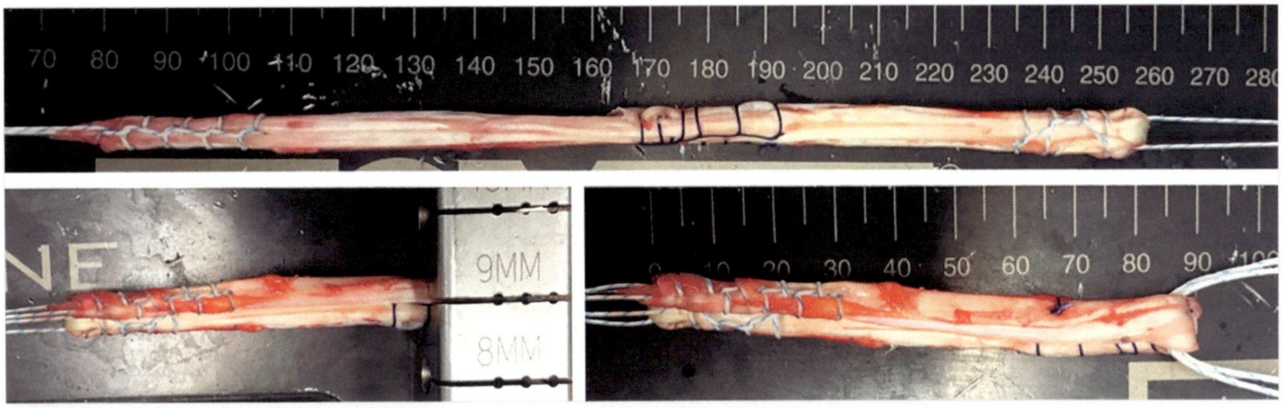

Fig. 22.4 Graft preparation.

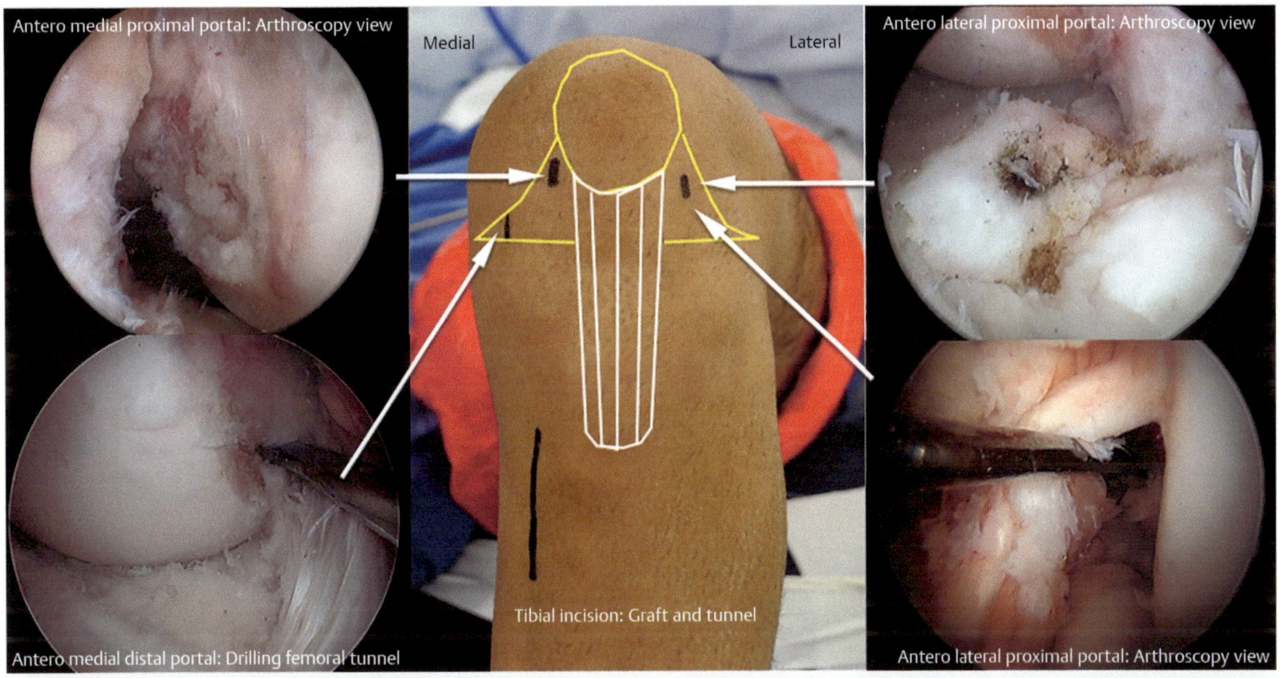

Fig. 22.5 Arthroscopic portals and resulting views.

leaving at least a 2- to 3-mm bone margin. The knee is then flexed 120 degrees (to ensure a femoral tunnel length between 36 and 42 mm deep) and a 2.3-mm guide pin is introduced all the way to the lateral cortex. Drilling the tunnel with flexion under 120 degrees can reduce the tunnel length and reduce the distance between the femoral tunnel and the lateral cortex of the femur risking the femoral cortical fixation. Drilling the femoral tunnel with the knee flexed at an angle over 120 degrees can cause the medial femoral tunnel to be damaged with the drill bit. Once the 2.3-mm guide pin is placed, a cannulated drill bit is introduced and a 30-mm femoral tunnel is drilled. Care must be taken to avoid damaging the proximal and posterior walls of the tunnel, which is very important if interference screw fixation is used. When cortical button fixation is used, a 4.5-mm tunnel is drilled all the way to the lateral femoral cortex with a 4.5-mm cannulated drill bit. The total length of the tunnel is measured, and the final drilling of the femoral tunnel is performed using a drill bit of the same size of the graft diameter, leaving at least 5 mm of distance from the condyle lateral wall to avoid violating the lateral femoral cortex. Fixation is performed with a cortical button (▸ Fig. 22.6).

22.10.5 Tibial Tunnel

With the camera through the anterolateral portal and the knee flexed at 90 degrees, the anatomical tibial reference points of ACL footprint are assessed. When the injury is recent, it is very useful to mark the full periphery of the footprint using an electrocautery or radiofrequency, as well as its central point, where the tunnel guide pin shall be placed. When there are no ACL stumps, to identify the tibial tunnel center, several reference points should be assessed, such as the posterior edge of the anterior horn of the lateral meniscus, the medial tibial spine, the posterior cruciate ligament (PCL), and the posterior horn of the

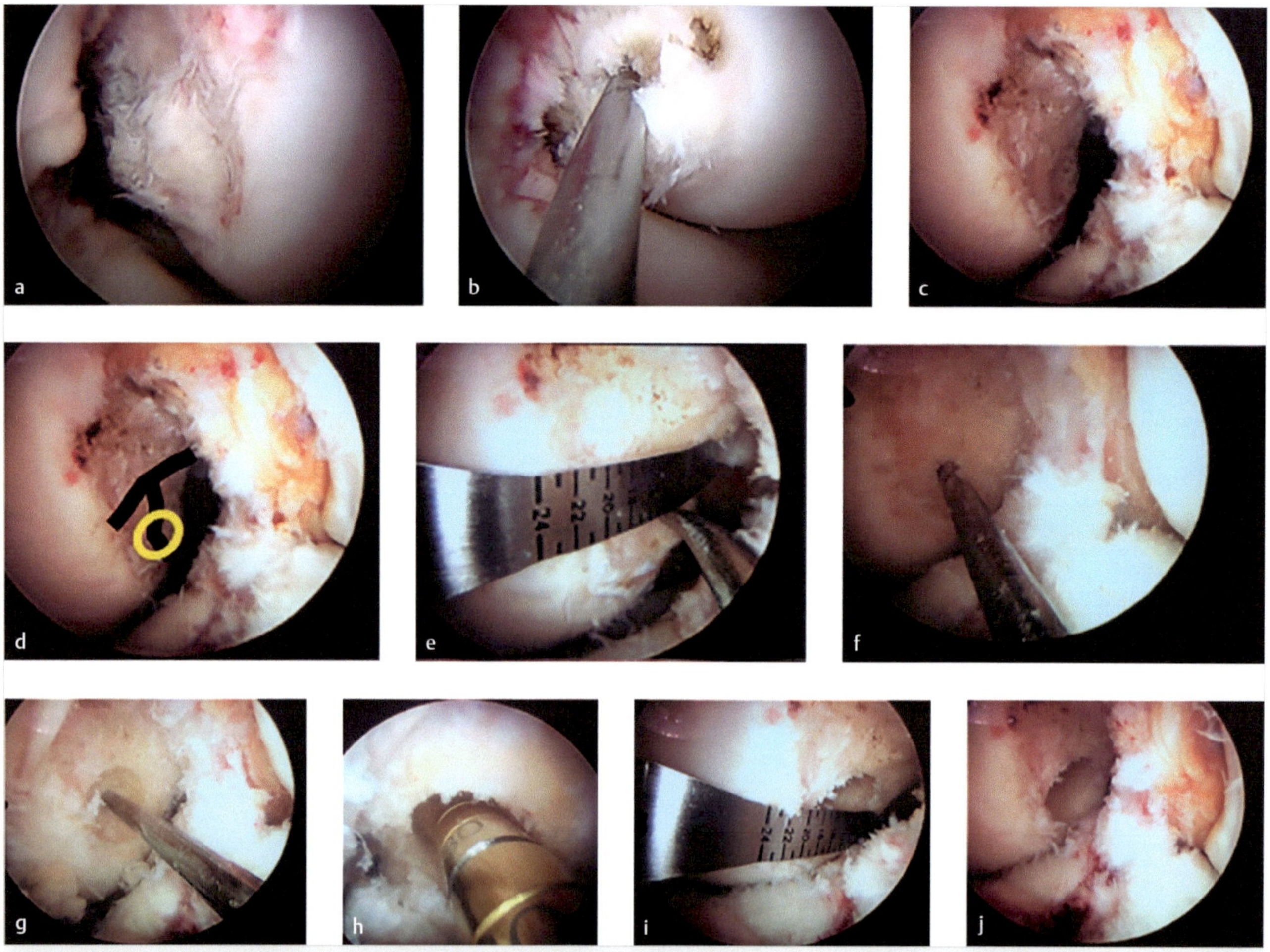

Fig. 22.6 (a–j) Femoral tunnel location and preparation.

lateral meniscus. In order to assess the correct position of the tibial tunnel, once the 2.3-mm guide pin is located at the center of the tibial footprint, a provisional drilling is performed with a cannulated drill bit 2 to 3 mm of less diameter than the final tunnel. The drill bit is brought into the joint through the tibial tunnel and the knee is brought to full extension checking that there is no impingement with the roof of the intercondylar notch, the lateral condyle, or with the PCL; if the assessed tunnel position is not ideal, the drill bit is removed and the 2.3-mm guide pin is inserted again and reoriented to where we would like to correct the tunnel position (anterior, posterior, medial, or lateral); it is placed by hammering it down and introducing it a short distance into the intercondylar fossa roof while the final tunnel is drilled, guaranteeing optimal anatomical position of the tibial tunnel in the footprint (▸ Fig. 22.7).

22.10.6 ACL Graft Passage

With the camera placed in the anteromedial portal, the femoral tunnel is visualized and through the accessory medial portal a 2.3-mm guide pin is introduced into the femoral tunnel; a #1 suture is passed through the tunnel leaving an intra-articular loop which is drawn through the tibial tunnel with a grasping clamp. In this way the #1 suture passes through both the tibial and femoral tunnels. Next the traction sutures on the graft are passed through the loop of the #1 suture and they are pulled into the tibial tunnel and into the femoral tunnel by pulling from the proximal ends of the #1 suture on the femoral side. It is very important to have accurate femoral and tibial tunnel diameters in order for the graft to fit as tight as possible in the tunnels to increase stability and to favor graft integration and healing 360 degrees around the tunnel walls.

22.10.7 Femoral Fixation

During fixation, tension on the graft must be maintained to guarantee a symmetrical fixation in the femoral tunnel. If femoral fixation is performed with an interference screw, a Nitinol guide is inserted through the accessory distal medial portal, placed between the anterior edge of the femoral tunnel and the graft; the interference screw (cannulated with blunt-atraumatic threads for soft tissue, with the same diameter than the tunnel or 1 mm wider for patients with poor bone quality) is screwed until it is sunk 2 to 3 mm deep into the femoral tunnel. If a cortical button fixation is chosen, during the introduction of the graft, the button should bypass completely the 4.5-mm tunnel to ensure fixation on the lateral cortex of the femoral condyle. Care must be taken not

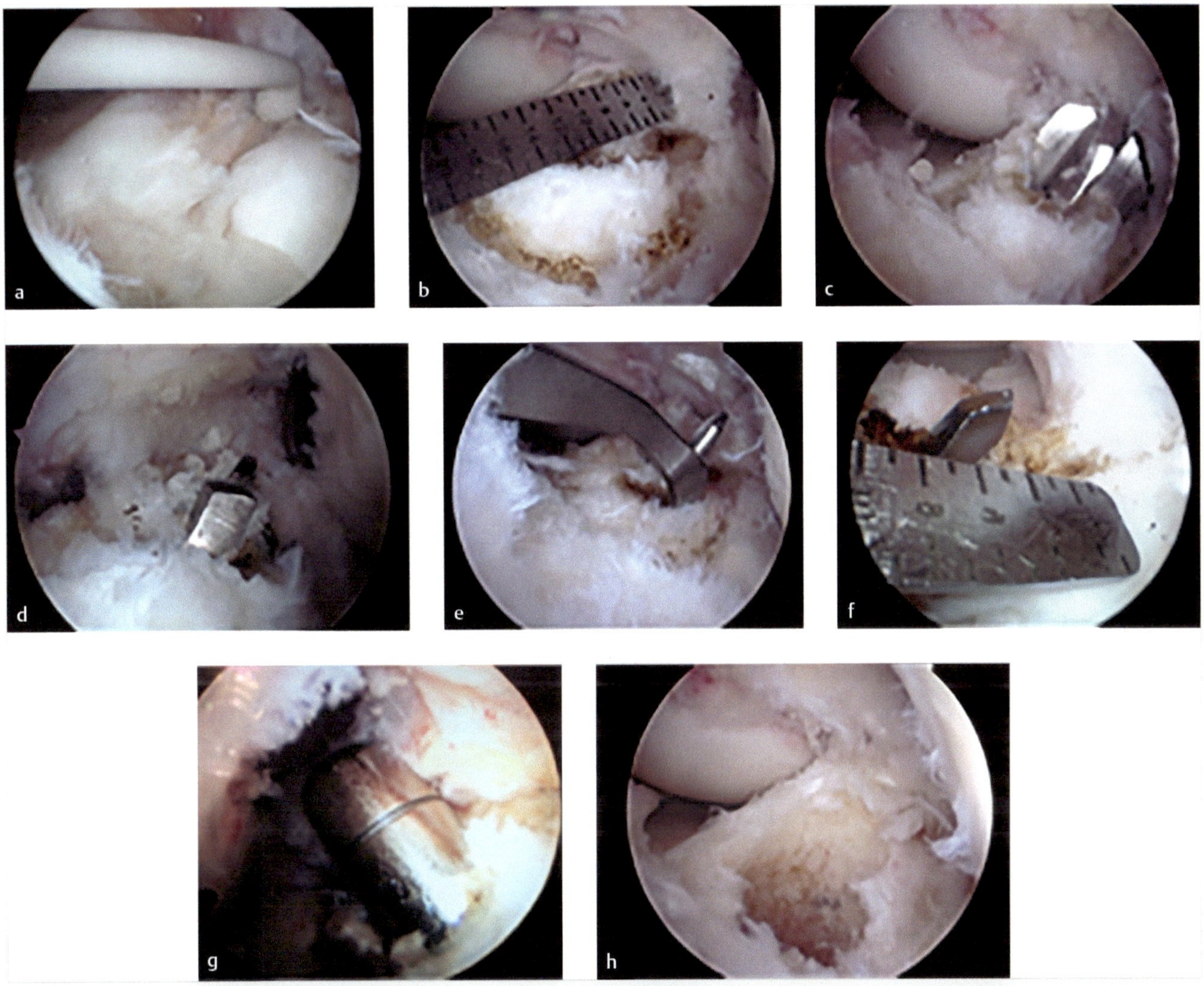

Fig. 22.7 (a–h) Tibial tunnel location and preparation.

to drive the button into the soft tissues of the thigh compromising the femoral fixation (▶ Fig. 22.8).

22.10.8 Graft Prestressing

With approximately 40 lb of traction on the graft, 20 repetitions of knee flexion and extension are made to prestress the graft. It is important to verify, particularly with adjustable cortical buttons, that the graft has not been pulled back in order to make the necessary corrections.

22.10.9 Tibial Tunnel Graft Tension and Fixation

With the knee flexed at 10 degrees, sustained traction of the graft is performed at approximately 40 lb of tension, and the graft is fixed at the tibial tunnel with an interference screw 1 mm or 2 mm wider than the tibial tunnel diameter. Additional fixation is performed on the tibia using the sutures in the distal ends of the graft over a 6.5-mm screw and washer. Partially threaded screws are preferred to avoid cutting the sutures while attaching them to the screw.

22.10.10 Final Checking and Wound Closure

At the end of the procedure, the graft position and adequate tension with no impingement are verified with arthroscopy; articular lavage is performed to remove debris generated by bone drilling and final hemostasis is obtained. Portals are closed with #3–0 nonabsorbable monofilament suture.

For postoperative analgesia, a cocktail is prepared with 20 mL of levobupivacaine 0.75% without epinephrine, 1 mg of hydromorphone or 5 mg of morphine; this mix is diluted in 50 mL of saline solution in order to obtain an adequate dilution of the anesthetic to avoid chondrocyte toxicity. The medial anterior wound is initially infiltrated, then the grafting zone, the sartorial fascia, the subcutaneous tissue, and the skin, with emphasis on the anatomical area of the saphenous nerve. Twenty mL of the mix is left for articular infiltration; once closure is done. The medial anterior wound is sutured by planes; initially, with separate stitches with a #0 absorbable suture, the sartorial fascia is reinserted into the periosteum over the graft donor site covering also the tibial tunnel area. Next, the subcutaneous tissue is closed with a #2 absorbable multifilament with separate

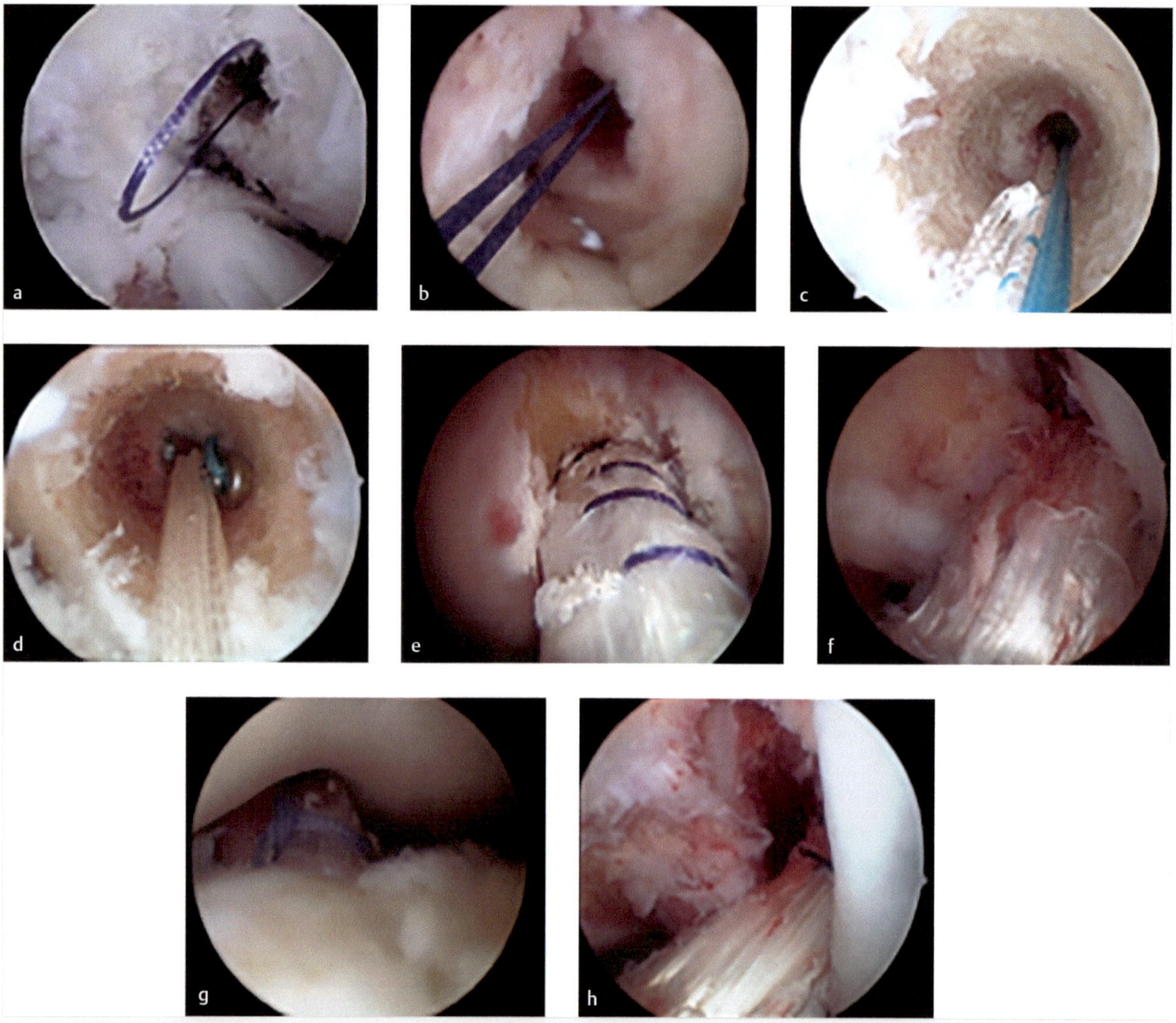

Fig. 22.8 (a–h) Graft path and femoral fixation.

sutures, and finally the skin with a subdermal suture with a # 3monofilament.

22.10.11 Postoperative Care

During the first week, ice is placed over the area. After the first day, muscle activation exercises, including isometrics, active range of motion, and walking with partial weight bearing on two crutches are initiated.

On the seventh postoperation (PO) day, the bandage is removed, wounds are checked—without removing the stitches, the patient is encouraged to continue with articular mobility, quadriceps isometric contraction, and gait exercises with progressive full weight bearing on two crutches. On the fourteenth PO day, skin suture stitches are removed and 0- to 90-degree range of motion is verified. After the second PO week, an accelerated rehabilitation protocol is initiated so that the patient can walk with full weight bearing, without aid by the third or fourth week, full articular maximum mobility by the sixth week, and proprioception exercises after the eighth week. After the fourth month, specific sport field work is initiated as long as the patient has achieved full range of motion, and recovered at least 80% extensor and flexor strength compared to the contralateral extremity, in order to reach competitive levels by the sixth to the ninth month.

22.11 Bailout, Rescue, Salvage Procedures

If the graft is amputated and is too short, the surgeon will either have to change to a different autograft source, or use an allograft to complete the ACL reconstruction.

22.12 Pitfalls

Care must be taken to avoid damage to the saphenous nerve during graft harvest.

23 Anterior Cruciate Reconstruction—Patellar Tendon Autograft

Marcio Albers and Freddie Fu†

23.1 Description

Anterior cruciate ligament reconstruction (ACLR) can be successfully performed using different graft options. The use of the patellar tendon autograft with bone blocks from the tibial tubercle and the patella, respectively, at the distal and proximal parts of the graft, has traditionally been called bone-tendon-bone (BTB) technique. The contemporary individualized anatomic ACLR technique allows for optimum utilization of this traditionally used graft, with the ultimate goal to restore knee function to preinjury levels. A thorough preoperative evaluation using radiographs and magnetic resonance imaging, as well as intraoperative evaluation of the native anterior cruciate ligament footprint and intercondylar notch morphology, warrants precise indication, thus yielding superior results and avoiding common complications.

23.2 Key Principles

The use of BTB autograft, when performing an individualized anatomic ACLR, yields favorable conditions for optimum graft integration, as bone-to-bone healing occurs. The intratunnel bone healing is responsible for decreased graft creep when the whole construct (fixation and graft) is considered. This combination allows for earlier return to play when compared to soft tissue-only graft options, with similar retear rates.

23.3 Expectations

The use of BTB graft is particularly instrumental in cases of competitive or high-demand athletes that would like to risk an earlier return to sports, after a minimum 6 months individualized rehabilitation program.

23.4 Indications

- Single bundle ACLR.
- Patella tendon sagittal thickness ≥ 5 mm (▶ Fig. 23.1a).
- Athletes who require medial stabilizers for sports-specific tasks (judo, sky, soccer).

23.5 Contraindications

- Kneeling-related sports activities or lifestyle.
- Narrow intercondylar notch.
- Graft length mismatch.
- Chronic patella tendon degeneration.
- Open physis.

23.6 Special Considerations

Detailed preoperative evaluation of the patient-specific needs and expectations, physical examination, flexion weight bearing and long cassette-standing radiographs, and magnetic resonance imaging (MRI) should be obtained. High-resolution ultrasound for quantitative and qualitative assessment of all the available graft options has been used systematically as part of the preoperative evaluation. The ACL tibial footprint sagittal length can be easily measured on the MRI. If it is longer than 18 mm, double-bundle ACLR should be considered (▶ Fig. 23.1b).

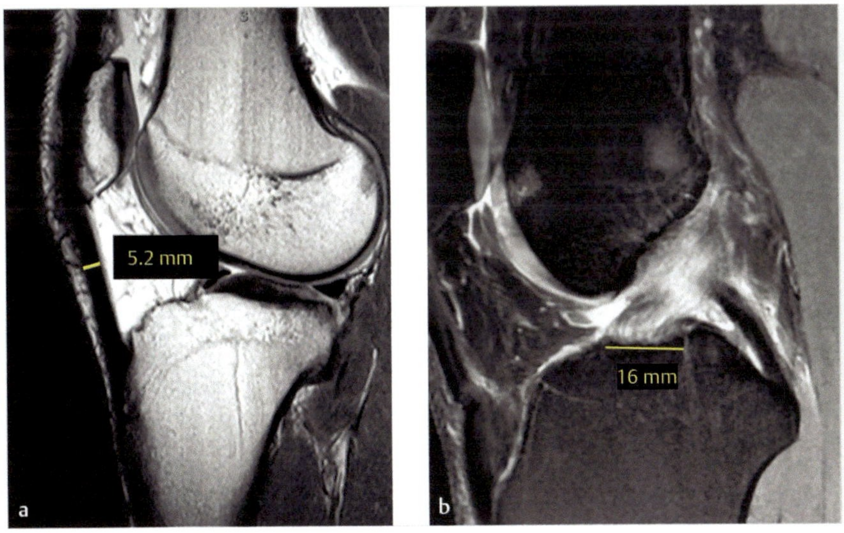

Fig. 23.1 **(a)** Preoperative magnetic resonance imaging (MRI) measurement of the patella tendon thickness on the sagittal plane, measured 15 mm distal to the inferior pole of the patella. **(b)** Preoperative MRI evaluation of the anterior cruciate ligament (ACL) tibial remnant showing a sagittal length of 16 mm.

† Deceased

23.7 Special Instructions, Positioning, and Anesthesia

- General endotracheal anesthesia with femoral and sciatic peripheral nerve blocks.
- Patient is positioned supine on the operating table.
- Operative knee is positioned in a leg holder allowing at least 120 degrees of flexion to full extension.
- Contralateral lower extremity is placed on a leg holder with the hip flexed and abducted to help prevent nerve injury.

23.8 Tips, Pearls, and Lessons Learned

The portals' placement is key for good arthroscopic visualization (▶ Fig. 23.2).

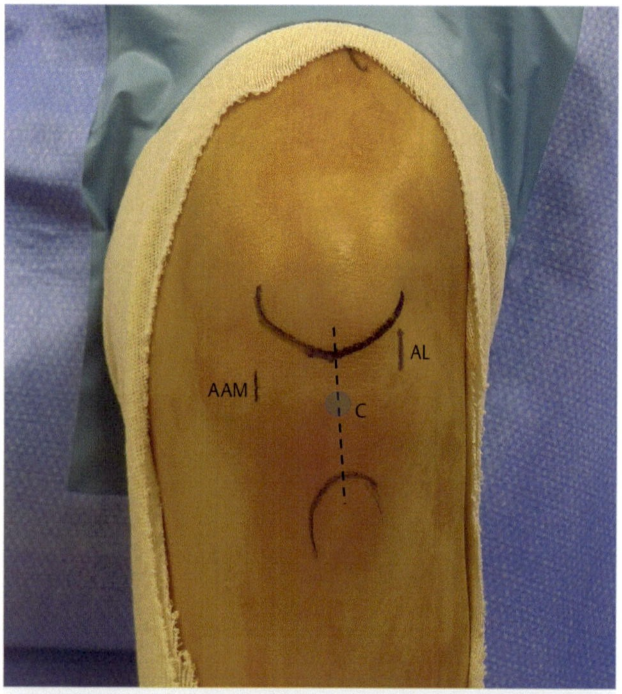

Fig. 23.2 Portals. The anterolateral portal (AL) is placed more proximally to allow optimum visualization of the tibial structures. The central portal (C) is placed through central portion of the patella tendon, while the accessory anteromedial portal is placed as medial as it is possible, ensuring that no damage to the medial femoral condyle will occur when drilling the femoral tunnels.

The high anterolateral portal allows for excellent visualization of the native tibial ACL footprint. The accessory anteromedial and central portals are ideally used as both visualization and work portals. The central portal should be done through the graft harvest site.

If the tibial remnant is not clearly demarcated, the tibial guide pin should be placed in line with the central portion of the anterior horn of the lateral meniscus. The ACL femoral native footprint (▶ Fig. 23.3) is better seen through the accessory anteromedial portal. In chronic cases, the bony landmarks should be used. The rotation of the camera by 90 degrees makes it easier to identify the residents' ridge (▶ Fig. 23.4).

23.9 Difficulties Encountered

During graft insertion via the tibial tunnel, the femoral-sided bone block may get stuck while flipping at the aperture of the tunnel. The use of the probe to aid the proximal bone block to achieve the correct orientation often warrants a smooth graft insertion. This may be particularly difficult in narrower intercondylar notches (▶ Fig. 23.4).

23.10 Key Procedural Steps

Graft harvesting aims to obtain 10 mm wide by 8 mm long bone blocks from the tibial tuberosity and distal patella. The bone plugs should be trapezoidal in shape which is easily achieved by slightly inclining the oscillating saw. Bone block preparation follows with the use of compression pliers that will create cylindrical bony plugs at each side of the graft. Excess bone is removed with a rongeur. The patella bone block is prepared for a button fixation device, while the tibial bone block is prepared with two strong sutures to allow adequate tension of the graft during fixation (▶ Fig. 23.5).

The ACL remnant is debrided to allow optimum visualization of both the tibial and femoral native footprints. With the knee in maximum flexion (over 120 degrees), femoral tunnel preparation is initiated at the center of the footprint with a microfracture awl. Flexible guide pins are used to protect the medial femoral condyle chondral surface and to allow for longer tunnels. The tunnel is drilled to the size of the bone block or 0.5 mm larger to avoid difficulties with the graft insertion. The tibial guide pins are then placed with the aid of a standard ACL guide at 55 degrees, aiming for the center of the native insertion site. After confirming the anatomic position, a coring reamer 1 to 2 mm smaller than the final tunnel diameter is used at first.

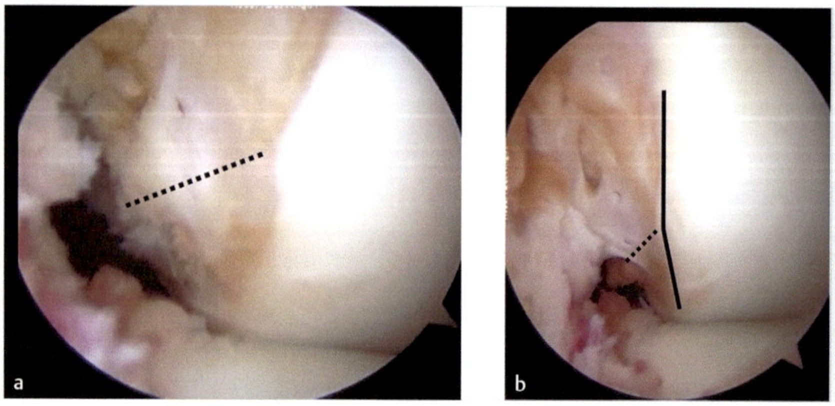

Fig. 23.3 **(a)** The femoral insertion site visualization is better achieved with the camera turned 90 degrees, as shown in **(b)**. The dotted line represents the residents' ridge, while the solid lines highlight the subtle inclination angle between the anterior cruciate ligament (ACL) native insertion site and the remainder of the lateral wall of the intercondylar notch.

Dilators are then used at 0.5-mm increments until the desired size. The bone cylinders recovered from the coring reamer are used to bone graft the defects at both the patella and the tibial tuberosity.

Insertion of the graft via the tibial tunnel is performed (▶ Fig. 23.6). The probe is used to help the femoral bone block insertion. Fluoroscopy is used to ensure the button is flipped.

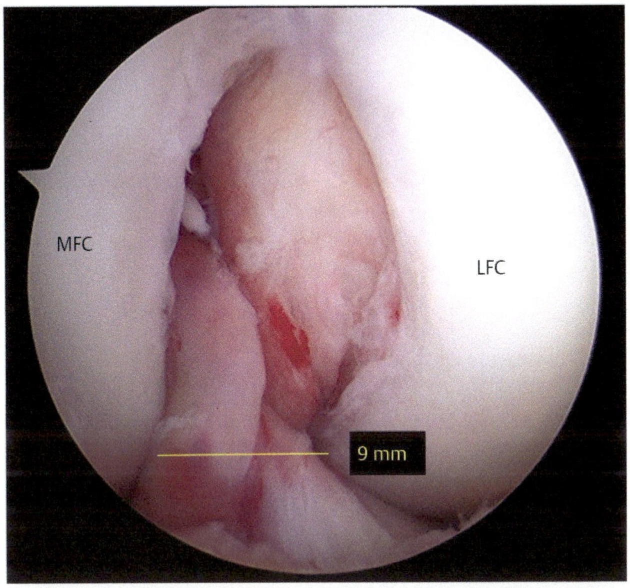

Fig. 23.4 Narrow intercondylar notches result in difficulties when inserting the graft in the femoral tunnel.

Tibial fixation with nonabsorbable interference screw (polyether ether ketone [PEEK]) is performed with the knee at 20 degrees of flexion. The bone chips recovered from the coring reamer are then used to fill in the donor areas of the patella and tibia.

23.11 Bailout, Rescue, and Salvage Procedures

If the bone blocks have different diameters, the graft can be prepared for insertion via the accessory anteromedial portal. In this case, strong sutures should be passed through the tibial bone block. The femoral bone block is inserted the standard way, being pulled by the button sutures, while the tibial bone block is inserted in a retrograde fashion.

23.12 Pitfalls

The femoral insertion of the graft can be difficult. Drilling the femoral tunnel 0.5 mm wider than the bone block and smoothing the border of the aperture with the shaver warrant a smoother insertion.

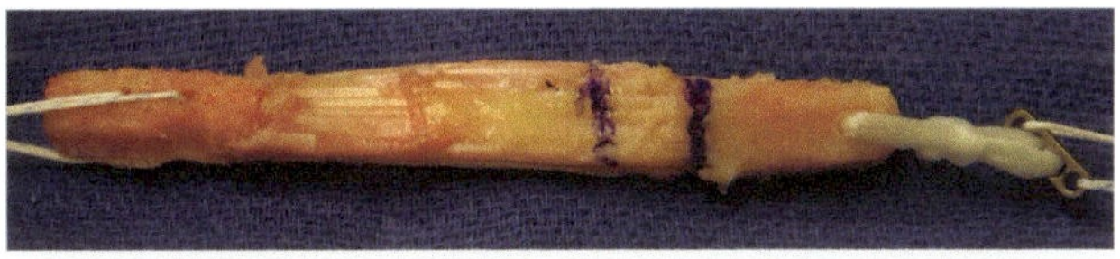

Fig. 23.5 Bone-tendon-bone (BTB) graft prepared with a closed loop button on the proximal end and two strong sutures on the distal end.

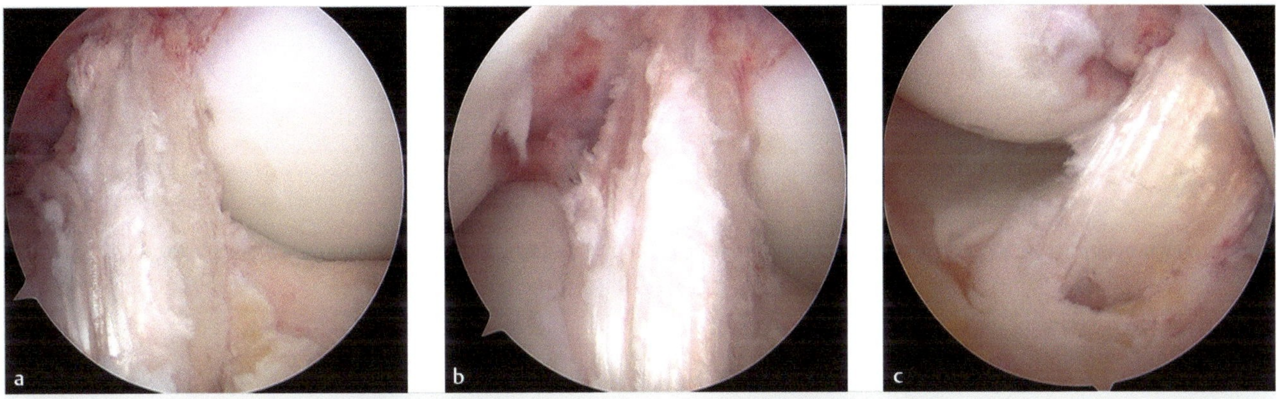

Fig. 23.6 The final aspect of the anatomic anterior cruciate ligament (ACL) reconstruction, views from the accessory anteromedial portal **(a)**, central portal **(b)**, and anterolateral portal **(c)**.

24 Anterior Cruciate Ligament Reconstruction—Pediatric Patient

Diego da Costa Astur and Moises Cohen

24.1 Description

The anterior cruciate ligament (ACL) is an important structure in the knee, as it resists anterior instability and internal rotation of the tibia. It does not heal following mid-substance tears, and surgical reconstruction is the standard treatment among active patients. Most ACL reconstruction techniques involve transphyseal tibial and femoral tunnels. In the pediatric population, transphyseal tunnels mean the possibility of causing a physeal injury, resulting in abnormal bone growth or angular deformities from the lower limb (▶ Fig. 24.1).

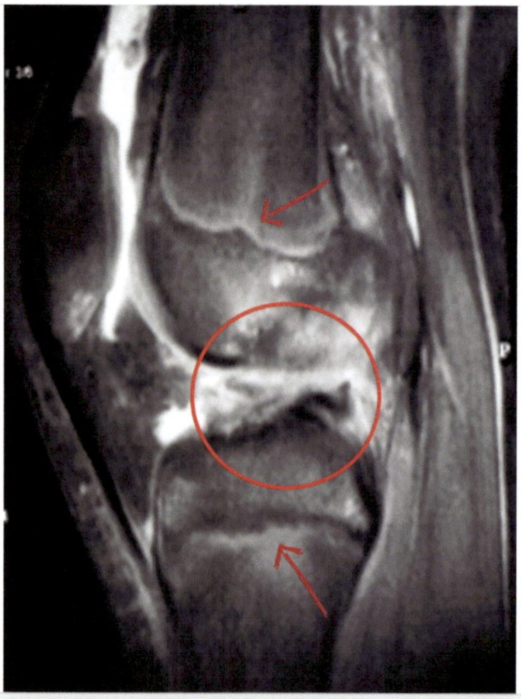

Fig. 24.1 Sagittal magnetic resonance image (MRI) with an anterior cruciate ligament (ACL) tear (*red circle*) in an open physis (*red arrow*) knee.

24.2 Key Principles

Improved understanding of the anatomy of the knee combined with the development of new surgical techniques minimizes the risk of physeal injury with ACL reconstruction. Respecting the growth potential of patients with open physes and choosing the most appropriate surgical technique have yielded high success rates without growth disturbances.

24.3 Expectations

- To stabilize the knee without causing a growth disturbance.
- Treat associated meniscal and chondral injuries.
- To allow return to sports and child's daily activities after treatment.

24.4 Indications

Traumatic ACL tear in an active pediatric patient with an unstable knee.

24.5 Contraindications

There are no contraindications to ACL reconstruction in the pediatric population. However, there are different surgical techniques, and the surgeon must choose the appropriate technique according to growth potential of the child. It can be measured using radiographic images (▶ Fig. 24.2) or physical characteristics that can classify these patients according to Tanner stages (▶ Fig. 24.3).

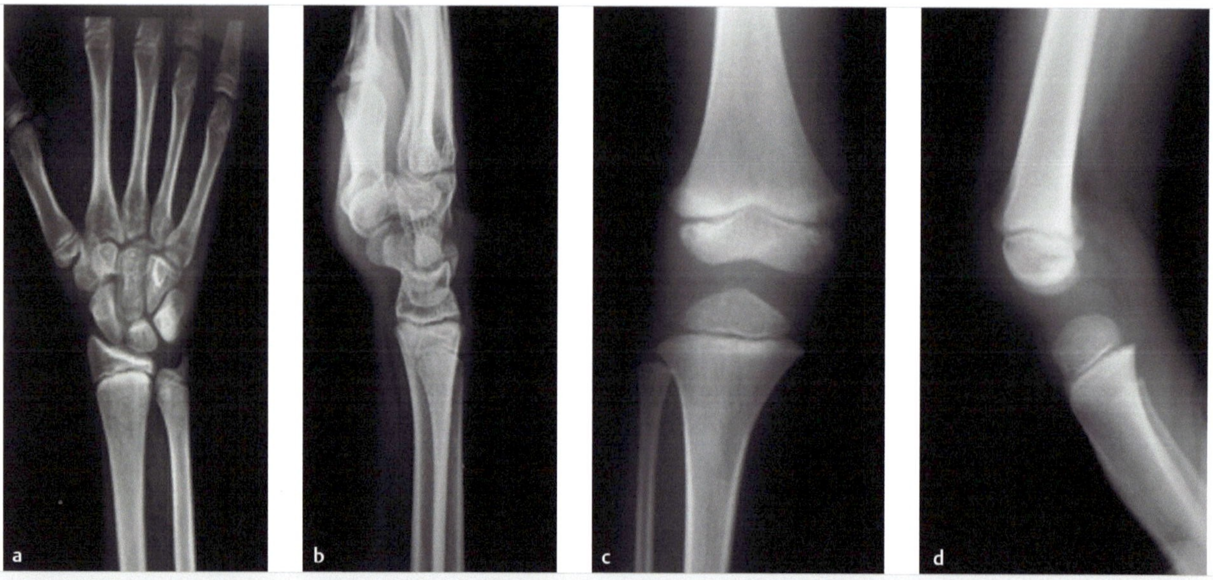

Fig. 24.2 X-ray images to estimate bone age. **(a,b)** Anteroposterior and lateral X-rays view from the wrist and **(c,d)** an open physis anteroposterior and lateral X-rays view from the knee.

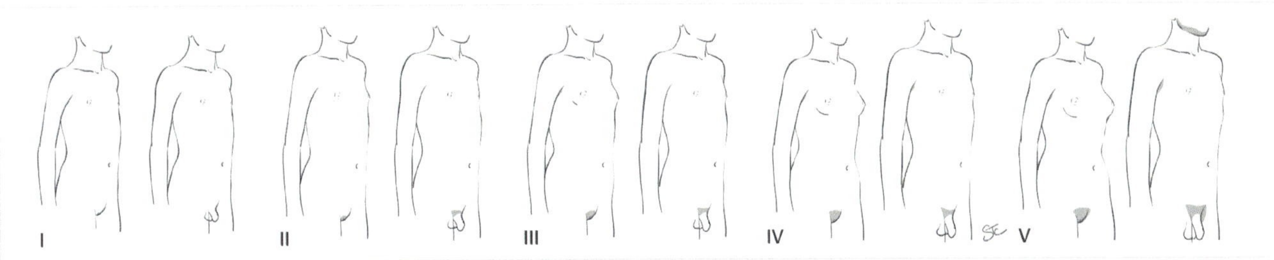

Fig. 24.3 Tanner stages described according to physical measurements of development based on external primary and secondary sex characteristics, such as testicular volume, development of pubic hair, size of the breasts and genitals.

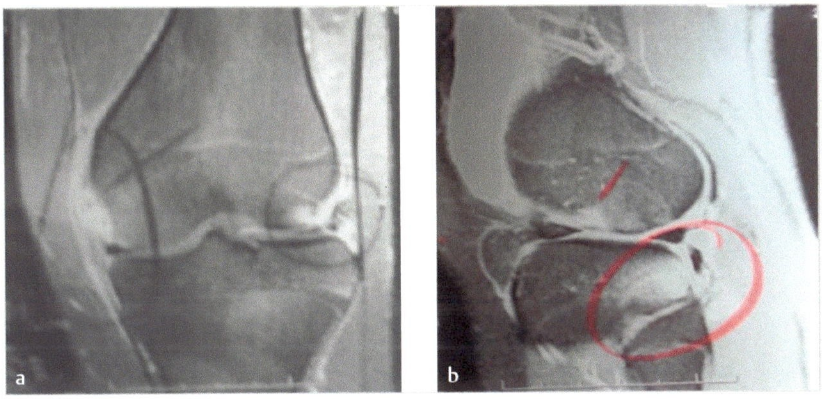

Fig. 24.4 (a,b) Meniscal injuries from a young patient who prefers not to do anterior cruciate ligament (ACL) reconstruction but return to her practice 3 months after injury.

24.6 Special Considerations

Classically, pediatric patients with an ACL injury were instructed to avoid sports and high-risk activities until sufficient bone maturity was achieved to perform conventional ACL reconstruction. Traditional surgical techniques include tibial and femoral tunnels that pass through the growth plate (transphyseal technique), risking a physeal injury in the pediatric population. Physeal injuries can result in lower limb deformities and abnormal bone growth. In practice, it is very difficult for pediatric athletes to avoid high-risk activities. In most cases of this conservative treatment method, the child develops associated meniscal or cartilage injuries resulting from the constant use of an unstable knee (▶ Fig. 24.4). Contemporary treatment recommendations reflect the belief that the risk of physeal injury is lower than the risk of associated intra-articular injuries of the knee in unstable patients. This has led to the recommendation of ACL reconstruction in patients with an open physis.

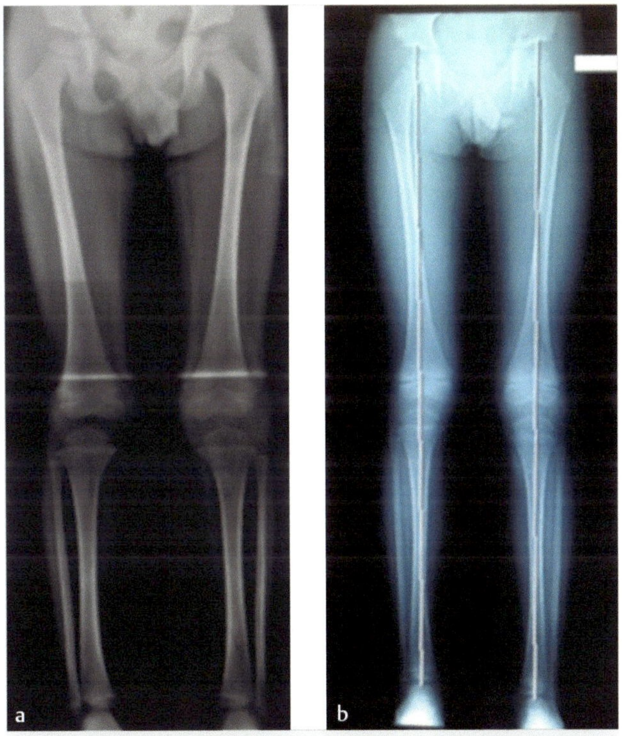

Fig. 24.5 (a,b) Lower limbs' radiographic scan is important before and after surgery to be sure that any growth disturbances resulting in leg-length discrepancies and angular deformities are happening.

24.7 Special Instructions, Positioning, and Anesthesia

ACL arthroscopic reconstruction with hamstring tendon autograft is the authors' preferred choice. Patients are positioned in a supine position and anesthesia varies from general to regional (spinal) anesthesia.

24.8 Tips, Pearls, and Lessons Learned

- A lower limb radiographic scan preoperatively demonstrating no limb length discrepancy or angular deformity is essential for comparison during follow-up (▶ Fig. 24.5).
- Associated injuries must be treated. Repair meniscal injuries if possible.
- Re-examine knee stability under anesthesia. Younger patients can adapt to their knee instability and to fool providers during preoperative evaluations.

24.9 Difficulties Encountered

The main difficulties are small bones, small epiphysis, and small graft size. These characteristics make it difficult to perform the technique and lead to a learning curve to obtain the best results.

24.10 Key Procedural Steps

Estimating the skeletal age of the pediatric patient and evaluating their clinical characteristics can help surgeons to decide the best treatment. The younger the skeletal age, the greater the risk of a growth disturbance as a result of ACL reconstruction. In our decision-making process, we use Tanner staging of sexual maturation. Tanner stage I and II patients are prepubescents, Tanner stage III are pubescents, and Tanner stage IV are postpubescents. We customize our ACL reconstruction techniques based on the patients' Tanner stage.

Tanner I: Patients are treated with surgical reconstruction using an extra-articular technique. A standard arthroscopic evaluation of the knee joint is done. Following this, a lateral approach is performed at the patients' thigh to dissect and harvest a portion of the iliotibial band. The graft is passed from the lateral condyle to the medial condyle through the anteromedial arthroscopic portal. After stitching one end of the graft at the posterior zone of the lateral femoral condyle, the loose end of the graft, located at the anteromedial approach, is pulled with forceps passing by the intercondyle notch, diving into the joint, heading to the proximal aspect of the tibia. The loose end of the graft is then fixed distal to the proximal tibial physis through anchor stitches (▶ Fig. 24.6 and ▶ Fig. 24.7).

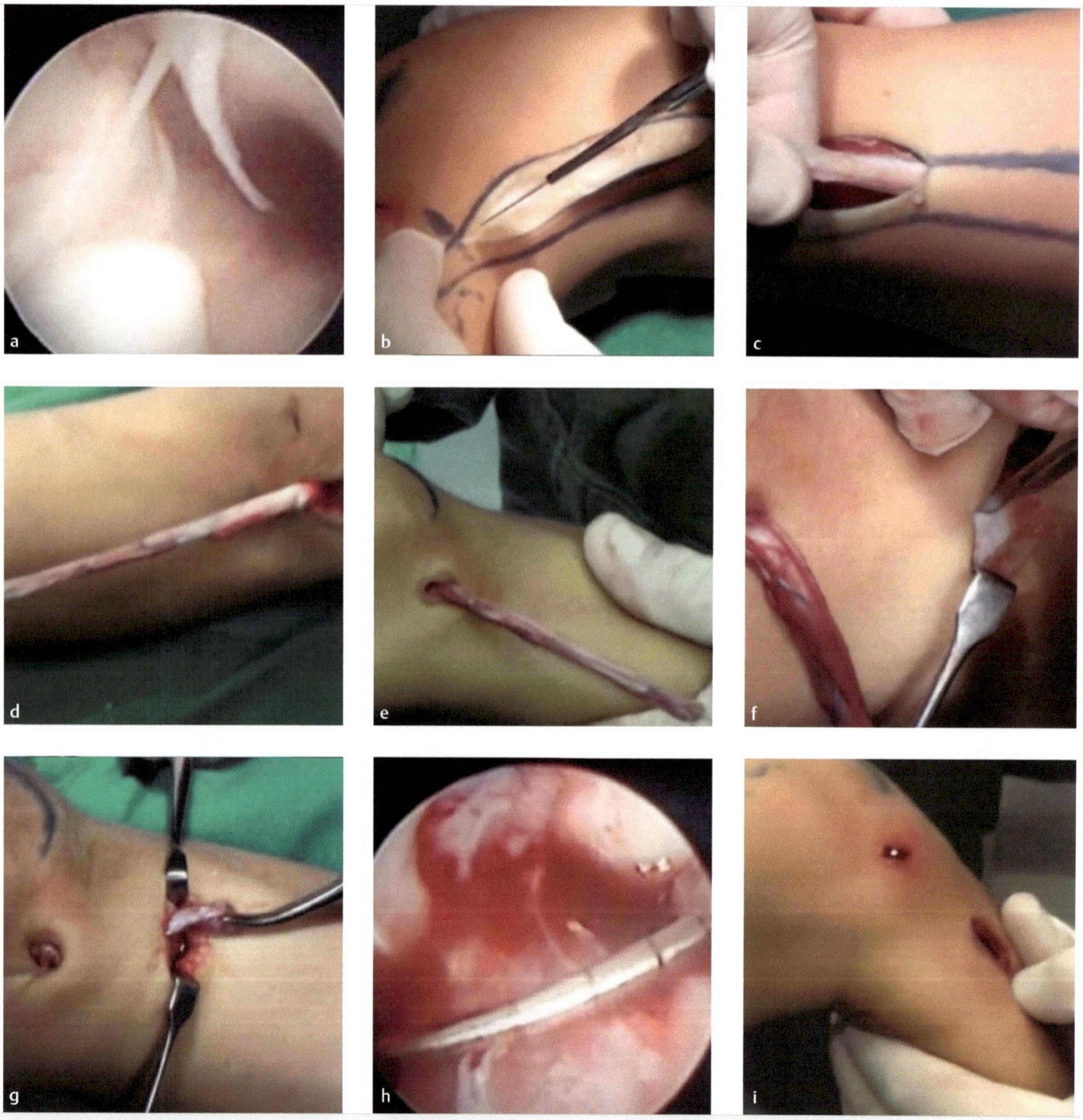

Fig. 24.6 Surgical procedure aspect of an extra-articular anterior cruciate ligament (ACL) reconstruction on the left knee **(a–i)**. **(a)** Arthroscopic visualization of the torn ACL. **(b)** Lateral approach to the thigh with visualization of the iliotibial band. **(c)** Isolation of the middle third of the iliotibial band. **(d)** Proximal detachment of the iliotibial band graft maintaining its distal insertion to Gerdy tubercle. **(e)** Tubulization of the graft. **(f)** Anteromedial proximal incision on the leg. **(g)** Graft is passed over-the-top, intra-articular from lateral to medial. **(h)** Arthroscopic view of the new-ligament. **(i)** Clinical evaluation with proved stability of the knee.

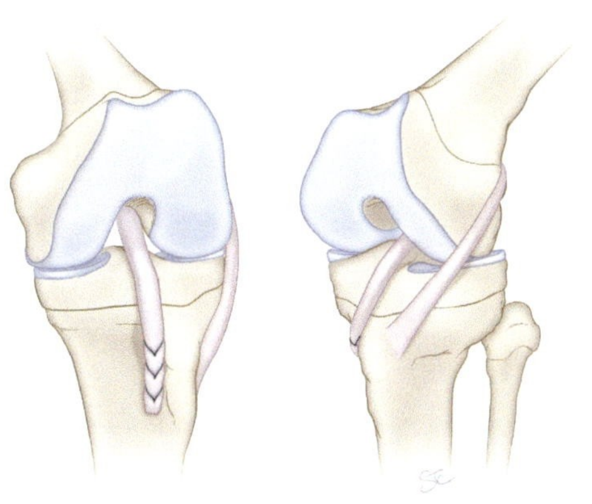

Fig. 24.7 Illustrative surgical technique (Kocher)—Physeal sparing, combined intra-articular and extra-articular reconstruction with use of an autogenous iliotibial band for prepubescent patients.

Tanner II: Intra-articular fixation of the graft is performed on the epiphysis of the femur and the tibia. It is possible to perform the femoral and tibial tunnel without damaging the growth plate, and the patient receives a more functional and anatomic reconstruction compared to extra-articular techniques (▶ Fig. 24.8, ▶ Fig. 24.9, ▶ Fig. 24.10).

Tanner III and IV: Transphyseal ACL reconstruction. After harvesting hamstring tendons, intra-articular arthroscopic examination is performed using standard methods. The tibial and femoral tunnels are drilled in the same way it is done in the adult patient. In order to avoid large femoral physis damage, it is recommended to ream the femoral tunnel more vertical than usual. Suspensory fixation is used on the femur with interference screw fixation on the tibia.

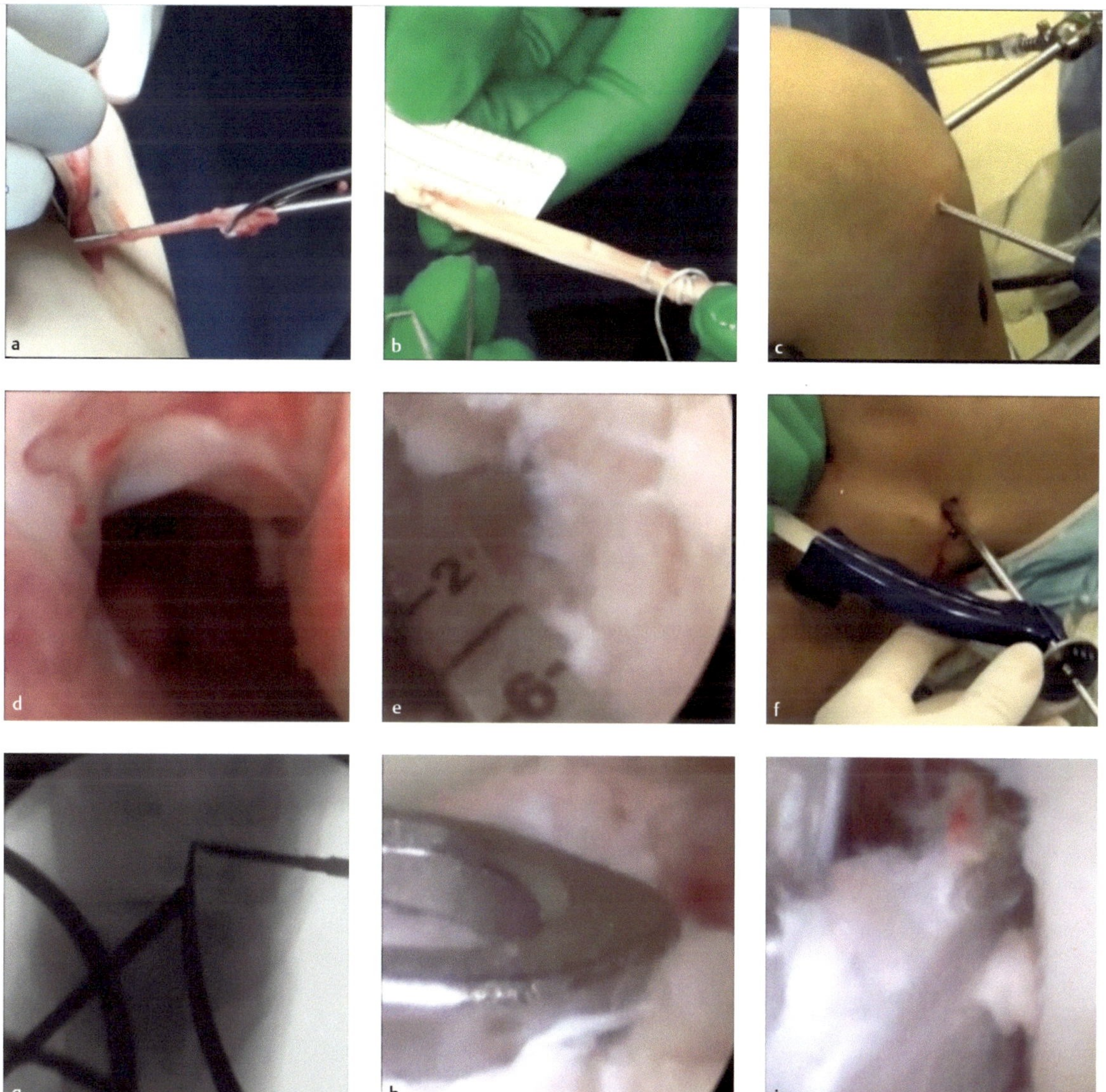

Fig. 24.8 A partial epiphyseal quadruple-hamstring anterior cruciate ligament (ACL) reconstruction. A 4-cm vertical incision made over the proximal medial tibia **(a)** to allow harvest of the gracilis and semitendinosus tendons in standard fashion **(b)**. Knee arthroscopy is performed through the standard anteromedial and anterolateral portals **(c)** and the remnants of the ACL are removed. **(d)** RetroDrill guide is inserted through the anterolateral portal and anatomic femoral footprint was defined. **(e)** A K-wire is placed percutaneously through the lateral femoral condyle from outside. **(f)** Intraoperative radiograph view is important to be sure physis are safe during K-wires and drill passage. **(g)** Tibial tunnel was prepared drilling through tibial physis because this patient was too young and epiphysis size was too small **(h)**. Final autograft view after tibial and femoral fixation with buttons **(i)**.

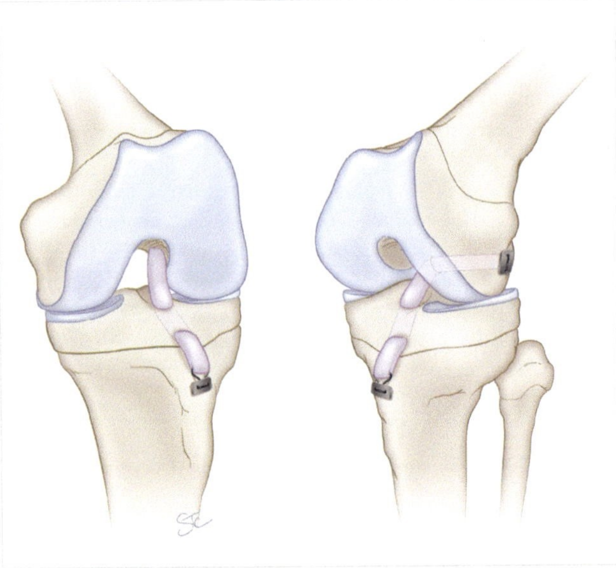

Fig. 24.9 Illustrative surgical technique–Trans epiphyseal ACL reconstruction technique. The physes of the distal femur and proximal tibia are not drilled, keeping them intact.

24.11 Bailout, Rescue, Salvage Procedures

The number of failures in pediatric ACL reconstructions is increasing. As this occurs, revision procedures may be necessary, making surgery more difficult and decreasing the number of good results.

Patients undergoing extra-articular techniques will need a standard intra-articular reconstruction after they reach maturity in most cases.

24.12 Pitfalls

- Cooperative Tanner I patients can be treated nonsurgically at the beginning of their treatment.
- Non-cooperative Tanner I patients will develop associated injuries in their knee with delayed surgical protocols. These injuries are a good indication for extra-articular ACL reconstruction, even as a temporary procedure.
- Sometimes, Tanner II patients submitted to trans-epiphyseal techniques don`t have sufficient tibial epiphysis for screw fixation. In these cases, it is possible to combine

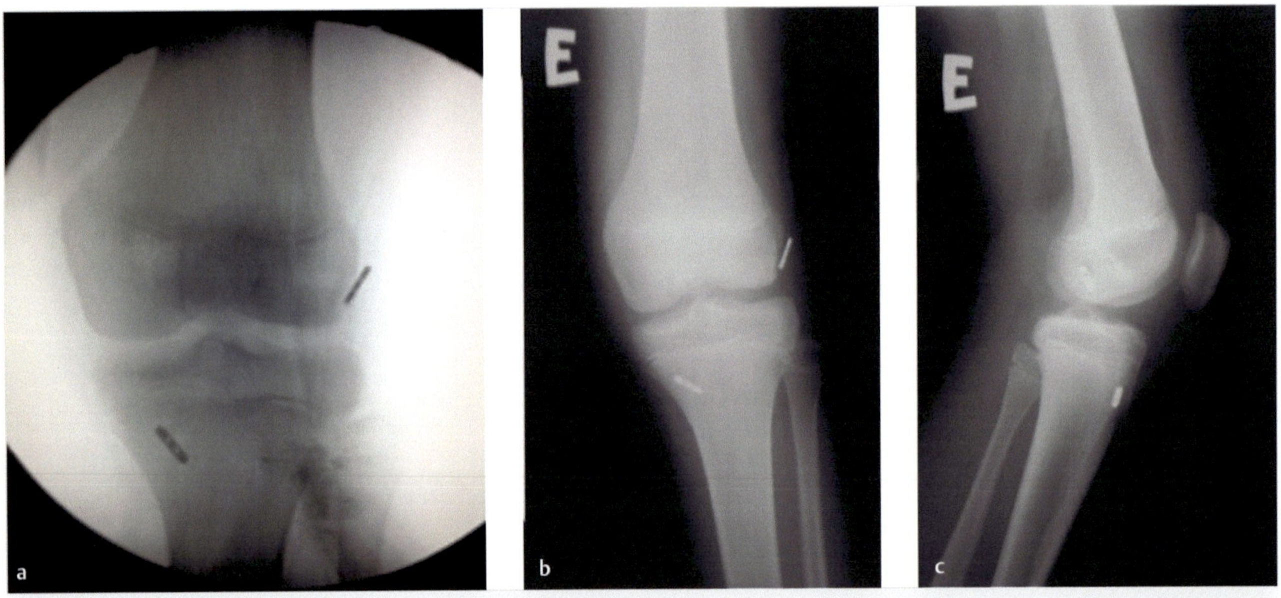

Fig. 24.10 (a–c) Intraoperative radiograph and anteroposterior and lateral x-rays view from the knee with tibial and femoral graft fixation with buttons.

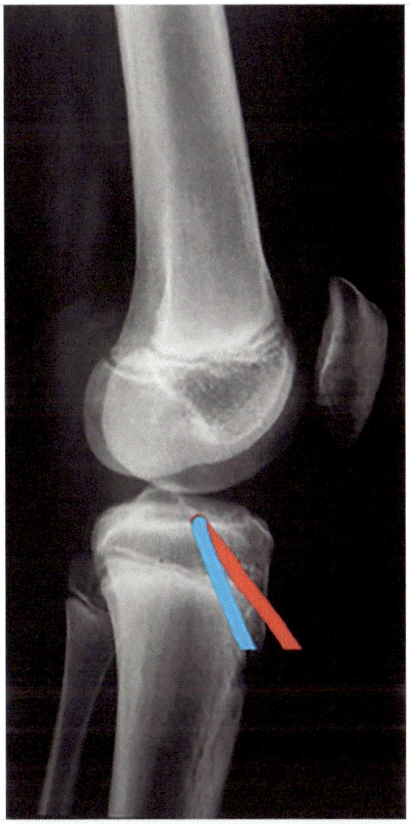

Fig. 24.11 More vertical for transphyseal anterior cruciate ligament (ACL) reconstruction in Tanner III and IV patients, to minimize physeal injuries during tunnel drilling.

trans-epiphyseal techniques to drill the femoral tunnel and transphyseal techniques to drill the tibial tunnel.

- Vertical tunnels can be done for ACL reconstruction in Tanner III and IV patients, minimizing the risk of physeal injuries during tunnel drilling (▶ Fig. 24.11).
- Drill at low speed with a smaller diameter drill.
- Avoid the peripheral portion of the tibial apophysis.
- Keep the tunnel clean to avoid bone fragments.
- Fill the tunnel with soft tissues.
- Avoid implants crossing the physis.

25 Anterior Cruciate Ligament—Tibial Avulsion

Elizabeth C. Truelove, Conor I. Murphy, Jeremy M. Burnham, Jan S. Grudziak, Volker Musahl, Joshua Pratt, and Rory McHardy

25.1 Description

Tibial spine or eminence avulsions, primarily a pediatric orthopaedic injury, are synonymous with anterior cruciate ligament (ACL) injuries. The attachment site of the ACL to the tibia is larger and more secure than its femoral site, making tibial-sided avulsions a rare subtype of ACL injury. While plain radiographs are often normal in ACL injuries without a segond fracture, tibial avulsion injuries can be apparent on plain films with the presence of a tibial eminence fracture. These injuries often occur in children with incomplete ossification of the tibial spine predisposing to it avulsion fracture rather than ACL failure. High-energy trauma with hyperextension, valgus, and external rotation forces less commonly result in these injuries in adults. Tibial avulsions have traditionally been classified according to the system described by Meyers and McKeever, with surgical intervention indicated for any amount of fracture displacement (Types II, III, and IV).

25.2 Key Principles

As with nearly all orthopaedic injuries, the key principles in treating tibial avulsion ACL injuries are patient history, physical examination, appropriate imaging, preoperative planning, and intraoperative preparedness. Thorough understanding of the anatomy is vital. Two prominences exist within the tibial eminence: the medial and lateral elevations. The ACL inserts onto the tibia at the medial elevation. The medial and lateral menisci also insert anteriorly at the tibial eminence, which may complicate repair of tibial eminence avulsions due to interposition at the fracture site. Special attention must be paid to the width, location, and status of the physis on radiographic analysis (▶ Fig. 25.1) as this will inevitably affect treatment and fixation.

A thorough physical exam must be performed to evaluate for any concomitant injuries. Examination in combination with review of appropriate radiographs guides indications for advanced imaging. Direct trauma is typically the cause of tibial avulsion injuries, whereas ACL tears are usually secondary to noncontact trauma. Computed tomography identifies concomitant bony injuries such as a tibial plateau fracture or tibial tuberosity injury, while magnetic resonance imaging (MRI) is required to evaluate associated soft tissue anatomy (▶ Fig. 25.2). Both imaging modalities may help to clarify the precise features of the injury as some avulsions have a substantial bony component while others are primarily cartilaginous. When there is not concern for other osseous injuries, MRI can generally provide adequate characterization of the injury while avoiding excessive radiation exposure in children.

Surgical treatment primarily incorporates either suture or screw fixation of the avulsion. Occasionally, temporary percutaneous Kirschner wires are utilized, although this is not the preferred fixation method as they lack long-term stability and must be later removed. The anatomical components of the avulsion will help dictate fixation methodology. Cartilaginous avulsions are more amenable to suture fixation, whereas larger bony avulsions will tolerate screw fixation. When operative management is appropriate, the treatment algorithm must include consideration of the patient's skeletal maturity and remaining skeletal growth through the proximal tibia physis. Anatomic reduction is best achieved under direct visualization and often requires retracting the medial meniscus, which can be torn or entrapped in the fracture.

25.3 Expectations

Establishing realistic expectations with the patient based on the severity of injury, need for surgical intervention, and his or her preoperative level of activity or competition is necessary. Traditionally, patients have good functional outcomes regardless of operative technique.

Loss of motion, specifically loss of extension, is the most common complication. This stiffness can be further exacerbated by arthrofibrosis, which is more common after surgical intervention compared with nonoperative treatment. The patient must understand that manipulation under anesthesia

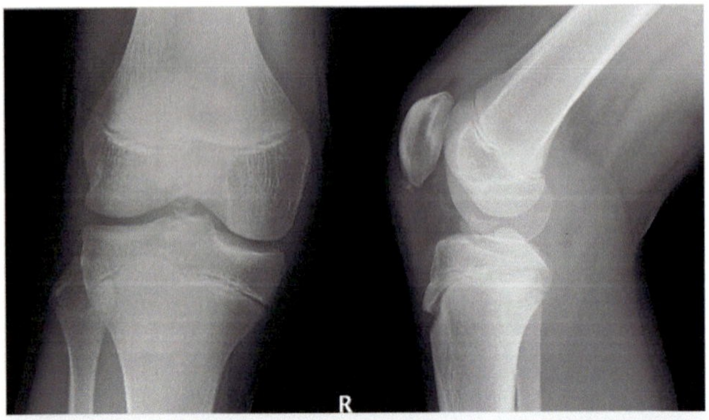

Fig. 25.1 Preoperative anteroposterior (AP) and lateral radiographs of the right knee of Patient A showing a displaced tibial eminence avulsion injury.

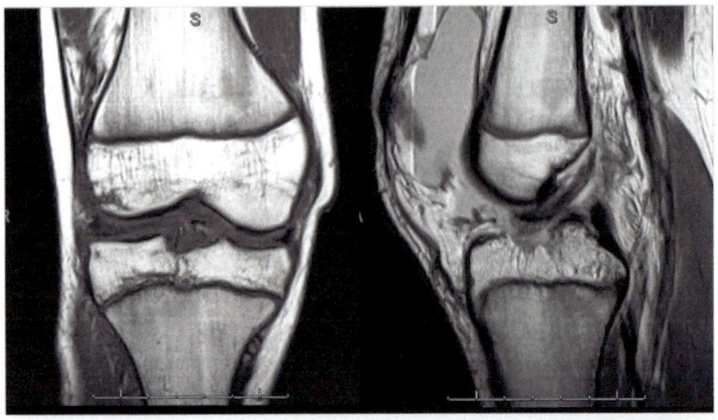

Fig. 25.2 Preoperative T1 coronal and turbo spin echo (TSE) sagittal magnetic resonance imaging (MRI) cuts of the right knee of Patient A showing an intact anterior cruciate ligament (ACL) and avulsion of the entire tibial eminence.

may be required if postoperative mobility is not regained or postoperative rehabilitation protocols are not followed.

In the pediatric population with ACL tibial avulsion injuries, the physis may be disrupted during surgery. This can potentially lead to growth arrest of the proximal tibia resulting in leg length discrepancy, and although uncommon, it must be discussed with the patient and parent or guardian.

Lastly, resultant ACL laxity may persist despite surgical treatment. Postoperative laxity is not always a direct outcome of surgical intervention. More often, the etiology is secondary to nonrecoverable strain and plastic deformation of the ACL at the time of injury secondary to a high amount of tension prior to failure of the tibial eminence. This laxity is often subclinical and has limited impact on functional outcomes, but at times, it may require that the patient undergoes delayed ACL reconstruction.

25.4 Indications

The most common classification system for these fractures was described by Meyers and McKeever in 1959. Type I injuries are nondisplaced or minimally displaced and best treated in a cast or splint with the knee in extension or slight flexion. Type II avulsions are those with superior displacement of the anterior aspect of the fracture with an intact posterior hinge, whereas type III injuries have complete detachment of the fragment. These are further divided into type IIIA injuries, those in which only the ACL insertion is involved, and type IIIB injuries, with avulsion of the entire tibial eminence. Some also describe Type IV lesions with fracture comminution.

Surgical treatment is indicated in all displaced fractures. This includes irreducible Type II injuries and all Type III and IV avulsions. Traditional management of Type II tibial avulsion injuries, or those hinged open anteriorly, includes an attempt at closed reduction by fully extending the knee. However, this is often unsuccessful in practice, as hyperextension of the knee will mechanically tension the ACL with a resultant net force potentially distracting the fracture.

25.5 Contraindications

Surgical management is not indicated for nondisplaced avulsion fractures. In addition, if the patient sustains a high-grade injury to the ACL itself, surgical fixation of the avulsion fracture is generally not adequate.

25.6 Special Considerations

The surgeon must prepare for both open and arthroscopic management of this injury. Although arthroscopic management should be attempted first and is the current standard surgical intervention, some injuries may not be amenable to an isolated arthroscopic approach, thus requiring greater surgical exposure through an open approach. Open surgical management can lead to issues such as soft tissue damage and a delay in rehabilitation due to appropriate time allotment for surgical incision healing. Arthroscopic treatment allows for direct visualization, anatomic intra-articular reduction, and the ability to address any other concomitant soft tissue injuries with minimal dissection.

Instrumentation for both suture fixation and screw fixation should be available in the operating room. In the pediatric population, it is often difficult to accurately assess the full extent of bony injury due to varying stages of ossification of the involved structures. Preoperative planning for the approach and fixation method may consequently be revised intraoperatively as initial imaging and physical exam are limited diagnostically compared to direct visualization of the injury in the operating room.

25.7 Special Instructions, Position, and Anesthesia

Supine patient positioning with the hip and knee flexed on a flat, radiolucent table is preferred. Conversion to open technique, should the need arise, is more easily performed with the patient supine as opposed to positioning the leg in a circumferential leg holder past the break in the table with the distal end dropped down. Furthermore, fluoroscopic examination of the knee after screw fixation is more feasible with supine positioning on a radiolucent table. Lastly, if the surgeon prefers postoperative immobilization with cylindrical casting, this is again logistically simplified with supine positioning.

The surrounding intra-articular soft tissues must be assessed arthroscopically prior to reduction and fixation. Often, the anterior horn of the medial meniscus or the intermeniscal ligament is interposed in the fracture site in displaced fractures and acts as a block to reduction (▶ Fig. 25.3). Final fixation and tightening prior to mobilization of the entrapped medial meniscus may result in further damage to the meniscus.

Meticulous anatomic reduction and initial fixation are paramount. The avulsed tibial fragment can be diminutive, preventing multiple attempts at fixation and purchase as one could potentially cause further comminution. Bailout options are limited in the setting of a severely comminuted avulsed fragment.

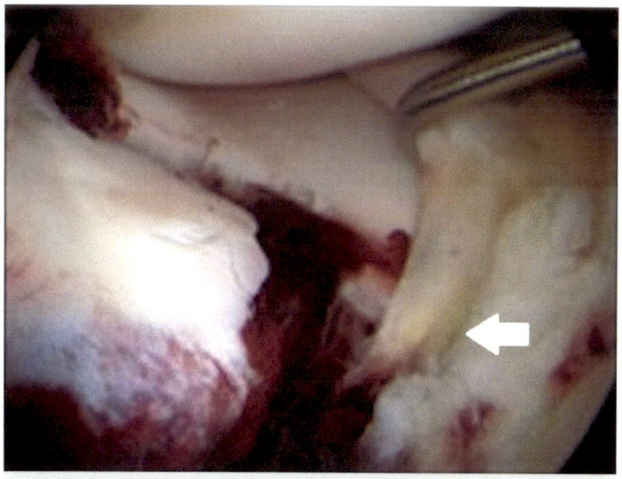

Fig. 25.3 Arthroscopic view through the anterolateral portal of Patient B showing medial meniscus entrapment within the tibial eminence avulsion fracture bed.

25.8 Tips, Pearls, and Lessons Learned

The typical pathogenesis of tibial avulsion injuries is traumatic, and patients will likely be in pain secondary to an acute hemarthrosis. Definitive management can often be delayed until 7 to 14 days after an injury, as immediate operative intervention before this window can be complicated by diminished visualization due to the hemarthrosis. Furthermore, allowing the acute inflammatory phase of this injury to resolve can decrease extravasation of arthroscopy fluid into the bone intraoperatively. During this waiting period, advanced imaging studies can be obtained while swelling and inflammation subsides.

Tensioning of the ACL and fixation can be difficult. During final tensioning, a posteriorly directed force on the tibia should be applied in order to shorten the distance between the ACL origin and its insertion on the tibial eminence. Over-reduction or countersinking the avulsed fragment within the fracture bed can help offset postoperative ligamentous laxity caused by plastic deformation of the ACL, as well. Nonrecoverable strain of the ACL prior to tibial eminence failure and avulsion is thought to be the cause of residual laxity after anatomic reduction and fixation. By countersinking the avulsed fragment within the fracture bed, adequate tensioning of the repaired ACL will limit postoperative laxity without overconstraining the joint.

25.9 Difficulties Encountered

If operative intervention is attempted arthroscopically, it can often prove challenging to achieve the appropriate trajectory for screw insertion. It is thus imperative that preoperative planning include deliberate portal placement and potentially the use of accessory portals to achieve adequate fixation.

When management is attempted through an open technique, the exposure must allow for direct visualization of all necessary structures. This can be difficult if the patient has preexisting patella baja or has had any prior surgeries that could lead to anterior scar tissue.

Finally, with either arthroscopic or open fixation, the surgeon has to be cognizant of any lateral meniscus involvement in addition to the medial meniscus and specifically address the anterior root of the lateral meniscus if it is an aspect of the injury complex.

25.10 Key Procedural Steps

25.10.1 Arthroscopic Technique

Standard arthroscopic portals for ACL reconstruction are used for tibial avulsion injuries. Typically, the anterolateral portal is used for visualization and diagnostic arthroscopy, the superomedial portal for outflow as needed, and the anteromedial portal for instrumentation and fixation.

The origin of the avulsion fracture should be debrided thoroughly down to a healthy subchondral base. All interposed tissues must be reduced from the fracture base and repaired as needed.

25.10.2 Open Reduction Internal Fixation

A medial parapatellar approach is the preferred open approach to tibial avulsion injuries. A midline or medial parapatellar skin incision will generally provide adequate access. Dissection is carried through the subcutaneous tissues and fat down to the retinaculum and medial border of the patella while leaving an adequate cuff of tissue to assist in repair upon closure. The patella and patellar tendon are then retracted laterally to allow access to the intercondylar notch, ACL, and tibial avulsion.

At this point, the avulsion base can be debrided and concomitant injuries addressed. After fixation, copious irrigation is necessary to flush all remaining intra-articular fragments and debris from the surgical site.

25.10.3 Suture Fixation

Suture fixation begins with a small incision just medial to the tibial tuberosity in order to properly seat the tibial drill guide. Suture fixation is achieved through two parallel transphyseal drill holes, one at the medial border and one at the lateral border of the tibial eminence avulsion. A tibial drill guide will orient the proper trajectory of the parallel drill holes, beginning just medial to the tibial tuberosity. The drill holes should be drilled with the oscillating function to avoid extensive damage to the physis. A suture is passed in an arthroscopic portal and through the base of the ACL as close to the tibial avulsion fragment as possible (▶ Fig. 25.4). A suture passer is then inserted through each drill tunnel to pass the individual ends of the now secured tibial avulsion.

At the time of fixation, it is essential to confirm that the medial meniscus, lateral meniscus, or intermeniscal ligament is not entrapped in the fracture site blocking reduction. After confirmation, the ends of the suture are tied over a bony bridge at the tibial tuberosity to secure fixation.

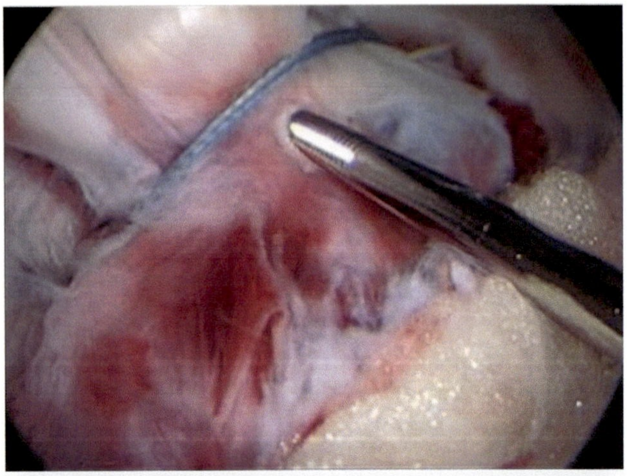

Fig. 25.4 Arthroscopic view through the anterolateral portal of Patient C showing suture fixation from medial to lateral around the base of the anterior cruciate ligament (ACL) at the site of the tibial eminence avulsion.

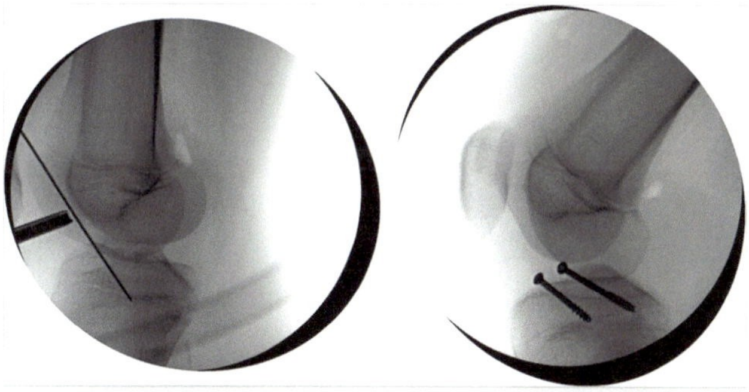

Fig. 25.5 Intraoperative fluoroscopic images of the right knee of Patient A showing guide pin placement and two 4.0-mm cannulated screws at the base of the tibial eminence.

25.10.4 Screw Fixation

Screw fixation is achieved over a guide pin directed through the base of the fragment into the epiphysis under fluoroscopic guidance (▶ Fig. 25.5). The trajectory is from anterior to posterior and superior to inferior. Special care must be taken not to disrupt the physis or protrude through the posterior cortex of the tibia into the nearby neurovascular structures adjacent to the posterior cortex. A second guide pin may be utilized to maintain reduction if the fragment has sufficient bone stock for fixation.

Either a 3.5-mm, 4.0-mm, or 4.5-mm cannulated screw is passed over the guide pin. Final tightening of the screw must be confirmed on fluoroscopic examination to ensure proper trajectory and length. A second screw can be placed over the additional guide pin if possible.

25.10.5 Hybrid Fixation

Hybrid fixation combines both suture and screw fixation techniques (▶ Fig. 25.6). Initially, the fracture is reduced and secured with suture fixation as described above. After tying the suture ends for final fixation, a 3.5-mm, 4.0-mm, or 4.5-mm cannulated screw is placed through the anterior base of the tibial avulsion over a guide pin as described above.

Tibial avulsion injuries are generally seen in the pediatric population, and surgical management is required for any fracture displacement. Both arthroscopic and open techniques are utilized to reduce and fix the fracture with sutures, screws, or a combination. It is important to identify any associated soft tissue injuries both preoperatively with advanced imaging as indicated and intraoperatively with visualization and address these injuries as appropriate. Possible complications postoperatively include stiffness and ACL laxity, but the majority of patients have good functional outcomes.

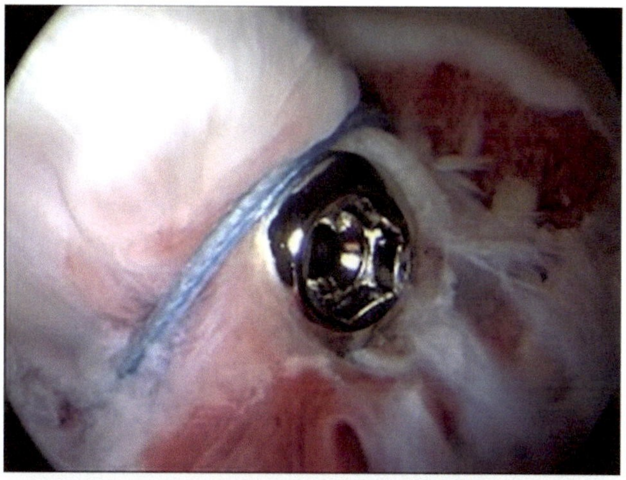

Fig. 25.6 Arthroscopic view through the anterolateral portal of Patient C showing hybrid fixation with a suture around the base of the anterior cruciate ligament (ACL) and a screw through the bony avulsion of the tibial eminence.

25.11 Bailout, Rescue, Salvage Procedures

If adequate fixation of a tibial avulsion injury cannot be achieved or if fixation fails postoperatively, ACL reconstruction with either autograft or allograft is the recommended salvage procedure. Again, it is important to consider the age and skeletal maturity of the patient when planning for reconstruction, and any existing hardware in the tibia must be taken into account regarding bone tunnel placement.

25.12 Pitfalls

An inability to adequately reduce the fracture fragment can lead to difficulties intraoperatively and complications postoperatively. This is sometimes due to a failure to remove any entrapped anterior medial meniscus from the fracture site, reinforcing the importance of direct visualization and anatomic reduction. High-grade injury to the ACL itself would likely require a different surgical strategy than tibial avulsion fixation with suture or a screw. A missed intrasubstance injury to the ACL could lead to a worse functional outcome. Finally, one must take care to avoid iatrogenic injury to the cartilage, especially as most patients are pediatric. The articular surface of the patella can easily be damaged during screw insertion; thus, portal placement and the use of accessory portals as needed to obtain a safe trajectory must be emphasized.

26 Posterior Cruciate Ligament Reconstruction: Achilles Tendon Allograft

James P. Stannard

26.1 Description

This chapter will describe both transtibial and tibial inlay posterior cruciate ligament (PCL) reconstruction using Achilles tendon allograft.

26.2 Key Principles

(1) The PCL functions biomechanically as a structure with two (double) bundles: the larger anterolateral bundle (AL) and the smaller posteromedial bundle (PM). (2) The AL bundle should be tensioned at 90 degrees of flexion and the PM bundle should be tensioned at full extension. (3) The AL bundle should be created using approximately 66% of the Achilles tendon and the PM bundle with the remaining 33% (▶ Fig. 26.1). (4) The Achilles tendon allograft is a strong graft source with bone available if needed for the inlay technique and outstanding results in patients of all ages. (5) I prefer the tibial inlay technique in morbidly obese patients and those with KD-IV dislocations (to decrease the issue of tunnel crowding). The ideal tibial placement for the bone allograft block is in the footprint of the insertion on the tibia approximately 1 to 1.5 cm distal to the articular surface and in the midline. (6) Both arms of the graft, AL and PM, are secured with suspensory fixation on the femur (GraftLink, Arthrex, Naples, FL) that can be tightened repetitively to eliminate the issue of graft loosening secondary to creep. (7) In case the transtibial technique is alternatively used, the transtibial tunnel should exit the tibia at least 1 to 1.5 cm below the joint line posteriorly (▶ Fig. 26.2). This places it in the exact same position as the tibial inlay graft and minimizes the "killer turn" and graft stretching and rupture.

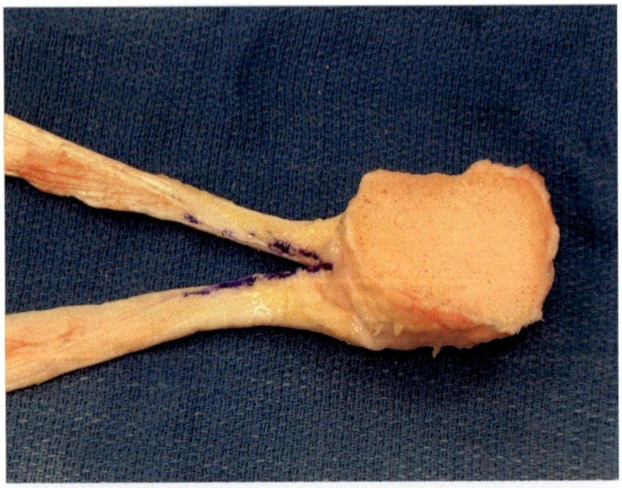

Fig. 26.1 Achilles tendon allograft divided for double bundle technique.

26.3 Expectations

PCL reconstruction using a double bundle technique with either the inlay or transtibial technique with a low posterior tibial tunnel exit can yield outstanding results with excellent stability and failure rates in the 4 to 8% range.

26.4 Indications

PCL reconstruction is recommended in most patients with a multiple ligament knee injury or dislocation. Isolated PCL injuries may be reconstructed in physiologically young patients and those who have failed conservative treatment with bracing and rehabilitation. Patients who are treated conservatively should be informed that they may develop posttraumatic osteoarthritis in their patellofemoral and medial compartments as a result of their instability.

26.5 Contraindications

PCL reconstruction should not be undertaken in patients with an isolated PCL tear and who are relatively inactive.

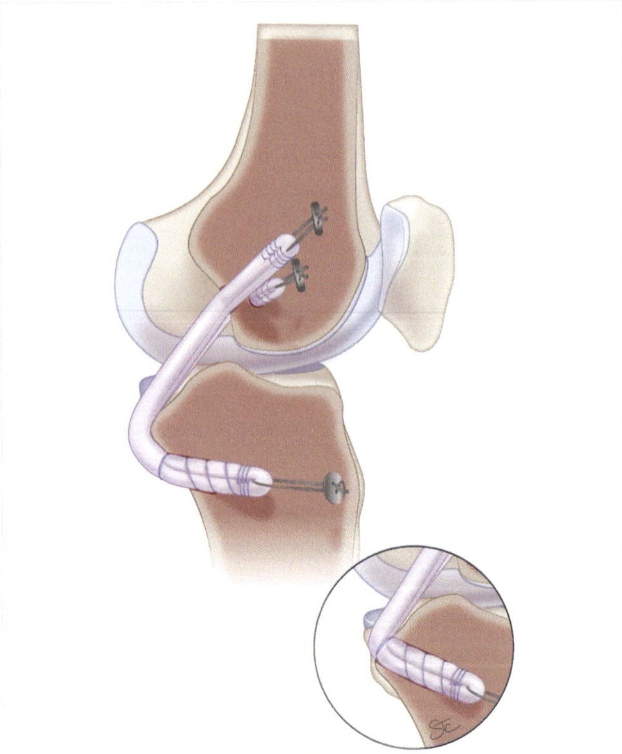

Fig. 26.2 Illustration showing importance of transtibial socket being placed low on the proximal tibia.

26.6 Special Considerations

PCL tears rarely occur in isolation. It is very important to perform a good neurovascular exam of any patient with an acute PCL tear and document the findings. It is also important to perform serial vascular exams over the first 48 hours because vascular occlusion can occasionally occur over the first couple of days secondary to swelling, bleeding, or large flow limiting intimal tears.

26.7 Special Instructions, Position, and Anesthesia

The patient should be placed supine with a lateral leg post to allow a full diagnostic arthroscopy. A tourniquet is left on the proximal aspect of the thigh but is not routinely used. If a tibial inlay is performed, it should be done by making a medial approach that is located along the posterior border of the tibia. The knee should be flexed approximately 90 degrees during the deep dissection to minimize risk to the neurovascular structures posteriorly (▶ Fig. 26.3). General anesthesia is most frequently used with a preoperative peripheral nerve block for pain control postoperatively.

26.8 Tips, Pearls, and Lessons Learned

26.8.1 Tibial Inlay

The bone block should be at least 10 mm thick to avoid fracture of the block when the lag screw is tightened. A trough is made using a ½ inch curved osteotome starting approximately 1 cm below the articular surface, in the center of the posterior aspect of the proximal tibia. A single drill hole is placed through the middle of the graft bone block with a 4.5-mm drill. Both the drill hole and the screw should be oriented slightly from posteromedial to anterolateral. This makes screw placement easier and assures the screw will not block a future tunnel for an anterior cruciate ligament (ACL) reconstruction. A 4.5-mm cannulated screw with a washer (Synthes, Paoli, PA) is used to affix the bone block in the trough (▶ Fig. 26.4).

26.8.2 Transtibial PCL

It is critical to make certain that the exit of the transtibial tunnel posteriorly is approximately 1.5 cm below the articular surface in the middle of the knee. Bruce Levy has designed a very accurate guide that will achieve this if you place it all the way down on the articular surface (Arthrex, Naples, FL). I make a socket rather than a full tunnel using an adjustable cutter that will allow reaming the tibial tunnel and both femoral tunnels with a single device (either Mitek, Raynam. MA or Arthrex, Naples, FL) in a retrograde fashion. I make certain I can visualize the cutting blades using the arthroscope prior to beginning to ream the posterior socked. The PCL guide can be used to "push" the neurovascular structures posteriorly and help protect them. If I am unable to visualize the cutting blades, I obtain a lateral fluoroscopic view prior to applying power to the reamer.

26.9 Difficulties Encountered

As already stated, PCL tears rarely occur in isolation. If the tear is part of a knee dislocation, great care must be taken to avoid the problems of tunnel crowding and overlap with potential damage to grafts when tunnels intersect. We already noted the importance of aiming the lag screw from posteromedial to anterolateral when using the inlay technique. This will avoid the screw crossing the path of the ACL tunnel. Similarly, the PM bundle femoral socket and the femoral socket of the posteromedial corner (PMC) reconstruction are frequently very close to each other on the medial femoral cortex. The tibial socket for the Posterior Oblique Ligament can also intersect with the tibial socket of the PCL reconstruction. Great care must be taken by the surgeon to avoid these high-risk areas for tunnel crowding and intersection.

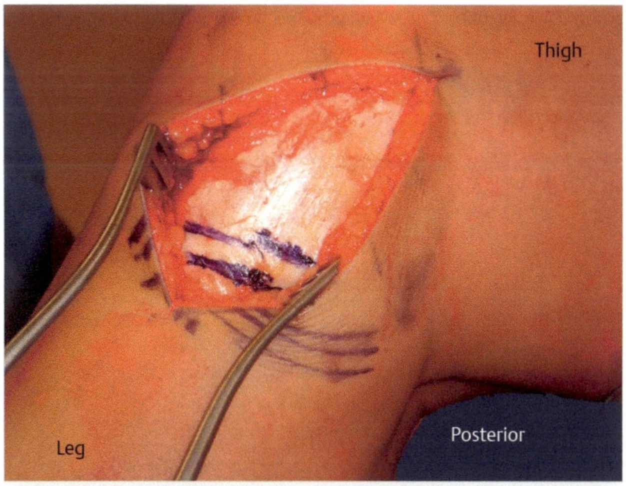

Fig. 26.3 Posteromedial incision for tibial inlay. The pes anserinus tendons are highlighted with the surgical marker.

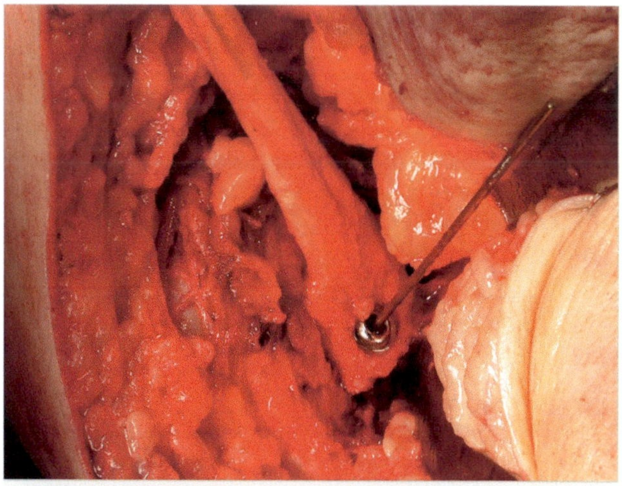

Fig. 26.4 Inlay graft held in place on the back of the tibia with a cannulated 4.5-mm screw.

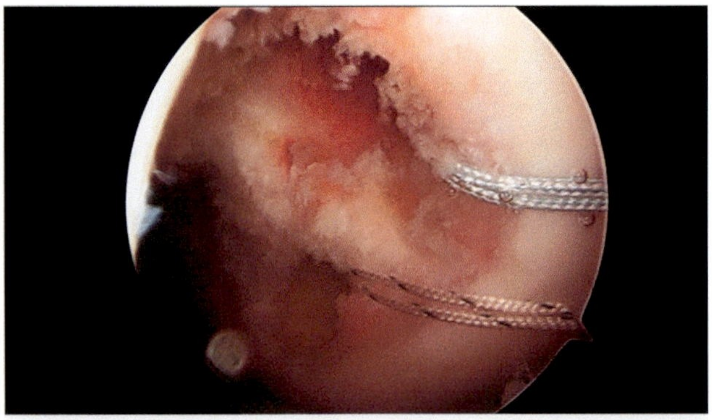

Fig. 26.5 Anterolateral (AL) and posteromedial (PM) sockets drilled with suture passed through them.

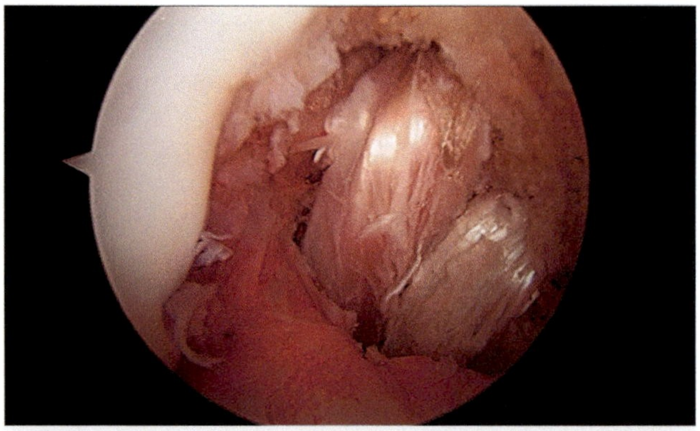

Fig. 26.6 Double bundle reconstruction arthroscopic view.

Another potential difficulty involves suture management when performing the double bundle PCL. We recommend pulling the FiberStick suture (Arthrex, Naples, FL) for the AL bundle out the anterolateral portal and the PCL and PM bundle sutures out the anteromedial portal. This simple step makes it easy to keep the sutures separated and minimizes the risk of tangling the sutures together in the knee.

26.10 Key Procedural Steps

We will divide this up into common steps that are performed in both the inlay and the transtibial reconstructions, followed by steps for the tibial inlay, and then steps for the transtibial PCL reconstruction.

26.10.1 Common Steps—Femoral Socket Preparation

- PCL femoral guide is used to drill a 10 to 11 mm adjustable retrograde cutter as high in the notch as possible and 10 mm from the articular cartilage to create the AL socket.
- Ream the AL socket to 25 mm, then pass suture through socket and out the lateral portal.
- Use PCL guide again to place PM socket directly below the AL socket and ream a 7- to 8-mm adjustable retrograde cutter to a depth of 25 mm. Pass the suture out the anteromedial portal to pull the PM bundle into the socket (▶ Fig. 26.5).
- After tibial socket preparation or placement of inlay (both described below), a Hewson suture passer is used, or a loop grasper is used to pull the PM bundle into the PM socket.
- Flip the button on the medial femoral cortex and pull the graft 15 mm into the PM socket.
- Grasp the AL suture in the back of the notch from the lateral side of the PM bundle, and pull it into the knee and into the AL socket.
- Flip the button on the medial femoral cortex and pull the graft 15 mm into the AL socket.
- Place knee in 90 degrees of flexion and retension both the tibial bundle and the AL bundle.
- Place the knee in full extension and tension the PM bundle.
- Place the knee through a full range of motion at least 8 to 10 times and retension grafts (▶ Fig. 26.6).

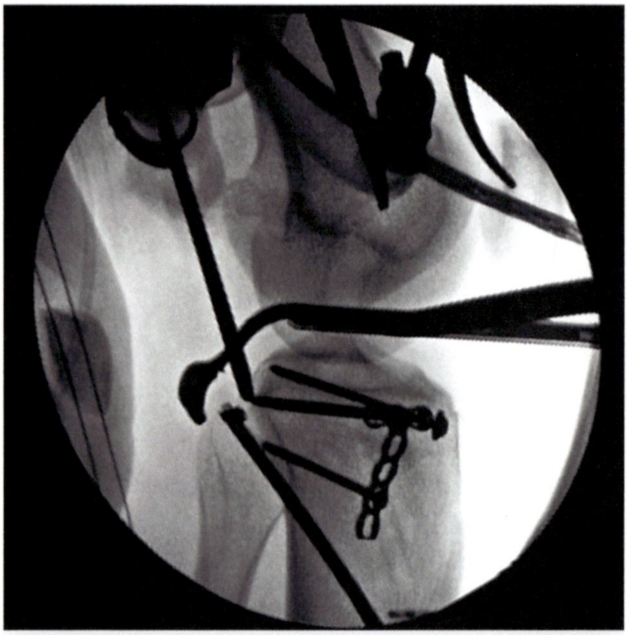

Fig. 26.7 Fluoroscopy shot with FlipCutter exiting low on the tibia prior to reaming socket.

26.10.2 Transtibial Tibia Socket Preparation

- Establish a posteromedial arthroscopy portal and debride the tibial insertion of the PCL off the back of the tibia.
- Place tibial PCL guide (Arthrex, Naples, FL) flat against the tibial surface of the notch with the guide as distal on the posterior tibia as possible.
- Drill the adjustable retrograde cutter through the guide and out the back of the tibia approximately 1.5 cm below the articular surface of the tibia (▶ Fig. 26.7).
- Ream a socket that is approximately a 12 mm diameter and at least a 40 mm length.
- Pass a suture through the socket and into the joint, using the posteromedial portal or the tibial PCL guide to assist if needed.

- Grasp the suture and pull it out the anteromedial arthroscopy portal.
- Pull the Achilles tendon soft tissue graft into the knee and into the tibial socket.
- Attach a button to the suture and tension the graft approximately 15 mm into the tibial socket. Pull the two femoral bundles into their sockets as described above.

26.10.3 Inlay Tibial Preparation

- Make a posteromedial approach to the knee beginning at the posterior crest of the tibia at the level of the insertion of the Pes Anserinus tendons. The knee should be flexed 90 degrees during the deep portions of the dissection.
- Make certain to stay directly on the posterior tibial bone surface with a Cobb elevator, then place a blunt Hohmann retractor in front of the popliteus muscle to protect the neurovascular structures.
- Continue the deep dissection proximally to the level of the joint, externally rotate the foot to improve exposure of the posterior tibia.
- Use a ½ inch curved osteotome to create a boney trough beginning 1 cm distal to the articular surface. The trough should be slightly wider than the osteotome and approximately 8 to 10 mm deep.
- Create an Achilles tendon allograft with two soft tissue bundles and a bone block that is 10 mm wide, 10 mm thick, and approximately 15 mm long.
- Drill a 4.5-mm hole in the middle of the bone block oriented slightly from posteromedial to anterolateral in direction.
- Place the bone block into the trough and impact it lightly but do not countersink.
- Drill a guidewire for a 4.5-mm cannulated screw and then place the 4.5-mm screw with a washer using a lag screw technique. Be careful not to overtighten the screw and fracture the bone block.
- Make a hole or passage in the posterior capsule with a hemostat or Kelly clamp in order to pass the graft bundles into the knee.
- Pass a Hewson suture passer through the anteromedial portal and out the back of the knee.
- Pull the PM suture in and out the anteromedial portal.
- Pass the Hewson suture passer again and make sure it goes lateral to the PM bundle.
- Pull the AL suture into the knee and out the anterolateral portal. Pull the two femoral bundles into the knee and continue with common steps as described above.
- Final tightening of the PM bundle should be performed with the knee in full extension and the AL bundle should be with the knee in 90 degrees of flexion.

26.11 Bailout, Rescue, and Salvage Procedures

One major problem that can occur is when the grafts are too long to allow tensioning. This will prevent successful reconstruction. The easiest salvage of this problem is to convert the sockets to full tunnels in the medial femoral condyle by removing the final 7 mm of bone. Fixation will require using the enlarged buttons that can then be attached.

26.12 Pitfalls

The most difficult part of the open procedure is passing the graft into the knee from posteriorly and making sure the AL bundle enters lateral to the PM bundle. One trick to avoid difficulties passing the grafts into the knee is enlarging the hole in the posterior capsule using a Kelly clamp or a similar device. This allows passing the two bundles smoothly and in the correct orientation. The second critical thing is to make certain to get the bone block to the middle of the tibia posteriorly. Two tricks to allow that are retraction with a Hohmann retractor slipped around the lateral border of the tibia posteriorly and rotating the knee externally (taking advantage of the multiligament injury) to provide the surgeon a good view to the middle of the posterior tibia.

The key to the arthroscopic procedure is the establishment of the posteromedial portal. Passing the graft from the tibia posteriorly into the knee can be difficult. We use the FiberStick (Arthrex, Naples, FL) to pass the suture. The footprint of the PCL guide or the open shaver can be used to pass the suture up into the knee.

27 Posterior Cruciate Ligament (PCL) Reconstruction—Autograft

Christopher D. Harner, Ryan J. Warth, and Jacob Worsham

27.1 Introduction

This chapter will cover posterior cruciate ligament (PCL) reconstruction with a quadriceps tendon autograft. The objective of this chapter will be to discuss indications and techniques for this reconstruction with specific attention to the quadriceps autograft. The senior author will also discuss his special considerations, pearls, and pitfalls that can happen while performing his reconstruction. This chapter will provide key procedural steps to performing a PCL reconstruction and will address specific difficulties encountered during reconstruction and bailout options.

27.2 Description

- Posterior cruciate ligament (PCL) injuries are highly variable in terms of degree (Grade I–III) of injury, isolated PCL versus combined (PCL plus other ligaments), and associated injuries to other structures such as meniscus and cartilage.
- Partial PCL (Grade I–II) tears can be treated nonoperatively with a possibility to heal and can remain asymptomatic for many years. Complete Grade III PCL injuries may also be treated nonoperatively but are more likely to develop instability and arthritis.
- In this chapter, we will focus on reconstruction of the PCL using autograft tissue. It is the senior author's preference in most PCL cases to utilize allograft but there are certain situations when autograft may be the only option (certain countries) or the surgeon and patient may prefer autograft (e.g., high-level athletes returning to their sports).

27.3 Key Principles

- Once the decision to perform PCL reconstruction is made, an anatomical restoration of the PCL is the goal.
- The PCL consists of three components; anterolateral (AL) bundle, posteromedial (PM) bundle, and meniscofemoral ligaments (MFLs). Each has specific insertion sites and a unique tensioning pattern with flexion and extension (▸ Fig. 27.1; **Video 27.1**). For single bundle reconstruction, the goal is to restore the AL component which is the largest and biomechanically the most important of the three components.

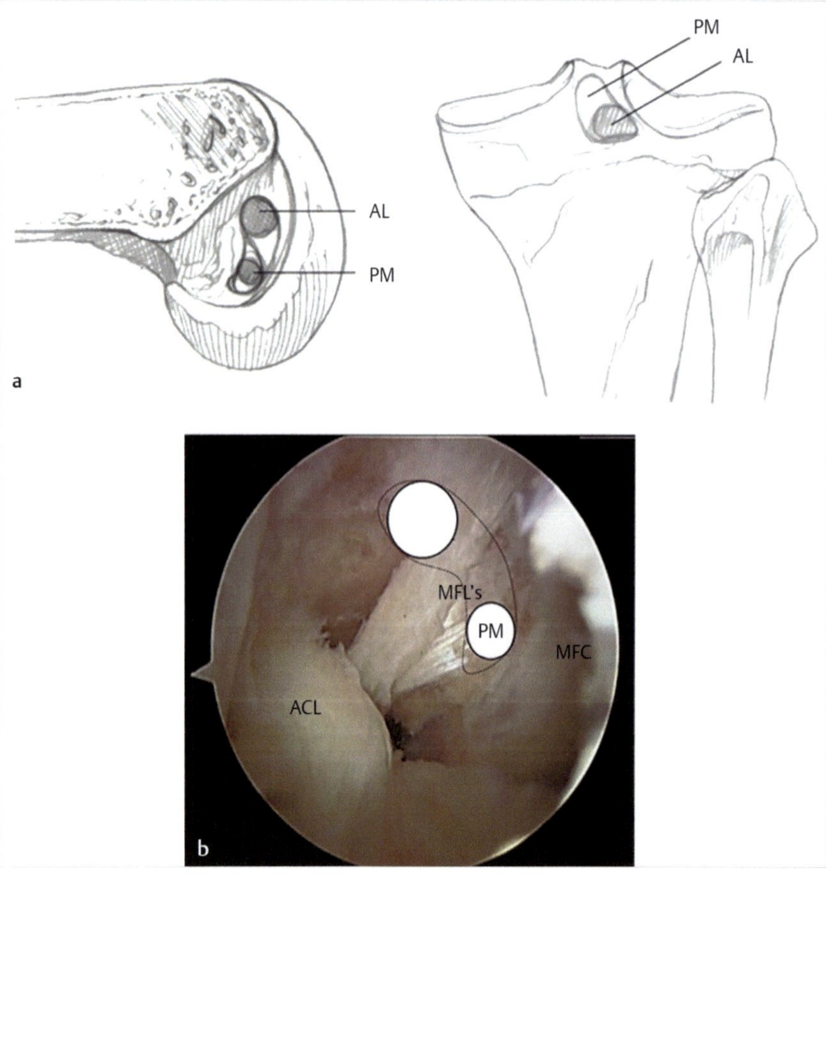

Fig. 27.1 Femoral and tibial insertion of the two bundles of the posterior cruciate ligament. **(a)** Line drawing. **(b)** Arthroscopic view of the femoral anterolateral (AL) and posteromedial (PM) insertion sites.

27.4 Surgical Indications

- Surgical decision-making for the PCL-injured knee can be challenging. Multiple variables must be considered, including functional status of the patient, grade of PCL injury, chronicity of injury, concomitant injury, and other knee pathologies (cartilage, meniscus, weight-bearing alignment).
- Grading and classifying the PCL-injured knee is critical to making the appropriate treatment decisions.
- The senior author prefers a classification system that includes the following:
  - Timing of injury (acute, chronic).
  - Anatomical classification of ligaments involved:
    - Isolated (PCL only).
    - Combined (other ligament involvement).
  - Location of injury (proximal, mid, distal).
  - Grade of injury to each ligament (Grade I–III).
- In general, most Grade III PCL injuries undergo surgical treatment, whether isolated or combined with other ligamentous injuries.

27.5 Contraindications

- Significant degenerative joint disease in any compartment.
- The most common compartments to have arthritis are the medial and patellofemoral:
  - If the medial compartment is significantly involved and there is varus malalignment, the PCL reconstruction is not recommended. In this case a biplanar osteotomy is recommended.
  - Grade I or II PCL injuries managed nonoperatively can have good long-term outcomes.
- In general, isolated grade I–II PCL injuries are treated with physical therapy and without surgery.

27.6 Special Considerations

- Graft options include autograft and allograft. We use allograft in approximately 80% of our cases (autograft in the remaining 20%).
- We prefer using autograft in high-level athletes and patients who do not want allograft.
- Certain countries in the world do not allow allograft (e.g., many countries in South America) and, therefore, autograft is the only option in these countries.
- If autograft is chosen, we prefer to use quadriceps tendon (with bone block) in 80% of cases and quadruple hamstring in the remaining 20%.
- When using allograft, we prefer Achilles tendon with bone block.
- One of the principles of PCL reconstruction using a transtibial technique is that the graft must be at least 9 to 10 cm in length.
- Graft diameter for the Achilles tendon allograft and quadriceps tendon autograft is 10 to 12 mm.

27.6.1 Quadriceps Tendon-Bone Autograft Harvest

- The graft harvest is performed with the knee flexed at 90 degrees.

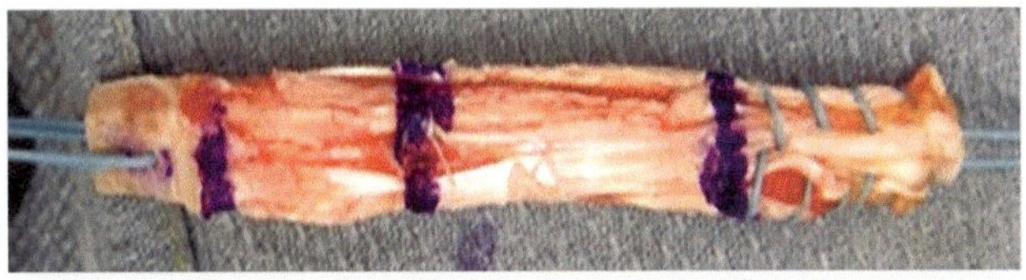

Fig. 27.2 Example of quadriceps tendon graft, bony portion to right sutured with #5 nonabsorbable suture, and the soft tissue component whip stitched with #5. Graft is marked at the bone tendon interface, then ideally at the 40-mm intra-articular portion of the graft, with ideal graft length being 9 to 10 cm.

- Incision is centered over superior pole of patella extending 5 to 10 cm proximally.
- Subcutaneous dissection to expose entire tendon and border of vastus medialis obliquus (VMO) at the level of its musculotendinous junction to adequately determine the thickness of tendon to be harvested.
- Layered dissection of quadriceps tendon from superficial to deep: rectus femoris, confluence of VMO and VLO, and the vastus intermedius.
- Care must be taken to avoid violating the suprapatellar pouch. If violated, it should be repaired.
- Excise 10 to 12 mm thickness from central portion of the quadriceps tendon with soft tissue harvester; the graft should be between 9 and 10 cm in length (including 2 cm bone block).
- Mark out the central third of the proximal patella, between 11 and 12 mm wide and 15 and 20 mm long.
- Cut the tendon first then the bone block second. Use an oscillating saw for the harvest.
- Occasionally, harvesting the bone block will require an osteotome to complete the removal.
- Superior patellar bone block is roughly 20 to 24 mm in length (equal to the width of tendon) and roughly 8 to 10 mm in depth (▶ Fig. 27.2).
- Two drill holes are made with a 2.0-mm drill to pass nonabsorbable suture. The soft tissue end of graft can be whip stitched with nonabsorbable #5 suture.
- The patellar bone defect can be grafted with bone tunnel reamings or demineralized bone matrix.
- Quadriceps tendon is meticulously closed using nonabsorbable #2 suture with the knee at 90 degrees of flexion.

27.6.2 Hamstring Tendon Autograft

- We will not dwell on the details of the hamstring harvest as it is already described in detail in multiple sources. Suffice it to say that the graft must be 9 to 10 cm in length when it is finished. When we utilize hamstring autograft, we use a quadruple construct.
- Graft diameter ranges from 8 to 10 mm which is not large enough for Grade III PCL laxity. We will only consider hamstring autograft in the rare case of a symptomatic Grade II PCL when PCL and MFL fibers remain attached to the femoral insertion.

27.7 Special Instructions, Position, and Anesthesia

- The senior author does not use a tourniquet.

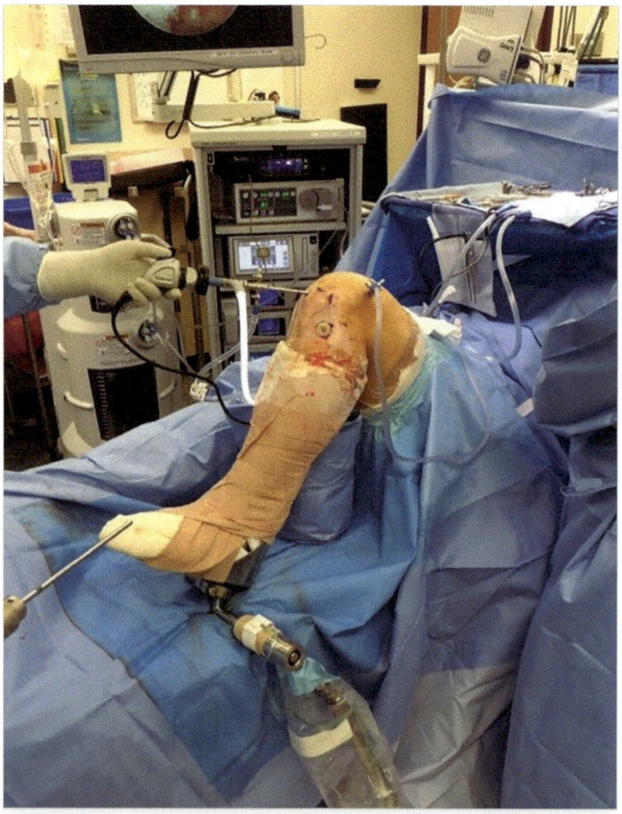

Fig. 27.3 Image shows example of pneumatic knee holder which allows for appropriate position of the knee during posterior cruciate ligament (PCL) reconstruction. Also visualized is the posterior calf bump to allow for anterior tibial translation during reconstruction.

- Adductor canal block is preferred over femoral nerve block for postoperative pain control.
- Examination under anesthesia is performed and the findings are critical to determine which ligaments are to be surgically addressed. For PCL grading, we utilize the posterior drawer exam (Grade I–III). Utilize intraoperative fluoroscopy to determine the final grade of patholaxity (measure the contralateral knee and compare side-to-side difference).
- We utilize a transtibial tunnel, a standard PCL guide, and a 70-degree arthroscope.
- Pneumatic leg positioner is helpful and preferred, but a simple post will allow the knee to be flexed at 90 degrees as well (▶ Fig. 27.3).

27.8 Tips, Pearls and Lessons Learned

- The skin incision used for hamstring autograft harvest can serve as a starting point for tibial tunnel drilling, thus avoiding the need for additional incisions and improving patient cosmesis.
- The bone plug on the quadriceps tendon autograft is always placed on the tibial side.
- The senior author prefers cortical fixation (rather than interference screw) on both the femur and tibia.
- Quadriceps graft diameter is 10 to 12 mm; Hamstring graft diameter is 8 to 9 mm.
- Placement of a soft "bump" behind the proximal tibia prevents posterior subluxation of the tibia during the procedure.

27.9 Difficulties Encountered

- Graft passage is always a challenge when utilizing a transtibial PCL tunnel. You should have available a threaded suture passer which will help facilitate graft passage.
- The PCL graft is passed from tibia to femur with the soft tissue limb being placed in the femoral tunnel.
- Our goal is to have 2 cm of graft within the femoral tunnel.
- If the graft is 8 to 10 cm in length, the tibial bone plug will be recessed into the tibial tunnel approximately 2 to 4 cm.
- When passing the graft, it is helpful to use a large right-angle clamp to push the sutures perpendicular to the tibial tunnel to facilitate graft passage. We do not utilize commercially available graft passers because they are expensive and can potentially erode the tibial tunnel.

27.10 Key Procedural Steps

27.10.1 Diagnostic Knee Arthroscopy and Tunnel Preparation

- Most of the procedure is done with the knee flexed to 90 degrees.
- Standard diagnostic knee arthroscopy is performed through anteromedial and anterolateral portals. An accessory PM portal is used to view and place working instruments for the PCL tibial tunnel.
- We first define the anatomy of the PCL femoral footprint. The femoral insertion of the fibers is intact in 90% of cases (▶ Fig. 27.4; Video 27.1).
- Our goal is to reproduce the AL portion of the PCL. We identify its insertion on the femur and clear the insertion site with an electrocautery device. An awl is then used to choose the exact insertion for the 3/32nd k-wire placement for subsequent femoral tunnel drilling. (See ▶ Fig. 27.4 and ▶ Fig. 27.5).
- Great care is taken to preserve the MFLs and the PM component of the PCL without injuring the ACL.
- The most challenging and time-consuming part of the surgery is developing visualization of the tibial footprint. We start by cleaning the synovial layer off the back of the tibia (▶ Fig. 27.6; Video 27.2). We start from the front of the knee and preserve the MFLs and ACL and then use the 70-degree scope to look down onto the tibial insertion.
- A PM portal is established and a shaver is brought through it to complete the cleaning of the PCL tibial insertion (see Video 27.2).
- Next we place a 30-degree scope into the PM portal to visualize the entire PCL tibial insertion (▶ Fig. 27.7; see Video 27.2).
- From the anteromedial portal (can also use the AL portal) a PCL guide is brought through the intercondylar notch (above the MFL and ACL) and placed distal and lateral on the tibial insertion (Video 27.3).

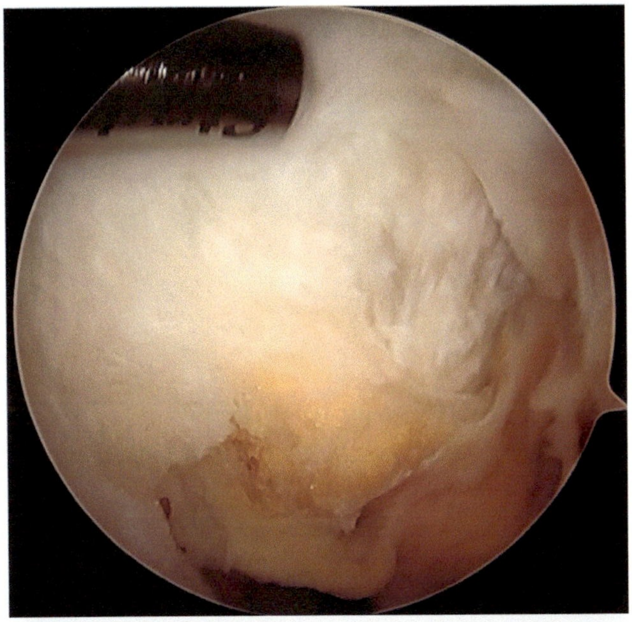

Fig. 27.4 Arthroscopic view from anterolateral portal showing the medial femoral condyle with all three components, anterolateral and posteromedial bundles and meniscofemoral ligaments, intact.

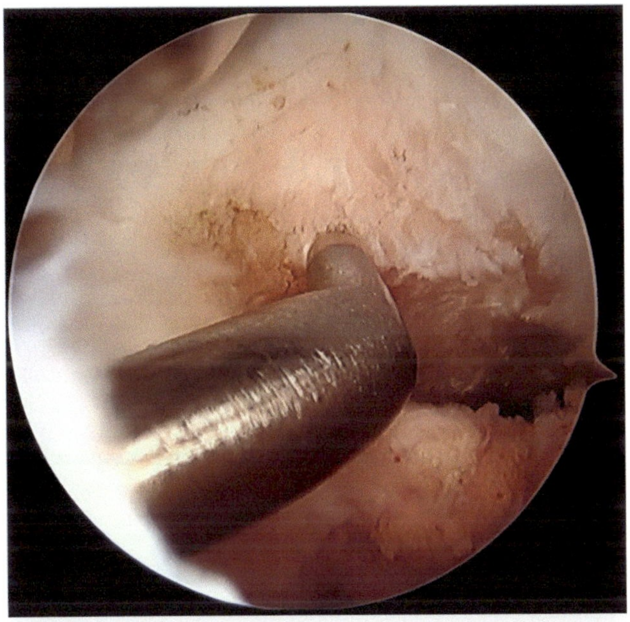

Fig. 27.5 Arthroscopic view from the anterolateral portal showing microfracture awl identifying proper anterolateral insertion. Superiorly one can see the articular cartilage of the medial femoral condyle and inferiorly the meniscofemoral ligaments.

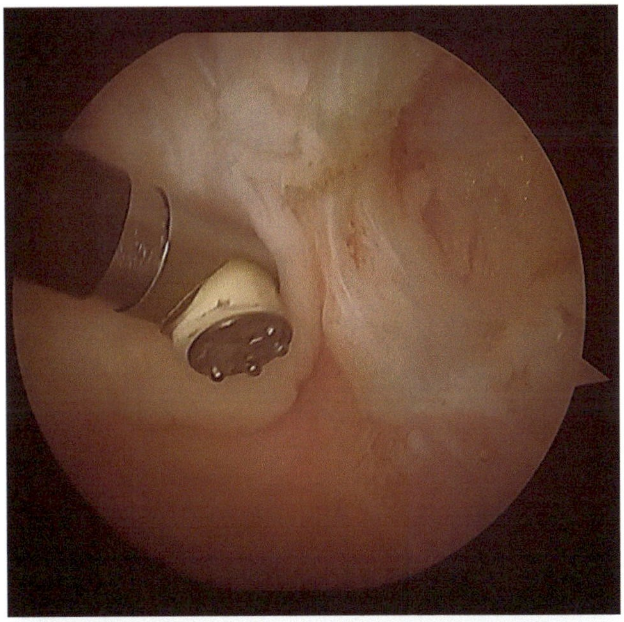

Fig. 27.6 Arthroscopic view from the anterolateral portal showing electrocautery inserted from the posteromedial portal; this is in preparation to clear off the posterior cruciate ligament (PCL) facet.

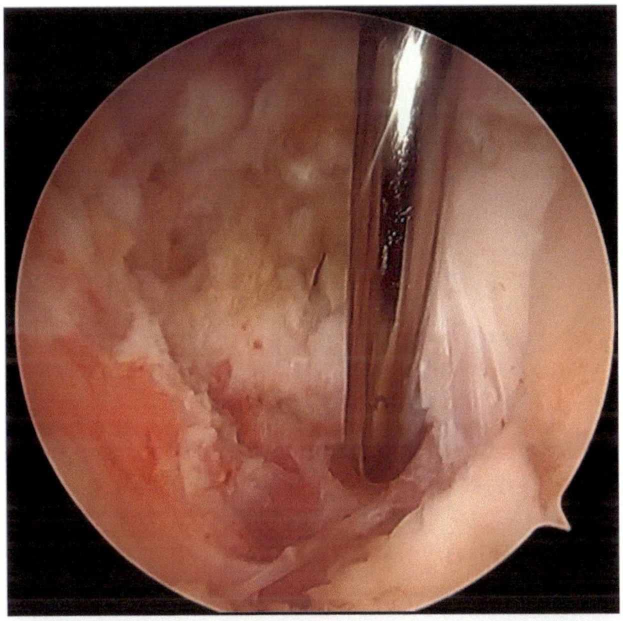

Fig. 27.7 View from the posteromedial portal viewing posterior cruciate ligament (PCL) footprint, and the PCL guide inserted from the anteromedial portal.

- A 3/32 Kirschner wire (K-wire) is drilled from anterior to posterior and intra operative fluoroscopy is always obtained to confirm correct placement as shown in ▶ Fig. 27.8 If the k-wire is not in a good position (which is usually too anterior) it can easily be readjusted with a parallel pin guide.
- If the K-wire is not where we want, a parallel pin guide is used to get correct placement.
- Drilling begins when the surgeon confirms appropriate PCL drill guide positioning both arthroscopically and fluoroscopically (▶ Fig. 27.9). Tunnel position is evaluated by frequent fluoroscopy to confirm appropriate position on the distal one-third of the PCL facet.
- After placing the guidewire, an appropriately sized reamer is used to overdrill the tunnel; tunnel length is confirmed using a graduated guide pin. Great care is taken to visualize tibial

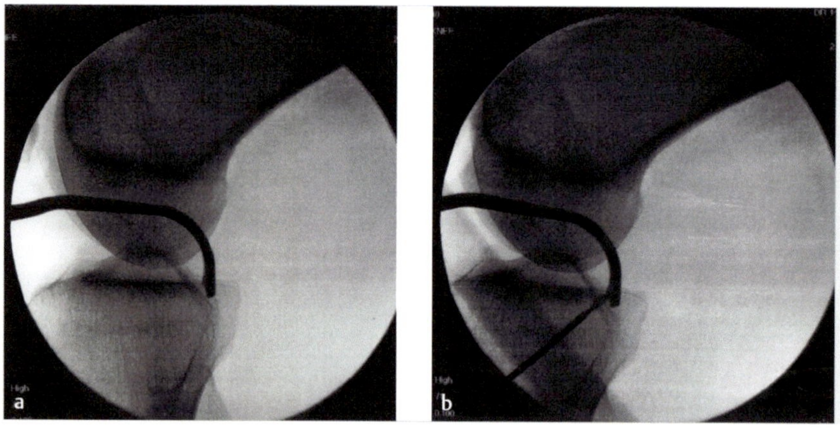

Fig. 27.8 (a,b) Lateral fluoroscopic views showing appropriate posterior cruciate ligament (PCL) guide placement and second confirming appropriate drill placement in the distal one-third of the PCL facet.

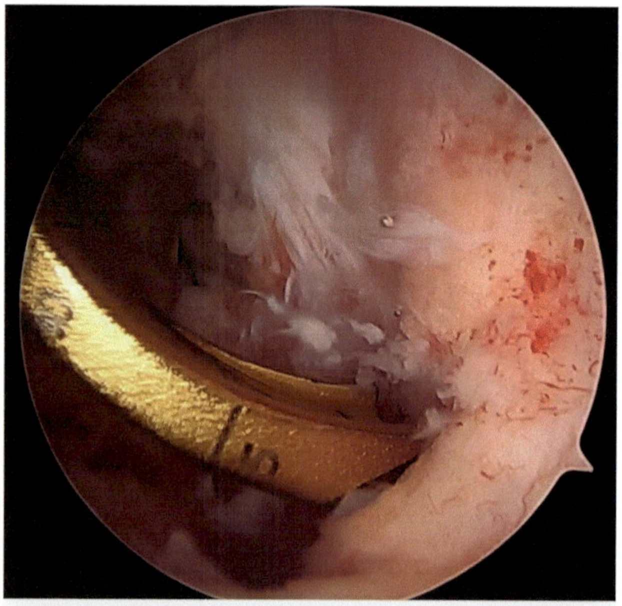

Fig. 27.9 Arthroscopic view through the posteromedial portal demonstrating appropriate posterior cruciate ligament (PCL) tibial guide placement. This is combined with fluoroscopic images in Fig. 27.8 to double check proper placement.

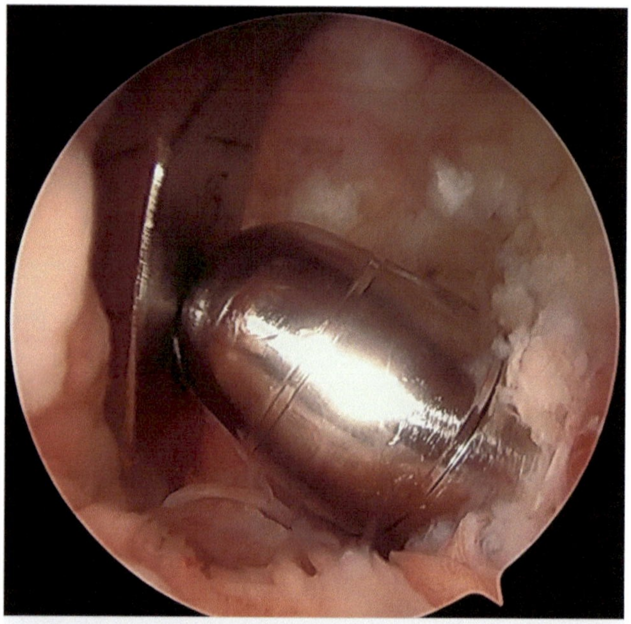

Fig. 27.10 Arthroscopic view from posterior medial portal shows posterior cruciate ligament (PCL) tibial tunnel dilation.

insertion and to protect the neurovascular structures during drilling. We start the drilling with power and switch to hand drilling to finish the tunnel.

- The tibia is reamed one size smaller than measured graft width; the tunnel dilator is used to expand the tunnel to the correct size (if 11-mm tunnel is desired, a 10-mm tunnel is drilled followed by 1-mm dilation) (▶ Fig. 27.10; Video 27.4).

27.10.2 Drilling the Femoral Tunnel (Inside Out)

- The goal of the graft placement is to reproduce the AL bundle.
- The AL footprint of the PCL is directly adjacent to the articular margin of the medial femoral condyle. The centroid of the AL insertion is in the anterior half of the femoral footprint (▶ Fig. 27.11).
- The center of the AL footprint is marked using an awl. A 3/32-mm guide pin is directed through the AL portal and situated over the marked location. The knee is flexed to 100 to 110 degrees. An acorn drill bit 10 mm in size is used to drill the tunnel. Great care must be taken to avoid injury to the patellar articular cartilage.
- The guide pin is then over-reamed with a low-profile acorn reamer while ensuring to avoid damaging the articular cartilage of the patella. Reamer size is determined by graft diameter using the same technique as described for the tibial tunnel (tunnel is drilled 1 mm smaller than measured graft size followed by 1-mm dilation) (Video 27.5).

27.10.3 Graft Passage and Fixation

Hamstring Graft Passage and Tensioning

- The hamstring quadruple graft is made. The free ends are whip stitched with #2 nonabsorbable suture. An appropriate length endobutton with its loop is attached. The goal is to have 2 cm of graft in the femoral tunnel. Total graft length is usually between 9 and 11 cm.

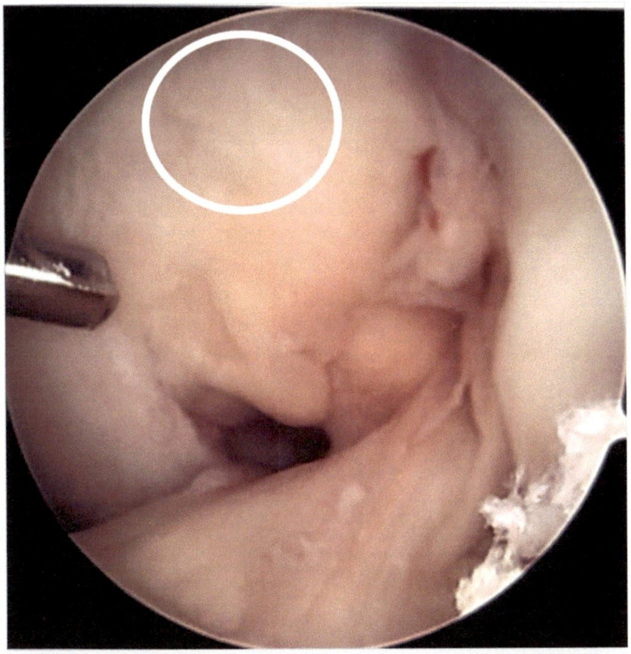

Fig. 27.11 Arthroscopic view from the anterolateral portal showing the medial femoral condyle. The white circle is the anatomic footprint for the anterolateral bundle of the posterior cruciate ligament (PCL). The arthroscopic shaver is entering from the anteromedial portal.

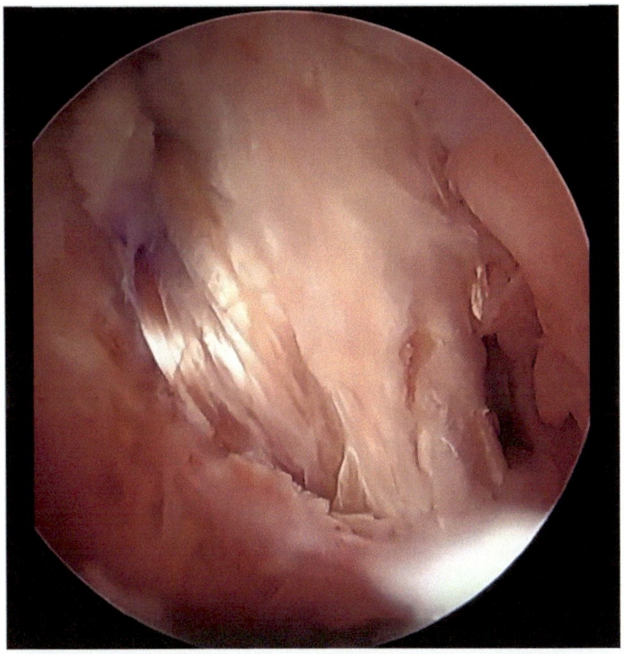

Fig. 27.12 View from the anterolateral portal showing posterior cruciate ligament (PCL) reconstruction with the knee at 90 degrees of flexion.

- After initial graft fixation, the knee is taken through full range of motion to confirm knee stability and appropriate graft tensioning.
  - Verify normal tibiofemoral translation at 90 degrees of knee flexion.
  - Graft tensioning occurs at 90 degrees of knee flexion where the AL bundle is tight.
- Tibial side is fixed with knee at 90 degrees of flexion with a 4.5-mm cortical screw and washer.

Quadriceps Tendon-Bone Graft Passage

- The quadriceps tendon graft has a 2-cm bone plug with 2 × #5 nonabsorbable sutures.
- The soft tissue end also has #5 nonabsorbable suture.
- The graft is passed from tibia to femur with the bone plug on the tibial side. This portion of the procedure can be technically demanding (**Video 27.6**).
- We recommend femoral fixation that is tied over a 6.5-mm cancellous screw with washer. A separate washer is required to achieve this fixation.
- After initial graft fixation, the knee is taken through a full range of motion to confirm knee stability and appropriate graft tensioning.
  - Verify normal tibiofemoral translation at 90 degrees of knee flexion.
  - Graft tensioning occurs at 90 degrees knee flexion where AL bundle is tight.
- Tibial side fixed with knee at 90 degrees of flexion, with a 4.5-mm cortical screw and washer.
- PCL tension is confirmed at 90 degrees of flexion using a nerve hook (▸ Fig. 27.12).

27.11 Bailout, Rescue, Salvage Procedures

- The senior author does not like to use interference fixation. He prefers cortical fixation. If there is any compromise of the suture being tied down, then an interference screw can be added as a backup.

27.12 Pitfalls

- Patella fracture from quadriceps tendon bone harvest.
- Loss of motion (loss of flexion is most common).
- Popliteal artery is 1 to 2 cm from the posterior capsular insertion. It can be injured with either the drill bit, K-wire, or arthroscopic shaver.
- Graft failure (secondary to poor graft position [technical failure], too aggressive or inappropriate postoperative rehabilitation, traumatic failure [secondary to major injury, e.g., fall, motor vehicle accident, sporting injury, etc.]).
- DVT is a very real possibility in these cases because of the longer surgical time, and conservative post op rehabilitation. We strongly recommend post op DVT prophylaxis in all patients undergoing PCL reconstruction and absolutely in all patients with increased risk factors (previous DVT, multiple ligament reconstruction, birth control in females, smoking, etc.)

28 Posterior Cruciate Ligament—Tibial Avulsion

Rodrigo Salim

28.1 Description

The posterior cruciate ligament (PCL) injury associated with a bone avulsion at the tibial insert is part of a spectrum of injury that can occur to this ligament. Clinical manifestation and progression to joint degeneration, if not adequately treated, is similar to other PCL injuries. The surgical treatment of this injury consists of reduction of the fracture and fixation.

28.2 Key Principles

There are several techniques for reinsertion of the PCL; however, none has been established as the "gold standard." These authors believe that precise restoration of the human anatomy provides the best surgical results. In this way, fracture reduction with stable fixation is the focal determinant for the treatment, and the avulsed fragment can be accessed either through open surgery or via arthroscopy.

28.3 Expectations

Arthroscopic treatment of the PCL avulsion is less invasive, though it is technically more difficult than the open procedure. In addition to a focus on the approach to treat the fracture, there have been discussions in the literature about the best method of fixation. Several implants have been proposed: conventional screws, toothed plate, anchors, and absorbable screws.

28.4 Indications

PCL avulsion with a displaced bone fragment is documented by imaging tests. On radiographs, the fragment is from the insertion site of the cranial PCL at the articular line on the lateral view. Displacement greater than 5 mm is usually considered significant. It is also frequently seen on computed tomography (CT) or magnetic resonance imaging (MRI) scans.

28.5 Contraindications

- PCL intrasubstance injury.
- Advanced tricompartmental arthrosis.

28.6 Special Considerations

The use of arthroscopic surgery in the reconstruction of PCL has been increasing over the past few decades. The avulsion fracture of the distal insertion of this ligament is a special type of PCL disruption. Descriptions of surgical techniques and fixation by arthroscopic techniques have appeared, are less invasive, and bring the possibility of treating associated joint injuries, such as cartilage or meniscus injury. However, these techniques require a long learning curve with challenges regarding reduction and fixation as well as the need of special instruments. Open surgery through a posteromedial safe access provides fragment exposure, allowing for absolute reduction with adequate fixation. This route can be used in hospitals that do not have in their arsenal all of the equipment needed for arthroscopic techniques.

28.7 Special Instructions, Positioning, and Anesthesia

28.7.1 Open Surgical Technique

- Epidural or general anesthesia.
- Prone position.
- Use of tourniquet in the proximal region of the thigh.
- Use of C-arm fluoroscopy.

28.7.2 Arthroscopic Technique

- Epidural or general anesthesia.
- Supine position.
- Use of tourniquet in the proximal region of the thigh.
- Need for posteromedial portal.
- Use of C-arm fluoroscopy.

28.8 Tips, Pearls, and Lessons Learned

28.8.1 Open Surgical Technique

After the positioning of the patient in prone position and with the use of a tourniquet and the knee flexed approximately 30 degrees, we perform an oblique incision of approximately 7 cm on the posteromedial aspect of the knee along the medial border of the medial head of the gastrocnemius muscle. We bluntly dissect the subcutaneous tissue to avoid damage to the saphenous vein and the sural nerve. After opening the deep fascia, we retract the medial head of the gastrocnemius to one side along with the neurovascular bundle, thus exposing the joint capsule safely. The capsule is opened longitudinally to expose the bone fragment. We perform debridement and irrigation of the injured area. After this, the reduction of this fragment is obtained easily by direct manipulation with a cushion on the anterior surface of the thigh and application of an anterior drawer. The fragment reduction can be checked by using fluoroscopy images. For fixation, we use a screw with a toothed washer or a plate depending on the size of the fragment and

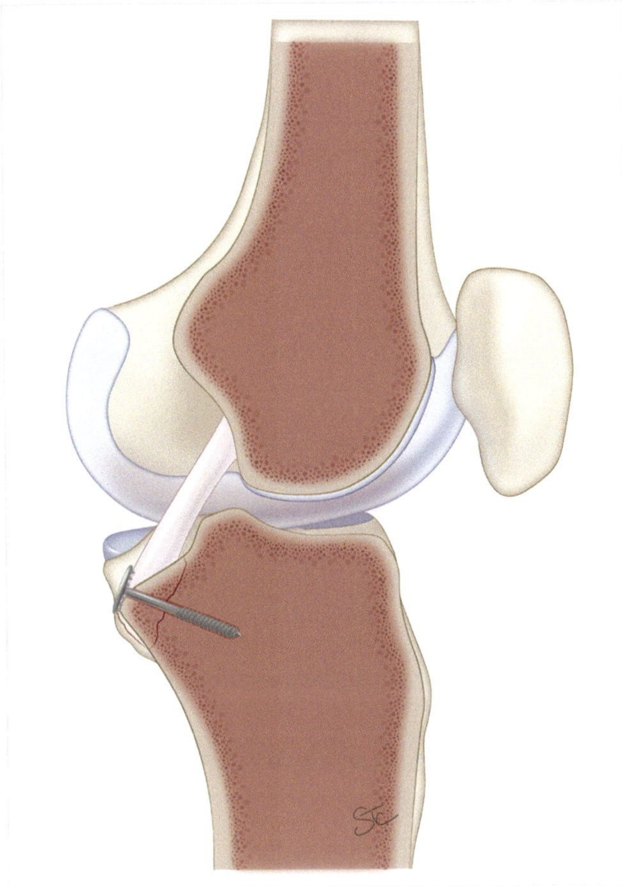

Fig. 28.1 Schematic diagram shows the fixation of a posterior cruciate ligament avulsion fracture with a toothed washer.

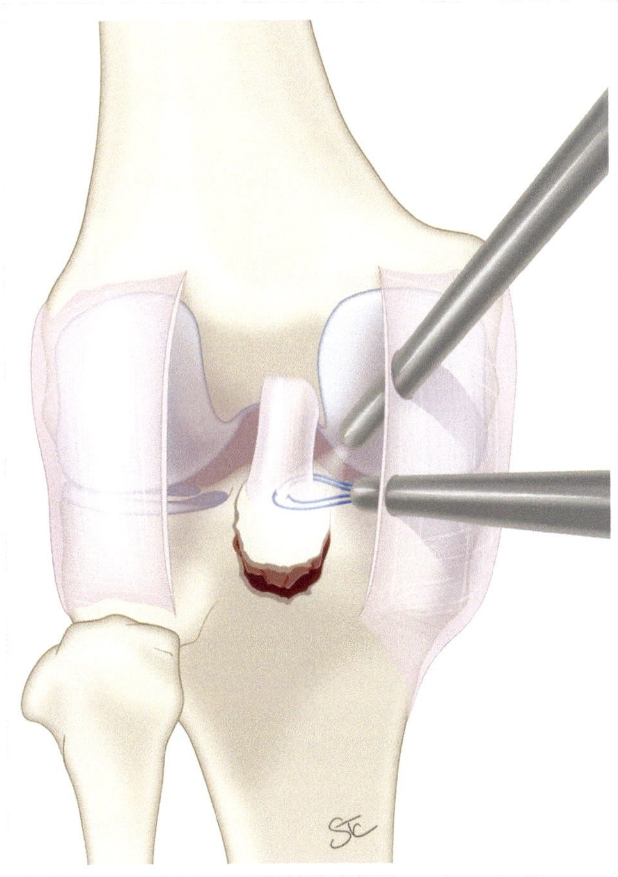

Fig. 28.2 Suture in the posterior cruciate ligament (PCL) above the avulsion bony fragment: illustration.

the degree of comminution (▶ Fig. 28.1). The wound is closed in layers without a drain.

28.8.2 Arthroscopic Technique

The patient is placed in the supine position with placement of a pneumatic tourniquet. The conventional anteromedial and anterolateral portals are made, and a diagnostic arthroscopy is carried out with the possibility of treatment of associated injuries to the meniscus and chondral cartilage. Two additional posteromedial portals are used for debriding the injury and placing suture, a high posteromedial portal and a low posteromedial portal (▶ Fig. 28.2). The portals are made 4 cm above the joint line and at the level of the joint line, respectively. Using the highest posteromedial portal to obtain the video images, we pass two suture strands of No.5 Ethibond in the PCL slightly cranial to their insertion from anterior to posterior by the anterolateral portal. These stitches are pulled and extracted from the capsule through the low posteromedial portal. After this, we perform an incision approximately 2 cm below the articular line on the medial face of the knee. Using the PCL guide at 55 degrees and the anteromedial portal, we create two bone tunnels with 4.5-mm-diameter cannulated drills, beginning on the medial tibia directing toward the insertion of the PCL, ensuring that there is no confluence between them. The previously passed sutures are pulled through the tunnels and tied together while applying an anterior drawer with the knee flexed at 70 degrees and tied over an anterior button (▶ Fig. 28.3). The fragment reduction and ligament tension are checked using the posteromedial portals.

28.9 Difficulties Encountered

We can perform the repair of the PCL detachment through the two techniques described above. The difficulties related to these procedures are:

- Open procedure—due to the proximity of the neurovascular bundle to the PCL insertion. Conventional "S" access to the popliteal fossa can cause serious iatrogenic injuries with permanent and severe complications. In the same way, posterolateral access can cause damage to the peroneal nerve.
- Arthroscopic procedure—this procedure requires a surgical learning curve, given the technical difficulty. In addition, the surgeon must have access to equipment to perform advanced arthroscopic procedures. The fixation and reduction of

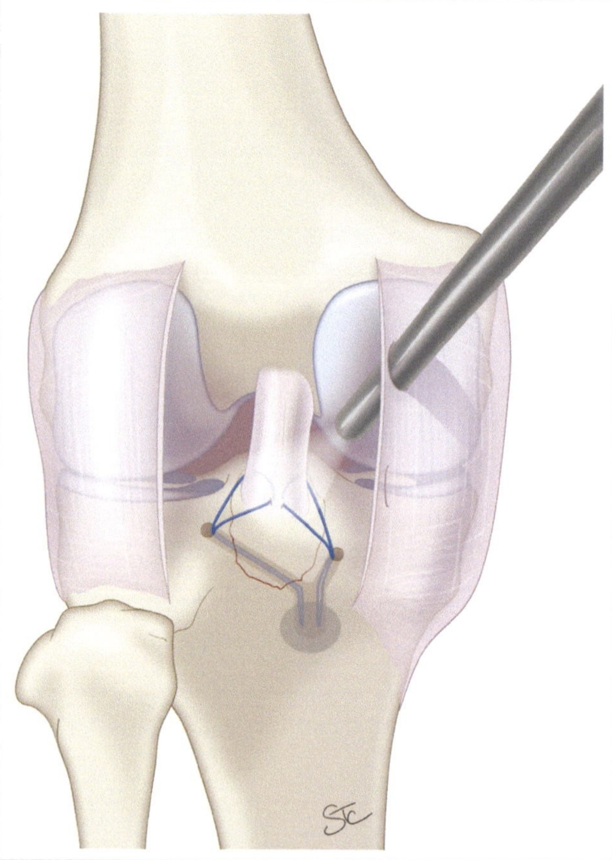

Fig. 28.3 Fixation of the suture after passing through the bony tunnels with anterior button.

fracture fragments are challenging in addition to the open surgery risks for neurovascular injuries.

28.10 Key Procedural Steps

PCL injuries with an avulsion fracture have an excellent prognosis. The outcome depends on fracture reduction and its fixation until consolidation. In this sense, having an adequate visualization of the fragment through open surgery, arthroscopy or even through the images of fluoroscopic equipment, is a crucial step. For fixation, some methods are described as absorbable or cannulated screws, sutures, anchors, and buttons. The arthroscopic route brings additional difficulty, since accessory portals are needed to fix the fragment. In the open route, we use screws with toothed washers to fix the fragment.

28.11 Bailout, Rescue, and Salvage Procedures

Surgical treatment of chronic injuries with a delayed diagnosis or nonunion of previous surgeries in PCL avulsion fracture is recommended when patients present functional disability and nonunion of the fracture. We recommend, in this situation, open surgery, since the debridement of the fibrous tissue is necessary. Sometimes, before the fixation, we chose to insert bone graft to fill the space created after the resection of the fibrous tissue. The fixation depends on the fragment(s). In case of large fragments, we give preference to screws with washers if they have sufficient size. Otherwise, we suture it by using anchors. Another salvage option in the failed open reduction and internal fixation (ORIF) of a PCL avulsion is switching to a PCL reconstruction.

29 Posteromedial Corner Knee Reconstruction

Robert Longstaffe and Alan Getgood

29.1 Description

Medial-sided knee injuries can often be treated successfully with nonoperative management. However, reconstruction should be considered in cases of multiligamentous injury or chronic valgus instability. Patients with valgus opening in extension and increased axial rotation undergo a posteromedial reconstruction entailing a superficial medial collateral ligament (sMCL) reconstruction with semitendinosus autograft and posterior oblique ligament (POL) reconstruction with gracilis autograft.

29.2 Key Principles

When considering a medial-sided reconstruction, it is crucial to determine when to address the POL along with reconstruction of sMCL. A detailed clinical evaluation is of paramount importance for diagnosing the extent of soft tissue damage to the medial side of the knee.

With the knee at 20 degrees of flexion, a valgus stress predominately isolates the sMCL. Increased external rotation in lower flexion angles is also indicative of a distal sMCL lesion. Excessive medial compartment opening in full extension indicates a more severe combined medial knee injury, and likely a combined cruciate ligament injury. Thus, valgus laxity at 20 degrees of flexion but not in extension indicates the POL is most likely intact.

To assess axial rotational stability, an anteromedial drawer test is performed with the knee flexed at 90 degrees along with external rotation of the foot at 15 degrees while applying an anteromedial force to the proximal tibia to assess anteromedial tibia rotation compared to the contralateral knee. Continued anterior translation with the tibia externally rotated is suggestive of anteromedial laxity, with deficiencies of either the deep medial collateral ligament (dMCL) or the posteromedial corner, the latter consisting of the posterior meniscotibial ligament, as seen damaged in a RAMP lesion of the meniscus. The dial test should also be performed. Previously thought to be pathognomonic for posterolateral corner injuries, the dial test has been shown to produce a positive test at both 30 degrees and 90 degrees of flexion with medial injury patterns too. A positive test is a sign of external rotation laxity; therefore, assessment of patients in both a supine and a prone position is important to interpret if excessive external rotation is a result of anteromedial opposed to posterolateral tibial rotation.

If the diagnosis is still in doubt, stress radiographs can be an extremely useful adjunct to clinical examination to identify the extent of the medial knee injury, particularly in chronic scenarios. Increased medial compartment gapping, greater than 3.2 mm compared to the contralateral knee on valgus stress radiographs, indicates a complete injury to the sMCL. If this increases to greater than 9.8 mm compared to the contralateral knee then a complete medial-sided knee injury is likely.

29.3 Expectations

A majority of posteromedial reconstructions are performed in combined injuries with cruciate reconstructions performed concomitantly. As such, the rehabilitation and recovery is somewhat slower than for isolated cruciate reconstruction. Due to the coronal plane rotational moments about the knee during weight-bearing, flat foot touch weight-bearing is initiated for the first 6 weeks postoperatively followed by progression to weight-bearing as tolerated thereafter. The knee is kept in a hinged brace allowing 0 to 90 degrees of motion for the first 2 weeks followed by full range of motion to prevent stiffness. From 6 to 12 weeks, patients will continue to wear their brace only when ambulating. Following 3 months, patients are fitted with a custom brace to be used during dynamic exercises and return to sport rehabilitation for at least one year.

29.4 Indications

- Acute medial knee injury associated with a multiligamentous knee injury/knee dislocation, where early range of motion is warranted.
- Chronic medial knee instability with normal alignment that has failed nonoperative management. This may include valgus laxity or a combination of valgus and rotational laxity in the anterior cruciate ligament (ACL) or posterior cruciate ligament (PCL) deficient knee.

29.5 Contraindications

- Extensive soft tissue injury that does not permit a safe incision or closure of wounds.
- Severe arthrofibrosis.
- Isolated sMCL injury that has not undergone a trial of nonoperative management.
- Malalignment (valgus) that would necessitate corrective osteotomy prior to soft tissue reconstruction unless performed as a concomitant procedure.
- Sepsis or active infection in proximity to incision.

29.6 Special Considerations

For patients presenting with chronic medial knee instability, it is imperative to assess their weight-bearing coronal plane alignment. Patients with valgus alignment should be considered for a corrective osteotomy to restore mechanical axis to neutral. The medial reconstruction can then be performed simultaneously or as a second procedure if they continue to have ongoing instability. In patients with valgus alignment and chronic medial knee instability, soft tissue reconstruction without limb alignment correction creates an inherent risk of graft failure due to the increased abduction moment creating undue stress to the soft tissue graft.

29.7 Special Instructions, Position, and Anesthesia

A general anesthetic is preferred, often augmented with a motor sparing adductor canal block of the femoral nerve. Patients are positioned supine on the operating table with a lateral thigh post and footrest to allow knee flexion to 90 degrees. An examination under anesthesia is performed, paying particular attention to medial compartment opening in 0 and 20 degrees of flexion to make final determination if a concomitant POL reconstruction is required. A well-padded high-thigh tourniquet is applied and inflated prior to commencement of surgery.

29.8 Tips, Pearls, and Lessons Learned

- In multiligamentous injuries, it is useful to perform the approach first, prior to arthroscopy. This allows for easier identification of medial structures prior to fluid extravasation. The egress of fluid from the incision can also help to mitigate the potential development of compartment syndrome.
- An ipsilateral bone-patellar tendon-bone or quadriceps tendon harvest can be performed through the same medial incision for posteromedial reconstruction if a cruciate ligament reconstruction is required (▶ Fig. 29.1a–c).
- Identification of adductor magnus tendon (AMT) and adductor tubercle (AT) allows for referencing important medial-sided structures.
- Tapping the cortical tibial bone tunnel prior to graft passage will allow for easier screw placement and less risk of graft damage during tibial interference screw placement.
- If a cruciate ligament reconstruction is required, this should be performed and tensioned first. If both cruciates are reconstructed, tension the PCL first, followed by medial side then ACL.
- Tension of the sMCL graft should be done at 20 degrees of flexion with a gentle varus force applied. Tensioning on the femoral side will provide a mechanical advantage by "pulling" the tibia into varus.
- If the medial knee is lax in full extension and adequate posterior capsule is present, the central arm of the POL can be imbricated and an augmentation of the POL can be performed with an extra-articular synthetic graft. If the posteromedial capsular tissue is deficient, a soft tissue graft, such as a gracilis autograft, is used to reconstruct the POL. In both cases, tension and fixation must be done in full extension and neutral rotation.

29.9 Difficulties Encountered

Severe medial-sided injuries can result in avulsion injuries to important medial structures and landmarks. The AMT and its insertion of the AT is a reliable landmark as it rarely is injured. However, given the importance of anatomic graft placement, if there is a difficulty in palpation of the adductor tendon and related soft tissue structures, intraoperative fluoroscopy should be considered to aid in proper tunnel placement.

One of the most difficult issues is that of tunnel coalition, particularly in multiligament reconstruction, and if performing double bundle PCL reconstruction. In these cases the ACL and PCL femoral tunnels are drilled first but grafts not passed. The medial tunnels are drilled and can be checked to ensure no communication. The use of anchors and a synthetic tape as an augment of the POL also assists in this issue by drilling sockets not tunnels.

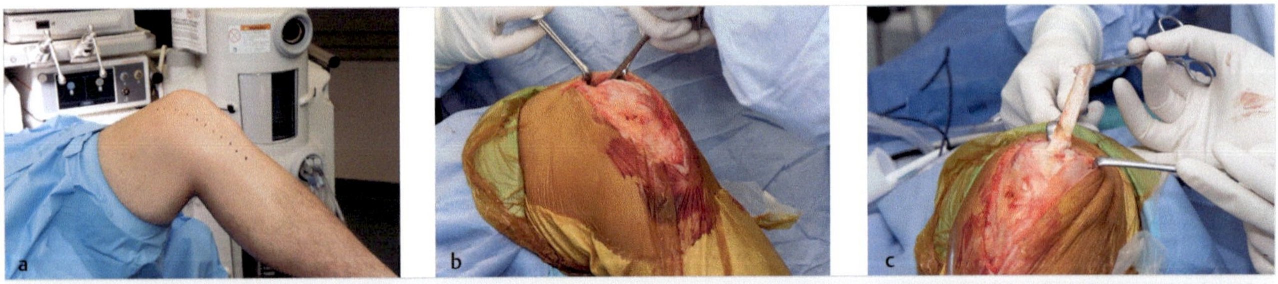

Fig. 29.1 (a) A medial longitudinal incision is made between medial border of patella and medial epicondyle carried from vastus medialis obliquus (VMO) to pes anserinus. **(b)** In cases of concomitant anterior cruciate ligament (ACL) or posterior cruciate ligament (PCL) reconstruction full-thickness soft tissue flaps can be elevated to allow exposure of patella and quadriceps for harvest. **(c)** A quadriceps graft has been harvested in this case for concomitant ACL reconstruction.

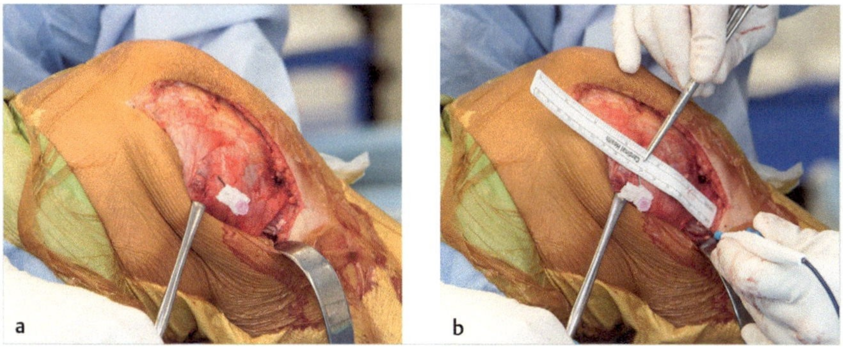

Fig. 29.2 **(a)** A spinal needle is used to identify the joint line. **(b)** The distal superficial medial collateral ligament (sMCL) is measured 6 cm from the spinal needle.

29.10 Key Procedural Steps

A longitudinal incision is made between medial border of patella and medial epicondyle carried from vastus medialis obliquus (VMO) to pes anserinus. Full-thickness flaps are developed, taking care to protect the saphenous nerve coursing 5 cm posterior to AT. The pes tendons are palpated and sartorial fascia is lifted and sharply dissected to identify the gracilis and semitendinosus tendons underneath. The tendons are harvested utilizing an open-ended tendon stripper.

A spinal needle is used to accurately identify the joint line. The distal insertion of the sMCL is measured 6 cm distal to the spinal needle (▶ Fig. 29.2a,b). Any remaining sMCL at its insertion is elevated off bone and an eyelet pin is inserted from posteromedial to anterolateral on the tibia. This is overdrilled with a drill size corresponding to the diameter of the doubled semitendinosus tendon to a depth of 25 mm. Due to the tough cortical bone at this point, the tunnel is tapped prior to inserting a passing suture to aid in placement of the interference screw.

The free ends of the gracilis tendon are whipstitched with a No. 1 Vicryl (Ethicon, Somerville, NJ). The semitendinosus tendon is passed through an Ultrabutton (Smith & Nephew, Andover, MA) and doubled (▶ Fig. 29.3). The free ends are whipstitched with a No. 1 Vicryl and passed into the tibial tunnel using the eyelet pin. The graft is fixed at its tibial insertion with Biosure PEEK interference screw (Smith & Nephew, Andover, MA).

Attention is turned to identification of the femoral attachments beginning with an incision through VMO fascia. The sMCL femoral insertion is identified, referencing approximately 12 mm distal and 8 mm anterior from the AT, just posterior and proximal to the medial epicondyle (▶ Fig. 29.4a,b). An eyelet pin is drilled from medial to lateral aiming slightly proximal and anterior (▶ Fig. 29.4c). The graft is wrapped around the pin and the knee is taken through a range of motion to ensure graft isometry. When dealing with the PCL-deficient knee, it is important to attempt to reduce the knee at this point if the PCL graft has not been passed. The posterior subluxation of the joint may alter the isometry of the sMCL graft and could result in abnormal graft placement. The pin is overdrilled with a 4.5-mm drill to and through the lateral cortex, with the tunnel length measured. The length of the Ultrabutton is adjusted accordingly to avoid the button being pulled through the iliotibial band. The medial cortex is then drilled with an appropriately sized drill based on graft diameter to allow placement of the graft.

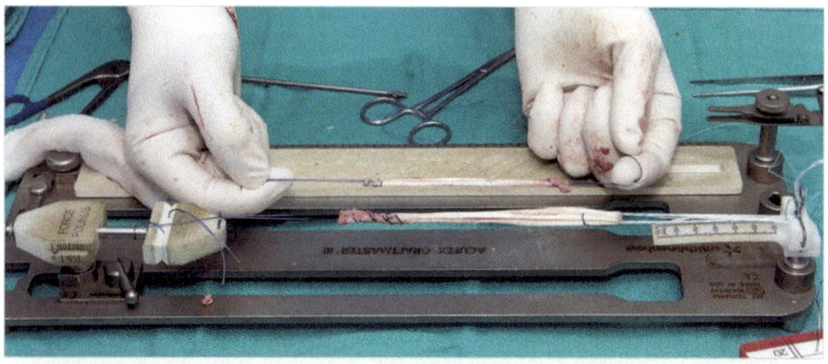

Fig. 29.3 Preparation of the semitendinosus and gracilis grafts. The gracilis graft has been whipped stitched on either end with a No. 1 Vicryl. At least 12 cm of length is required for reconstruction of posterior oblique ligament (POL). The semitendinosus tendon has been double and passed through the Ultrabutton (Smith & Nephew, Andover, MA). The free ends have been whipstitched together with a No. 1 Vicryl. At least 16 cm of length is required for reconstruction of superficial medial collateral ligament (sMCL).

Following this, the femoral and tibial attachments of POL are identified. Insertion of semimembranosus (SM) and location of medial head of gastrocnemius are identified. The posteromedial capsule is found just posterior to the remnant of sMCL (▶ Fig. 29.5a). The femoral attachment of the central arm of POL is identified approximately 8 mm distal and 3 mm anterior of gastrocnemius tubercle (▶ Fig. 29.5b). An eyelet pin is drilled through the lateral cortex followed by an appropriate-sized drill through the medial cortex to a depth of 25 mm. The tibial attachment of the central arm of POL is found slightly anterior to the direct arm attachment of the SM. An eyelet pin is again placed aiming toward Gerdy tubercle. This is overdrilled with an appropriate-sized drill to a depth of 25 mm (▶ Fig. 29.5c). Shuttling sutures are placed into both tunnels and attention is turned back to fixation of the sMCL femoral attachment.

The semitendinosus graft is tunneled underneath the sartorial fascia proximally toward the femoral tunnel. The graft

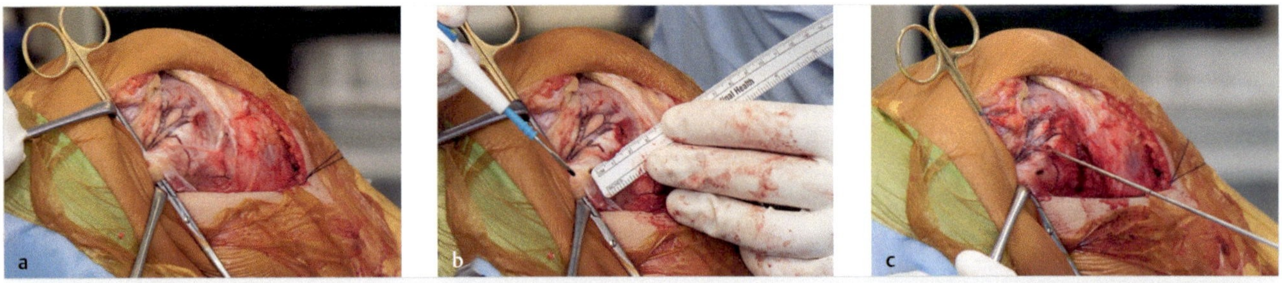

Fig. 29.4 (a) Metzenbaum scissors have been placed beneath adductor magnus tendon allowing for identification of adductor tubercle. (b) The femoral insertion of superficial medial collateral ligament (sMCL) is measured 12 mm distal and 8 mm anterior to adductor tubercle. (c) The eyelet pin is drilled from medial to lateral aiming slightly proximal and anterior.

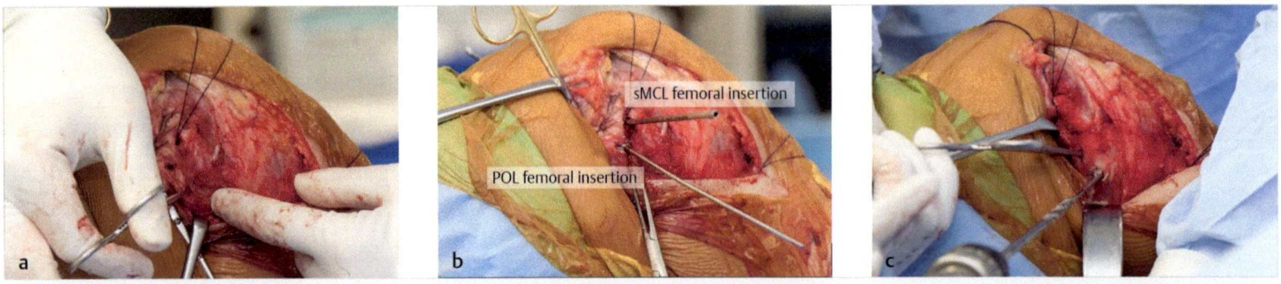

Fig. 29.5 (a) The redundant posteromedial capsule can be seen with the use of an Alice forceps applying traction (b) An eyelet pin and 4.5-mm drill demonstrate the femoral insertions for both the superficial medial collateral ligament (sMCL) and posterior oblique ligament (POL). (c) The tibial insertion of central arm of POL is found slightly anterior to the direct arm attachment of the semimembranosus (SM) and is drilled toward Gerdy tubercle.

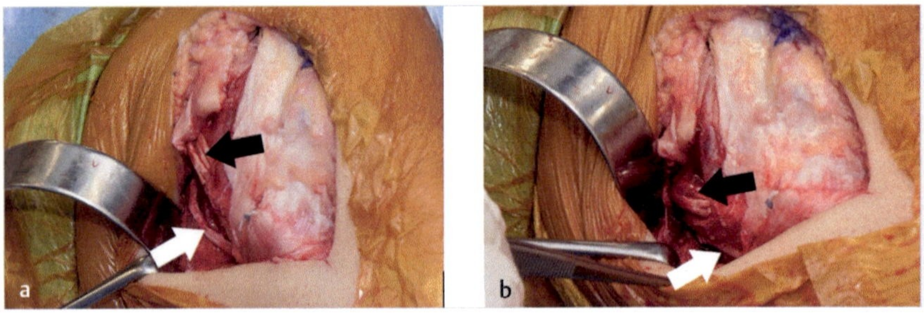

Fig. 29.6 (a) With the knee flexed, the posterior oblique ligament (POL) reconstruction (*white arrow*) should be lax. (b) With the knee extended, the POL reconstruction (*white arrow*) should be taut. The superficial medial collateral ligament (sMCL) reconstruction (*black arrow*) should remain isometric through range of motion.

is shuttled into the femoral tunnel and the Ultrabutton is flipped and provisionally tensioned at 20 degrees of flexion. The knee is again cycled to eliminate any remaining creep in the graft and retensioned through the adjustable loop with the knee at 20 degrees of flexion and a gentle varus force applied. Again, referencing off the joint line, the proximal tibial insertion of sMCL is identified 14 mm distal to the joint. A 4.5-mm Twinfix suture anchor (Smith & Nephew, Andover, MA) is inserted anterior to the distal insertion of the central arm of POL. The sutures are passed through the anterior limb of the graft and tied in a mattress fashion at 90 degrees of flexion. This ensures that an intact limb of the graft is present from femoral origin to proximal and distal tibial insertions of the sMCL.

The gracilis graft is shuttled into the tibial tunnel and fixated with a Biosure PEEK interference screw. The graft is then shuttled into the femoral tunnel and again secured with a Biosure PEEK interference screw with the knee in full extension and neutral rotation. If appropriately placed, the gracilis graft should be taut in extension and lax in flexion (▶ Fig. 29.6a,b). A final check of stability is performed with a gentle valgus force at both 0 and 20 degrees of flexion. ▶ Fig. 29.7 depicts the two graft reconstruction of the posteromedial corner.

In cases where there is adequate posteromedial capsule, an augmentation repair can be performed. A horizontal incision is made through the posteromedial capsule at the level of the joint. A "pants-over-vest" suture pattern is utilized to imbricate the POL utilizing #2Ethibond. The central arm of POL is further

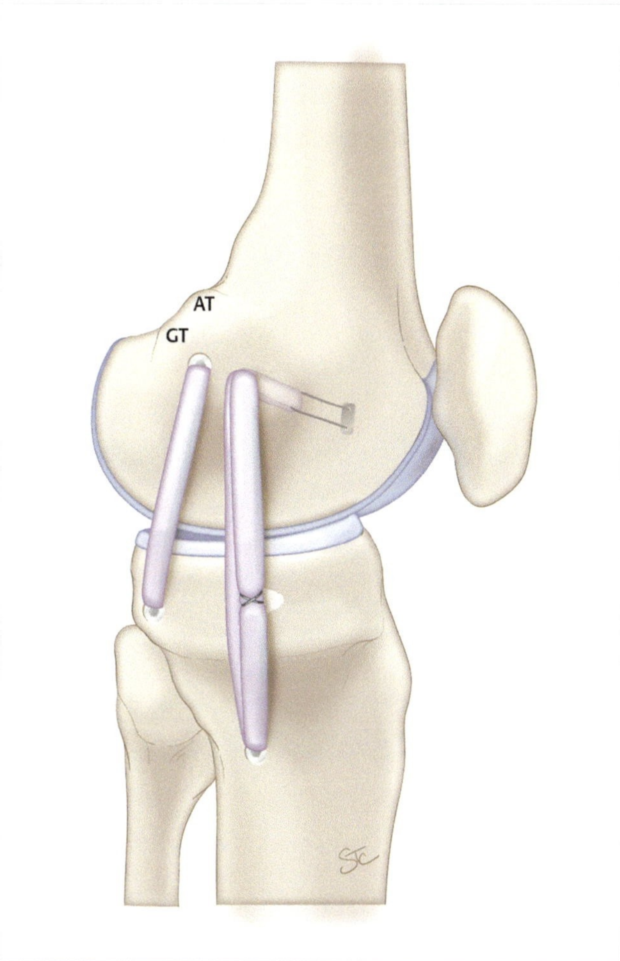

Fig. 29.7 Drawing of two graft anatomic reconstruction of the posteromedial corner.

augmented with the use of FiberTape fixated at both insertion and origin with a 5.5-mm SwivelLock anchor (Arthrex, Naples, FL). The FiberTape is fixated initially on the tibial side then inserted into the femoral side, tensioned with the knee in full extension and neutral rotation.

29.11 Bailout, Rescue, and Salvage Procedures

Premature graft amputation during hamstring harvest is a commonly feared complication. At least 16 cm of semitendinosus is required to reconstruct the sMCL and 12 cm of gracilis for POL. If premature graft amputation results in less than required length, consideration should be made for use of an alternative graft. Options include harvesting the contralateral semitendinosus or the use of allograft. Several surgical techniques have been described utilizing allograft that have reported good results. Alternatively, a single strand of ST may be used.

29.12 Pitfalls

- Do not tension sMCL graft in more than 20 degrees of flexion as the loop will not slacken and may capture the knee, resulting in an extensor lag.
- Do not base decision to reconstruct the medial side of knee based on the examination following fixation of ACL graft. This will lead to reduced valgus stress laxity although all the stress will be placed on the ACL graft.
- Do not use medial epicondyle for femoral tunnel placement as it will lead to excessive tightness of sMCL graft in flexion and capture the knee.
- Making an incision too posterior can place the saphenous nerve at risk.

30 Posterolateral Corner Reconstruction

Robert F. LaPrade and Samantha L. LaPrade

30.1 Description

Acute grade III and chronic posterolateral corner (PLC) injuries have a low likelihood of healing without intervention and lead to morbidity. A PLC reconstruction of the three main static stabilizers, the fibular collateral ligament (FCL), popliteus tendon, and popliteofibular ligament (PFL) (▶ Fig. 30.1), anatomically restores the knee structures in order to reproduce the native anatomy and biomechanics of the knee.

30.2 Key Principles

The PLC structures are important for static and dynamic stabilization of the knee. The PLC also provides a secondary restraint for concurrent anterior cruciate ligament (ACL) and posterior cruciate ligament (PCL) injuries. If the PLC is not repaired or reconstructed in these cases, there are higher failure rates of ACL and PCL reconstruction grafts.

30.3 Expectations

Prompt diagnosis and treatment of PLC injuries are essential. The outcomes for treatment of acute PLC injuries are significantly better than for chronic PLC injuries.

30.4 Indications

- Acute grade III PLC injury (within the first few weeks of injury) or chronic PLC injury.

30.5 Contraindications

- Acute grade I or grade II PLC injury amenable to nonoperative treatment.
- Significant comorbidities which preclude being able to follow proper postoperative rehabilitation.

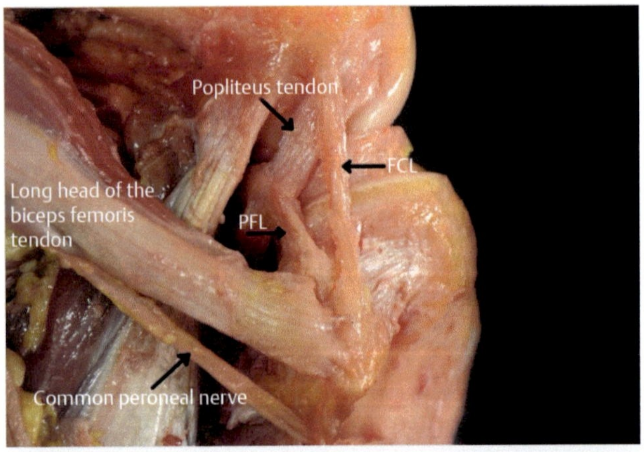

Fig. 30.1 Dissection demonstrating the posterolateral corner (PLC) structures of a right knee. The fibular collateral ligament (FCL), popliteofibular ligament (PFL), and popliteus tendon are identified.

30.6 Special Considerations

Appropriate diagnostic imaging should be performed including anteroposterior and varus stress radiographs to objectively evaluate varus gapping indicative of a PLC injury. Additional imaging including magnetic resonance imaging (MRI) may be warranted to evaluate for concomitant injuries, such as to the ACL, PCL, menisci, and associated fractures. In patients with a chronic PLC injury with varus malalignment, a proximal tibial osteotomy is required prior to PLC reconstruction because there is a high risk of PLC reconstruction failure with an uncorrected malalignment. In addition, 40% of patients with a first-stage osteotomy may not require a second-stage ligament reconstruction. Reassessment of PLC laxity and the patient's symptoms after proximal tibial osteotomy is therefore indicated. Reconstruction is required for midsubstance acute and chronic PLC injuries, whereas repairs may be appropriate if the PLC injury was an acute avulsion with no midsubstance injury.

30.7 Special Instructions, Position, and Anesthesia

- Operating table with removable ends or the ability to flex down the end of the bed.
- Arthroscopy tower and equipment available as well as instruments for ACL and PCL reconstructions, meniscal inside-out and root repairs, and microfracture treatment.
- Supine position with tourniquet in place on the proximal thigh of the surgical leg, and distal thigh secured with a leg holder and nonsurgical leg is secured out of the surgical field in an abduction stirrup.
- Surgical leg hangs at approximately a 70-degree angle.
- General anesthesia, epidural, or spinal anesthesia per the surgeon and patient preference.
- Standard skin preparation and sterile draping.
- Anatomic reconstruction of the FCL or popliteus tendon is performed using an autogenous hamstring graft when one is torn in isolation from the other; however, if torn concurrently, a complete PLC reconstruction with a split Achilles tendon allograft is recommended.

30.8 Tips, Pearls, and Lessons Learned

Concomitant injuries needing repair should be treated concurrent with the procedure. If the patellar tendon autograft is being harvested, position the PLC approach incision more posteriorly in order to maintain a minimum 6-cm skin bridge between the two incisions.

The distance between the reconstruction tunnel guide pins for the femoral attachments of the FCL and popliteus tendon should be 18.5 mm. Any significant variation from the 18.5-mm distance indicates either nonanatomic positioning or misidentification of femoral attachments.

30.9 Difficulties Encountered

The common peroneal nerve may be encased in scar tissue or displaced, especially in the case of biceps femoris avulsions off the fibular head.

Chronic posterolateral knee injuries may have heterotopic ossification of the lateral capsule which complicates identification of anatomic attachment locations.

Revision PLC surgeries may require intraoperative fluoroscopy to aid in proper tunnel placement.

30.10 Key Procedural Steps

An examination under anesthesia is performed initially to confirm the suspected pathology. A standard lateral superficial hockey stick incision is made beginning along the posterior midportion of the iliotibial (IT) band and extending across the knee to the anterior compartment, crossing the knee at the level of Gerdy tubercle (▶ Fig. 30.2). The incision is then carried through the subcutaneous tissue to the IT band.

A step-by-step open dissection of the posterolateral knee is performed to identify PLC injuries needing repair versus reconstruction. First, identify the long and short heads of the biceps femoris. Identify the common peroneal nerve 2 to 3 cm distal to the long head of the biceps femoris (▶ Fig. 30.3), or palpate it 2 cm distal to the fibular head, and perform a neurolysis. If avulsed from the fibular head, place a tag stitch in the distal aspect of the biceps tendon and release it from proximal scar tissue to allow repair.

Assess structures in order of attachment to the fibula, femur, tibia, and lateral meniscus and plan for repair or reconstruction and the graft(s) to be used. Evaluate the distal FCL attachment by making an incision through the anterior arm of the long head of the biceps femoris through the biceps bursa; place a tag stitch at the distal aspect of the remnant ligament. The FCL requires reconstruction if there is evidence of midsubstance tearing or substantial intrasubstance stretch injuries (▶ Fig. 30.4). Identify the insertion of the PFL on the posteromedial aspect of the fibular head. Reconstruction of the PFL is required if there is substantial intrasubstance stretch injury, midsubstance tear, or musculotendinous avulsion. Consider direct repair of the PFL if the popliteus tendon is intact, the

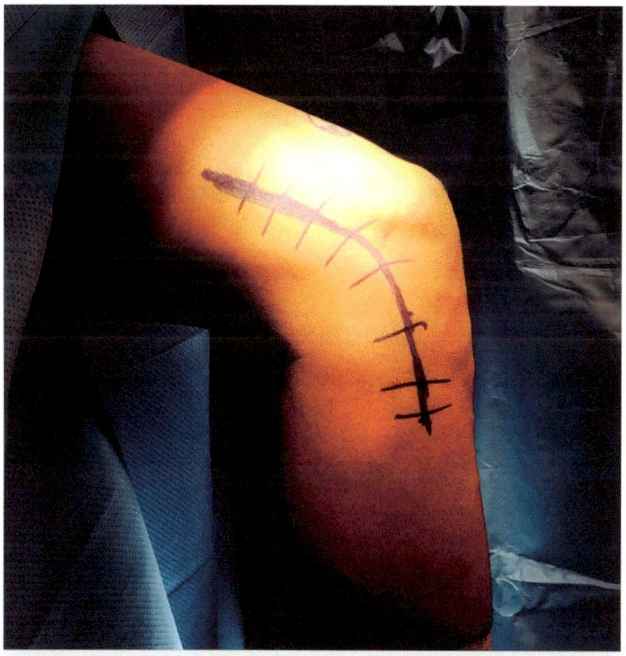

Fig. 30.2 A right knee with a standard lateral hockey stick incision outlined from the posterior midportion of the iliotibial (IT) band across the knee to over the anterior compartment.

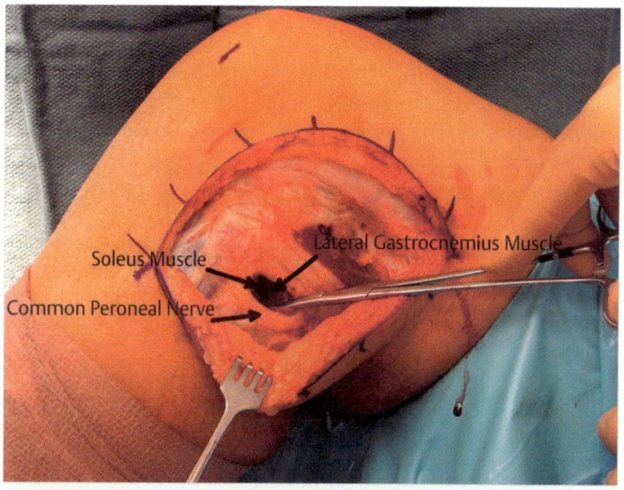

Fig. 30.3 Lateral view of a left knee showing a hemostat in the interval between the lateral gastrocnemius muscle and soleus muscle; the common peroneal nerve is located below the hemostat and the long head of the biceps tendon.

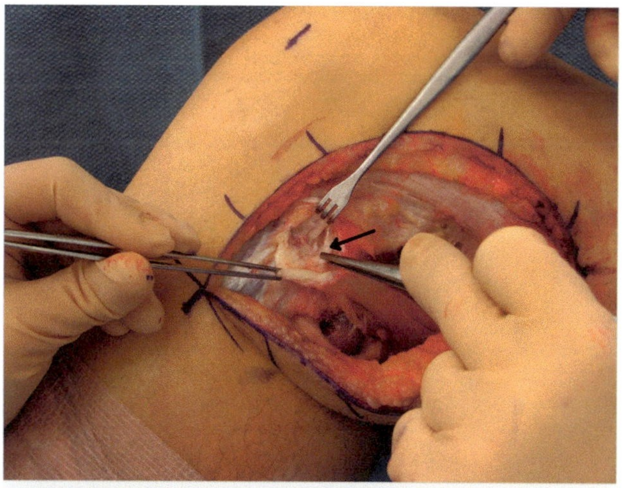

Fig. 30.4 Lateral view of a left knee with a torn fibular collateral ligament (FCL) within the biceps bursa (*arrow*).

PFL is avulsed from the fibular head, and the tissue is amenable for approximation via suturing.

Drill the fibular head tunnel reconstruction beginning directly at the lateral attachment of the FCL and continuing through to the posteromedial downslope of the fibular styloid. A guide pin is placed along this path using a cruciate-aiming device and a retractor is inserted posterior and medial to the fibular head to protect the neurovasculature structures while drilling. Ream the fibular head tunnel using a 7-mm reamer and place a passing suture through the fibular tunnel for future graft passage.

Next, preparation for reaming of the tibial tunnel is conducted with identifying Gerdy tubercle following dissection of the distal attachment of the superficial layer of the IT band. A small flat area is found medial and distal to Gerdy tubercle, and adjacent to the lateral aspect of the patellar tendon. Dissection of this area to bone is performed and the soft tissue is removed using a rongeur to expose the site for the anterior aperture of the tibial tunnel to exit. At the posterior aspect of the tibia, identify the musculotendinous junction of the popliteus tendon between the gastrocnemius-soleus complex. The tibial tunnel will exit about 1 cm medial and 1 cm proximal to the fibular tunnel exit point and at the level of the musculotendinous junction. A guide pin is placed from the previously identified flat area on the anterior tibia to the exit site using an ACL-aiming device. A retractor is again used to protect the neurovasculature of the posterior knee from the guide pin. A 9-mm reamer is then used to ream the tibial tunnel.

The femoral attachments of the PLC are now evaluated via a splitting incision in line with the fibers of the IT band, just anterior to the lateral epicondyle and extending distally to Gerdy tubercle. The FCL attachment site is found slightly proximal and posterior to the lateral epicondyle. The popliteus tendon attachment site is in the anterior aspect of the popliteus sulcus, approximately 18.5 mm anterodistal to the FCL attachment, and the popliteus tendon is directly palpated at this site. A vertical incision through the lateral capsule of the knee allows for visualization of the femoral popliteus attachment.

Reaming of the femoral tunnels is performed after identification of both femoral attachment sites. One guide pin is passed through the FCL attachment anteromedially across the knee and through the medial thigh, avoiding the intercondylar notch, saphenous nerve, and potential cruciate ligament femoral tunnels. Another guide pin begins at the anterior insertion of the popliteus tendon attachment and is placed parallel to the FCL guide pin. The distance between guide pins is measured and should be 18.5 mm apart. After confirmation of this distance, the tunnels are reamed using a 9-mm reamer to a depth of 25 mm for both the popliteus and FCL tunnel. Passing sutures are passed into both tunnels at this time.

Arthroscopic assessment of the knee is performed while an assistant prepares the PLC reconstruction grafts. If only the FCL or popliteus tendon is torn in isolation from each other, a hamstring autograft may be used; however, if both are torn concurrently an Achilles tendon allograft is recommended for a complete anatomic posterolateral knee reconstruction. Arthroscopic assessment for gapping of the lateral compartment, injury to the coronary ligament and attachment to the lateral meniscus posterior horn, integrity of intra-articular portion of the popliteus tendon, popliteomeniscal fascicles, and meniscofemoral portion of the posterior capsule is conducted. Perform a meniscal tear repair versus partial meniscectomy as indicated. Evaluate the cruciate ligaments and perform reconstructions as needed; secure cruciate ligament grafts in the femoral tunnels but delay fixation of cruciate ligament grafts in the tibial tunnel(s) until PLC femoral graft fixation is completed.

Repair or reconstruction of PLC injuries is performed in order of attachment site starting with first at the femur, second at the lateral meniscus, third at the tibia for lateral capsule repairs, fourth at the fibula, and finally on the tibia for the reconstruction graft fixation. The bone ends of the grafts are placed into the femoral tunnels. From the bone plugs, passing sutures are placed in the looped passing sutures (▶ Fig. 30.5). Confirm that the graft and bone plugs fit tightly and secure with screw fixation using a 7-by-20-mm cannulated titanium screw. The guide pin should be positioned between the tunnel edge and bone plug so that the screw may fit between the tunnel wall and bone plug. Verify graft fixation with a firm tug laterally. The popliteus tendon graft may now be passed distally along the popliteal hiatus to exit the knee between the lateral gastrocnemius and soleus. Pass the FCL graft distally and deep to the superficial IT band and lateral to the long head of the biceps femoris aponeurosis. The FCL may now be passed into the fibular head tunnel.

Popliteomeniscal fascicle and coronary ligament tears from the lateral meniscus posterior horn are now repaired with vertical mattress sutures. Tears of the superficial layer of the IT band from Gerdy tubercle and the meniscofemoral and meniscotibial portions of the midthird lateral capsular ligament are also repaired with suture anchors.

Perform PCL tibial graft fixation as needed prior to securing the FCL in the fibular tunnel with the anterolateral bundle fixed at 90 degrees, followed by the posteromedial bundle at 0 degree. After PCL fixation, the FCL graft may be secured with a 7-mm bioabsorbable screw while pulling on the graft end proximally and applying valgus force with the knee in 20 degrees of flexion. An exam should be performed at this time to ensure correction of varus instability. The remaining popliteus tendon and

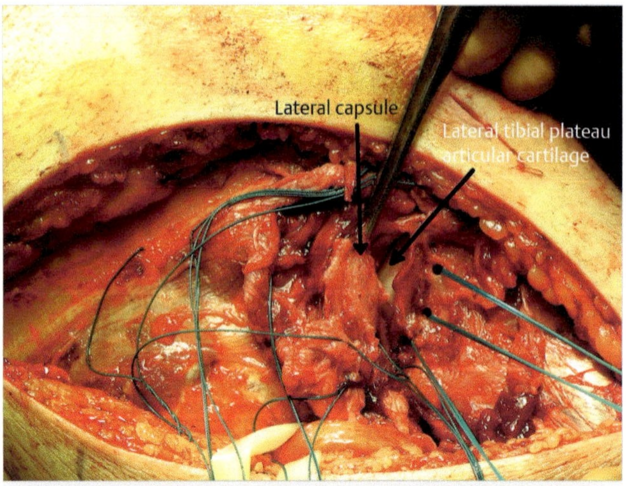

Fig. 30.5 Lateral view of a right knee with a complete grade III posterolateral knee injury showing the placement of suture anchors in the tibia and the torn lateral capsule.

PFL grafts are passed from posterior-to-anterior through the tibial tunnel. Ensure that there is no residual laxity and proper tension is applied. Fix PLC grafts in the tibial tunnel while the knee is flexed to 60 degrees in neutral rotation and sufficient tension applied to the grafts using a 9-mm bioabsorbable screw. Repair avulsions of the biceps femoris with suture anchors to the anatomic attachment site on the fibular head and styloid while the knee is in full extension; if there is not adequate tissue length for repair, proximal release of the long head of the biceps from adhesions and scar tissue may be necessary.

Fixation of ACL graft in the tibial tunnel may now be performed. A re-examination under anesthesia is now conducted to evaluate for restoration of knee stability. The safe zone for arc of motion postoperatively may now also be assessed.

30.11 Bailout, Rescue, and Salvage Procedures

In the case of fibular head avulsions or intraoperative fractures, consider dropping the fibular head tunnel distally on the fibular shaft. Alternatively, place cerclage nonabsorbable sutures to secure the fracture and consider a more conservative rehabilitation program.

30.12 Pitfalls

- Be cautious of peroneal nerve injuries and malposition with biceps femoris avulsions off the fibular head.
- It is important to always assess for varus alignment in chronic PLC injuries because this can lead to PLC reconstruction graft failure if the malalignment is not corrected.
- Reconstructions over repairs should be considered for acute PLC injuries, while chronic injuries should always undergo reconstructions.
- Failure to perform proximal release of the long head of the biceps femoris when there is not adequate length for repair of biceps femoris avulsions may result in failure of the repair when the knee is placed in full extension. There may also be a need for immobilization of the knee in flexion postoperatively until the knee is healed.
- Avoid iatrogenic fibular head fractures by thoroughly palpating the fibular head guide pin position prior to reaming the fibular reconstruction tunnel.

31 Knee Dislocation: Reconstruction

Gregory C. Fanelli and Matthew G. Fanelli

31.1 Description

The multiple ligament injured (dislocated) knee is a severe injury that may also involve neurovascular injuries, fractures, and other systemic injuries which can all impact the surgical treatment of the knee dislocation. This chapter will discuss my surgical technique for combined posterior and anterior cruciate ligament, medial and lateral side reconstructions in acute and chronic multiple ligament injured knees with global laxity.

31.2 Key Principles

The goals of surgery are to correct pathologic laxity in the anterior posterior, varus-valgus, and axial rotation planes. A mechanical graft-tensioning device is helpful with cruciate ligament tensioning. Some low-grade medial side injuries may be amenable to brace treatment, while high-grade medial side injuries require combined surgical repair-reconstruction. Lateral posterolateral injuries are most successfully treated with combined surgical repair-reconstruction. Surgical timing in acute multiple ligament injured knees depends upon the ligaments injured, injured extremity vascular status, skin condition of the extremity, degree of instability, and the patient's overall health. Allograft tissue is preferred for these complex surgical procedures. Delayed reconstruction of 2 to 3 weeks may decrease the incidence of arthrofibrosis. It is important to address all components of the instability.

31.3 Expectations

Surgical treatment offers good functional results documented in the literature by physical examination, arthrometer testing, stress radiography, and knee ligament rating scales.

31.4 Indications

Acute knee dislocations with multiple ligament knee instability in the anterior-posterior, varus-valgus, and axial rotation planes, and chronic multiple ligament injured knees with functional instability.

31.5 Contraindications

Contraindications to ligament reconstruction include arterial injuries, deep venous thrombosis, open wounds, poor skin conditions, and multiple system injuries. When delayed or staged reconstruction techniques are used, documentation of maintained reduction of the tibiofemoral and patellofemoral articulations with serial radiographs is required.

31.6 Special Considerations

Chronic bicruciate multiple ligament knee injuries often present to the orthopaedic surgeon with functional instability, and some degree of posttraumatic arthrosis. Considerations for treatment require the determination of all structural injuries, and planes of instability. These structural injuries may include various ligament injuries, meniscus injuries, bony malalignment, articular surface injuries, and gait abnormalities. Surgical procedures under consideration may include proximal tibial or distal femoral osteotomy, ligament reconstruction, meniscus transplant, and osteochondral grafting.

31.7 Special Instructions, Positioning, and Anesthesia

The procedure is performed in an outpatient or inpatient operating room setting. The patient is placed on the operating room table in the supine position. A tourniquet is applied to the upper thigh of the operative extremity. The well leg is supported by the fully extended operating room table which also supports the surgical leg during medial and lateral side surgery. A lateral post is used to control the surgical extremity. An arthroscopic leg holder is not used. Preoperative and postoperative antibiotics are given. Allograft tissue is prepared prior to bringing the patient into the operating room.

31.8 Tips, Pearls, Lessons Learned

31.8.1 Posteromedial Safety Incision (PMSI)

The posteromedial safety incision establishes a plane between the capsule of the knee joint anterior to the surgeon's finger, and the medial head of the gastronomies muscle and neurovascular structures posterior to the surgeon's finger. The PMSI protects the neurovascular structures, confirms the accuracy of the posterior cruciate ligament (PCL) tibial tunnel, and facilitates the flow of the surgical procedure.

31.8.2 PCL Tibial Tunnel

The transtibial PCL tibial must be placed posterior and inferior in the proximal tibia to ensure that the PCL graft tissue will approximate the anatomic tibial insertion site of the PCL. This mimics the tibial inlay technique of PCL reconstruction.

31.8.3 PCL Femoral Tunnel

The PCL femoral tunnel is made from inside to outside which allows a more accurate positioning of the femoral tunnel in both single- and double-bundle reconstructions. The inside-out PCL femoral tunnel orientation also provides a greater margin of safety between the tunnel and the medial femoral condyle articular surface decreasing the chance of articular surface damage or medial femoral condyle fracture.

31.8.4 Single- and Double-Bundle PCL Reconstruction

Single- and double-bundle PCL reconstructions are both successful in multiple knee ligament reconstructions and knee dislocations in my experience. There is no statistically significant difference in the acute and chronic setting with respect to static stability evaluated by stress X-ray (SB 2.56 mm, DB 2.36 mm), KT 1000 (SB 2.11 mm, DB 2.94 mm) side to side difference measurements, or return to preinjury level of function (SB 73%, DB 84%).

31.8.5 Transtibial ACL Reconstruction

Transtibial femoral tunnel anterior cruciate ligament (ACL) reconstruction allows accurate placement of the ACL tibial and femoral tunnels, avoids hyper flexion of the knee during femoral tunnel drilling, and prevents lateral femoral condyle crowding during posterolateral reconstruction.

31.8.6 Mechanical Graft Tensioning

Mechanical graft tensioning using the tensioning boot (Biomet Sports Medicine, Warsaw, Indiana, USA) has improved postoperative posterior drawer testing in knee dislocation surgery from 46% normal posterior drawer to 87% normal posterior drawer.

31.8.7 Posterolateral Reconstruction (PLR)

Fibular head-based (FHB) PLR combined with a posterolateral capsular shift is effective for most cases. A popliteus bypass graft through the proximal tibia is performed in conjunction with the FHB PLR and posterolateral capsular shift when there is asymmetrical hyperextension, excessive posterolateral drawer, proximal tibia fibula joint injury, and revision PLR. Peroneal nerve decompression and lateral-posterolateral capsular surgery (shift or reattachment) are performed in every case. Screw-and-washer fixation is used because it allows graft retensioning if necessary.

31.8.8 Posteromedial Reconstruction (PMR)

Posteromedial capsular shift corrects axial rotation instability and mild valgus laxity. Free graft superficial medial collateral ligament reconstruction (SMCLR) is required for higher grade valgus laxity. Screw-and-washer fixation is used on the tibial side. Passing the graft around the adductor magnus (AM) insertion site on the distal medial femur, and sewing the graft back on itself and to the AM insertion site prevents medial femoral condyle crowding with hardware and sockets.

31.9 Difficulties Encountered

31.9.1 Fractures

Tibial plateau fractures require anatomic reduction and secure fixation to allow accurate determination of instability patterns, and to prevent persistent instability despite ligament reconstruction due to incongruous articular surfaces.

31.9.2 External Fixation

External fixators are to be applied with the pins as close to the knee as possible without violating the surgical field. Accurate reduction and maintained accurate reduction are to be documented with serial radiographs since redislocation can occur with an improperly applied fixator.

31.10 Key Procedural Steps

31.10.1 Posterior Cruciate Ligament Reconstruction (PCLR)

An extracapsular extra-articular posteromedial safety incision is made by creating an incision approximately 1.5 to 2 cm long starting at the posteromedial border of the tibia approximately one inch below the level of the joint line and extending distally (▶ Fig. 31.1). An interval is developed between the medial head of the gastrocnemius muscle and the nerves and vessels posterior to the surgeon's finger, and the capsule of the knee joint anterior to the surgeon's finger. The curved over-the-top PCL

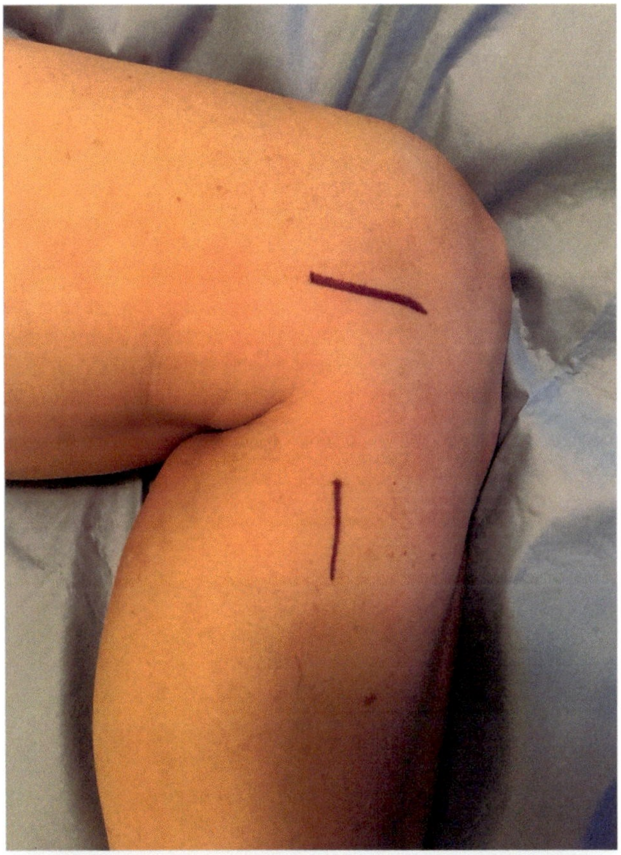

Fig. 31.1 Posteromedial safety incision protects the neurovascular structures, confirms the accuracy of the posterior cruciate ligament (PCL) tibial tunnel, and facilitates the flow of the surgical procedure. The posteromedial safety incision is the vertical line, and the horizontal line is the medial joint line.

instruments (Biomet Sports Medicine, Warsaw, Indiana) are used to sequentially lyse adhesions in the posterior aspect of the knee, and elevate the capsule from the posterior tibial ridge. This will allow accurate placement of the PCL/ACL drill guide, and correct placement of the tibial tunnel.

The arm of the PCL/ACL guide (Biomet Sports Medicine, Warsaw, Indiana) is inserted through the inferior medial patellar portal. The tip of the guide is positioned at the inferior lateral aspect of the PCL anatomic insertion site. This is below the tibial ridge posterior and in the lateral aspect of the PCL anatomic insertion site. The bullet portion of the guide contacts the anteromedial surface of the proximal tibia at a point midway between the posteromedial border of the tibia and the tibial crest anterior at or just below the level of the tibial tubercle. This will provide an angle of graft orientation such that the graft will turn two very smooth 45 degree angles on the posterior aspect of the tibia. The tip of the guide, in the posterior aspect of the tibia, is confirmed with the surgeon's finger through the extracapsular extra-articular posteromedial safety incision. Intraoperative anteroposterior (AP) and lateral X-ray may also be used; however, I do not routinely use intraoperative X-ray. When the PCL/ACL guide is positioned in the desired area, a blunt spade-tipped guide wire is drilled from anterior to posterior. The surgeon's finger confirms the position of the guide wire through the posterior medial safety incision.

The appropriately sized standard cannulated reamer is used to create the tibial tunnel. The surgeon's finger through the extracapsular extra-articular posteromedial incision monitors the position of the guide wire. When the drill is engaged in bone, the guide wire is reversed, with blunt end pointing posterior, for additional patient safety. The drill is advanced until it comes to the posterior cortex of the tibia. The chuck is disengaged from the drill, and completion of the tibial tunnel is performed by hand.

The PCL single-bundle or double-bundle femoral tunnels are made from inside out using the double-bundle aimers, or an endoscopic reamer can be used as an aiming device (Biomet Sports Medicine, Warsaw, Indiana). The appropriately sized double-bundle aimer or endoscopic reamer is inserted through a low anterior lateral patellar arthroscopic portal to create the PCL anterior lateral bundle femoral tunnel. The double-bundle aimer or endoscopic reamer is positioned directly on the footprint of the femoral anterior lateral bundle PCL insertion site. The appropriately sized guide wire is drilled through the aimer or endoscopic reamer, through the bone, and out a small skin incision. Care is taken to prevent any compromise of the articular surface. The double-bundle aimer is removed, and the endoscopic reamer is used to drill the anterior lateral PCL femoral tunnel from inside to outside. When the surgeon chooses to perform a double-bundle double femoral tunnel PCL reconstruction, the same process is repeated for the posterior medial bundle of the PCL. Care must be taken to ensure that there will be an adequate bone bridge (approximately 5 mm) between the two femoral tunnels prior to drilling.

A Magellan suture retriever (Biomet Sports Medicine, Warsaw, Indiana) is introduced through the tibial tunnel into the joint, and retrieved through the femoral tunnel. The traction sutures of the graft material are attached to the loop of the Magellan suture retriever, and the graft is pulled into position. The graft material is secured on the femoral side using two-stacked 19-mm polyethylene ligament fixation button for cortical suspensory fixation.

The cyclic dynamic method of graft tensioning using the Biomet graft-tensioning boot is used to tension the posterior and anterior cruciate ligament grafts. Tension is placed on the PCL graft distally using the Biomet graft-tensioning boot. Tension is gradually applied with the knee in zero degrees of flexion (full extension) reducing the tibia on the femur. This restores the anatomic tibial step off. The knee is cycled through a full range of motion multiple times to allow pretensioning and settling of the graft. The process is repeated until there is no further change in the torque setting on the graft tensioner. The knee is placed in 70 to 90 degrees of flexion, and fixation is achieved on the tibial side of the PCL graft with a bioabsorbable interference screw, and backup fixation with a bicortical screw and spiked ligament washer or polyethylene ligament fixation button.

31.10.2 Anterior Cruciate Ligament (ACL) Reconstruction

With the knee in approximately 90 degrees of flexion, ACL reconstruction is performed using the transtibial femoral tunnel endoscopic surgical technique. The arm of the drill guide enters the knee joint through the inferior medial patellar portal. The bullet of the drill guide contacts the anterior medial proximal tibia externally at a point midway between the posterior medial border of the tibia and the anterior tibial crest just above the level of the tibial tubercle. A 1-cm bone bridge or greater exists between the PCL and ACL tibial tunnels. The guide wire is drilled through the guide and positioned so that after creating the ACL tibial tunnel, the graft will approximate the tibial anatomic insertion site of the ACL. A standard cannulated reamer is used to create the tibial tunnel.

With the knee in approximately 90 to 100 degrees of flexion, an over-the-top femoral aimer is introduced through the tibial tunnel, and used to position a guide wire on the medial wall of the lateral femoral condyle to create a femoral tunnel approximating the anatomic insertion site of the ACL. The ACL graft is positioned, and fixation achieved on the femoral side using two-stacked 15-mm polyethylene ligament fixation buttons for cortical suspensory fixation.

The cyclic dynamic method of tensioning of the ACL graft is performed using the Biomet graft-tensioning boot. Traction is placed on the ACL graft sutures with the knee in zero degrees of flexion, and tension is gradually applied reducing the tibia on the femur. The knee is then cycled through multiple full flexion and extension cycles to allow settling of the graft. The process is repeated until there is no further change in the torque setting on the graft tensioner, and the Lachman and pivot shift tests are negative. The knee is placed in approximately thirty degrees

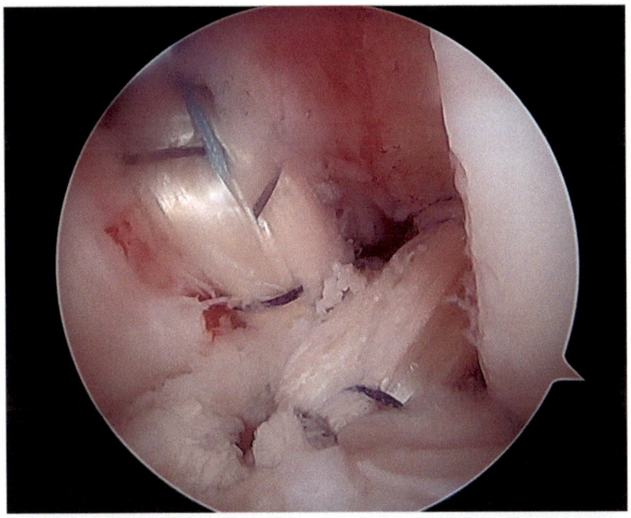

Fig. 31.2 Combined posterior cruciate ligament (PCL) and anterior cruciate ligament (ACL) reconstruction in knee dislocation using Achilles tendon allografts.

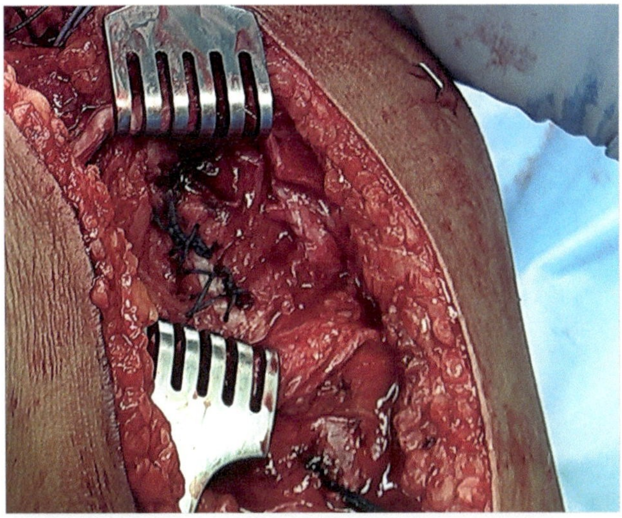

Fig. 31.3 Posterolateral capsular shift. A longitudinal incision is made parallel to the posterior border of the fibular collateral ligament in the interval between the midlateral and posterolateral capsule. Number two permanent braided suture in horizontal mattress fashion is used to perform the posterolateral capsular shift with the knee in 90 degrees of knee flexion.

of flexion, and fixation is achieved on the tibial side of the ACL graft with a bioabsorbable interference screw, and backup fixation with a 15 mm polyethylene ligament fixation button (▶ Fig. 31.2).

31.10.3 Fibular Head-Based Posterolateral Reconstruction

A curvilinear incision is made in the lateral aspect of the knee extending from the interval between Gerdy tubercle and the fibular head to the lateral epicondyle and then proximal following the course of the iliotibial band. A peroneal nerve decompression/neurolysis is performed, and the peroneal nerve is protected throughout the procedure. The fibular head is identified and a tunnel is created in an anterolateral to posteromedial direction at the area of maximal fibular head diameter. The tunnel is created by passing a guide pin followed by a standard cannulated drill 7 mm in diameter. The peroneal nerve is protected during tunnel creation, and throughout the procedure. The free tendon graft is passed through the fibular head drill hole.

An incision is made in the iliotibial band in line with the fibers exposing the lateral femoral epicondyle area of the distal femur. A longitudinal incision is made parallel to the posterior border of the fibular collateral ligament in the interval between the midlateral and posterolateral capsule. Number two permanent braided suture is used to perform the posterolateral capsular shift with the knee in 90 degrees of knee flexion (▶ Fig. 31.3).

The graft material is passed medial to the iliotibial band for the fibular collateral ligament limb, and medial to the common biceps tendon and iliotibial band for the popliteus tendon popliteofibular ligament limb. The limbs of the graft are crossed to form a figure of eight with the fibular collateral ligament component being lateral to the popliteus tendon component. A 3.2-mm drill hole is made to accommodate a 6.5-mm-diameter fully threaded cancellous screw that is approximately 40 mm to 45 mm in length. The drill hole is positioned in the lateral epicondylar region of the distal lateral femur so that after seating a 17- to 20-mm washer with the above-mentioned screw, the washer will precisely secure the two limbs of the allograft tissue at the respective anatomic insertion sites of the fibular collateral ligament and popliteus tendon on the distal lateral femoral condyle. This drill hole is approximately 1 cm anterior to the fibular collateral ligament femoral insertion. The graft material is tensioned at approximately 40 to 45 degrees of knee flexion, secured to the lateral femoral epicondylar region with a screw and spiked ligament washer at the above-mentioned point. The anterior and posterior limbs of the figure-of-eight graft material are sewn to each other proximal to the washer to create a closed loop, and also to the midlateral and posterolateral capsule to reinforce and tighten the construct.

31.10.4 Two-Tailed Posterolateral Reconstruction

A 7- or 8-mm drill hole is made over a guide wire approximately two centimeters below the lateral tibial plateau. A tibialis anterior or other soft tissue allograft is passed through this tibial drill hole and follows the course of the popliteus tendon to its anatomic insertion site on the lateral femoral epicondylar region. Nerves and blood vessels must be protected. The allograft is

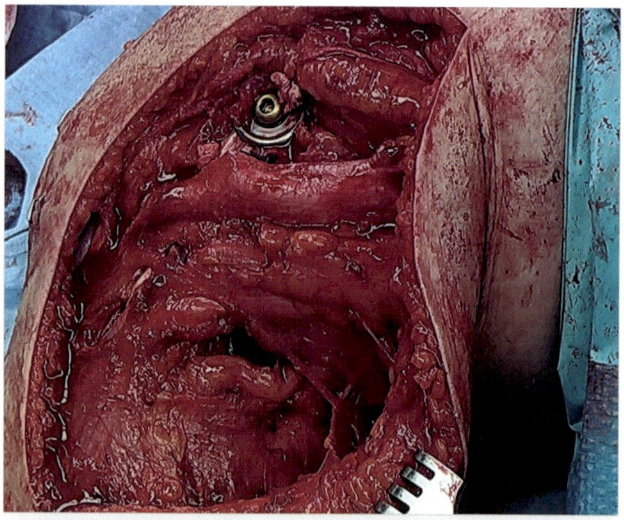

Fig. 31.4 Two-tailed posterolateral reconstruction (PLR). A tibialis anterior allograft is used to perform the popliteus bypass component of the PLR, while a semitendinosus allograft is used to perform the fibular head-based figure-of-eight component of the PLR. Peroneal nerve decompression is always performed and the nerve protected throughout the procedure.

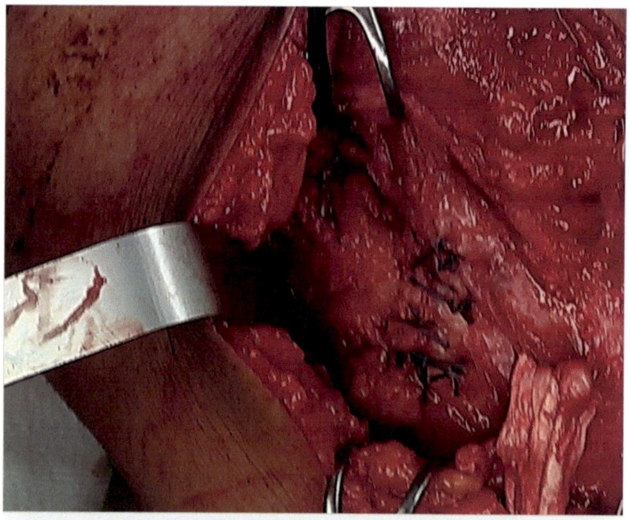

Fig. 31.5 Posteromedial capsular shift. A longitudinal incision is made parallel to the posterior border of the superficial medial collateral ligament (MCL), and in the interval between the posterior oblique ligament and the superficial MCL. The semimembranosus tendon is identified and protected. The meniscocapsular junction is sharply separated and with the knee in approximately 40 to 45 degrees of flexion, posteromedial capsular shift performed with three #2 permanent braided sutures in horizontal mattress fashion tied with the knee in 40 to 45 degrees of flexion. The meniscocapsular junction is repaired with a #2 permanent braided suture. That suture line is then reinforced with a running #2 permanent braided suture.

secured with a suture anchor, and multiple #2 braided nonabsorbable sutures at the popliteus tendon anatomic femoral insertion site. The knee is cycled through multiple sets of full flexion and extension cycles, placed in 90 degrees of flexion, the tibia slightly internally rotated, slight valgus force applied to the knee, and the graft tensioned, and secured in the tibial tunnel with a bioabsorbable interference screw, and polyethylene ligament fixation button. The FHB reconstruction and posterolateral capsular shift procedures are then carried out as described above (▶ Fig. 31.4).

31.10.5 Posteromedial Reconstruction (Posteromedial Capsular Shift)

The surgical extremity was placed on the fully extended operating room table in a supported figure-of-four position. Medial curvilinear incision is made and dissection carried down to the Sartorius fascia. Neurovascular structures are protected throughout the procedure. The Sartorius is incised in line with its fibers and the superficial MCL identified along with the patulous and redundant posteromedial capsule. A longitudinal incision is made parallel to the posterior border of the superficial MCL, and in the interval between the posterior oblique ligament and the superficial MCL. The semimembranosus tendon is identified and protected. The meniscocapsular junction is sharply separated, and with the knee in approximately 40 to 45 degrees of flexion, posteromedial capsular shift performed with three #2 permanent braided sutures in horizontal mattress fashion. Those were tied with the knee in 40 to 45 degrees of flexion. The meniscocapsular junction was repaired with a #2 permanent braided suture. That suture line was then reinforced with a running #2 permanent braided suture (▶ Fig. 31.5).

31.10.6 Posteromedial Reconstruction (Free Graft)

The posteromedial capsular shift procedure or capsular reattachment is performed first as outlined above. The AM tendon is identified at its insertion into the distal medial femur and a passing suture is looped around the AM tendon. A 3.2-mm drill hole is made in the center of the superficial MCL tibial approximately 4 to 5 cm distal to the joint line, and a 6.5 × 30 mm fully threaded cancellous screw and a 20-mm spiked ligament fixation washer are placed in that drill hole. A semitendinosus allograft is looped around that screw-and-washer assembly and the two tails passed proximally to the AM insertion site deep to the sartorius fascia. The screw and washer assembly are tightened. With the knee in approximately 45 degrees of flexion, a posteromedial capsular shift was performed as outlined above.

The tails of the semitendinosus graft are passed deep to the Sartorius fascia and are looped around the AM tendon, one tail from posterior to anterior, the other from anterior to posterior and then tensioned against the AM tendon and the tails sewn back into the body of the graft, and into the AM insertion site with #2 permanent braided suture (▶ Fig. 31.6).

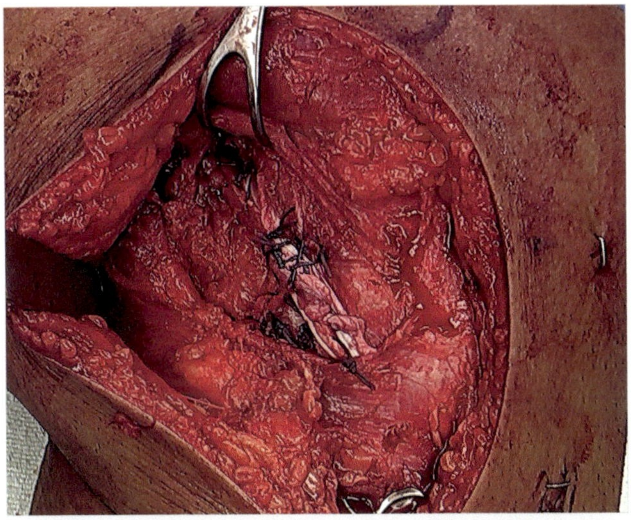

Fig. 31.6 Superficial medial collateral ligament (MCL) reconstruction. A semitendinosus allograft is looped around that screw-and-washer assembly and the two tails passed proximally to the adductor magnus insertion site deep to the sartorius fascia. The tails of the semitendinosus graft are passed deep to the sartorius fascia and are looped around the adductor magnus tendon, and then tensioned against the adductor magnus tendon. The tails sewn back into the body of the graft, and into the adductor magnus insertion site with #2 permanent braided suture. This is performed in combination with the posteromedial capsular shift.

31.11 Bailout, Rescue, and Salvage Procedures

Improperly positioned PCL tibial tunnels can be addressed by using the tibial inlay PCL reconstruction surgical technique. Inability to position the transtibial ACL femoral tunnel in the proper position can be addressed by using the outside-in method of ACL femoral tunnel creation. Osteopenic bone that will not provide secure screw-and-washer fixation can be addressed with transosseous suture fixation.

31.12 Pitfalls

Knee dislocations may be accompanied by ipsilateral femoral or tibial fractures with retained hardware that prevents optimum tunnel positioning. Alternate methods of reconstruction may need to be utilized as outlined in section 30.11. Hardware removal prior to ligament reconstruction may be required which may alter surgical timing.

32 Patellofemoral Instability—Medial Patellofemoral Ligament Reconstruction

Gilberto Luis Camanho and Marco Kawamura Demange

32.1 Description

We describe a technique for reconstructing the medial patellofemoral ligament (MPFL) using a strip of the medial third of the patellar tendon in cases of acute patellar dislocation.

32.2 Key Principles

A complete understanding of the anatomy and biomechanics of the MPFL is essential. The MPFL has a very consistent origin at the transition between the proximal and middle thirds of the patella. The femoral insertion may vary regarding its width and size. It attaches to a location close to the medial femoral epicondyle and the adductor tubercle. Our biomechanical studies demonstrated that the MPFL's tensile strength is around 80 N, and its patellar insertion is the only one that did not fail under axial traction.

32.3 Expectations

There is controversy in the literature about the best treatment protocol for acute patellar dislocations. In our initial clinical series, comparing surgical versus nonsurgical treatments, we found that recurrent dislocation occurred in 50% of the patients treated conservatively. In contrast, it did not occur in patients who underwent surgery. In a subsequent randomized clinical trial comparing nonoperative treatment (20 patients) and MPFL reconstruction (21 patients) performed using a 5-mm strip of the medial third of the patella ligament (patellar tendon), we observed better results in the surgical group. After a minimum of 2-year follow-up, there was no recurrence of patella instability in the surgical group. We have also analyzed predisposing factors as high patella and signs of a flat trochlea on true lateral and axial radiographs. In these two groups, representing 41 patients, the presence of predisposing factors did not affect the results, with regard to recurrence of dislocation or complaints of instability. Patients treated surgically had better Kujala scores. We also observed that patients with predisposing factors, especially flat trochlea presented inferior final Kujala scores.

32.4 Indications

We consider that active patients with acute dislocation of the patella should be treated surgically. The preferred surgical treatment is an MPFL reconstruction, provided there are no other predisposing factors to the dislocation, which may require associated surgical indication. In cases of MPFL avulsion at the patella site, observed in the magnetic resonance imaging (MRI), surgical reinsertion may also be considered.

32.5 Contraindications

- Patients who are not eligible for orthopaedic surgical treatment.
- Patients that are noncompliant with postoperative rehabilitation protocols.
- Patients with comorbidities that may compromise the outcomes of the surgery—as diseases of the collagen tissue.
- Elderly and nonactive patients that may not benefit from the surgical intervention.

32.6 Special Considerations

Authors diverge regarding the ideal femoral attachment site for the the patellofemoral ligament graft during surgical reconstruction. The MPFL presents an anisometric biomechanical pattern during flexion and extension. Inadequate placement of the graft may significantly increase the pressures in the patellofemoral joint, especially in the medial facet of the patella. It is also essential not to overtighten the patellofemoral joint. The medial vastus muscle presents insertional fibrous bands to the normal MPFL, accounting for its dynamic influence in the MPFL tension. Reconstruction techniques should consider this anatomical aspect. Postoperative rehabilitation is an essential step of treatment and begins right after surgery. We prescribe a knee brace in extension for 3 weeks, during which isometric exercises are performed, and electrostimulation is provided. Analgesic medications, as well as cryotherapy, are recommended. We initially advise patients to use a pair of crutches and bear weight as tolerated. The patients will have a toe touch weight-bearing right after surgery and increase the weight-bearing status progressive according to their pain tolerance. The knee is maintained in extension for the first week. In between the first and the third week, we begin a progressive range of motion until the patient reaches 90 degrees of flexion. We remove the use of a knee brace after the third week when the patient begins using a stationary bicycle. After 6 weeks postop, we start closed kinetic chain exercises and gradually progress to open kinetic chain exercises. Our aim is that patients should be able to return to their preoperative sports activities after approximately 12 weeks.

32.7 Special Instructions, Position, and Anesthesia

General or regional anesthesia techniques are our preferred choices. The patient is placed supine on the operative table. An exam under anesthesia is performed, confirming patellofemoral instability. A tourniquet is left on the proximal aspect of the thigh and is not routinely used in our cases. We perform a detailed arthroscopic inventory of the joint, aiming to

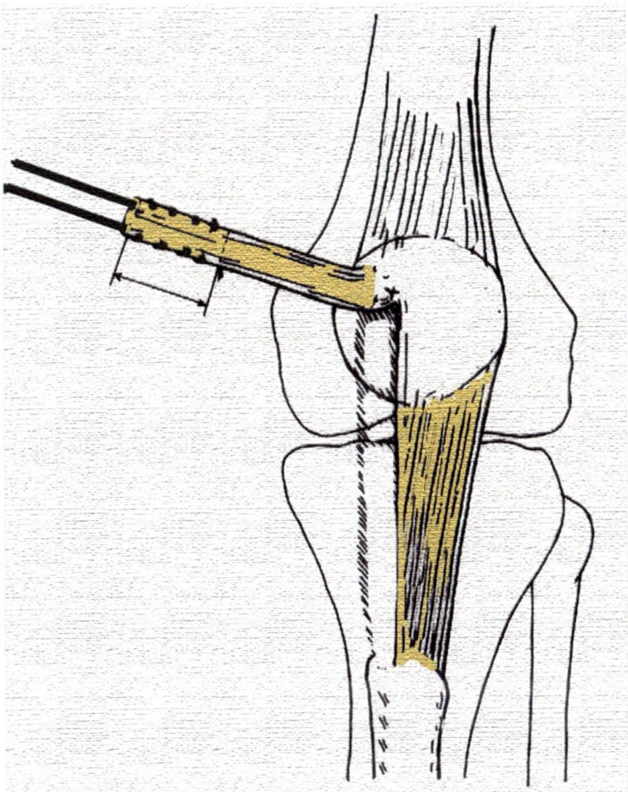

Fig. 32.1 Harvesting the graft. The medial third of the patellar tendon is elevated from the anterior tibial tubercle and dissected subperiosteally on the anterior surface of the patella, until the proximal third of its patellar attachment. The free end of the graft is prepared with nonresorbable Krackow stitches.

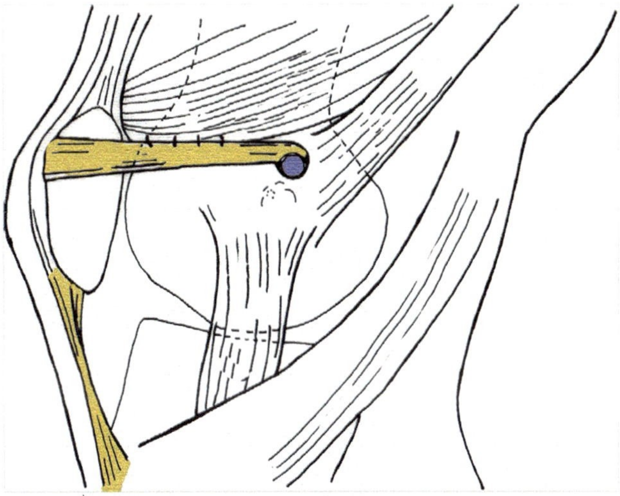

Fig. 32.2 Attaching the graft. The patellar autograft is fixed to the medial femoral condyle, posterior and proximal to the medial femoral epicondyle. Observe that it is also sutured to the fibers of the vastus medialis oblique. An interference screw (*blue*) is utilized when the graft is long enough to be docked to the femur. Otherwise, anchors are applied to fix the graft to the medial femoral condyle.

address associated cartilage injuries. We do not perform any lateral retinaculum release. The landmarks for our surgical incision are the medial edge of the patella and the medial femoral epicondyle. A longitudinal incision is placed medially to the medial edge of the patella. This incision begins at the level of the superior and medial borders of the patella. It extends itself toward the medial aspect of the anterior tibial tubercle, incorporating the anteromedial arthroscopic portal. We incise the peritendon in line with the medial edge of the patellar tendon. We measure the width of the patellar tendon with a ruler. We mark a width corresponding to the medial one-third of the tendon. We incise the tendon fibers at the junction between its middle and medial thirds. We elevate the tendon with a periosteal sleeve at its attachment on the tibial tubercle. We flip the tendon strip superiorly and then perform a subperiosteal elevation of the tendon. We elevate it up to the junction between the middle third and superior third of the patella (▶ Fig. 32.1). The strip is secured to the patella with nonabsorbable sutures, avoiding that it peels off from the anterior surface of the bone. We apply sutures to the free end of the graft using a Krackow technique.

We identify the site for the femoral attachment of the graft. It corresponds to a broad area, which is posterior and proximal to the medial epicondyle. We then make a small incision over this area. We measure the distance between the patellar attachment of the graft and its desired femoral attachment. If the graft is too short, we dock it to the femoral site using anchors. If the graft is long enough, we drill a tunnel at the femoral site and fix the graft to the femur with a resorbable interference screw (▶ Fig. 32.2). We fix the graft with the knee flexed at approximately 45 to 60 degrees of flexion. The femoral insertion for MPFL reconstruction may be checked intraoperatively with fluoroscopy. We advise the use of the landmarks described by Schottle et al[1], recommending an anatomical and radiographic femoral attachment site located 1.3 mm anterior to the posterior cortex extension, 2.5 mm distal to a perpendicular intersecting the origin of the posterior medial femoral condyle, and 3 mm proximal to a perpendicular intersecting the posterior point of the Blumensaat line on a lateral view with the posterior condylar margin overlapped. It is essential to be concerned about testing the full range of motion and patella stability to ensure the fixation method is adequate. We advance and suture the vastus medialis over the graft, adding a dynamic component to this reconstruction (▶ Fig. 32.3).

We close the peritendon using 3.0 Vicryl and then close the derm layer using undyed 4.0 Monocryl. We use local anesthetics at the time of closure and apply dry dressings to the surgical wound. A long knee immobilizer is applied to the lower limb.

Postoperative radiographs are obtained to document proper height of the patella and isometric insertion of the femoral anchor/screw (▶ Fig. 32.4).

32.8 Tips, Pearls, and Lessons Learned

- The correct preparation of the graft is of critical importance. The sutures applied to the patellar attachment of the graft prevent the graft from peeling off.
- Incorporating the vastus medialis to the reconstruction is essential, as it adds a dynamic component to the construct.

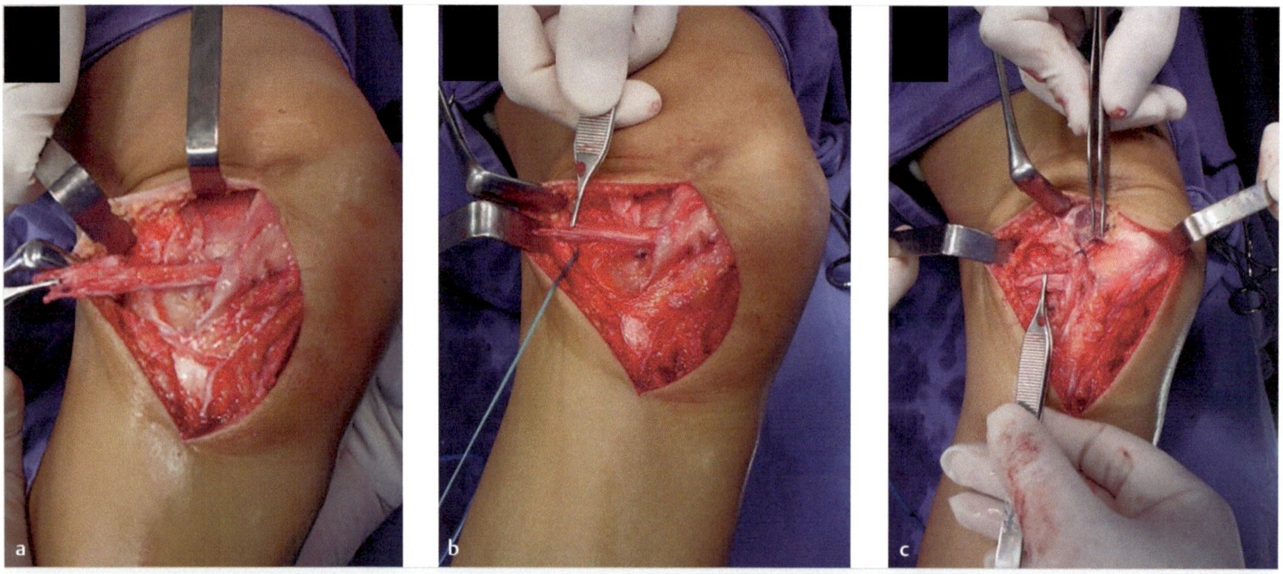

Fig. 32.3 Intraoperative images. **(a)** Harvesting of the medial third of the patellar tendon, which is tilted toward the femoral insertion of the medial patellofemoral ligament; **(b)** preparation of the free end of the patellar autograft with nonresorbable stitches; **(c)** final aspect of the new medial patellofemoral ligament, which is attached to the patella and to the medial femoral condyle.

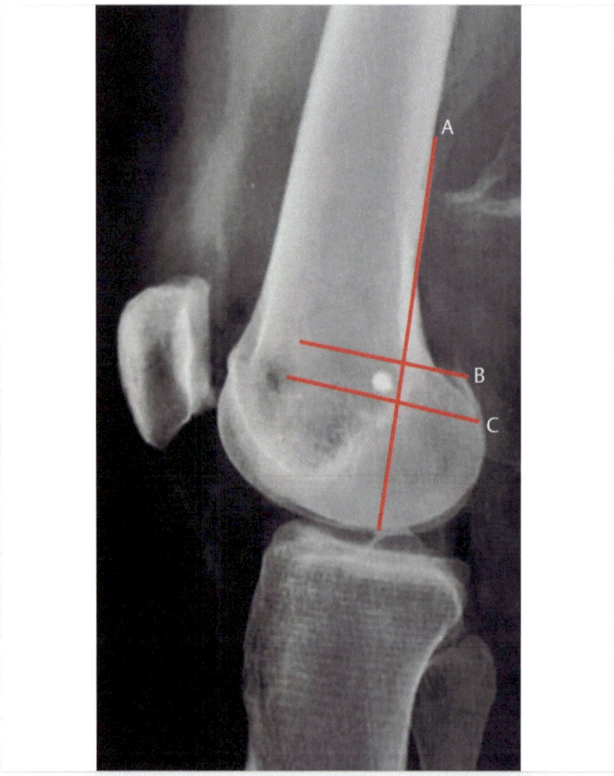

Fig. 32.4 Postoperative radiograph—lateral projection. The femoral positioning of the medial patellofemoral ligament (MPFL) is demonstrated by the radiographic location of the metallic fixation anchor. The ideal fixation site should be approximately 1 mm anterior to the posterior cortex line (A) and just proximal to the crossing point between line A and Line C, the latter being a perpendicular line to the most posterior aspect of the Blumensaat line, as described by Schottle et al.

- The graft should act as a "seat belt" and should not be over tightened. Otherwise, the pressures in the patellofemoral joint rise, and the patient will have pain.
- The MPFL reconstruction should not be seen as the only procedure to be performed in the set of recurrent patellar dislocation. It should be an adjuvant to more complex three-dimensional bony realignment procedures.

32.9 Difficulties Encountered

Predisposing anatomical factors for patellofemoral instability may pose an additional threat to good outcomes in cases of acute patellar dislocations. Some of these patients will require additional procedures to address the instability, avoiding its recurrence.

Significant quadriceps atrophy may prevent patients from recovering quickly. We should encourage patients to adhere to the rehabilitation protocols. Early weight-bearing and isometric quadriceps exercises should be adopted right after surgery.

Lack of compliance to physical therapy is a significant factor preventing full recovery and good outcomes.

32.10 Key Procedural Steps

- We consider it critical to identify the proper femoral attachment for the MPFL. Fluoroscopy and surgical examination are used to assist in this identification.
- The adjustment of the tension of the MPFL is essential. Tight constructs are associated with pain, lack of function, and increased pressures in the patellofemoral joint.
- Graft fixation should be tested intraoperatively. It should be stable enough to allow for early postoperative motion.
- Compliant rehabilitation is a requirement for the success of this treatment.

32.11 Bailout, Rescue, and Salvage Procedures

Intraoperatively the surgeon should be prepared to use an alternative graft if the use of the patellar tendon does not work. Causes for intraoperative failure could be the inadequate length of the tendon or graft's peel off from the patella. A possible alternative in those cases could be the use of the gracilis tendon.

If there is significant pain and knee stiffness in the postoperative set, a revision procedure should be considered. A comprehensive evaluation of predisposing factors should be carried out. The graft should be released. If needed, we revise the graft and also address bony predisposing factors for patellofemoral instability.

Cartilage damage should be addressed simultaneously, mainly if the lesions are located in the medial facet or the central portion of the patellar articular surface.

32.12 Pitfalls

- Not recognizing associated predisposing factors for patellofemoral instability.
- Not using anatomical landmarks to attach the graft to the femur.
- Not suturing the graft to the patella before attaching it to the femur.
- Overtightening of the construct.
- Using the MPFL as the only tool in the management of patellofemoral instability, especially in the set of associated predisposing factors.

Reference

[1] Schöttle PB, Schmeling A, Rosenstiel N, Weiler A. Radiographic landmarks for femoral tunnel placement in medial patellofemoral ligament reconstruction. Am J Sports Med. 2007 May;35(5):801–4.

33 Proximal Realignment: Lateral Retinaculum Lengthening

Andrew J. Garrone, Betina B. Hinckel, Riccardo Gobbi, and Seth L. Sherman

33.1 Description

Tightness of the lateral patellofemoral (PF) soft tissues is associated with many disorders of PF maltracking including lateral patellar compression syndrome, lateral patellar instability, and PF arthritis. Lateral retinaculum lengthening is an effective method of soft tissue balancing performed by lengthening the retinaculum through its deep and superficial layers. This technique corrects patella tilt and relieves excessive lateral soft tissue tension without the morbidity or potential complications associated with full-thickness lateral release.

33.2 Key Principles

- Lateral retinaculum lengthening is performed in isolation only in selected cases of lateral patellar compression syndrome.
- In other PF disorders (PF instability, cartilage lesions, and arthritis) it should be performed as an adjunct to other procedures.
- Tightness of the lateral retinaculum is identified by a combination of the physical exam maneuvers and imaging studies. This is confirmed with examination under anesthesia and arthroscopic evaluation.

33.3 Expectations

With appropriate surgical indications and meticulous technique, lateral retinaculum lengthening assists in soft tissue balancing for the PF joint.

33.4 Indications

Lateral retinaculum lengthening is performed in isolation only in selected cases of lateral patellar compression syndrome that have failed extensive conservative treatment options (NSAIDS, physical therapy, taping, bracing, injections, weight loss). In other PF disorders (PF instability, cartilage lesions, and arthritis), it should be performed as an adjunct procedure when there is concomitant lateral retinaculum tightness diagnosed by clinical exam/imaging studies and confirmed with exam under anesthesia (EUA) and arthroscopy. In these cases, the indications for surgery correspond to the major underlying diagnosis (i.e., recurrent patella instability, failed conservative treatment of chondral lesion).

Clinical signs of lateral tightness are decreased medial patella translation and excessive nonreducible lateral patella tilt. Patellar glide and tilt tests are the most direct evaluation of lateral retinaculum. Medial displacement less than one quadrant is consistent with tight lateral retinaculum and greater than three quadrants is consistent with laxity. In full extension, patellar glide test evaluates exclusively the soft tissue restraints; at 30 degrees of flexion, it also assesses PF engagement and morphology. Patellar tilt test measures the lifting up of the lateral edge of the patella in relation to the ground line. Elevation between zero and 20 degrees is normal, whereas lack of patellar tilt reduction means lateral retinaculum is tight and > 20 degrees means it is loose.

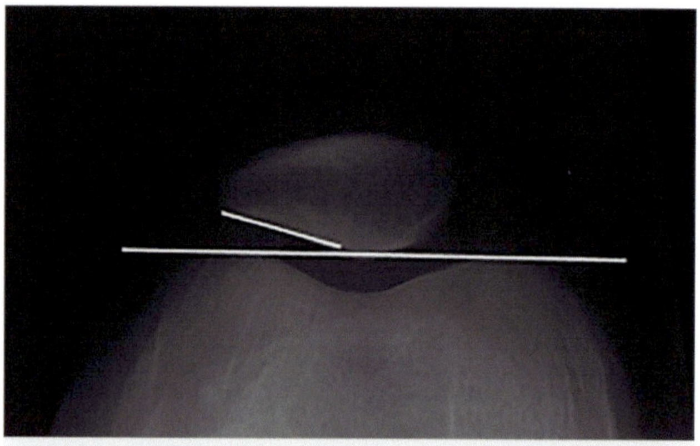

Fig. 33.1 Lateral patellofemoral angle in the Laurin view. Formed by the line tangent to the anterior points of the medial and lateral trochlear facets and the line tangent to the lateral patellar facet.

Imaging evaluation relies on the degree of patellar tilt that can be assessed by axial or lateral radiographs, computed tomography (CT), and magnetic resonance imaging (MRI).

On the axial radiograph at 20 degrees of flexion (Laurin view), the lateral PF angle can be evaluated. It is formed by the line tangent to the anterior points of the medial and lateral trochlear facets and the line tangent to the lateral patellar facet (▶ Fig. 33.1). In normal knees, this angle opens laterally. Images with progressive flexion can be very useful to verify reduction of patellar tilt. The lack of reduction during early flexion suggests lateral tightness.

On CTs and MRIs, the patellar tilt angle (formed by a line joining the medial and lateral edges of the patella and a line drawn tangent the posterior femoral condyles; ▶ Fig. 33.2) > 20 degrees is increased and abnormal.

Decision making is based on the combination of the physical exam and imaging. While excessive lateral patellar tilt can be recognized on imaging, the contribution of lateral tightness must be verified by the physical exam (i.e., restraint to medial patellar displacement and lack of neutral patella tilt).

When considering lateral lengthening for treating patellar pain, taping and patellar unloading braces can simulate the lateral unloading result and preview the outcomes. Patients that respond well to those therapies have a higher likelihood of improvement if they fail conservative treatment and require surgery.

33.5 Contraindications

- Lateral retinacular laxity or normal lateral restraint as demonstrated by physical examination/imaging studies and confirmed by EUA/arthroscopic evaluation.
- Lateral retinaculum lengthening is **NEVER** indicated as the sole treatment of PF instability.

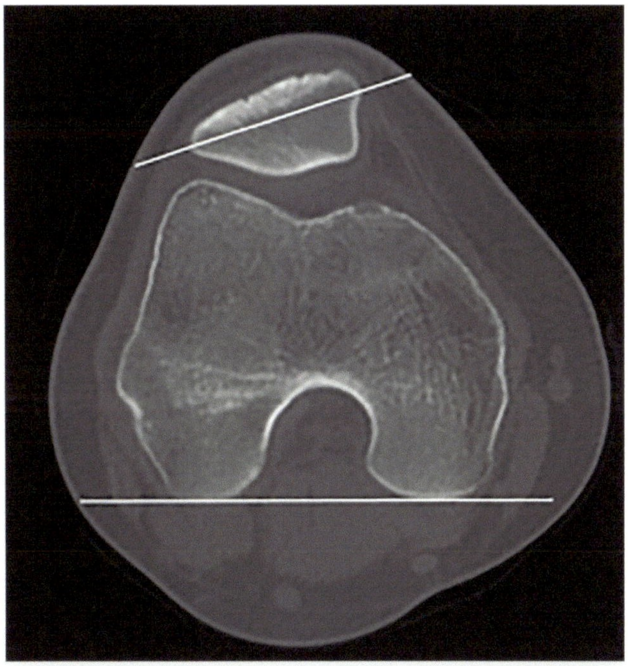

Fig. 33.2 Patellar tilt angle. Formed by a line joining the medial and lateral edges of the patella and a line drawn tangent the posterior femoral condyles.

33.6 Special Considerations

Lateral retinacular soft tissue balancing should not be considered an all-or-nothing procedure. It should be quantified to avoid either excessive release resulting in iatrogenic pain and/or medial instability or insufficient release resulting in maintenance of excessive tightness and associated symptoms. Therefore, arthroscopic lateral release should be rarely, if at all, performed because it completely releases the capsule and both deep and superficial retinaculum layers. Outcomes for lateral lengthening are generally superior to complete lateral release, considering both function and pain, because it allows fine adjustment of soft tissue balancing. Furthermore, complete release lowers the ability of the patella to resist lateral displacement, which is of critical importance when treating PF instability patients.

33.7 Special Instructions, Position, and Anesthesia

The patient is positioned supine on the operating table. A tourniquet is placed but generally not used. General anesthesia is performed and adductor nerve block may be used. Examination under anesthesia of both the involved and contralateral sides is performed prior to sterile prep and draping. Arthroscopic evaluation is performed prior to the open portion of the case. The approach for isolated lateral retinacular lengthening is described below. In combined cases, lateral lengthening should be performed prior to medial patellofemoral ligament (MPFL) reconstruction to ensure appropriate soft tissue balance. Lateral lengthening is also performed as an adjunct to realignment tibial tubercle osteotomy (anteromedialization, medialization, or distalization) and is often the preferred approach to access the patella or trochlea for cartilage restoration.

For an isolated procedure, a 3-cm to 5-cm incision is performed along the lateral edge of the patella. An anterior incision is usually the best option, especially when other procedures are associated. Subcutaneous dissection in a posterior and lateral direction is performed reaching the posterior border of the iliotibial band. The junction between the anterior border of the iliotibial band and the vastus lateralis is identified, and those structures are separated by blunt dissection. The iliotibial band is a reference for the superficial layer. With a sharp scalpel or electrocautery, an incision initially about the patellar length (can be extended proximally and distally as needed) is performed close to the lateral patellar edge. The depth of the incision equals the thickness of the superficial layer of the retinaculum (identified by oblique fibers that come from the iliotibial band). The superficial layer is peeled from the deep layer (identified by transverse fibers that attach to the vastus lateralis proximally, running from the deep portion of the iliotibial band to the patella along with the lateral PF ligament). The deep transverse retinacular layer is then incised near its attachment on the iliotibial band. Typically, this results in 15 mm to 22 mm of lengthening. The underlying synovial layer may be preserved or incised depending on surgeon preference and if joint access is required. The knee is then moved through a full range of motion to identify the flexion angle in which the incised edges are farthest apart (this is the degree of flexion it will be tightest), typically between 30 and 60 degrees of flexion. The cut edges of the superficial oblique and deep transverse fibers are then sutured together using absorbable suture with the appropriate amount of lengthening to remove excess tension in the lateral structures while keeping lateral soft tissue integrity (▶ Fig. 33.3).

All-arthroscopic lateral release techniques cut the lateral retinaculum from inside-out using electrocautery. This technique is more aggressive as it requires initial release of the capsule and deep transverse layer in order to access, adequately expose, and release the superficial layer. Soft tissue balancing is an all-or-none event in this situation and essentially irreversible. In addition, the vastus lateralis is vulnerable during the approach and often violated causing unnecessary morbidity to the soft tissue envelope. As stated above, the lateral retinaculum is a secondary restraint to lateral patella translation. Complete violation of these structures through lateral release may accentuate lateral patella instability and/or cause iatrogenic medial instability and release site pain. Adequate hemostasis is also more challenging through arthroscopic surgery. For these reasons, the authors do not recommend arthroscopic lateral release as an isolated or concomitant procedure at this time.

33.8 Tips, Pearls, and Lessons Learned

Identification of the Layers

- Identification of the superficial and deep layers of the retinaculum is very important. Finding the iliotibial band proximally and following it distally helps. Superficial fibers are oblique and deep fibers are transverse.

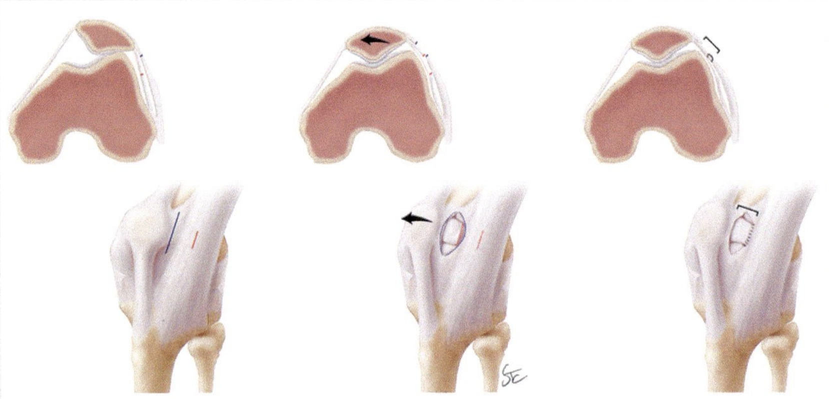

Fig. 33.3 Illustration of lateral retinaculum lengthening technique. Blue line represents the incision in the superficial layer and the red line the incision in the deep layer. (Reproduced with permission from © University of Missouri.)

33.8.1 Hemostasis

- Open procedure, performed with meticulous hemostasis and without an inflated tourniquet, decreases the risk of hematomas and related pain.

33.8.2 Medial and Lateral Balance

- Be aware that Z-plasty lengthening technique can provide at maximum approximately 20 mm of lengthening. Goal is to obtain 1 to 2 patellar quadrants of medial and lateral patellar glide in extension and a neutral patellar tilt. Perform a full range of motion to ensure patella stays centered on the trochlea. The lateral retinaculum should be set to length with the knee around 30 to 60 degrees of flexion.

33.9 Pitfalls

33.9.1 Identification of the Layers

- Inadequate dissection of the layers can result in insufficient lengthening and/or inadequate preservation of lateral soft tissue.

33.9.2 Hemostasis

- Inadequate hemostasis can result in hematomas and pain.

33.9.3 Medial and Lateral Balance

- Undercorrection or overly aggressive release: excessive release may result in iatrogenic pain and/or medial instability whereas insufficient release may result in maintenance of excessive tightness associated with symptoms.

33.10 Difficulties Encountered

In cases with flexion instability, chronic patellar dislocation, and extreme bony dysplasia, or both, the resulting gap between the lateral structures may be too great and lengthening is not possible. A standard lateral release may be performed instead. If desired, this gap can be closed using a strong collagen structure, such as an allogenic fascia lata tissue or a dermal allograft patch.

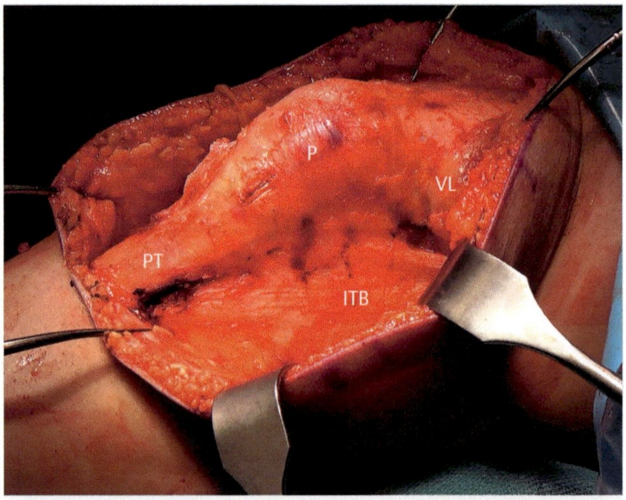

Fig. 33.4 Anatomy of the lateral retinaculum. Identification of the iliotibial band and the vastus lateralis prior to beginning the lengthening procedure. Abbreviations: ITB, iliotibial band; VL, vastus lateralis; P, patella; PT, patella tendon.

33.11 Key Procedural Steps

- Identify the iliotibial band and the vastus lateralis (▶ Fig. 33.4).
- Incise the superficial oblique layer at the patella border.
- Separate superficial and deep retinaculum layer and dissect posteriorly (▶ Fig. 33.5 and ▶ Fig. 33.6).
- Incise the deep transverse layer.
- Balance lateral soft tissue and repair the lengthening with absorbable suture (▶ Fig. 33.7 and ▶ Fig. 33.8).

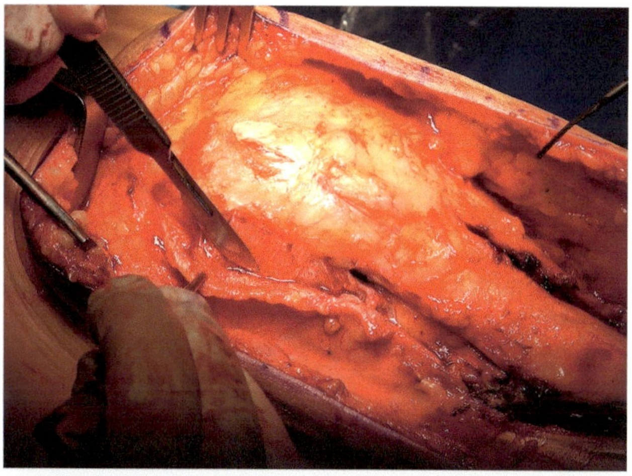

Fig. 33.5 Dissection between the superficial and deep layers of the lateral retinaculum. A 10-blade scalpel is used to section the superficial layer close to the patella. Superficial layer is dissected of the deep layer of the lateral retinaculum.

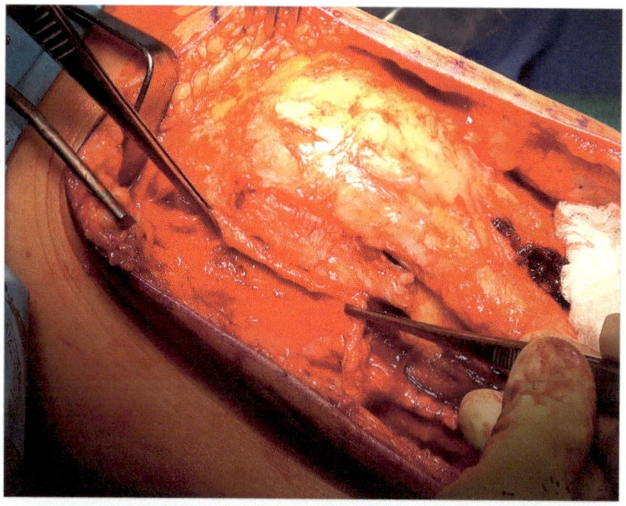

Fig. 33.7 Lengthening of the lateral retinaculum. The posterior edge of the superficial layer is brought close to the anterior edge of the deep layer of the lateral retinaculum.

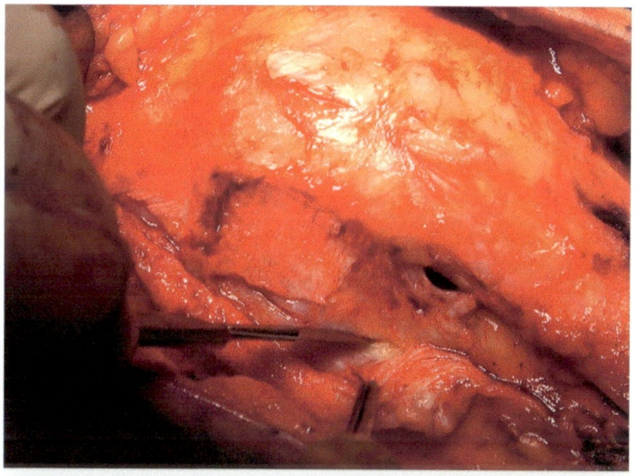

Fig. 33.6 Section of the deep layer of the lateral retinaculum. With a 10-blade scalpel, a posterior incision is made in the deep layer of the lateral retinaculum with the amount of lengthening desired (up to 22 mm).

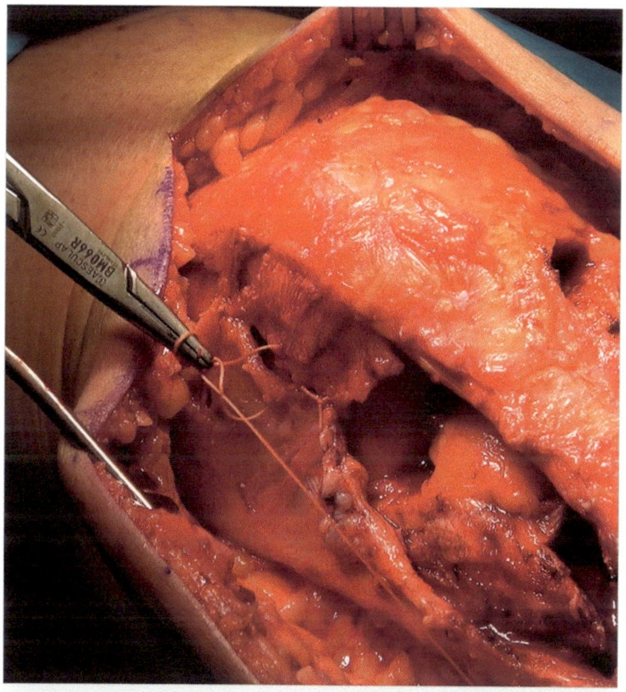

Fig. 33.8 Suturing of the superficial and deep layers. The edges of the superficial and deep layers of the lateral retinaculum are sutured with absorbable sutures.

33.12 Bailout, Rescue, and Salvage Procedures

Medial instability (medial patellar dislocation and medial patellar subluxation) is an iatrogenic condition that can result from excessive lateral release, with no reports of that condition after lateral lengthening. It is a consequence of loss of lateral restraint and muscle atrophy, probably associated with the extent of the release and section of vastus lateralis tendon. Treatment options are closure of the lateral retinaculum and reconstruction of the lateral PF ligament or lateral patellotibial ligament. Open lateral retinaculum closure provides successful outcomes and should be

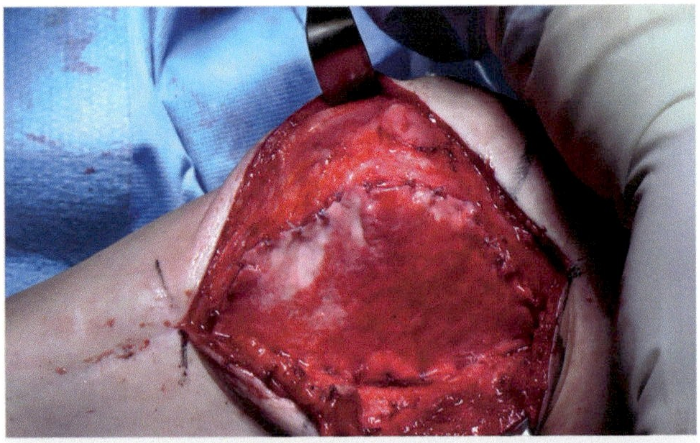

Fig. 33.9 Soft tissue augmentation. Dermal allograft (ArthroFLEX, Arthrex) is sutured over the remnant lateral soft tissue for augmentation in a case of iatrogenic medial instability from aggressive prior lateral release.

attempted first. When lateral retinaculum closure is precluded by inadequate lateral soft tissue—when closure will lead to lateral subluxation or when medial instability persists after lateral retinaculum closure—lateral soft tissue reconstructions are indicated. Medial instability, differently than lateral instability, is an iatrogenic consequence of lateral soft tissue disruption. The anatomy, morphology, and alignment favors patellar lateralization. Therefore, it is the author's opinion that restoring the lateral soft tissue integrity is sufficient and has less chances of overconstraint compared to lateral ligaments reconstruction. The soft tissue quality can be enhanced by allografts such as fascia lata or decellularized dermal tissue (▶ Fig. 33.9). If lateral PF ligament reconstruction is considered, it should be as isometric as possible to avoid tightness. The patellar insertion should be in the proximal or middle third and the femoral insertion close to the lateral epicondyle. Lateral patellotibial ligament reconstruction should respect the normal function of the structure and be tighter in flexion.

34 Recurrent Patellofemoral Dislocation—Distal Realignment

Richard Ma and Seth L. Sherman

34.1 Description

Distal realignment or tibial tuberosity osteotomy (TTO) is a well-described surgical treatment for a broad range of patellofemoral joint disorders including patellofemoral instability, chondral lesions, and arthritis. Customization of the osteotomy can correct lateralized patellar tracking, patellar height abnormalities, or reduce patellofemoral stress to unload focal chondral lesions. Medialization/anteromedialization (AMZ) or distalization (DTZ) of the tibial tubercle is typically considered for recurrent lateral patellofemoral instability. While TTO may be performed in isolation, it is typically combined with medial soft tissue patellar stabilization procedures (medial patellofemoral ligament reconstruction) +/–. lateral retinaculum lengthening in the setting of patellofemoral instability.

34.2 Key Principles in Tibial Tubercle Osteotomy for Recurrent Patellofemoral Dislocation

- Careful scrutiny of the patient's history and clinical exam is necessary to determine the chief patellofemoral complaint (instability, pain, or both). This will impact the orientation of TTO in order to produce the desired effect. The rationale to include TTO in patellofemoral instability is based upon patient-specific factors, biomechanical abnormalities, and the presence/location of any patellofemoral cartilage lesion. Patients with bony malalignment and other risk factors including bilateral recurrent instability, underlying trochlear dysplasia, low-energy dislocations, large focal cartilage lesions, failed prior soft tissue repair/reconstruction are generally candidates for concomitant TTO.
- In cases of recurrent lateral patellofemoral instability, preoperative imaging is important to assess patellar height (i.e., WB lateral X-ray), lateralized force vector (i.e., axial computed tomography/magnetic resonance imaging [CT/MRI] to measure tibial tubercle-trochlear groove distance [TT-TG]), and cartilage lesions (MRI) (▶ Fig. 34.1).
- Values for TT-TG vary between CT and MRI and no single value should guide the surgeon toward or against osteotomy. In general, the goal of a medialization-type TTO for patellar instability is to normalize the TT-TG within a range of 10 to 15 mm. In the setting of chondral lesions, adding anteriorization of 10 to 15 mm can reduce patellofemoral contact forces by approximately 20%. DTZ-type TTO can normalize the Caton-Deschamps ratio closer to 1:1 in the setting of patella height abnormalities (normal ratio range 0.6–1.3; patella baja: < 0.6; patella alta: > 1.3). Preoperative planning allows one to calculate the angle of the TTO in order to determine the amount of tubercle medialization, anteriorization, and/or DTZ required to reduce lateralized force vector, patella alta, or to decrease patellofemoral contact stress, respectively (▶ Table 34.1).

34.3 Expectations

- Excellent outcomes have been reported for AMZ or DTZ when appropriately indicated as an adjunct procedure in the setting of recurrent patellar instability. Outcomes of TTO are more predictable for patellofemoral instability than for patients who present with both pain and instability. Poorer outcomes are associated with patients who have untreated Outerbridge III/IV pan-patella, central, or medial patellofemoral lesions, as TTO may add additional stress to these regions. The addition of tubercle DTZ (disruption of the distal osseous hinge) may be associated with increased risk of postoperative complications including nonunion of the osteotomy and fixation failure.

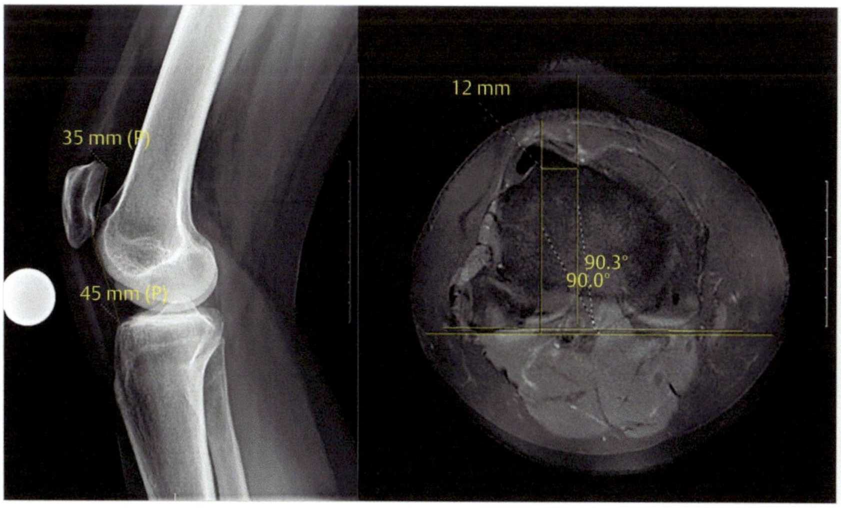

Fig. 34.1 Measurement of Caton-Deschamps index which is the ratio of the distance between the lower pole of the patella and upper limit of the tibia and the length of the patellar articular surface (left). The tibial tubercle-trochlear groove (TT-TG) is the distance between perpendicular lines drawn at the deepest point of the trochlear groove and the center of the tibial patellar tendon attachment (right).

Table 34.1 Reference guide for osteotomy slope

Osteotomy slope angle							
45 degrees	Anteriorization (mm)	10	11	12	13	14	15
	Medialization (mm)	10	11	12	13	14	15
60 degrees	Anteriorization (mm)	10	11	12	13	14	15
	Medialization (mm)	5.8	6.4	6.9	7.5	8.1	8.7

34.4 Indications

- TTO is indicated for skeletally mature patients with bony malalignment in the setting of documented recurrent patella dislocation events. Patients with recurrent subluxation events who fail conservative treatment (i.e., patellar bracing, McConnell taping, closed chain exercises, core strengthening, proprioceptive training, balance training, and gait training) may also be surgical candidates.
- In general, AMZ is considered in patients with TT-TG > 20 mm and DTZ is considered with Caton-Deschamps index > 1.3. These threshold values are only a guide and may vary based on patient-specific factors (number of dislocations, underlying trochlear dysplasia, rotatory abnormalities, prior failed soft tissue surgery, presence of chondral lesion, age and activity).

34.5 Contraindications

- Skeletal immaturity.
- For AMZ, untreated significant arthrosis of the medial patellofemoral facet or proximal patella (if not combined with cartilage restoration procedure). AMS of the tibial tubercle increases patellofemoral contact forces on the medial and proximal patellofemoral articulation.
- General contraindications for osteotomy (i.e., smoking, inflammatory arthropathy, osteoporosis, morbid obesity).
- Patient noncompliance.

34.6 Special Considerations

- A diagnostic knee arthroscopy should be performed to evaluate patellofemoral tracking and to investigate for contraindications to osteotomy prior to the open approach. Size, depth, and location of chondral lesions should be carefully documented as this may alter the planned degree of anteriorization or medialization. The camera can be placed at the inferomedial or superolateral portal to assess intraoperative patellar tracking and patella tilt. The latter may be corrected with combined soft tissue balancing (lateral retinaculum lengthening) during the open portion of the case.

34.7 Special Instructions, Positioning, and Anesthesia

- For TTO, place the patient in a supine position with a lateral hip post and a diagnostic knee arthroscopy set-up. The C-arm is typically positioned to come in from the operative side, particularly if a medial soft tissue repair or reconstruction will be performed, since more medial based exposure/drilling/implant placement will be needed. A thigh tourniquet is placed, but rarely utilized. If the thigh tourniquet is inflated, it should be released before skin closure in order to obtain hemostasis. Intraoperative transamenic acid (TXA) is also administered to limit perioperative bleeding.
- A peripheral nerve block can be placed preoperatively to assist with postoperative pain control (typically one time motor sparing block of the adductor canal). We typically avoid popliteal blocks, given the need to monitor lower leg compartments following the osteotomy.
- Bone marrow may be aspirated from the proximal tibia or distal femur and concentrated. The bone marrow concentrate can be mixed with scaffold and placed around the osteotomy in order to facilitate bony integration and healing, particularly for higher risk osteotomies (DTZ or revision).

34.8 Tips, Pearl, and Lessons Learned

- The surgical exposure for TTO is relatively straightforward. The proximal cut beneath the patellar tendon insertion is made easier by clearly identifying the distal aspect of the patellar tendon in terms of both of its medial and lateral borders as it inserts onto the tibial tubercle and placing a retractor under it to lift it out and away from the proximal tibia. Care is taken to avoid excessive dissection around the fat pad to minimize arthrofibrosis.
- Commercial cutting guides (Arthrex T3 System, Arthrex Inc., Naples, FL, and Tracker AMZ Guide System, DePuy/Synthes Inc., Raynham, MA) are available to help make the bone cut for the length of the osteotomy (authors' preference). The key is to design an appropriate bone pedicle (~7 cm), which increases the bone surface area for healing and screw fixation. Alternatively, a series of evenly spaced K-wires can be placed across the tibia at the desire angle and the osteotomy then completed with an osteotome if a cutting guide is not available (▸ Fig. 34.2). An anterior cruciate ligament (ACL) guide can be used in this instance for reproducible placement of the K-wires.
- Once the osteotomy is complete and the desired correction is achieved, secure the osteotomy with K-wire(s) to help maintain the correction during drilling for screw fixation of the osteotomy.
- If concomitant DTZ of the pedicle is performed, careful contouring of the distal aspect of the pedicle is performed so as to maximize congruity to help facilitate bony healing in this area after surgery. Periosteal flap may be elevated before the cut and sutured over the top of the "at-risk" distal portion of the osteotomy site (▸ Fig. 34.3).

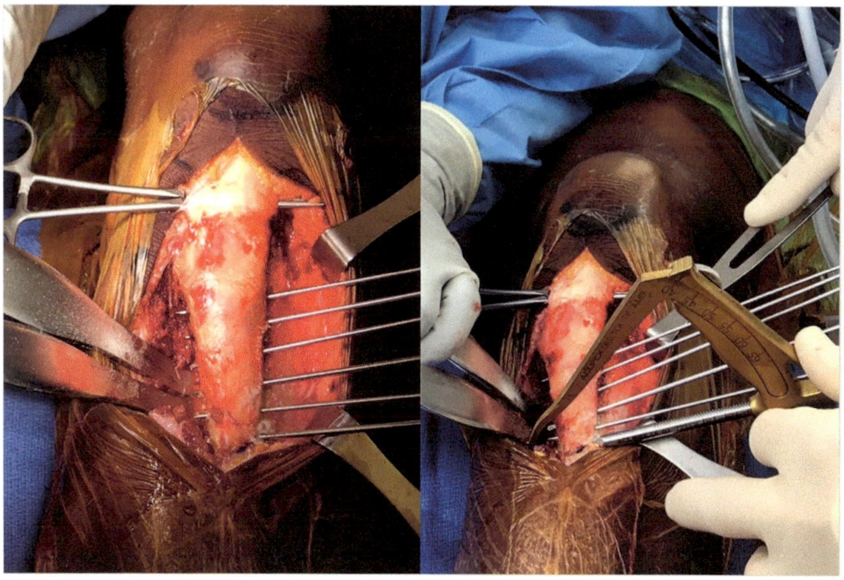

Fig. 34.2 A series of evenly spaced K-wires can be placed across the tibia at the desired angle with the help of an ACL guide and then the osteotome is used to complete the osteotomy between the K-wires.

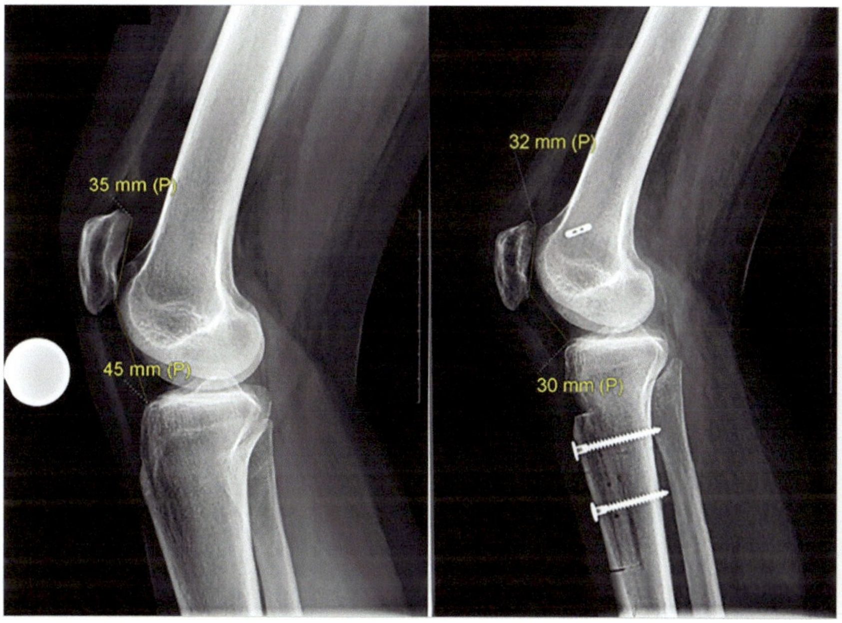

Fig. 34.3 Recurrent patellar dislocation with patella alta and medial patellofemoral ligament (MPFL) deficiency. Patient was treated with concomitant anteromedialization (AMZ) + distalization (DTZ) and MPFL reconstruction with normalization of patellar height.

34.9 Difficulties Encountered

- Once the angle of the osteotomy is chosen and the desired correction is achieved, K-wires are used to maintain provisional fixation until cortical screws are placed. Loss of the correction can occur during compression of the cortical screws. Having additional K-wire(s) out of the plane of the screws can help maintain correction during screw placement.

34.10 Key Procedural Steps

- After induction of general anesthesia, the patient is positioned supine with a lateral hip post and fluoroscopy on the operative side.
- TXA and antibiotics are given prior to initial skin incision.
- Examination under anesthesia is performed, comparing to the opposite limb, prior to sterile preparation and draping.
- A diagnostic knee arthroscopy is first performed to assess patella tracking and to determine the size, location, and depth of any chondral lesions. Chondroplasty and/or synovectomy may be performed.
- A straight longitudinal incision is made starting at the lateral arthroscopic portal and extending 7 cm distal to the tibial tuberosity, just lateral to the tibial crest (▶ Fig. 34.4).
- The anterior tibial crest, along with the medial and lateral borders of the patellar tendon, is exposed and defined (▶ Fig. 34.4). The fat pad is protected.
- The anterior compartment fascia is then incised and subperiosteal dissection is performed to expose tibial bone along the length of the osteotomy. The posterior soft tissue is carefully elevated and a retractor is placed to protect the

anterior compartment musculature and the deep peroneal nerve and anterior tibial artery (▶ Fig. 34.4).

- The medial border of the tibial crest is then demarcated extending from the medial border of the patellar tendon proximally and extending to the distal end of the pedicle. If an AMZ without DTZ is desired, the shingle is triangular shaped with it tapering distally and exiting near the anterior cortex of the tibia. Alternatively, if DTZ is desired, the pedicle is designed so it does not exit anteriorly and a vertical cut is done distally to release the pedicle. The pedicle length is usually 7 to 10 cm. Once the cutting guide is placed at the desired angle slope based on preoperatively planning, two reference pins are placed to secure the cutting guide into place (▶ Fig. 34.5).
- A sagittal saw is then used to complete the osteotomy with the lateral retractor in place to protect the posterior neurovascular structures (▶ Fig. 34.5). A straight osteotome, saw, or metal ruler can be used to make sure the osteotomy is complete from medial to lateral. The proximal osteotomy cuts are made with a straight osteotome with a retractor protecting and pulling the patellar tendon anteriorly.
- For AMZ, the distal attachment of the shingle is left intact. Once the osteotomy is complete, a slow firm force with an osteotome is used to displace the shingle and deform the distal anterior tibial crest bone hinge (▶ Fig. 34.6). For DTZ, a vertical cut is made at the distal end of the shingle to release it. A second distal cut into the shingle proximal to the first cut is then made based on the amount needed to normalize the patellar height. Fluoroscopic imaging can be used to judge the patellar height correction achieved, as it is important avoid iatrogenic patella baja with an overaggressive correction.

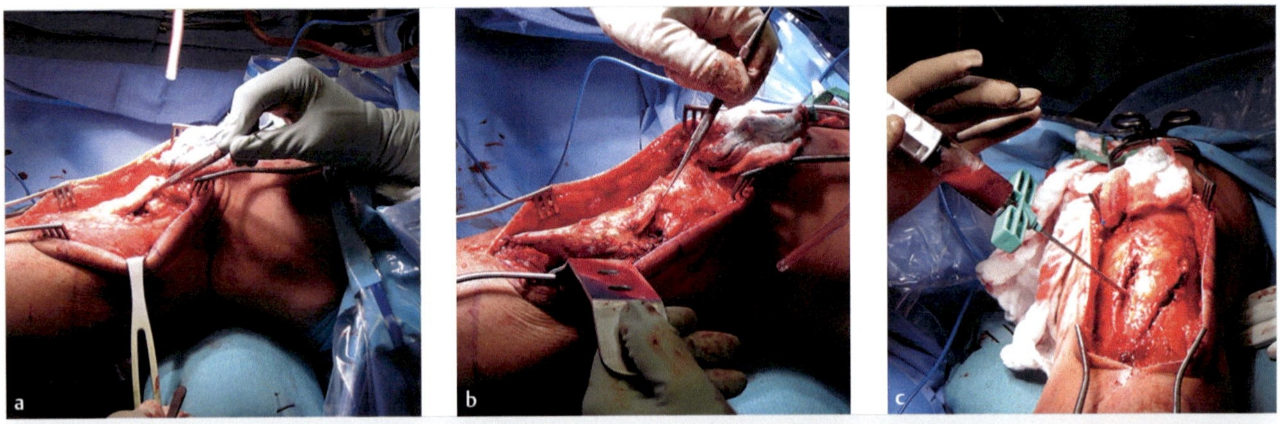

Fig. 34.4 A midline incision is made with the distal insertion of the patellar tendon isolated and protected **(a)**. The anterior muscle compartment is elevated and posterior neurovascular bundle protected with retractor **(b)**. Bone marrow aspirate can be collected from the proximal tibia for bone graft at the end of the osteotomy **(c)**.

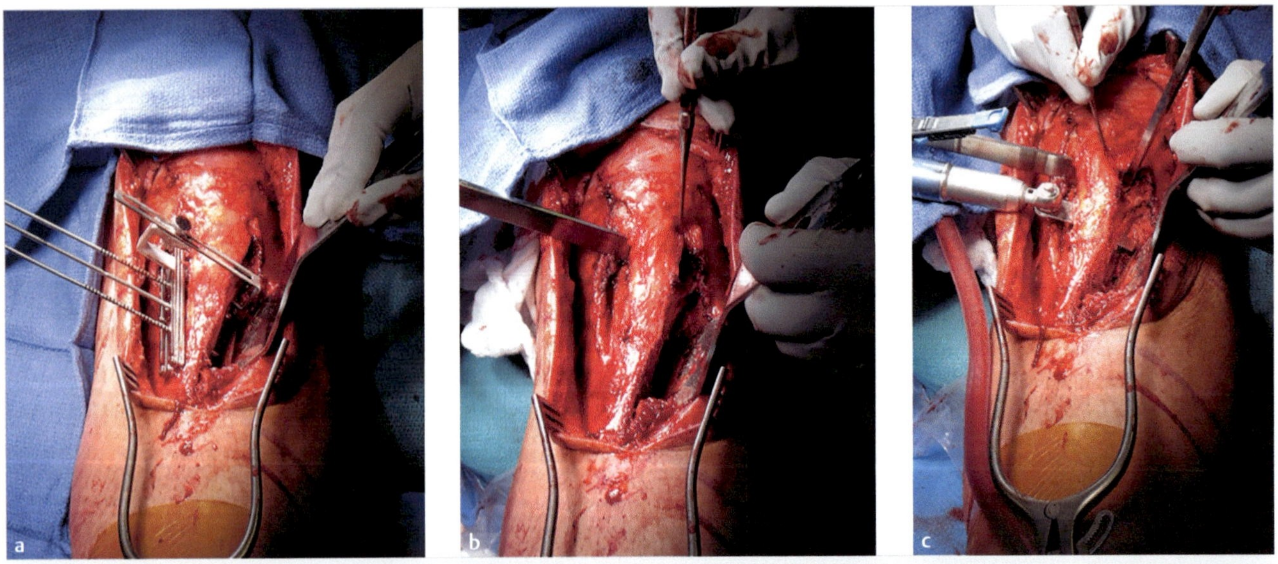

Fig. 34.5 Anteromedialization (AMZ) without DTZ. The cutting guide is placed at the desired slope along the anteromedial tibia and pinned into place (Arthrex T3 System, Arthrex Inc., Naples, FL) **(a)**. The saw blade exit indicator shows where the saw blade will exit along the posterolateral tibia. Proximal cuts beneath the patellar tendon is completed with osteotome with the patellar tendon protected **(b)**. Final check to make sure all cuts are complete for the AMZ **(c)**.

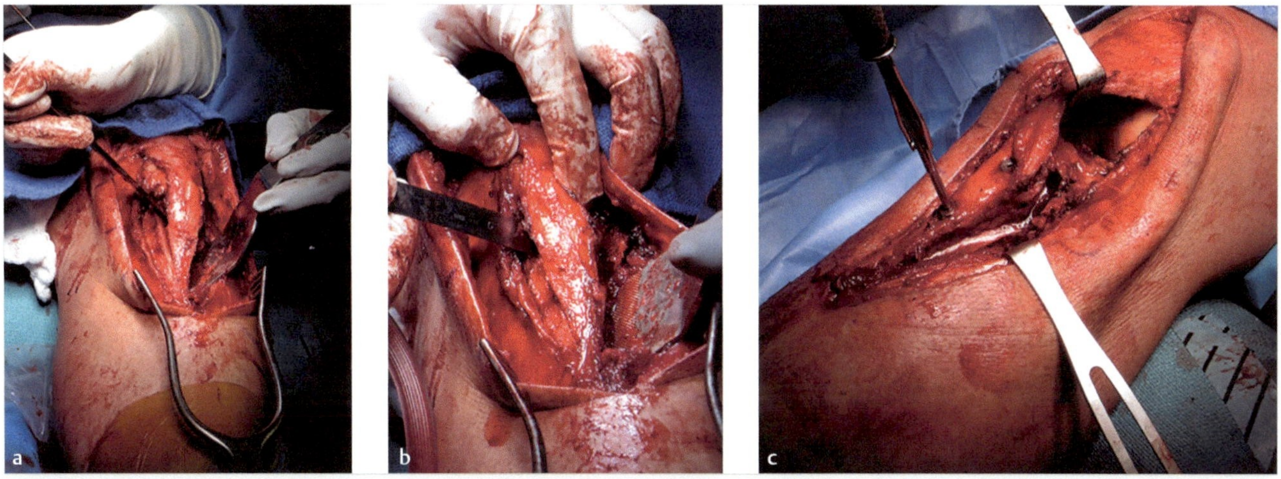

Fig. 34.6 (a) Once all the osteotomy cuts are complete, the shingle is lifted with an osteotome applying a gentle steady force (b) and the tubercle is transposed anteriorly and medially the desired distance based on preoperative planning. (c) Two 4.5-mm cortical screws are used to fix the osteotomy into place.

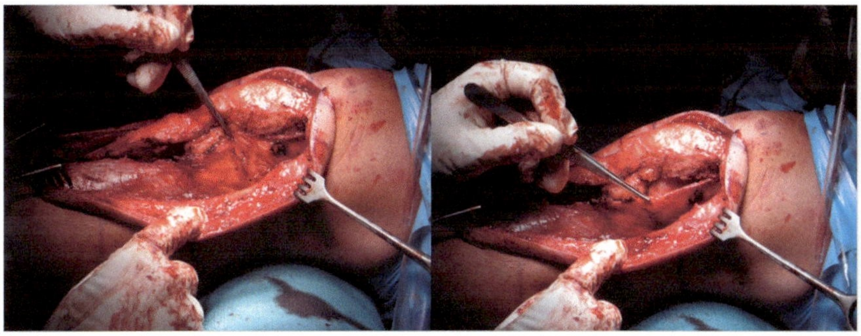

Fig. 34.7 The incision can be extended proximally to perform an open lateral retinacular lengthening. The first layer of the lateral retinaculum (forceps) is released directly off the patella. The lateral patellofemoral ligament (second layer) is then released 2 cm away from its patellar attachment and the first layer is sutured to the lateral patellofemoral ligament in a lengthened state.

- Once the appropriate amount of anteriorization, medialization, and/or DTZ has been achieved, K-wires are used to hold the shingle in place. The knee is ranged at this point and intraoperative assessment of patellar tracking is performed. Adjustment can be made at this point. If the lateral retinacular structures are tight, a lateral lengthening procedure can be performed to ensure the patella is centered on the trochlea without undo force (▶ Fig. 34.7). Once satisfactory, two or three appropriate length 4.5 mm cortical screws are placed to secure the shingle (▶ Fig. 34.6). The screw holes within the shingle are overdrilled to achieve interfragmentary compression.
- The medial overhang of the pedicle from the medialization can then be contoured with a rasp or saw blade and bone graft/BMAC can be used to pack around the shingle and tibia to assist with bone integration.
- A medium hemovac is typically used and placed deep to the fascia of the anterior compartment to minimize postoperative hematoma and to mitigate the potential for compartment syndrome. The anterior muscle fascia is repaired back to the proximal tibia. A compartment release or pie crusting the compartment fascia with a No. 11 blade can be performed to further minimize the potential for compartment syndrome postoperatively.

34.11 Bailout, Rescue, and Salvage Procedures

- Early fixation failure after distal realignment can occur with aggressive therapy or weightbearing. These cases can often be remedied with revision of the fixation either using larger screws in the same screw holes (6.5-mm screws) or drilling new screw holes after preparation of the bony healing interface (▶ Fig. 34.8). In cases where screw fixation is not optimal, plating of the osteotomy can be achieved. Plate fixation is also a good option if an intraoperative fracture of the shingle occurs during screw fixation.
- Proximal tibia fracture can occur after TTO particularly if weightbearing is initiated before radiographic healing occurs or in older individuals with poor bone quality. Open reduction and internal fixation of the proximal tibia fracture can salvage those challenging scenarios (▶ Fig. 34.9).

34.12 Pitfalls

- The medial patellofemoral ligament (MPFL) acts as the primary checkrein to lateral patella translation. MPFL

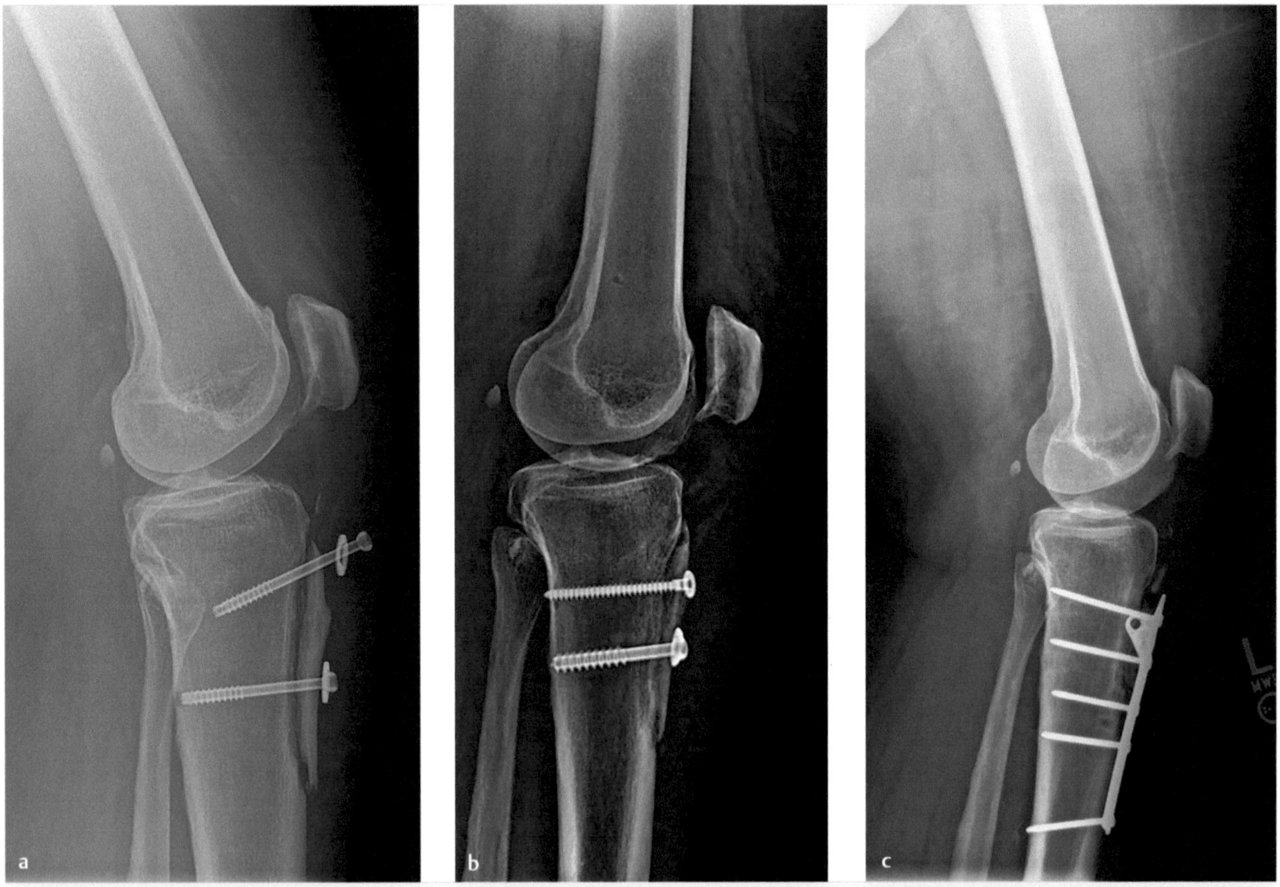

Fig. 34.8 **(a)** Early fixation failure can occur with excessive activity after surgery. **(b)** This was revised with different 4.5-mm cortical screw proximally and a 6.5-mm screw distally. **(c)** In instances where screw fixation is not possible, compression plating can be used (clover plate, DePuy/Synthes Inc., Raynham, MA).

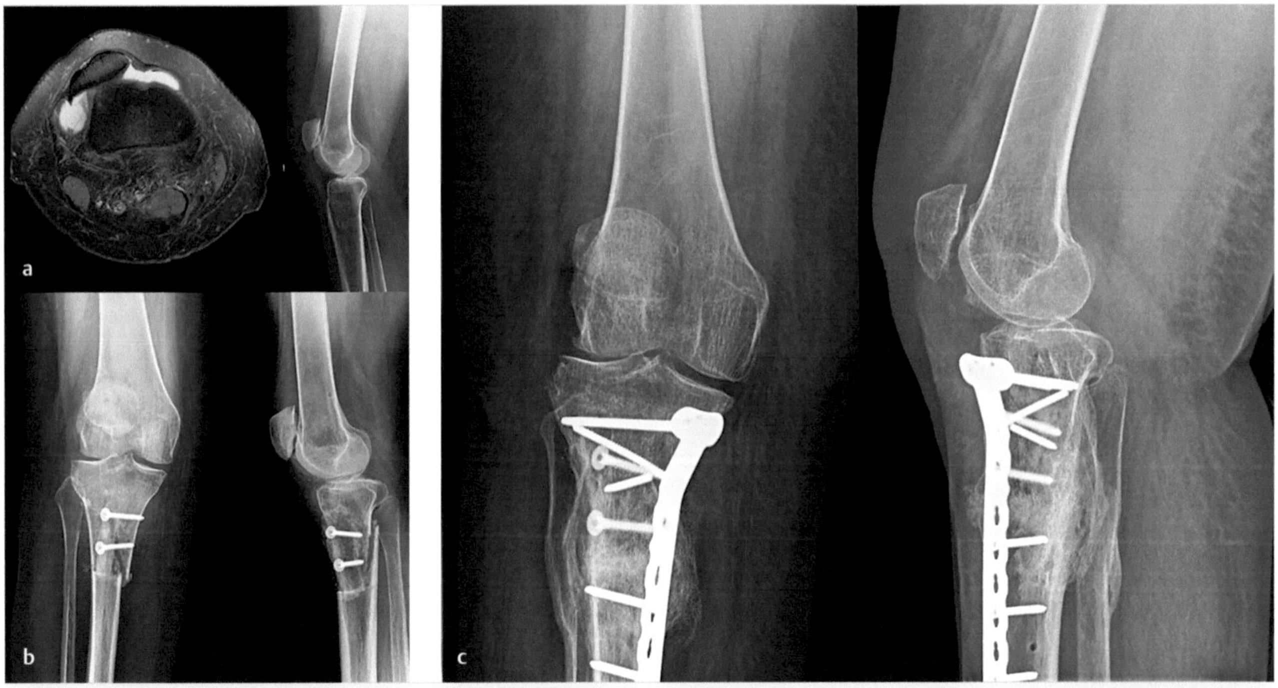

Fig. 34.9 **(a)** Preoperative images of a patient with patellofemoral instability. The MRI image confirms a lateral maltracking of the patella. The radiograph on lateral projection depicts a patella alta; **(b)** Early postoperative images after a tibial tuberosity osteotomy. The radiographs reveal a proximal tibial fracture. **(c)** Posteoperative images after open reduction and internal fixation of the proximal tibia revealing complete fracture healing.

reconstruction is typically performed in every case of patella instability. TTO is an adjunct procedure in select cases to help normalize forces and to center the patella on the trochlea prior to soft tissue stabilization. If malalignment remains uncorrected and the MPFL reconstruction is utilized improperly to “pull” the patella into the trochlea, this will likely lead to abnormal joint pressures and overconstraint, with eventual graft failure and/or arthritis.

- Overmedialization of the tibial tubercle can be detrimental by leading to increased medial patellofemoral stress. One should aim to achieve a final TT-TG of 10 to 15 mm with the TTO.
- Overanteriorization (> 15 mm) of the tibial tubercle can result in skin necrosis. Elevation of 12.5 mm reduces the patellofemoral contact forces with further elevation providing less benefit.
- Weightbearing too early can lead to fracture of the proximal tibia if the patient is returned to full weightbearing prior to radiographic healing.

35 Meniscal Tears and Principles of Partial Meniscectomy

Wilson Mello Jr. and Marco Kawamura Demange

35.1 Description

Meniscal tears are very common and can be didactically classified as traumatic and nontraumatic. The traumatic tears usually occur in young people. The nontraumatic tear usually occurs above age of 50 years old, presenting different patterns as a radial tear (also named fatigue meniscal tear), root tear, flap tear (with or without osseous impact), and degenerative tears. Root tears in the nontraumatic scenario usually happen in the medial meniscus. In contrast, traumatic root tears in younger patients usually occur on the lateral side and are frequently associated with ligament lesions (▶ Table 35.1).

35.2 Key Principles

Understanding the pattern of the meniscal tear, the patient expectations, the healing capacity of the menisci, the patient physiologic age and activity demands, and the nonsurgical treatment results are mandatory before considering surgical treatment.

Menisci are fundamental in decreasing load transmission, shock absorption, knee stability, cartilage lubrication and nutrition, and proprioception. They decrease the contact stress and increase the contact area while improving joint congruity.

Partial meniscectomy and meniscal repair are the most common options. The healing capacity of the meniscus for a repair is related to its vascularity (based on the localization of the tear and the patient's age), tear pattern, and chronicity. Meniscus healing is also enhanced with biological stimulation when combined with anterior cruciate ligament surgery, patient adherence to the rehabilitation protocol, and adequate repair technique. The more peripheral the meniscus tear, the higher the healing capacity as the outer third has good vascularity (red zone) and the inner third has virtual no-vascularity (white zone). Regarding patient age, it is well known that children may have almost-total meniscus vascularity while adults above 50 have vascularity in only the peripheral quarter.

In this chapter, we are going to focus on partial meniscectomy principles.

35.3 Expectations

Meniscal preservation is one of the main goals when surgically approaching a meniscus tear. In this way, partial meniscus resection should involve the minimal possible resection for each case. During surgery, surgeons should distinguish between a normal meniscus with a localized tear and a degenerative meniscus with several tears. Whenever approaching a normal meniscus, the surgical principle rests on removing the tear while obtaining a "normal"-shaped residual meniscus. On the other hand, in a degenerative tear, surgeons should avoid trimming the meniscus all the way to normal tissue as it may result in a total meniscectomy.

In patients with nontraumatic acute onset type of meniscus tears, especially root tears or complete radial tears, it is important to explain the risk of osteoarthritis progression or subchondral insufficiency fracture following the lesion (either with or without surgery).

35.4 Indications

In the traumatic tear, partial meniscectomy is indicated in symptomatic patients whenever successful repair is not possible. This includes but not limited to the following.

- Inner-third (white zone) tears.
- Chronic tears.
- Isolated flap tears.
- Isolated nonreducible buckle tears.
- Complex pattern tears.

In the nontraumatic tear group, nonsurgical care is routinely performed. Flap tears causing osseous impact and partial radial tears usually benefit from surgical treatment if a 6- to 12-week attempt at nonsurgical treatment fails to resolve symptoms. Patients with degenerative tears may benefit from a longer course of nonsurgical treatment. Clinically, partial radial tear patients and osseous-meniscal impact flap tear patients often present with acute nontraumatic (or minimal trauma) onset of symptoms. In the first, magnetic resonance imaging (MRI) usually presents a radial or vertical flap tear in the body to posterior horn junction of the medial meniscus with normal (or almost normal) cartilage. The patients with flap tears causing osseous overload usually present pain with bone palpation during physical exam and bone marrow overload edema on the MRI (▶ Table 35.1).

Root tears may progress to insufficiency fracture or SPONK, and these usually do not benefit from surgical partial meniscectomy, in order to prevent osteoarthritis progression, following meniscectomy (▶ Fig. 35.5).

Table 35.1 Meniscus tear patterns with regards to mechanism of injury and expected clinical presentation

Meniscus Tears				
Traumatic	Nontraumatic or minor trauma			
Bucket handle Longitudinal Radial Flap (▶ Fig. 35.1) Ramp lesions Meniscal root avulsion	Acute pain onset			Chronic degenerative (▶ Fig. 35.4)
	Radial tear (▶ Fig. 35.2)	Root tear	Flap tear (▶ Fig. 35.3)	

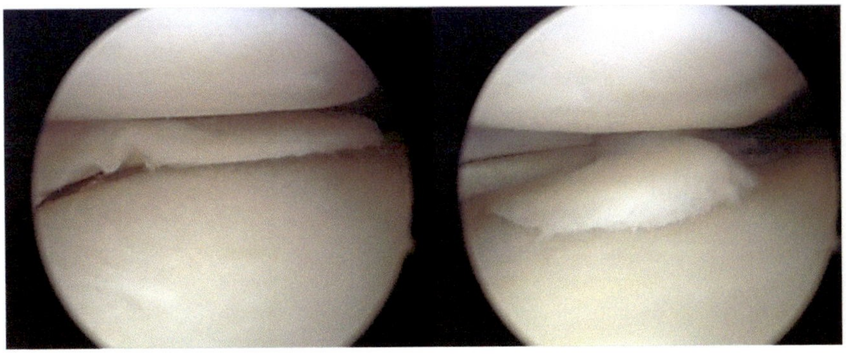

Fig. 35.1 Meniscus flap tear.

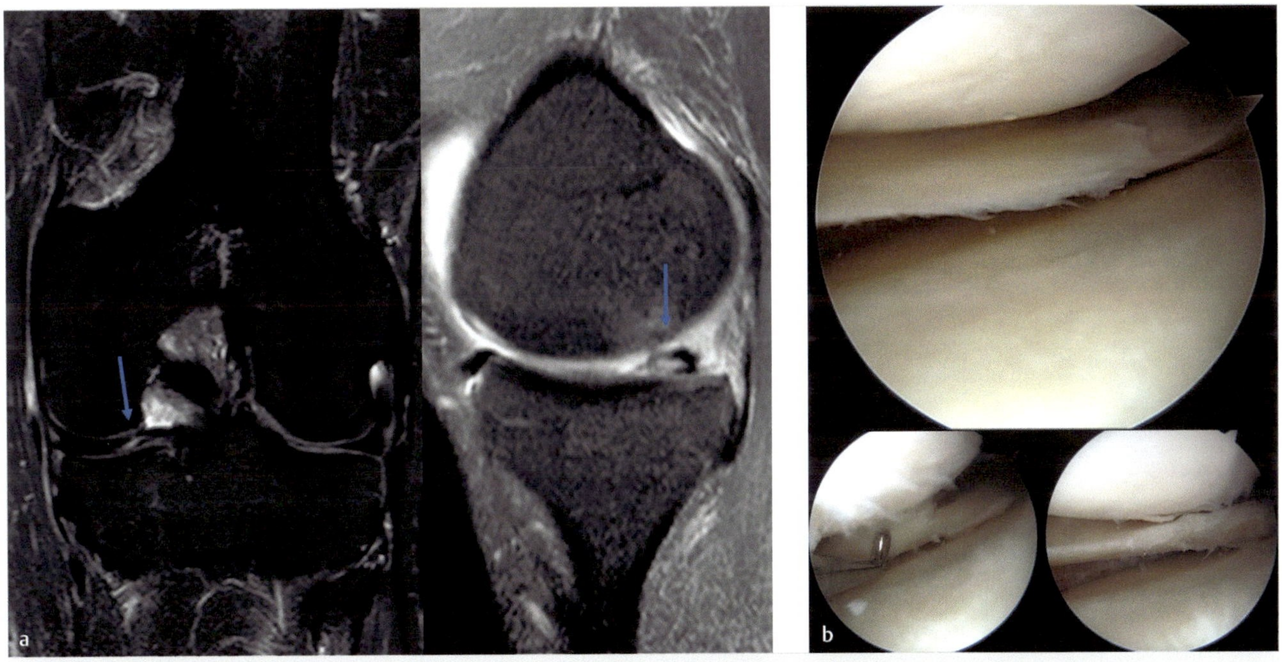

Fig. 35.2 Nontraumatic meniscus partial radial tear. **(a)** Magnetic resonance imaging (MRI) and **(b)** arthroscopy images.

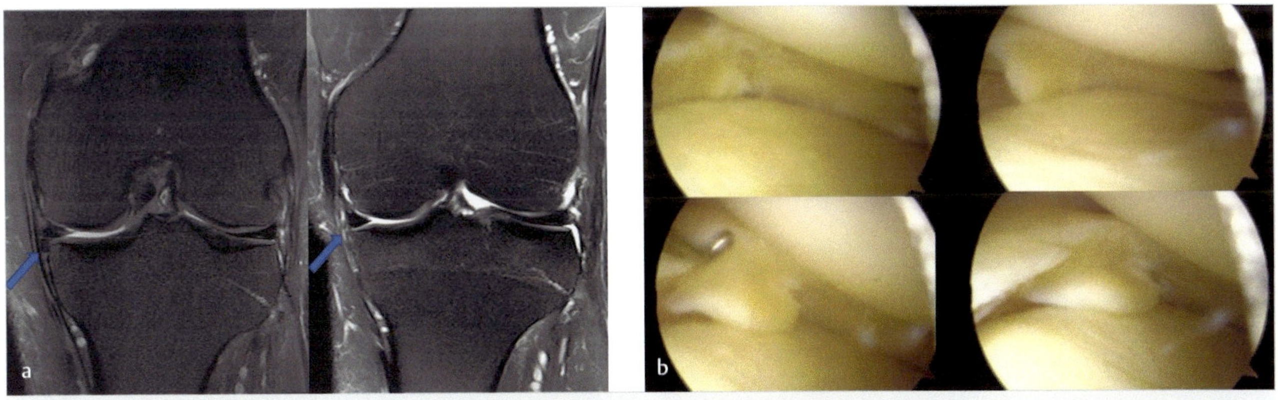

Fig. 35.3 Nontraumatic flap tear causing osteomeniscal impact in the tibia. Note in the **(a)** magnetic resonance imaging (MRI) coronal T2 image the presence of increased signal in the tibia corner (*arrow*). **(b)** Note the flap, in that the flap is not seen initially and after pulled with the probe.

35.5 Contraindications

Patients with knee osteoarthritis should avoid surgical meniscectomy.

Surgeons should avoid meniscectomy in patients with meniscal extrusion, complete radial tears, or root tears.

These should be seen as a relative contraindication.

35.6 Special Considerations

Knee alignment should be evaluated regarding the risk of overloading the compartment. The presence of meniscus extrusion and subchondral bone edema is associated with worse prognosis. Subchondral bone fracture (insufficiency fracture or SPONK) may occur after partial meniscectomy, particularly in patients above the age of 50 years.

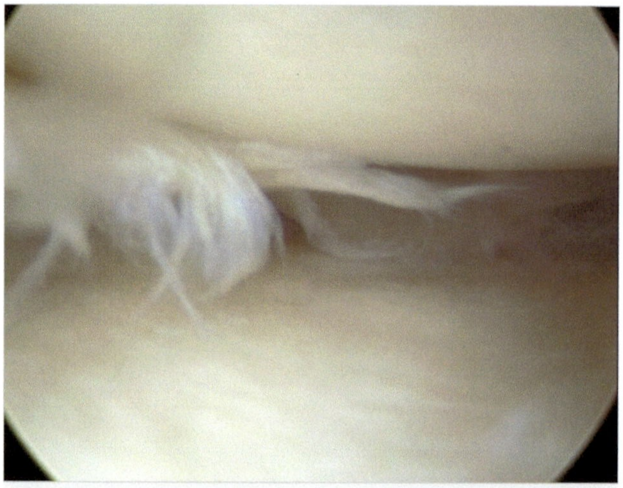

Fig. 35.4 Degenerative meniscus tear.

Always evaluate the subchondral bone before performing a partial meniscectomy.

35.7 Special Instructions, Position, and Anesthesia

Surgeon should employ preoperative planning and determine if partial meniscectomy or meniscus repair is intended to be the primary goal for the procedure. Patient position will be different among these procedures.

Medial meniscectomy is usually performed with the knee near extension (up to 40 degrees of flexion) and lateral meniscectomy may be performed with the knee in a "figure-of-4" position. Having a "leg holder" or a pole to contain lateral movement of the knee may facilitate valgus opening for partial medial meniscectomy procedures (▶ Fig. 35.6).

Meniscus repair patient positioning will not be described in this chapter.

To perform a good partial meniscectomy procedure, surgeons should preserve maximum meniscus remnant and avoid injury to the hyaline cartilage during arthroscopy. In this way, having adequate instruments such as small arthroscopy basket (straight, curved to the left, curved to the right, and elevated baskets) and arthroscopic scissors is very helpful (▶ Fig. 35.7).

Partial meniscectomy may be performed with a spinal anesthesia or with local + intra-articular + general anesthesia (laryngeal mask). The later protocol allows patients to recover more quickly from the procedure. The use of a tourniquet is optional. Intra-articular injection of a local anesthetic with epinephrine or the use of a saline infusion pump improves visualization if a tourniquet is not used.

Surgeons should also consider local anesthetics' chondrotoxicity when choosing which one to infuse. We prefer the use of ropivacain based on experimental research available in the literature.

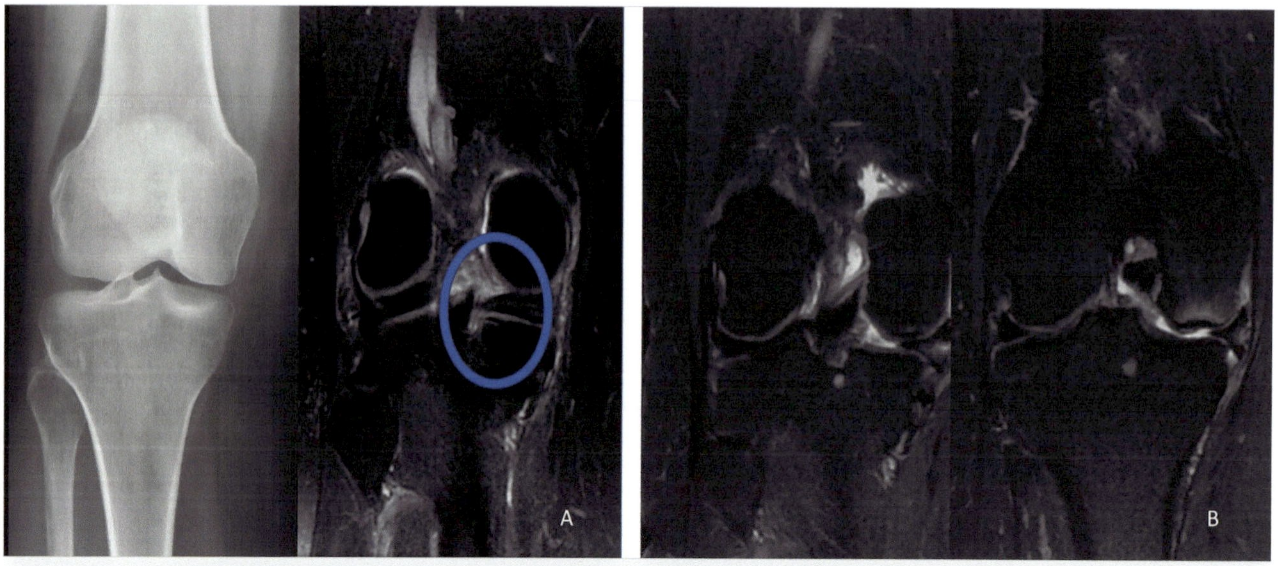

Fig. 35.5 Magnetic resonance imaging (MRI) of an insufficiency fracture or SPONK after a root tear.

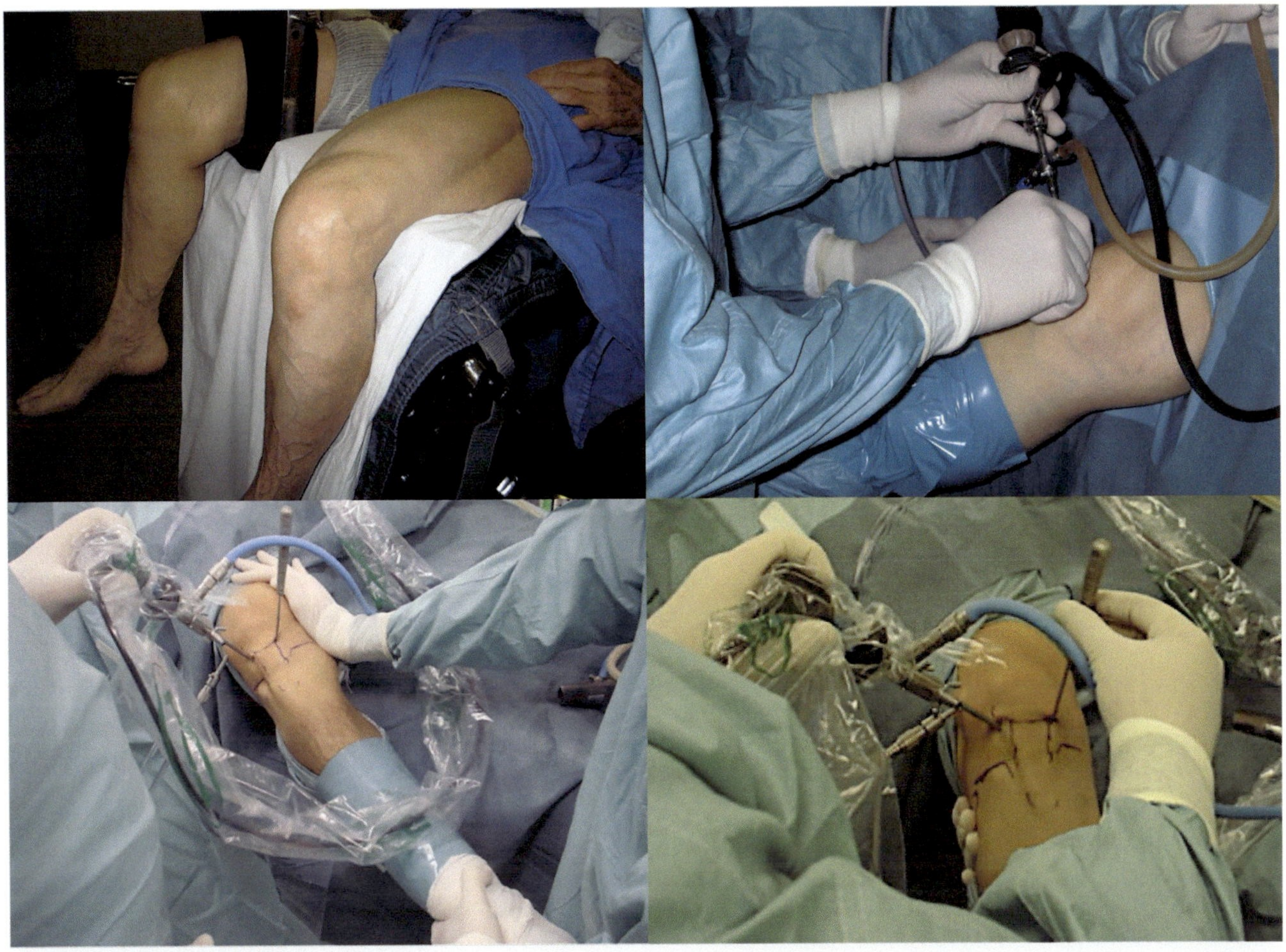

Fig. 35.6 Patient positioning for surgery.

35.8 Tips, Pearls, and Lessons Learned

It is important to have a complete set of instruments including a good probe, different angle basket punches, adequate grasper devices, and small arthroscopic scissors. Also, select a shaver with a diameter that fits into the medial or lateral compartment without damaging the articular cartilage.

Whenever approaching displaced bucket handle tears, reduce the meniscus fragment before performing a partial meniscectomy if that is required. Initially we cut 90% of the posterior portion of the meniscus tear with an arthroscopy scissor. Then we switch the portals to have a direct access to the anterior portion of the tear. We then cut the anterior portion of the tear. Finally, with a grasper we pull out the torn portion of the meniscus. If the remaining bridge of tissue between the cuts is too wide to allow us to pull the fragment out, then we make a third arthroscopic portal to cut the bridge with an arthroscopy scissor.

When performing a partial meniscectomy in older patients, we advise being very careful with the rehabilitation protocol. Respecting the "knee envelope of function" principle, as proposed by Dr. Scott Dye, allows the patient to reestablish normal function.

35.9 Difficulties Encountered

In some cases, especially in the medial compartment, approaching an isolated posterior tear may be difficult in tight knees. In those cases, consider minimal release of the medial collateral ligament with a pie-crust technique. Always avoid iatrogenic cartilage injury during surgery.

Changing portals during arthroscopy may be very helpful to approach anterior horn medial meniscus tears.

35.10 Key Procedural Steps

- Before deciding if surgery is indicated, consider factors such as patient's age, level of activity, knee alignment, knee stability, and expectations.
- Always perform a complete joint visualization in the beginning of the arthroscopy. Analyze the global aspect of the joint, especially regarding the cartilage status. Presence of large cartilage defects or osteoarthritis may change the indicated surgical approach.
- Evaluate the meniscus considering whether it is normal or significantly degenerative.
- Perform a partial meniscectomy with the goal of removal of the minimum amount of meniscal tissue possible to allow an

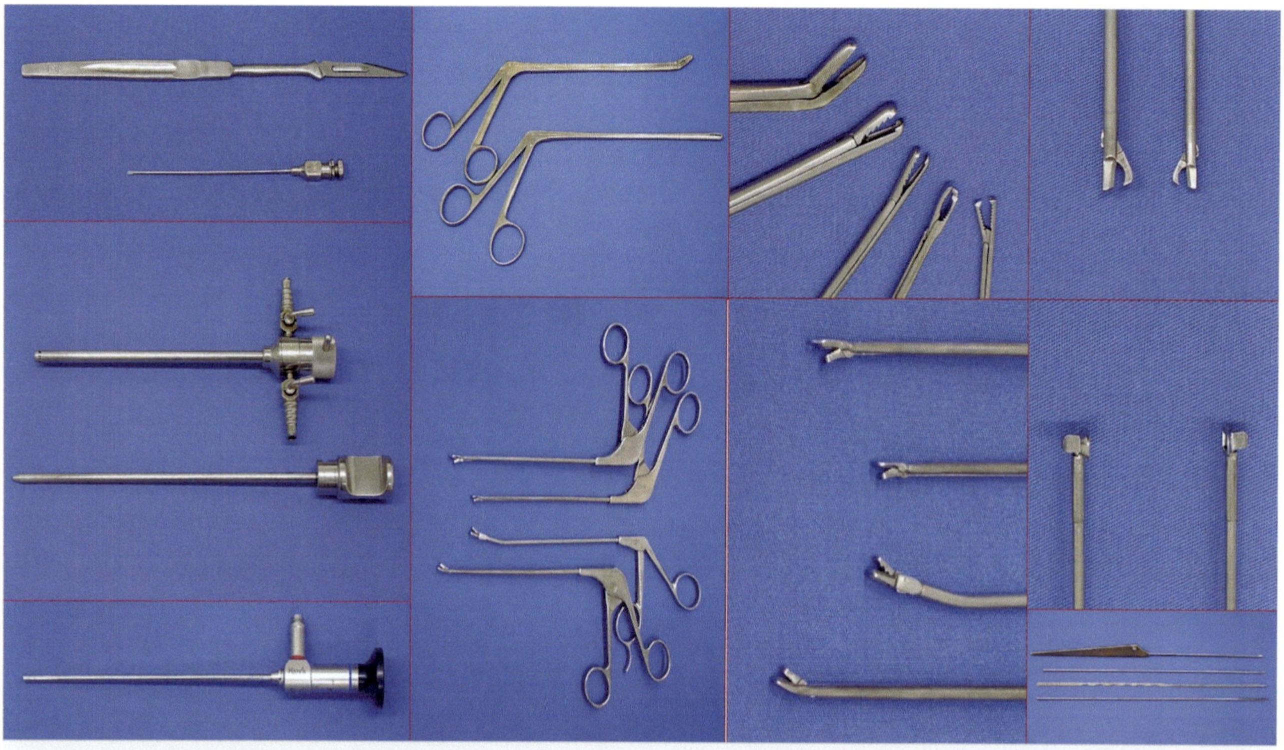

Fig. 35.7 Set of instruments for partial meniscectomy.

adequate or near normal shape in the remnant meniscus. Also, whenever facing a degenerative meniscus, remove only meniscus tissue that may cause symptoms. Avoid extensive tissue removal.

35.11 Bailout, Rescue, Salvage Procedures

In the young patient, excessive meniscus removal may cause severe symptoms as well as progressive cartilage damage. Whenever these conditions occur, alignment surgery (osteotomies), meniscus transplant, or both may be needed.

In elderly patients, subchondral insufficiency fracture may occur. The treatment of a subchondral fracture varies from unloading the joint to partial arthroplasty.

35.12 Pitfalls

- Meniscus lesion size may be underestimated as magnetic resonance imaging (MRI) cuts have space in between the images. Small radial tears and ramp lesions may be missed on MRI scan.
- Even when you are scheduling a partial meniscectomy in a young patient, you must be prepared to perform a meniscal repair if needed.
- Minor traumas between the time of the MRI and surgery may be sufficient to cause lesion progression.

36 Meniscus Repair

Carlos Eduardo Franciozi, Sheila J. McNeill Ingham, and Rene Jorge Abdalla

36.1 Description

This chapter will outline technical notes to address meniscal lesions by the inside-out technique. Root tears will be addressed in the next chapter.

36.2 Key Principles

Save the meniscus. A meniscus repair leads to improved long-term outcomes, including clinical outcome scores, and less radiographic degenerative changes when compared with partial meniscectomy.

36.3 Expectations

This chapter intends to review the current indications and contraindications for meniscus repair considering the technical advancements and biological augmentations available. Also, the surgical technique for the gold-standard inside-out meniscus repair will be described and explained in addition to the author's tips and pearls.

36.4 Indications

- Traumatic unstable tears in all zones. Repairs to the avascular zone should be biologically enhanced.
- Vertical longitudinal tears > 10 mm.
- Horizontal tears in young patients.
- Radial tears involving more than 90% of the meniscus.

36.5 Contraindications

- Degenerative tears in middle-aged and older patients.
- Ligament-deficient unstable knee if the ligament will not also be addressed.

36.6 Special Considerations

Meniscus lesions in children should always be considered for repair.

Lateral meniscus lesion in high-demand athletes requires special attention and higher efforts for repair as a lateral meniscectomy in this type of patient can lead to chondrolysis and return to sports at a decreased level or no return at all.

36.7 Special Instructions, Position, and Anesthesia

The patient is placed in a supine position with a proximal thigh tourniquet. A lateral thigh post is used to create an opening valgus stress to the medial compartment and the figure-of-4 position is used to create an opening varus stress to the lateral compartment. The traditional anterolateral and anteromedial portals are made. A spinal needle can be used to optimize the anteromedial portal position in order to better access the desired medial or lateral compartment.

The meniscus tear is debrided with a shaver and/or a meniscal rasp over its edges. Also, the rasp is used at the perimeniscal capsular synovium over the lesion intending to cause bleeding and vascular infiltration stimulation. Tears at the posterior horn and meniscus body are addressed by the inside-out (the senior author's preference), all-inside, or hybrid techniques, while tears at the anterior horn are addressed by the outside-in technique.

36.7.1 Medial Meniscus Inside-Out Technique

A posteromedial incision is made with the knee in flexion. Transillumination helps to determine its placement and also to visualize the saphenous vein. A 3.5-cm incision is made posterior to the medial collateral ligament. One-third of the incision is placed above the joint line and two-thirds distal to it as the needles often bend downward after exiting at the joint capsule. The sartorius fascia is identified deep to the subcutaneous tissue and dissected from proximal to distal using a Metzenbaum scissor. The surgeon works at the interval anterior to this fascia. Retracting the hamstrings posteriorly protects the saphenous nerve which is located posteromedial to the tendons. The interval between the medial gastrocnemius and the joint capsule is bluntly dissected with a Metzenbaum scissor and the surgeon's finger from proximal to distal. The authors use a small- or medium-sized speculum to retract and protect the neurovascular structures also deflecting the needles once they exit the capsule (▸ Fig. 36.1).

Single- or double-lumen cannulas are used, entering from the anterolateral portal or a secondary anterolateral portal. This portal is frequently located more superiorly and medially. Ten-inch flexible needles preloaded with a No. 2.0 Ethibond suture or high-strength braided suture, such as No. 2.0 Ultrabraid, are used to accomplish the repair. The cannula is positioned at the desired location and the first needle is passed into the meniscus while an assistant recovers it with a needle driver at the posteromedial incision. The second needle is inserted preferably creating a vertical mattress pattern. Oblique and horizontal patterns can also be used, although they are biomechanically inferior. Multiple sutures are inserted from posterior to anterior, 3 to 5 mm apart. Typically, a bucket-handle tear or a horizontal tear involving the body and one horn is sutured using 8–14 sutures. Meniscocapsular tears are addressed by passing the first needle through the meniscus and the second through the capsule near the tear. Sutures may be inserted at the femoral or tibial side of the meniscus. Normally, the femoral-sided sutures are inserted first, as they are easier to place. However, it can sometimes create a pucker appearance with meniscal tissue folded superiorly. This pucker can be corrected by the placement of tibial-sided sutures. The sutures can be tied immediately after cutting the needle out or tagged with a clamp and

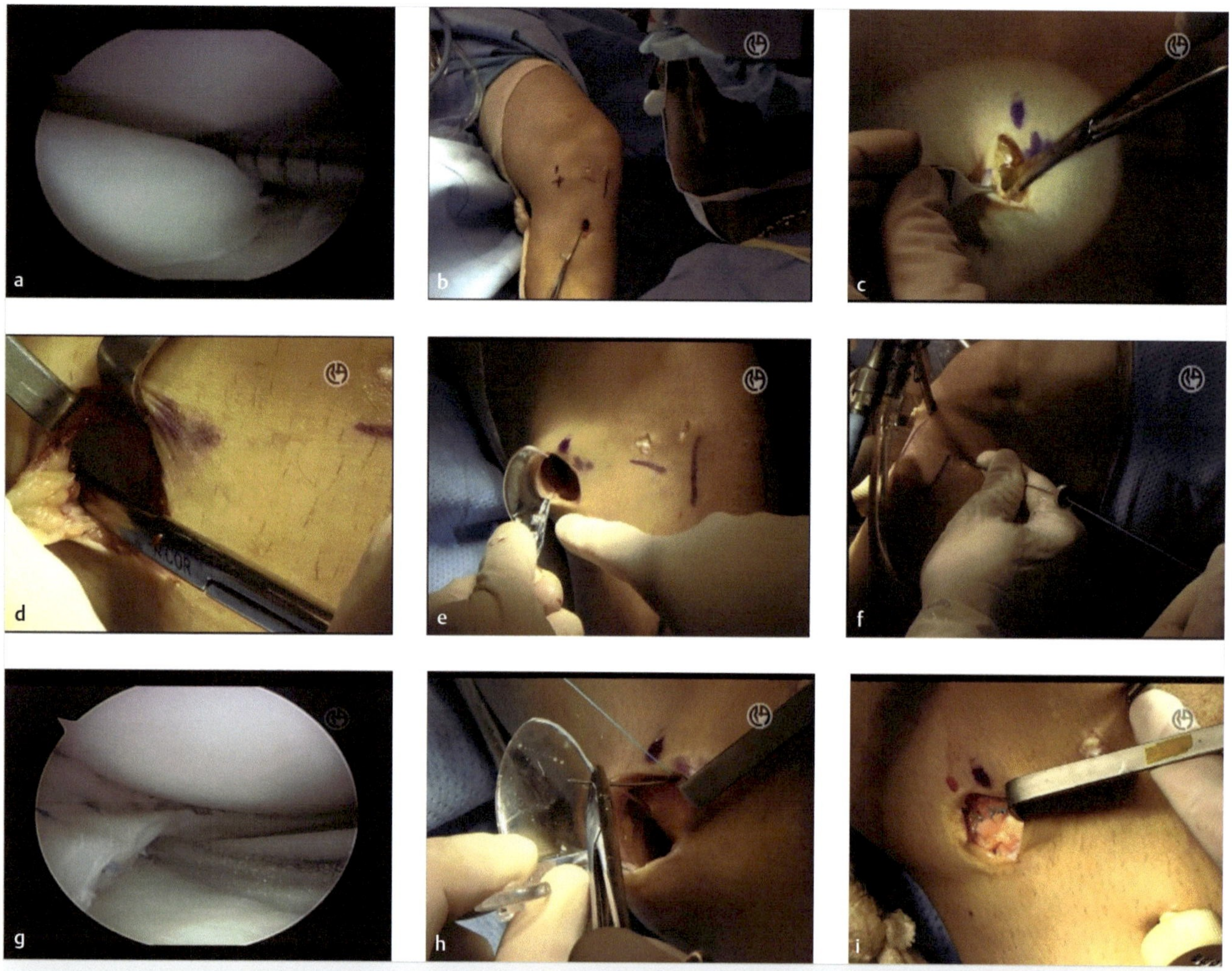

Fig. 36.1 Medial meniscus inside-out technique. **(a)** Arthroscopic view of a bucket-handle tear of the medial meniscus in a patient that also requires an anterior cruciate ligament (ACL) reconstruction. **(b)** Reference points demarked. **(c)** Skin incision made posterior to the medial collateral ligament with one-third above the joint line and two-thirds distal to it; subcutaneous dissection. **(d)** The sartorius fascia is identified and dissected from proximal to distal using a Metzenbaum scissor, while the surgeon will work at the interval between the medial gastrocnemius and the joint capsule bluntly dissected with Metzenbaum scissor and the surgeon's finger from proximal to distal. **(e)** Speculum placed anterior to the medial gastrocnemius. **(f)** Suture preloaded needle passing through the arthroscopic cannula from the anterolateral portal. **(g)** Arthroscopic view from the anteromedial portal of a tibial-sided suture placement using the cannula inserted from the anterolateral portal; a total of 10 sutures were used. **(h)** The suture preloaded needle is retrieved by the assistant using a needle driver at the posteromedial incision. **(i)** Final aspect of the suture knots tightened over the medial capsule.

tied as group after the passage of them all. They are normally tied at slight flexion without overtensioning in order to avoid a flexion contracture.

36.7.2 Lateral Meniscus Inside-Out Technique

An incision is made with the knee in 90 degrees of flexion. Transillumination helps to determine its placement. A 3.5-cm incision is made posterior and parallel to the lateral collateral ligament. The interval between the iliotibial band and biceps tendon is dissected and the surgeon must remain anterior to the biceps to avoid the peroneal nerve. One-third of the incision is placed above the joint line and two-thirds distal to it as the needles often bend downward after exiting at the joint capsule. The interval between the lateral gastrocnemius and the joint capsule is bluntly dissected with a Metzenbaum scissor and the surgeon's finger. The authors normally use a small- or medium-sized speculum to retract and protect the neurovascular structures also deflecting the needles once they exit at the capsule (▸ Fig. 36.2).

Single- or double-lumen cannulas are used, entering from the anteromedial portal or an additional anterolateral portal. Ten-inch flexible needles preloaded with a No. 2.0 Ethibond suture or high-strength braided suture, such as No. 2.0 Ultrabraid, are used for the repair.

The cannula is put at the desired location and the first needle is passed into the meniscus while an assistant recovers it with a needle driver at the posterolateral incision. The second needle is inserted preferably creating a vertical pattern. Oblique and horizontal patterns can also be used, although they

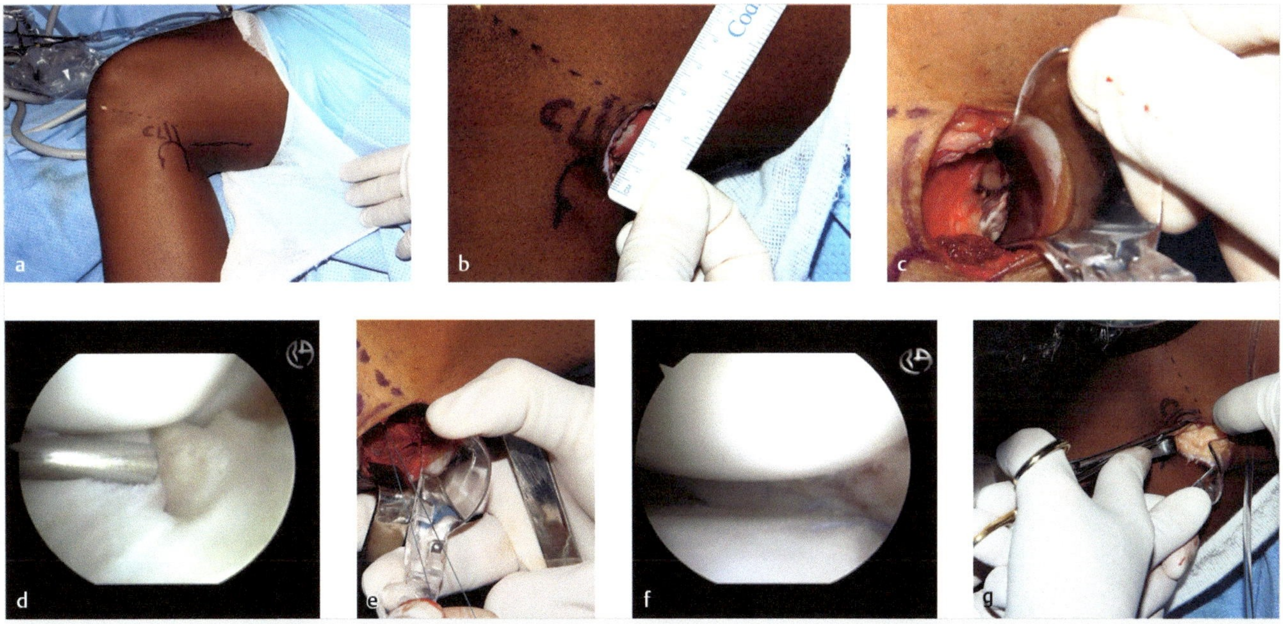

Fig. 36.2 Lateral meniscus inside-out technique. (a) Reference points demarked. (b) A 3.5-cm skin incision made posterior to the lateral collateral ligament with one-third above the joint line and two-thirds distal to it. (c) Speculum placed anterior to the lateral gastrocnemius after dissection of the interval between the iliotibial band and biceps tendon. (d) Arthroscopic view of cannula placement for suture preloaded needle insertion at the anterior portion of a bucket-handle tear of the lateral meniscus in a patient that will be also submitted to anterior cruciate ligament reconstruction with patellar tendon bone tendon; posterior sutures have already been placed. (e) The suture preloaded needles are retrieved by the assistant using a needle driver at the posterolateral incision leaving just the nonabsorbable suture. (f) Final aspect arthroscopic view of the inside-out repaired bucket-handle tear of the lateral meniscus; a total of eight sutures were used. (g) Needle driver retrieving suture-loaded needle; the suture knots will be tied over the lateral capsule.

are biomechanically inferior. Multiple sutures are inserted from posterior to anterior, 3 to 5 mm apart. Typically, a bucket-handle tear or a horizontal tear involving the body and one horn is sutured using 8–14 sutures. Meniscocapsular tears are addressed passing the first needle through the meniscus and the second through the capsule near the tear. The popliteus tendon ideally should be avoided. However, sutures can be passed through it if necessary. Sutures may be inserted on the femoral or tibial side of the meniscus. Normally, the femoral-sided sutures are inserted first, as it is easier to do so. However, femoral-sided sutures can sometimes create a pucker appearance with meniscal tissue folded superiorly. This pucker can be corrected by the placement of tibial-sided sutures. The sutures can be tied immediately after cutting the needle out or tagged with a clamp and tied as group after the passage of them all. They are normally tied at slight flexion without overtensioning in order to avoid a flexion contracture at the medial side.

36.7.3 Biologic Augmentation

If a ligament reconstruction is not performed simultaneously to the meniscus repair, a marrow vent procedure is made. Four to five microfracture awls are made into the lateral aspect of the intercondylar notch to release bone marrow elements into the joint [1]. A fibrin clot can also be used. Thirty milliliters of venous blood is harvested from the patient. A 3-mL syringe is cut open with a scalpel blade to be used as a cannula and the blood is aspirated into it and left for 15 minutes to form a clot. The clot is inserted into the meniscus lesion through the syringe piston gentle push, by a grasper or by a pull-through suture entering from one of the standard arthroscopic portals before the sutures are made. Suturing the tear will hold the fibrin clot in place.

36.8 Tips, Pearls, and Lessons Learned

- For a tight lateral compartment: a wrapped sterile fabric drape is used like a cushion under the foot during the figure-of-4 position to increase the heel height and optimize varus stress enhancing lateral compartment opening.
- For a tight medial compartment: percutaneous medial collateral ligament release can be made in a pie-crust-like fashion. Under a controlled valgus force applied by the surgeon or assistant, a beveled 14-gauge needle is inserted at the posterior third of the superficial medial collateral ligament proximal to the medial meniscus. Once the needle perforates the ligament, there is a difference in resistance. From this point on, the surgeon stops penetrating the needle and moves it from anterior to posterior in a see-saw movement using the bevel and a controlled valgus force to gradually release the medial compartment until enough space is available. This maneuver facilitates the meniscus repair creating more room and diminishes iatrogenic cartilage injury by the surgical instruments. If used in a pie-crust manner, normally four punctures with a 16-gauge needle are enough.

- Additional portals may be necessary to access posterior tears or optimize the attack angle. In addition, a central transpatellar portal can be very useful.
- Bucket-handle: access and debridement of the posterior edge is easier with the meniscal fragment displaced anteriorly.
- If a longitudinal tear is difficult to reduce or keeps dislocating back, one can use the inside-out cannula to reduce it at the middle dislocated fragment, normally at the transition of the posterior horn and meniscus body. After the passage of the first suture, it can be used to maintain the meniscus reduced, keeping it tensioned.
- Radial and horizontal tears can also successfully heal after suture.
- For radial tears, horizontal sutures are placed closing the edges, followed by diagonal oblique crossing sutures.
- For horizontal tears, vertical sutures are first placed at each meniscus leaf separately. After that, vertical sutures involving both leaves are placed in order to close the edges wrapping the lesion.

36.9 Difficulties Encountered

- Tight lateral compartments.
- Hypertrophic tibial spines.
- Fibromyalgia patients.
- Chronic complex lesions that evolved to degenerative lesions in young and middle-aged osteoarthritic patients that preclude suturing. Sometimes it is difficult to define the tissue quality threshold to allow meniscus repair over resection.

36.10 Key Procedural Steps

- Incision location, anatomical dissection respecting the planes and intervals, and proper retractor placement.
- Adequate number of sutures in order to stabilize the lesion.
- Trained surgical team.

36.11 Bailout, Rescue, and Salvage Procedures

All meniscus lesions in children and all lateral meniscus lesions in high-demand athletes should be considered for repair, despite avascular zone location or complex pattern, in order to avoid cartilage degeneration and performance loss. A biologic augmentation may be added if no concomitant intra-articular ligament reconstruction is planned.

36.12 Pitfalls

- Iatrogenic cartilage lesion due to tight medial compartment or inadequate lateral compartment opening.
- Iatrogenic fibular nerve or arterial lesion during the inside-out technique for lateral meniscus tears if the space anterior to the biceps and lateral to the lateral gastrocnemius is not respected and protected by a retractor such as a Henning retractor, a curved spoon, or a speculum.
- Iatrogenic saphenous nerve damage during the inside-out technique for medial meniscus tears if the incision is made too posterior or if the sartorius fascia is not elevated and a retractor is not placed anterior to it. Making the incision before the suture passage helps to avoid this complication and nerve entrapment.
- Flexion contracture may occur if the medial sutures are overtightened in flexion.

37 Meniscus Repair—Root Tears

Patrick A. Smith

37.1 Description

Meniscal root avulsions are common in two clinical scenarios that are distinctly different for the medial and lateral meniscus. Specifically, lateral meniscal root tears are typically seen with anterior cruciate ligament (ACL) tears in a younger patient population. Medial meniscus root tears are generally seen in older individuals, particularly females, who likely have some associated medial joint degenerative change. Although medial root tears can be related to a traumatic episode, they more commonly present insidiously.

My approach for either a medial or lateral meniscal root repair is with a minimally invasive arthroscopic technique based on anatomic attachment of the torn root with secure suture fixation to the bone through creation of a bone socket (▸ Fig. 37.1). The concept of the bone socket is to stimulate good blood flow from the bone, which further enhances healing of the root reattachment. Ultimately, with creation of only a 6.0-mm diameter socket, very little meniscal tissue is actually pulled into the bone with the repair. New technology has greatly facilitated meniscal root repair as detailed in the procedural steps below.

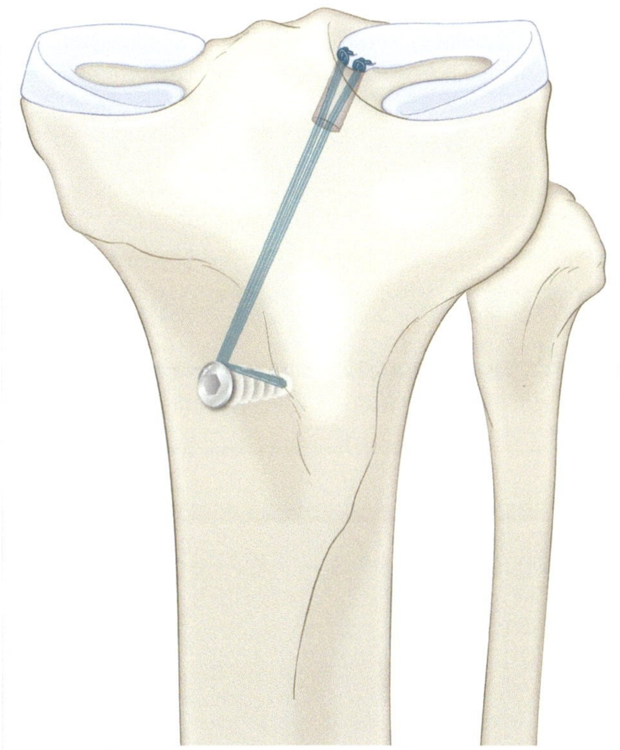

Fig. 37.1 Schematic of lateral meniscus root repair. Two cinch configuration sutures are placed in the root of the meniscus and anchored through a bone socket in the tibial with an absorbable fixation anchor on the tibia.

37.2 Key Principles

The loss of attachment at the root of the meniscus impairs the ability to maintain hoop strain when the tibiofemoral joint is loaded. This loss of hoop strain is responsible for increased pressure on the articular cartilage, thereby increasing the risk for arthritic development.

37.3 Expectations

Stable root repairs in patients translate clinically into restoration of normal meniscal biomechanics to minimize the risk of the development of arthritis in the involved compartment.

37.4 Indications

Root tears of the medial meniscus are usually straightforward to diagnose on magnetic resonance imaging (MRI). On coronal T2 images, the normal root attachment centrally will not be seen and generally, some degree of meniscal extrusion will occur along with bowing of the superficial medial collateral ligament if there is significant excursion. On the sagittal images, there may be a "ghost sign" (▸ Fig. 37.2) with absence of the normal posterior horn of the medial meniscus compared to the intact anterior horn.

Root tears of the lateral meniscus can be difficult to diagnose preoperatively on MRI, especially if the meniscofemoral ligaments

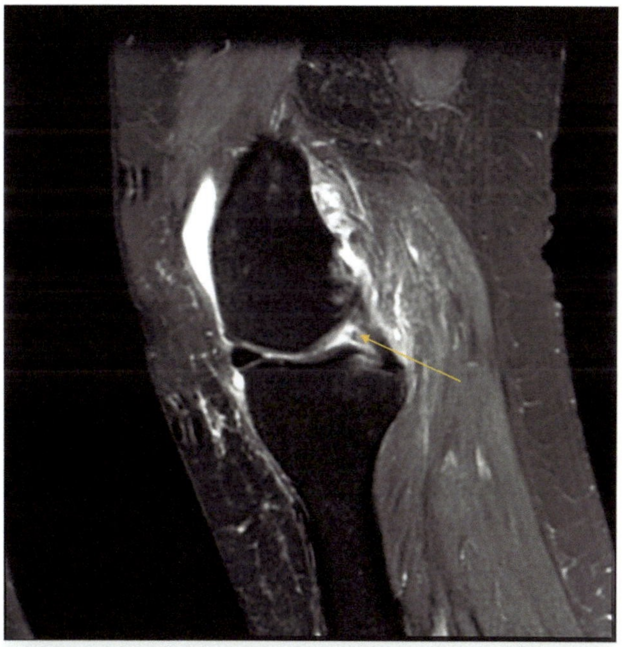

Fig. 37.2 T2 sagittal magnetic resonance imaging (MRI) of right knee with "ghost sign" representing absence of the posterior horn of the medial meniscus, due to root tear.

are intact. However, on some occasions, the lateral root tear is seen nicely on the coronal views on MRI. Lateral root avulsions are more common with ACL tears, so one must carefully probe the lateral meniscal root at the time of ACL surgery.

37.5 Contraindications

The primary contraindications for root repair relate to the medial meniscus. Specifically, on preoperative assessment, meniscal extrusion greater than 5 mm is generally a contraindication. In addition, it is critical to assess standing alignment preoperatively with a long cassette film; if in varus more than 5 degrees, a concomitant valgus tibial osteotomy should be strongly considered. Then, at the time of surgery, if a patient has medial joint articular cartilage degenerative changes more severe than early grade 3 isolated on the femur or tibia, root repair should *not* be done. Bipolar articular cartilage disease more than grade 2/3 is also a contraindication.

37.6 Special Considerations

Relative to the lateral meniscus, in patients with acute ACL tears, I frequently encounter a root tear "variant" which is the oblique tear where just a small portion of the root of the meniscus is still attached to bone centrally but is completely detached from the rest of the meniscus (▶ Fig. 37.3). In that setting, it is frequently difficult to do a good side-to-side suture repair. Instead, I will do a bone socket repair of the free portion of the posterior horn of the lateral meniscus close to the remaining flap of meniscus that is still attached to the root.

Similarly, on the medial side, a root tear "variant" is seen when there is a radial meniscus tear approximately 5 mm from the true root attachment. In that setting, a bone socket can be drilled to the posterior medial tibia for meniscus reduction at that point, as reattachment to the true root is not indicated.

37.7 Special Instructions, Position, and Anesthesia

For this surgical technique, the patient is in the supine position to allow easy manipulation of the affected joint. General anesthesia is preferred. A foot-holding mechanism is recommended to keep the knee at the desired degree of flexion during the procedure. For medial root repair, a lateral post along the distal femur is essential to enhance valgus stress for medial exposure.

Critical instrumentation necessary includes use of the Knee Scorpion device (Arthrex Inc., Naples, FL), which facilitates intra-articular suture passage, and the FlipCutter (Arthrex Inc., Naples, FL) device to easily create the anatomic bony attachment through a bone socket, retrocutting from inside the joint.

37.8 Tips, Pearls, and Lessons Learned

One helpful tip is to use a PassPort Cannula (Arthrex, Inc., Naples, FL) to facilitate suture passage and management to avoid soft tissue entrapment from the portal site. In terms of suture placement in the detached root of the meniscus, it is important to place the sutures close to the root to restore the normal anatomy. If the sutures are placed too far within the body of the posterior horn, this could alter normal meniscus anatomy and overtension the meniscus, thus putting it at risk for a tear in a different location from the root.

37.9 Difficulties Encountered

For the lateral meniscus root repair, I generally pass sutures from the medial portal without difficulty. Occasionally, I can be "blocked" to good access to the meniscus from the lateral tibial spine. In that situation, I change my viewing portal to medial and come in laterally with the Scorpion device. If need be, I just transfer the suture in the meniscus through the portal with the PassPort Cannula. The key "pearl" for medial meniscus root repair relates to exposure, as frequently, the joint is "tight." In that setting, I routinely "piecrust" the medial collateral ligament above the meniscus with an 18-gauge spinal needle while applying valgus stress and generally the medial joint opens up very nicely.

37.10 Key Procedural Steps: Lateral Root Tear

This illustrated case was a lateral meniscus root tear in association with an ACL tear (▶ Fig. 37.4). First, an arthroscopic curette

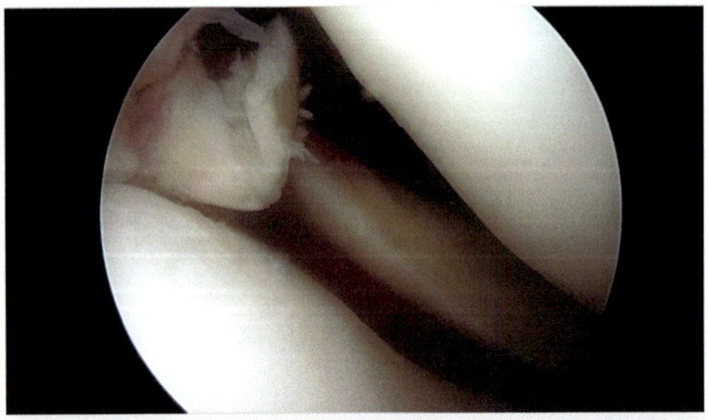

Fig. 37.3 Left knee. Viewing from anterolateral portal. Root variant tear of the lateral meniscus.

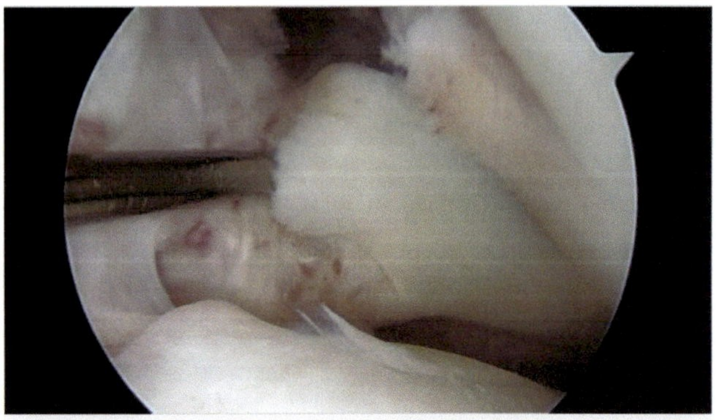

Fig. 37.4 Left knee. Viewing from anterolateral portal. Lateral meniscus root tear.

is utilized to debride the normal root attachment site on the posterolateral tibia for the lateral meniscus, and the posteromedial tibia for the medial meniscus. This is helpful both to stimulate a good healing response and to create a nice "landing area" for the drilling guide. Sutures in the root of the lateral meniscus can be placed from either a standard lateral or medial parapatellar portal because pathologic elevation of the root of the lateral meniscus following a tear makes suture placement just as accessible from the medial portal. However, if the lateral tibial spine makes it difficult for suture passage, then it is appropriate to change the approach to the lateral portal. The first step in suturing the root of either the lateral or medial meniscus is placement of a PassPort Cannula through the chosen portal for suture passage; this facilitates suture management to avoid inadvertent development of a soft tissue bridge with suture passage, which can be very frustrating. In this case, the cannula was placed in the medial parapatellar portal. Suturing is done with a Knee Scorpion device. An 0-FiberLink (Arthrex, Inc., Naples, FL) is loaded into the lower jaw of the device. Partially deploying the needle with the trigger "captures" the suture, thus preparing it for passage. This suture makes it very easy to create a cinch or "luggage tag"-type stitch in the root of the meniscus.

The Knee Scorpion is brought through the medial portal via the PassPort Cannula for the first suture pass; the lower jaw of the opened Knee Scorpion is placed under the root of the meniscus near its normal bony attachment. The trigger of the Knee Scorpion is deployed, and the upper jaw then captures the suture so that pulling the Knee Scorpion out of the joint brings the 0-FiberLink suture out of the PassPort Cannula as one simple step of both passing and retrieving the suture (▶ Fig. 37.5). Firing the Knee Scorpion trigger again outside of the joint releases the 0-FiberLink suture, and the free end of the suture is passed through the suture-loop, thereby creating a "cinch" configuration as the free end is pulled to slide the cinch down to the posterior horn of the meniscus. A second 0-FiberLink cinch suture is placed the same way, 3 mm lateral to this first suture (▶ Fig. 37.6).

Next, attention is directed toward the creation of a tibial bone socket to reduce the lateral meniscus root securely to bone. This requires drilling from the tibia up into the joint, which necessitates anterior tibial exposure. Since this root repair is being done concomitant with an ACL reconstruction, a 2-cm medial tibial incision is made medial and just proximal to the tibial tuberosity, which can also be utilized to create the tibial tunnel for the ACL reconstruction. The periosteum is mobilized to expose the bone. Retrodrilling from inside the joint is done with a 6.0-mm FlipCutter—a 3.5-mm-diameter pin that converts to a 6.0-mm reamer. An ACL tibial aiming device is positioned through the medial portal with the tip of the guide intra-articularly at the normal anatomic attachment for the lateral meniscus root, which has been prepared with an arthroscopic curette. Viewing laterally with the arthroscope and holding the ACL aiming guide sleeve securely to the proximal tibia (▶ Fig. 37.7), the 3.5 mm FlipCutter pin is drilled up into the joint exiting out the posterior central lateral tibia at the point of the ACL tibial aimer (▶ Fig. 37.8). For hard tibial bone, this hole for the FlipCutter can be predrilled with a 3.5-mm drill bit to make for easier passage of the 3.5-mm FlipCutter pin. The ACL

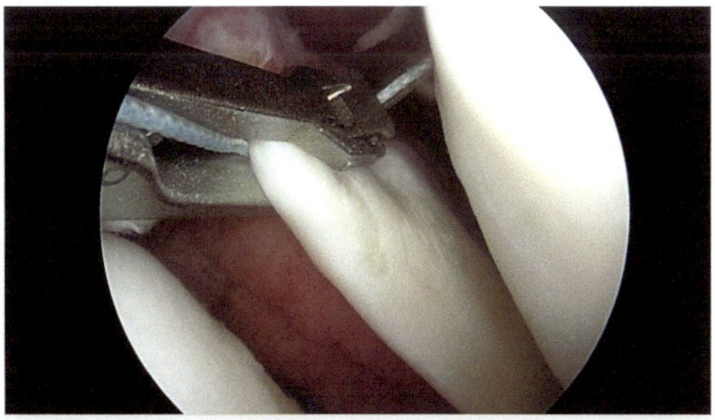

Fig. 37.5 Left knee. Viewing from anterolateral portal. Knee Scorpion passing 0-FiberWire suture through the root of lateral meniscus. The suture is captured in the upper jaw and then retrieved out of the joint.

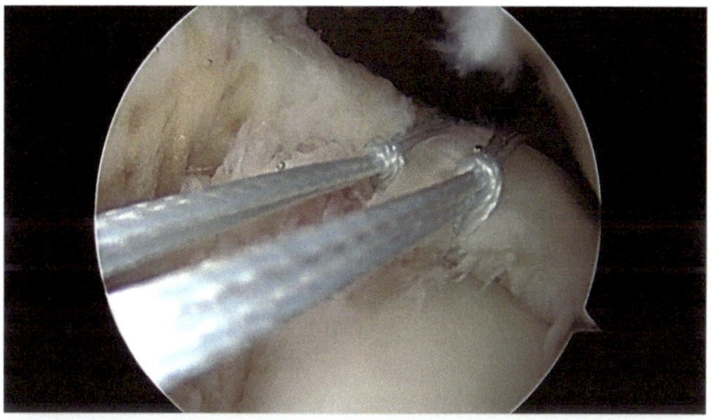

Fig. 37.6 Left knee. Viewing from anterolateral portal. Two 0-FiberWire sutures in place in lateral meniscus root tear.

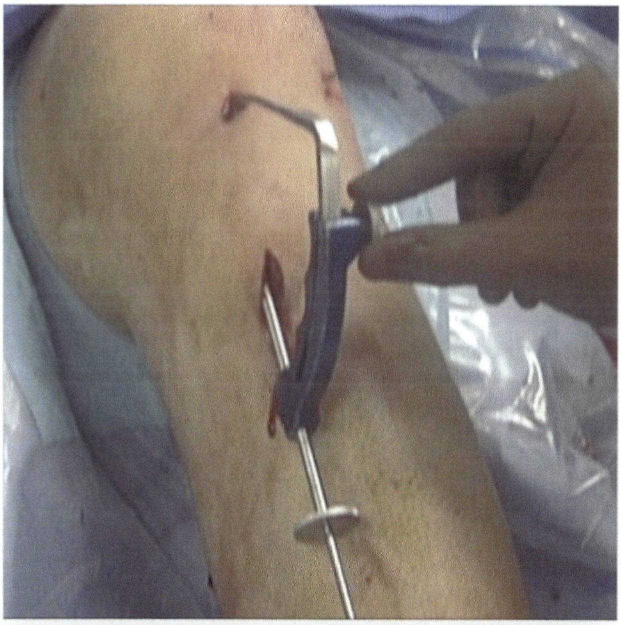

Fig. 37.7 Left knee. Anterior cruciate ligament (ACL) aiming guide in position with tip of guide intra-articularly at anatomic tibial attachment point of lateral meniscus root. FlipCutter is drilled to this point. Guide sleeve is tapped 7 mm into the tibial bone to maintain this position after FlipCutter removal for ease of suture passage into joint to serve as shuttle for root repair sutures.

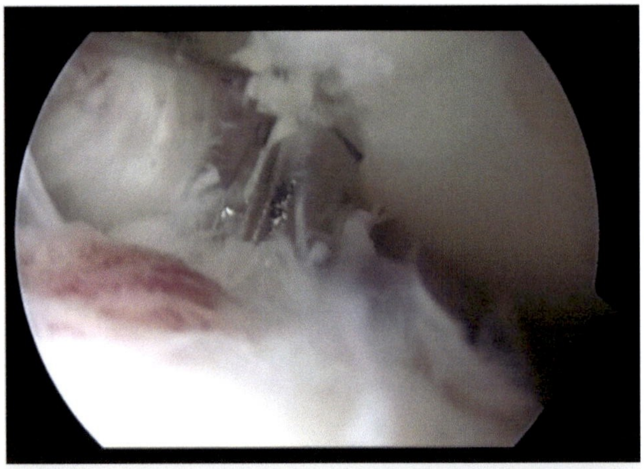

Fig. 37.8 Left knee. Viewing from the anterolateral portal. FlipCutter drilled as straight pin into joint at tibial anatomic attachment point for lateral meniscus root. It will then be deployed for retrodrilling the tibial socket.

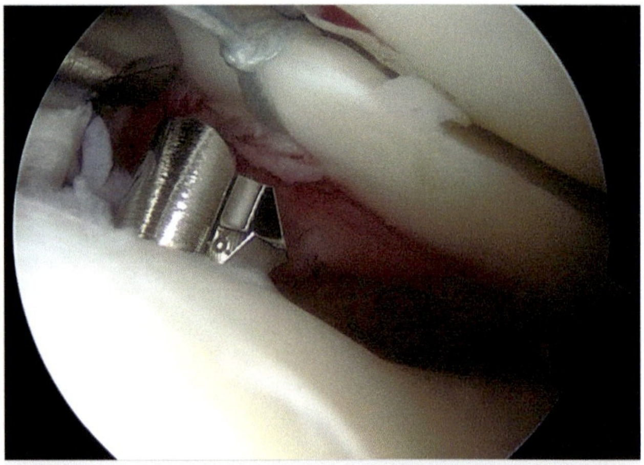

Fig. 37.9 Left knee. Viewing from anterolateral portal. 6.0-mm FlipCutter is deployed to retrodrill the tibial bone socket for root repair.

tibial aimer can be removed through the PassPort Cannula, leaving the FlipCutter in place. The guide sleeve is then tapped 7 mm into the bone of the proximal tibia, marked by a hub at that point. This ensures access to this drill hole in the tibia. The FlipCutter device is then deployed as a 6.0-mm reamer from a straight pin by squeezing the button on the proximal end of the FlipCutter (▶ Fig. 37.9). Drilling in forward, a socket is retrodrilled to a depth of 10 to 12 mm in the posterior tibia with the FlipCutter. Still drilling in forward, the FlipCutter is brought back into the joint. During the drilling process, the arthroscope can be moved to the medial portal so an arthroscopic shaver can be used from the lateral portal to remove bone debris from creating this tibial socket. The FlipCutter is then converted back to a straight pin by squeezing the button, so that it can then be removed through the guide sleeve in the proximal tibia.

A #2 FiberStick suture (Arthrex, Inc., Naples, FL) in its red plastic sheath is used as a suture shuttle for the two 0-FiberWire cinch sutures in the posterior horn of the lateral meniscus with retrieval of the #2 FiberStick on the joint side. This is prepared by folding the #2 FiberStick suture in half and passing the folded end in the sheath. This is facilitated by the fact that half of the suture is prestiffened to where the folded loop is just coming out the end of the plastic sheath. This sheath is then passed through the tibial guide sleeve into the joint. Viewing laterally, a looped suture grasper passed from PassPort Cannula in the medial portal is used to retrieve this loop of the #2 FiberStick suture below the posterior horn of the meniscus and pull it out the cannula. This suture loop is then used to shuttle the two 0-FiberWire cinch sutures in the root of the meniscus into the created tibial socket to secure the root of the lateral meniscus to bone with ultimate fixation on the proximal tibia. Pulling on the two cinch sutures out the small hole from the proximal tibia securely reduces the root to the bone socket to enhance bony reattachment of the root (▶ Fig. 37.10).

Secure cortical fixation of the two cinch sutures in the root of the lateral meniscus is done on the tibia with a BioComposite 4.75-mm SwiveLock anchor (Arthrex, Inc., Naples, FL). A 4.5-mm stepped reamer is drilled a distance of 20 mm to accept the

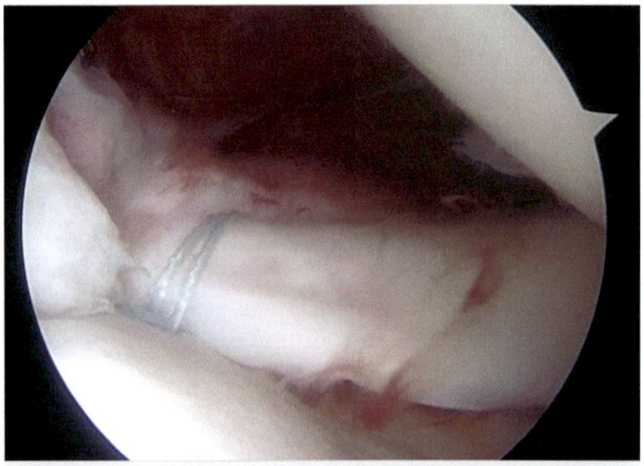

Fig. 37.10 Left knee. Viewing from anterolateral portal. Repaired lateral meniscus root tear using two 0-FiberWire sutures into tibial bone socket.

19.1-mm long SwiveLock anchor. The tibial cortex is always tapped with a 4.5-mm tap since this bone is generally hard. Watching arthroscopically to confirm that the meniscal root is reduced, with the knee usually at approximately 45 degrees of flexion, the free ends of the two cinch sutures are passed through the eyelet of the SwiveLock anchor, pulled tight, and secured in the reamed hole by holding the paddle of the SwiveLock anchor and turning the knob of the handle clockwise until the SwiveLock anchor is flush to the bone. The sutures are then cut.

37.11 Key Procedural Steps: Medial Root Tear

For the medial meniscus, frequently, exposure to pass sutures in the root can be difficult if the knee is "tight." Rather than removing bone and performing a "reverse notchplasy," I prefer "piecrusting" the medial collateral ligament with an 18-gauge needle to gain good exposure. I always bring the Scorpion device for suturing in through the medial portal. Furthermore, I drill from the medial tibia more centrally toward the midline so the FlipCutter is oriented posterior and medial to the medial femoral condyle in the notch to avoid iatrogenic damage to the articular cartilage as it is brought into the joint. Suture passage through the meniscus, socket drilling, and suture fixation on the tibia is done the same way as described above for the lateral meniscus.

37.12 Bailout, Rescue, and Salvage Procedures

If there is suture pullout from the medial meniscus root with loss of fixation with this socket technique, the best salvage procedure is to establish a posteromedial portal for suturing access to the posterior aspect of the root with a lasso-type device while viewing through the notch. Then, from the posteromedial portal, fixation could be accomplished with a PushLock device punching a hole toward the more posterior bony root attachment point. On the lateral side, that bailout would be technically more difficult if there was a problem with the bone socket approach. Conceivably, since the ACL is usually torn with the lateral root repairs, sutures could be passed even more centrally in the root tissue and passed through the ACL tibial tunnel and fixated separately on the tibia with a SwiveLock.

37.13 Pitfalls

When placing the aiming guide to drill the FlipCutter into the joint, be sure to not be too anteriorly positioned for either the medial or lateral attachment site. Otherwise, due to the angle of drilling from the medial tibia which tends to be a bit acute, you may exit onto the tibial plateau's articular surface. Using the arthroscopic curette to make a "home" on the bone at the anatomic attachment point as a starting point for the tip of the aiming guide to engage can be very helpful in that regard. In addition, a starting point on the tibia closer to the midline helps ensure a proper entrance point in the joint for the lateral meniscus root attachment to both avoid the central lateral tibial plateau articular surface and to make sure the FlipCutter does not hit the lateral femoral condyle by coming into the notch area. Since lateral root repairs are more common with ACL tears, the same medial incision used to drill the tibial tunnel can be used for the root repair drilling. For a medial root repair, starting position on the tibia should also be closer to the midline for the same reason to avoid violating the medial tibial plateau and also the medial femoral condyle with the FlipCutter.

38 Meniscal Allograft Transplantation (Medial and Lateral)

Jacob Worsham and Walter R. Lowe

38.1 Description

- Meniscal transplantation is a procedure used in a physiologically young patient with symptomatic meniscal deficiency.
- The goals are to restore joint stability and load-bearing function, and provide chondroprotective effects and overall decrease in patient's symptoms.
- Alignment must be assessed and addressed prior to or at the time of meniscal transplantation.
- Communications and expectations are key. I counsel patients with meniscal transplant that they need to commit 12 months to doing the right rehabilitation for optimal results.

38.2 Key Principles

- Candidates for meniscal transplant must have or achieve stable knee ligaments, normal limb alignment, and no (or treatable) full-thickness articular cartilage lesions.
- If combined with anterior cruciate ligament (ACL) revision surgery, the previous ACL tunnels and their potential interference with the bony insertions of the meniscal transplant must be critically evaluated. Computed tomography (CT) scan is most useful for this assessment (▸ Fig. 38.1).
- Appropriate postoperative rehabilitation is critical for success.

38.3 Surgical Indications

- Indications for medial meniscus transplant: (1) Symptomatic medial compartment with meniscus deficiency and minimal degenerative chondral changes in that compartment. Stability in revision ACL surgery with medial meniscal deficiency.
- Indications for lateral meniscal transplant: symptomatic lateral compartment with meniscal deficiency (often associated with prior discoid meniscus). (2) Revision ACL surgery with absent lateral meniscal root deficiency from pervious excision.
- There is controversy regarding operative treatment of meniscal deficiency. Multiple variables must be considered prior to undertaking this salvage procedure.
- Controversial patients include:
  - Skeletally immature, discoid variants.
  - High BMI.
  - Elite athletes wishing to return to full competition.
  - Young, asymptomatic patients.
  - Patients with focal chondral lesions.
  - Physiologically/Chronologically older patients.

38.4 Contraindications

- Advanced osteoarthritis in any compartment.
- Inflammatory arthritis.
- Advanced patient age.
- Muscle atrophy.
- High BMI.
- Uncorrected varus or valgus malalignment, ligament stability, or cartilage lesions.
- Limited range of motion or arthrofibrosis.

38.5 Special Considerations

- Graft preparation is an essential part of the case. Acquiring grafts from an accredited American association of tissue bank facility is desired.

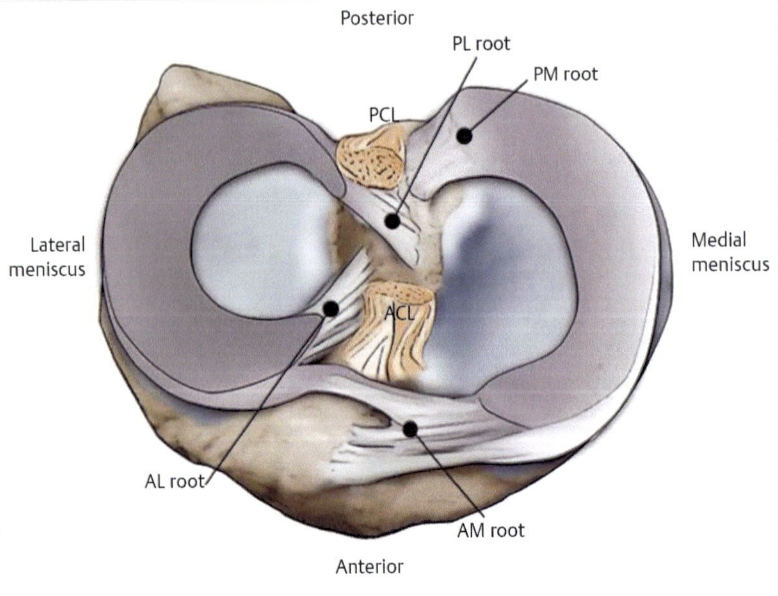

Fig. 38.1 Axial overview of the anatomy of the meniscal root attachments and the proximity to other important structures.

- Appropriate graft size is determined by radiographs and MRI measurement—these imaging techniques can underestimate appropriate graft size (▶ Fig. 38.2—MTF Measurement Chart, and ▶ Fig. 38.3—MTF Algorithm).

38.5.1 Medial Meniscal Graft Preparation

- Allograft checked for appropriate sizing prior to starting procedure (▶ Fig. 38.4).
- 2.4-mm guide pin drilled into anterior and posterior horn attachment sites, at the angle planned for the drilled tunnels in the tibia.
- Retrograde ream with cannulated coring reamer to subchondral bone.
- With a microsagittal saw, make four cuts around each side of the meniscal horns to form a 1 × 1 × 1 centimeter box at the same angle as the retrograde drilled coring reamer.
- Tubularize bone plugs with ronguers to fit the holes to be drilled. Anterior horn 9 × 10 millimeters (mm) and posterior 8 × 8 mm. Mark depth on bone plugs to know when graft is appropriately seated (▶ Fig. 38.5).
- Using a 2.4-mm drill, drill a path for suture from anterior to posterior in each bone block.
- Make sure to mark the graft with anterior and posterior labels to avoid confusion, and use different colored or patterned suture to allow for appropriate orientation.

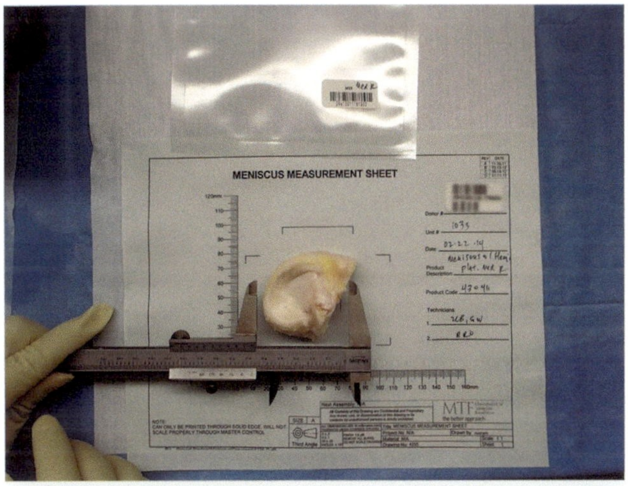

Fig. 38.2 Imaging showing Musculoskeletal Transplant Foundation (MTF) Measurement Chart for Meniscal Transplant.

- Pass suture through posterior bone plug using a modified Kessler or horizontal mattress to incorporate meniscal tissue.
- Pass sequential vertical mattress sutures from posterior to anterior. Starting with posterior horn 5 mm from posterior bone plug use a 2–0 blue fiberwire, then 5 to 10 mm medial from the last vertical mattress place a 2–0 green ethibond in vertical fashion and then one more vertical mattress thrown with 2–0 prolene into the body of the meniscus (▶ Fig. 38.6).
  - Colors of suture are important here for suture management in future steps of this case. The colors corresponding to the graft will be used when the lasso passes them through the meniscocapsular tissue in the host.
  - It is important for the last suture to be in the body of the meniscus to prevent the graft from flipping over intra-articularly while drilling anterior socket in flexion.

38.5.2 Lateral Meniscal Graft Preparation (▶ Fig. 38.7)

- Preparation of the lateral meniscus allograft is complex.
- Allograft checked and evaluated for appropriate sizing prior to starting procedure.
- Bone block trimmed of excess bone and soft tissue.
- Arthrex Dovetail Meniscal Allograft Workstation allows cuts made to fit graft length similar to A-P cut of tibia.
- Gross vertical and parallel saw cuts made in bone block to establish desired length.
- Trapezoid rasp for tibial slot preparation, outline this dovetail shape on end of the bone block. Make sure bone is cut 1 cm from articular surface and in line with each root.
- Vertical cut made on midline and angled cut made on lateral side of bone plug.
- Position allograft upside down in guide allowing meniscus to hang free from bone block.
- Align medial edge of dovetail with vertical face of the holding posts. Ends are secured into the workstation graft holding posts shown.
- Make three modular cuts starting with inferior, parallel cut, followed by medial vertical cut and subsequently the angled lateral cut forming the dovetail.
- Rounger edge of bone to remove loose pieces and assess for appropriate fit.
  - Do not rasp or change the angled lateral cut—it can pose problems with fit.

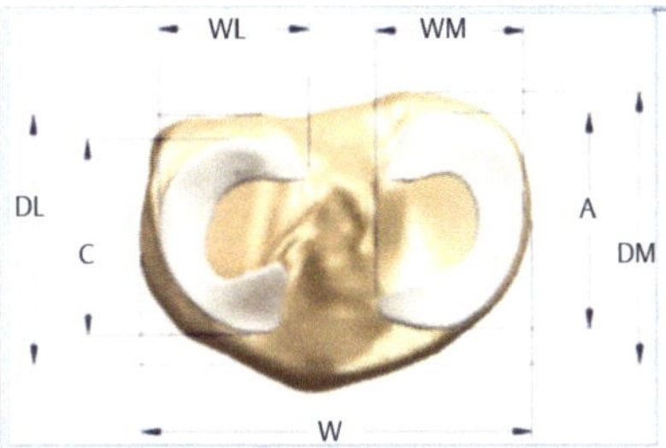

W' – Medial/lateral measurement of the entire tibial plateau taken at the maximum width of the articular surface
A – A/P measurement taken at the longest point anteriorly and longest point posteriorly of the meniscus
C – A/P measurement taken at the longest point anteriorly and longest point posteriorly
DM – Depth of the articular surface on the medial side from anterior to posterior
DL – Depth of the articular surface on the lateral side from anterior to posterior
WM – M/L measurement of the medial meniscus
WL – M/L measurement of the lateral meniscus

Fig. 38.3 Musculoskeletal Transplant Foundation measurement guide for appropriate sizing of meniscal allograft.

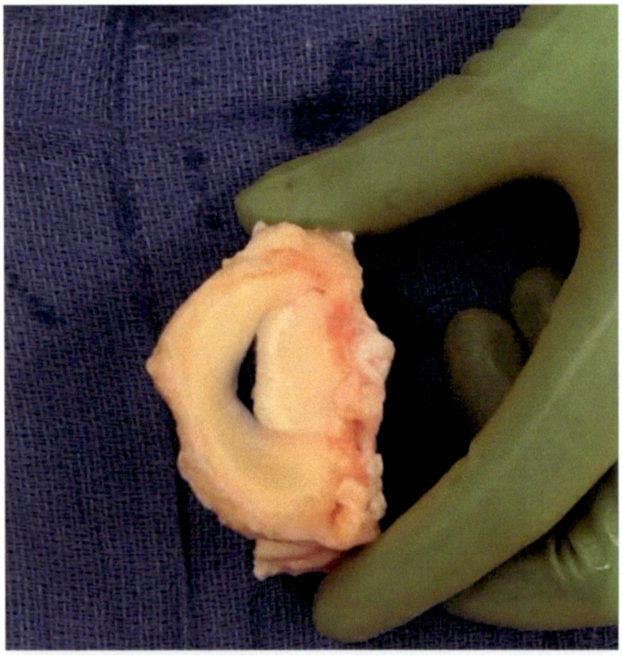

Fig. 38.4 Allograft meniscus with bone block.

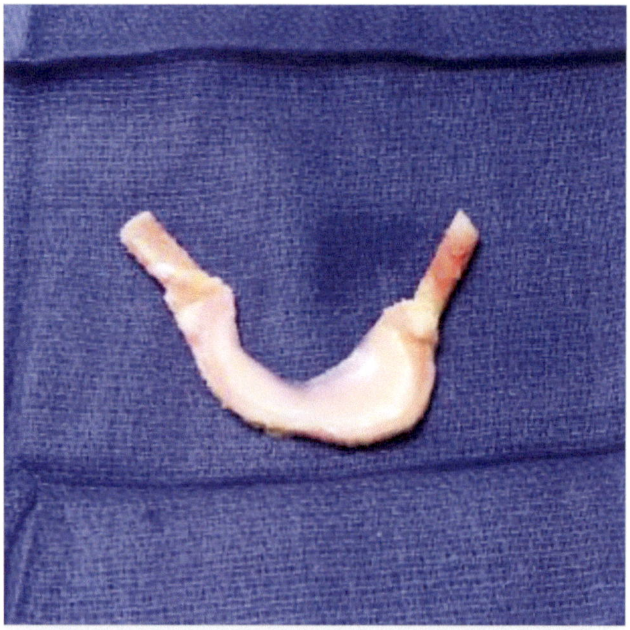

Fig. 38.5 Meniscus preparation after performing coring reaming method and tubularization of bone blocks.

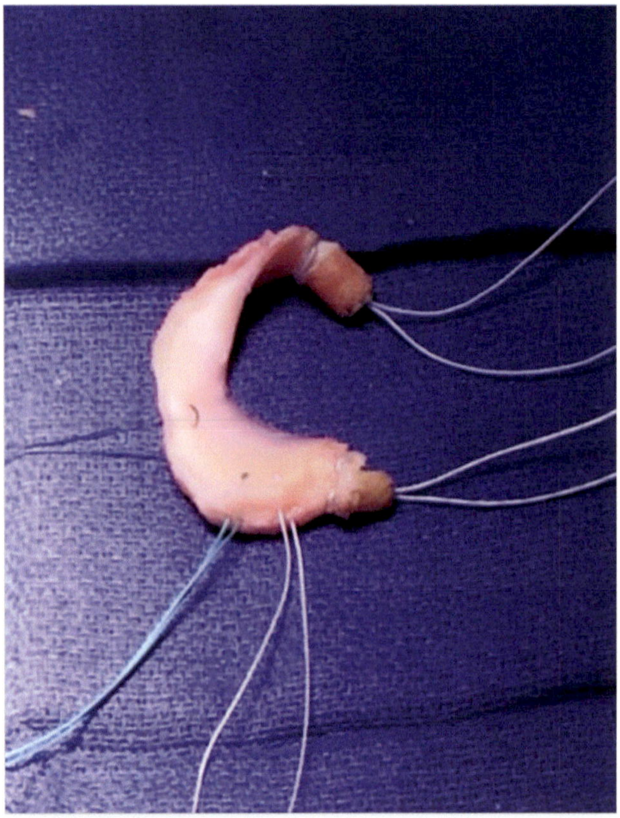

Fig. 38.6 Final meniscal graft preparation showing appropriate suture placement as described in text.

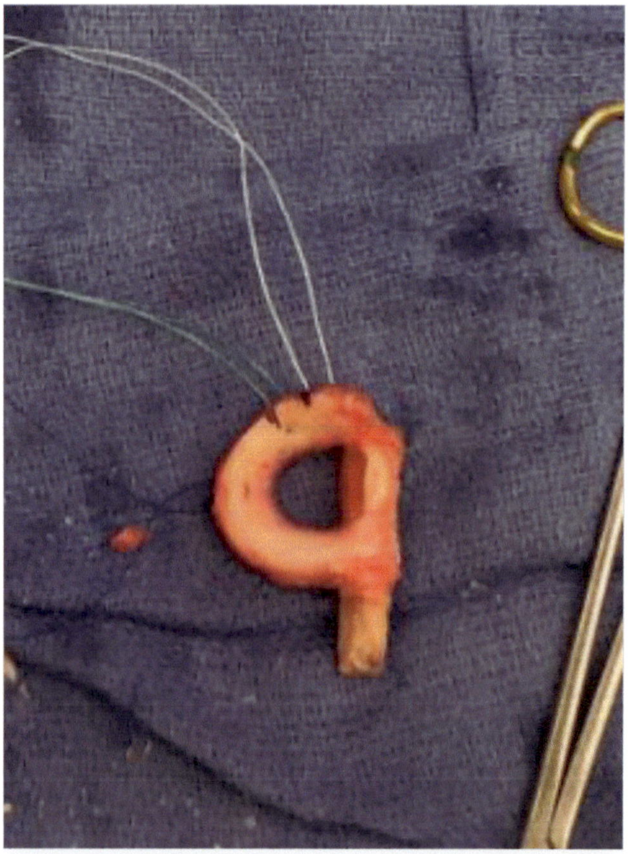

Fig. 38.7 Final lateral graft.

38.6 Special Instructions, Position and Anesthesia

- Medial and lateral meniscal transplant are highly technical procedures with many steps and therefore these should not be performed by novice surgeons without previous training.
- Patient position is supine with a post (not knee holder) in meniscal transplants.
- Anesthesia can be the surgeon's choice.

38.7 Tips, Pearls, and Lessons Learned

- Protect medial insertional fibers of ACL on medial transplant.
- Use differently colored sutures.
- Make sure one suture is in meniscal body to prevent graft flip into joint.
- Mark allograft to ensure accurate placement:
  - Superior edge of bone plug (proper depth).
  - Anterior to posterior orientation.
- With revision ACL, follow this order:
  - Place posterior horn.
  - Pass/secure ACL.
  - Place anterior horn plug.
  - Suture meniscus to capsule (inside-out).

38.8 Difficulties Encountered

- Graft passage.
- Suture management.

38.9 Key Procedural Steps

38.9.1 Medial Meniscal Allograft Transplant (Video 38.1)

- Medial compartment preparation—debriding remaining meniscal tissue to a bleeding rim in preparation for suture passage.
- Use a combination of electrocautery and burr to develop the anatomic posterior footprint of the medial meniscus—clearing structures that inhibit posterior root bone block passage (i.e., tibial spine, medial femoral condyle). This is considered a "sub-PCL notchplasty" and technically makes graft passage less difficult.
- Extension of anteromedial portal to 3 cm open approach to medial compartment:
  - Ethibond can be used to retract anterior meniscocapsular structures.
  - Remove retropatellar fat for visualization.
- Posterior medial capsular exposure for medial approach to the knee:
  - 3 cm posterior medial incision.
  - Protect infrapatellar branch of saphenous nerve.
  - Identify semimembranosus and medial head of gastrocnemius.
  - Using blunt dissection create interval for popliteal retractor, protecting neurovascular structures while passing suture in posterior medial compartment.
  - Anatomic position of the posterior horn of the medial meniscus identified just off edge of posterior medial cartilaginous area just behind the tibial eminence.
- Tip-to-tip guide used at a 70-degree angle and a 2.4-mm guide pin is drilled to confirm appropriate position, important to find the anatomic site for posterior meniscal root.
  - Sequential a 4.5 mm and then an 8 mm retrograde reamer used to create an appropriate tunnel for the posterior medial horn. Arthroscopic shaver to clean off tunnel for positioning. A flip cutter can be used for this sequence as well.
  - Using a grasper make sure to hold on to guide pin while reaming, this prevents any excessive excursion of the pin and avoids any neurovascular injury.
  - Prepare tunnel with shaver and electrocautery for ease in graft passage. This is crucial to being able to seat the bone block appropriately.
- Using a suture lasso, pass three sutures through the residual meniscal rim and meniscocapsular structures. The passage of these three sutures will correspond to the position of the sutures passed in the graft. Make sure to use same colored suture as in graft and start posterior and work anterior.
  - Starting with posterior horn use a 2–0 blue fiberwire (most lateral), then 5 to 10 mm medial from the last throw a 2–0 green ethibond in and then one thrown with 2–0 tiger wire into the meniscus rim where the body of the meniscus used to be.
  - The tiger wire will be exchanged for the corresponding prolene on the allograft.
- Using a fiber stick, pass suture into joint and allow for posterior bone block passage.
- Pass graft into joint and start passing suture with posterior root bone block.
- Using arthroscopic and visual guidance, pass:
  - 2–0 Blue Fiberwire (closest to bone block) to corresponding suture in patient.
  - 2–0 Green Ethibond (middle) to corresponding suture in patient.
  - 2–0 prolene (meniscal body) to tiger wire—This stitch is important to keep meniscus from flipping in the joint, obstructing visualization.
- Hemostat might be required to orient bone block. Once bone block is seated, secure both limbs of suture to medial tibia with hemostat to keep bone block in proper position.
- Once complete, tie down the blue and green sutures, leaving the meniscal body free.
- Keeping the knee flexed to 90 degrees, find anatomic position of anterior meniscal root and drill 2.4-mm drill guide in the center of the anterior meniscal root.
- Using a 9-mm acorn reamer drill, drill tunnel for the 9 mm x 10 mm anterior bone plug.
- Drill through the center of bone tunnel out to medial tibia and pass a fiber stick suture to secure the bone plug suture in the anterior tunnel.
- Pass graft with careful suture management and tension on the bone plugs.

- Once bone plug is seated in anterior tunnel with tension on suture, press-fit bone plug into tunnel and secure suture with hemostat against anterior tibia with hemostat.
- Tie the anterior and posterior bone plug sutures over appropriate size cortical buttons. This must be done prior to inside-out suture repair to prevent extrusion of the transplant.
- Move knee from 90 degrees to appropriate valgus orientation and Tie prolene suture.
- Confirm position of meniscal allograft, then start passing zone-specific sutures until meniscus seats comfortably in joint. This will incorporate arthroscopic visualization while "catching" sutures in the posterior medial approach performed previously.
- Zone-specific 2–0 sutures should be placed on the superior and inferior surfaces of the meniscus to balance repair and ensure contact of entire meniscus rim with medial capsule.

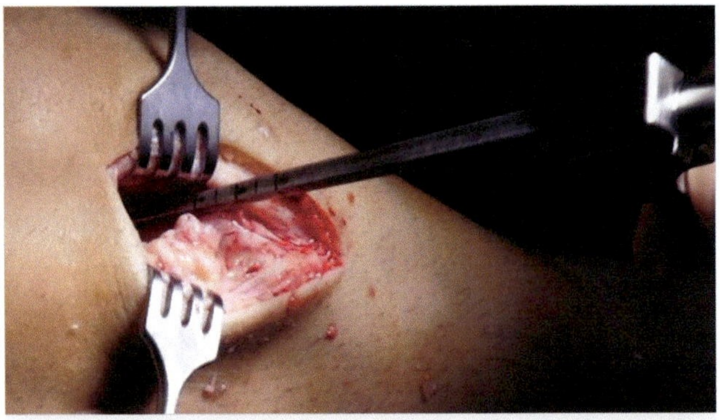

Fig. 38.8 Graduated guide, measuring anterior-to-posterior distance of lateral tibial plateau.

38.9.2 Lateral Meniscal Allograft Transplant (Video 38.2)

- Anterior lateral arthroscopy portal made in line with anterior horn attachment of lateral meniscus—position will be important for lateral arthrotomy.
- Figure four position and debridement of meniscal remnant (leave small amount).
- With the knee at 90 degrees of flexion, start the posterolateral approach to the knee:
  - 3-cm incision immediately posterior to LCL.
  - Identify interval between short head of biceps and iliotibial band.
  - Separate posterolateral capsular attachments from short head biceps.
  - Develop space between posterolateral capsule and lateral gastrocnemius bluntly with cobb.
  - Place popliteal retractor for suture passage and management during inside-out repair of the meniscal allograft.
- Make a lateral parapatellar incision incorporating anterolateral portal.
- Using a motorized burr, the lateral tibial spine is flattened and debridement of anterior and posterior horns is performed making a trough for reference during tibial preparation.
  - This will be the guide for pin placement/drilling of trough for the dovetail bone block. It is critical this is placed in line with the anatomic lateral meniscal roots.
- Use a measuring stick to estimate of the anteroposterior (AP) dimension of the tibial plateau (▸ Fig. 38.8).
- Using a drill sleeve, place two, 2.4-mm drill guides parallel to the trough made above.
- Make sure the guide wires are not passed through the posterior cortex. Use arthroscopic visualization to confirm and make sure guide pins are in appropriate anatomic position.
- Once both guide pins are in appropriate position, ream a 7-mm tunnel over the distal guide wire and a 6-mm tunnel over the proximal wire—Do not plunge through posterior cortex.
- Remove guide wires once reaming is complete and identify the appropriate dilating rasp.
- Insert rasp into slot created by reamers, with top of rasp flush with articular surface.
- Dilate with combination of hand rasping and malleting until the slot is trapezoidal and is clear all the way to the posterior cortex of the tibia. It is important that the trapezoidal slot is clear of debris that could prevent appropriate allograft position and seating.
- Evaluation of the trough arthroscopically and use of burr to clean up edges is often necessary to assure appropriate graft fit. Key step for success in passing graft.
- Returning to the figure four position, the lateral compartment is prepared similar to the medial meniscal transplant mentioned earlier.
  - Starting with posterior horn use a 2–0 blue fiberwire (most medial), then 5 to 10 mm lateral from the last, throw a 2–0 green ethibond in and then one thrown with 2–0 tiger wire into the meniscus rim where the body of the meniscus used to be.
  - The tiger wire will be exchanged for the corresponding prolene on the allograft.
  - Colors of suture are important for suture and graft management, and posterolateral approach to the knee performed for passage of sutures.
  - Suture shuttling can be seen with similar colored suture, exchanging those placed with the lasso to those attached to the graft.
- Position the bone block portion of the graft into the slot prepared, pass the sutures through the graft and sequentially start from posterior to anterior:
  - The posterior horn of the graft must clear the femoral condyle before the bone plug will fully seat.
  - Care must be taken to advance the bone block; any resistance could lead to fracture of the allograft.
- Once graft is fully seated, zone-specific sutures are used to tether the lateral meniscal allograft to the meniscal remnant of the host.

38.10 Bailout, Rescue, and Salvage Procedures

- With graft preparation especially of a medial transplant the bony attachment of the meniscal root can be damaged leaving no residual bone to fix to tibial tunnel. Make sure transplant graft has been prepared successfully prior to drilling any bone tunnels. If significant bone damage occurs it can be salvaged by doing a meniscal root repair.
- Inability to drill posterior tunnel in medial transplant is due to inadequate visualization. Salvage by burring down the medial tibial eminence and doing a sub-PCL notchplasty.
- Posterior tibial tunnel that extends medially into the articular surface is a risk. Causes include inadequate angle of drill guide (drill guide pin at 70-degree setting) or too medial a starting point on proximal tibia. This tunnel position causes failure and should be bone grafted with core from an allograft femoral head and a new more vertical tunnel drilled.
- Passing the meniscal allograft can also be a problem. An adequate notchplasty and excision of tibial eminence will allow the posterior bone plug to pass through the notch to its attachment site for docking. To avert difficulty passing the posterior bone plug, use a 9-mm OATS sizing device to assure room to pass the posterior bone plug.
- The sutures that pass through the posterior bone plug can cut through the bone plug creating an oblique pull of the suture through the posterior bone plug which prevents seating the bone plug in its tunnel. To prevent this situation do not pull on these sutures till the bone plug is seated within the tunnel. I pass the plug through the notch with a hemostat and dock in tunnel before pulling on the sutures. If this happens you can attempt to pass plug into tunnel with a hemostat and press into tunnel with a small bone tamp.
- The medial compartment may be very tight even without medial compartment arthritis. This should be recognized prior to passing the graft. This can be solved with limited release of deep MCL done with an 18-gauge spinal needle and controlled valgus pressure.
- Extrusion of the meniscal allograft is a significant postoperative problem and dooms the transplant. Attaching capsule to the meniscus not the meniscus to the capsule averts this complication. This requires the anterior and posterior bone plugs of a medial meniscal transplant to be seated in their respective tunnels and fixed securely in their tunnels before the inside-out suture repair of the medial meniscus.
- The biggest technical issue with lateral transplant is establishing the bone slot in tibia too lateral. When this occurs, it creates a size mismatch of lateral meniscal body and extrusion of transplant with suture fixation. If this problem occurs it can be salvaged by widening the bone slot medially with a burr and fixing the bone slot with small interference screws on the lateral side of the slot, medializing the transplant.
- Postoperative tear or failure of transplant can be addressed with revision transplant without significant difficulty, provided there has been healing of bony attachments.

38.11 Pitfalls

- Appropriate patient selection is critical to success and ignoring malalignment or compartment degeneration will lead to failure.
- Arthrofibrosis.
- Neurovascular injury—Medially the infrapatellar branch of saphenous nerve is at risk as is the peroneal nerve laterally. Popliteal retractors should be used passing inside-out sutures.
- Graft failure—Revision transplant is the solution to the failure of the transplant.
- Deep vein thrombosis/pulmonary embolism (DVT/PE).
- Inappropriate graft size—It is very unusual to have an inadequately sized graft. Grafts that don't appear to fit during the repair usually are the result of surgical errors. Medially the pulling of the posterior bone plug deep into the tunnel will make the graft appear too small. The posterior tunnel for medial transplant that is too medial on medial tibial plateau will make the graft seem too large. As discussed above a bone trough that is too lateral for lateral meniscal transplant will make transplant appear too large.

39 Anterolateral Ligament Reconstruction

Patrick A. Smith

39.1 Description

The recently named anterolateral ligament (ALL) corresponds to the previously described middle third capsular ligament. It is commonly torn along with the anterior cruciate ligament (ACL), as are the capsulo-osseous deep fibers of the iliotibial band (ITB). Both structures play an important role in controlling pivot shift instability. In some cases of isolated ACL reconstruction, normal knee kinematics is not restored, resulting in residual laxity that ALL reconstruction may help correct. The ultimate goal with an ALL reconstruction is to decrease rotational stress on an ACL graft and minimize the risk of a graft re-tear. My operative approach is done in a minimally invasive fashion with use of a tendon graft. The end goal is to reproduce both the ALL and the capsulo-osseous ITB fibers with an extra-articular reconstruction, which I term an anterolateral reconstruction (ALR) to be described as such in this chapter.

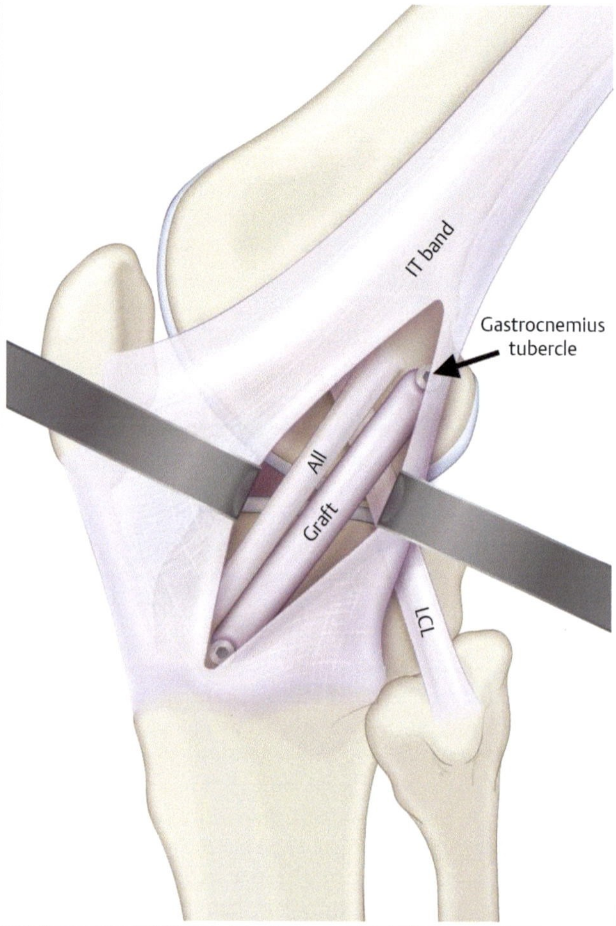

Fig. 39.1 This is an illustration of positioning for an anterolateral reconstruction (ALR) graft to recreate both the anterolateral ligament (ALL) and the deep iliotibial (IT) band capsulo-osseous fibers. The graft is attached proximally to the lateral gastrocnemius tubercle and distally halfway between the center of the fibular head and Gerdy's tubercle.

39.2 Key Principles

Both the ALL and capsulo-osseous ITB fibers are torn to some extent with a rotational ACL tear; however, in many cases, spontaneous healing may occur in these extra-articular structures. Therefore, extra-articular reconstruction is only necessary in a small subset of patients. Graft position is based on a femoral position posterior and proximal to the lateral epicondyle, which has been shown to be the normal attachment point for the ALL. In addition, this position also recreates the orientation of the important capsulo-osseous deep fibers of the ITB. The constant reproducible surgical landmark is the lateral gastrocnemius tubercle in this location (▶ Fig. 39.1). A graft placed here is close to the origin of the deep ITB capsulo-osseous fibers and is also fairly parallel to the normal course of the ALL. Importantly, this location is well away from the femoral attachment of the lateral collateral ligament helping avoid iatrogenic injury. Tibial fixation is at the anatomic ALL attachment halfway between Gerdy tubercle and the center of the fibular head, which also corresponds to the normal tibial attachment of the capsulo-osseous fibers.

39.3 Expectations

The goal with an extra-articular reconstruction is to optimize rotational joint stability with a concomitant ACL reconstruction. In turn, this hopefully protects the ACL graft to minimize the risk of a graft re-tear, which too frequently occurs in young, active patients.

39.4 Indications

Indications for ALR include patients with a 3 + positive pivot shift, MRI evidence for significant ALL or capsulo-osseous injury, or X-ray showing either a large impaction fracture of the lateral femoral condyle consistent with a major rotational injury or a Segond fracture off the lateral tibia directly indicative of an ALL tear (▶ Fig. 39.2). In addition, patients deemed "high risk" for an ACL graft re-tear are appropriate ALR candidates. Examples include patients with excessive knee hyperextension greater than 10 degrees and athletes such as young female soccer players or young males involved in vigorous cutting sports. In addition, revision ACL reconstruction patients tend to be more unstable, thus warranting a situation in which adding an extra-articular ALL would be appropriate.

39.5 Contraindications

In patients with a 2 + or less pivot shift without the indications for ALR noted above, ALR should not be done as that could lead to internal rotation overconstraint of the joint. Also, if a patient has undergone a significant lateral meniscectomy, there could

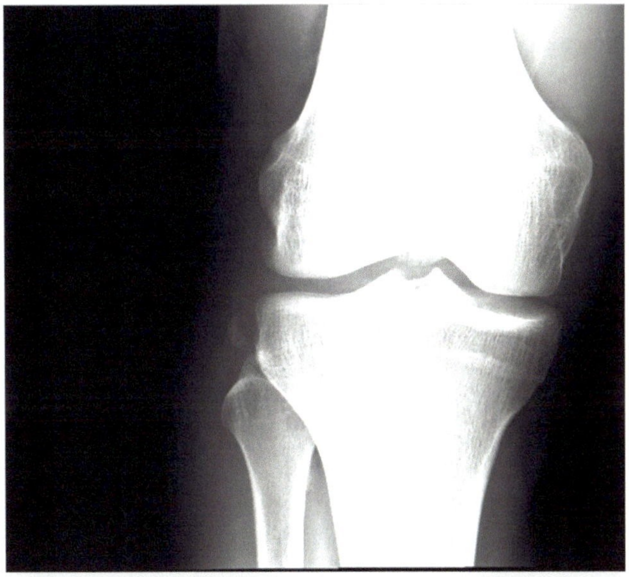

Fig. 39.2 A Segond bony avulsion off the lateral tibial plateau.

be an increased potential for lateral compartment overload and resultant degenerative arthritic development with an ALR.

39.6 Special Considerations

Patients who present with a Segond fracture represent an avulsion of the ALL off its tibial attachment. In those cases, I generally prefer an open reduction and internal fixation (ORIF) of the fracture fragment itself to restore ALL integrity. The fragment is usually too small for a screw, and so I utilize an absorbable 3.0-mm biocomposite SutureTak (Arthrex Inc., Naples, FL) anchor with two attached #2 FiberWire sutures (Arthrex Inc., Naples, FL) to reattach the bony fragment anatomically.

39.7 Special Instructions, Position, and Anesthesia

This procedure is typically done after ACL reconstruction has been completed. Therefore, the patient will remain in the supine position under general anesthesia. It is helpful to have a device attached to the operating table with a foot support, in combination with a thigh support device to maintain appropriate flexion angles during the procedure.

39.8 Tips, Pearls, and Lessons Learned

After splitting the ITB, there is typically prominent soft tissue on the femoral side near the lateral gastrocnemius tubercle landmark related to the deep ITB fibers which are carefully taken down—including the capsulo-osseous fibers—and preserved. To facilitate finding the key landmark of the lateral gastrocnemius tubercle through this small incision, palpate the distinct, distal extent of the lateral intermuscular septum. Just distal to that point is the prominence where the lateral gastrocnemius tendon attaches. A guide pin is drilled here, and after reaming with the 4.5-mm bit, it is helpful to use electrocautery to fully define the created bone socket here to make it easier to insert the graft with the SwiveLock anchor (Arthrex Inc., Naples, FL). The goal is for a nonisometric graft that lengthens in extension and loosens in flexion. If you have a shortening pattern in extension, move the femoral pin more posteriorly. There is more "forgiveness" with socket position on the tibial side, so I typically only change the femoral pin to obtain the desired nonisometric pattern. The retained #2 FiberWire suture in the femoral SwiveLock anchor is used to reattach the critical capsulo-osseous fibers after graft placement.

39.9 Difficulties Encountered

Generally, ALR is a straightforward procedure. One technical challenge relates to the tibial fixation. First of all, the socket is drilled in flexion, but fixation is done in extension or hyperextension, making exposure a bit more challenging. Also, with the forked SwiveLock anchor used here for fixation, the fixation point on the graft has to be adjusted to ensure adequate graft is inserted into the socket with ultimate optimal tension. This requires a bit of finesse through the small tibial incision with skin retraction.

39.10 Key Procedural Steps

Either a soft tissue allograft or a gracilis autograft can be used for the ALR as a graft diameter in the range of 4 to 5 mm is appropriate. I prefer allograft tissue so I do not have to harvest autograft tissue in addition to the ACL graft. The graft is prepared placing a #2 FiberLoop suture (Arthrex Inc., Naples, FL) in a locking SpeedWhip fashion over 20 mm on one end of the graft. If an allograft is used, I pretension it at 75 N for 15 minutes to eliminate creep in the tissue. Again, ALR is always performed following the ACL reconstruction.

The first step is exposure on the femur. The lateral epicondyle is palpated and marked, and approximately 1.5 cm posterior and proximal a 2-cm skin incision is made. This is carried down to the ITB, which is then split in the line of its fibers. The deep ITB fibers are carefully taken down including the capsulo-osseous fibers for later reattachment. Next, the lateral intermuscular septum is palpable; just distal is the reproducible palpable landmark of the lateral gastrocnemius tubercle. A 2.4-mm guide pin is drilled at this point parallel to the joint line (▶ Fig. 39.3).

Next, on the tibia, the lateral joint line is marked along with the center of Gerdy tubercle and the center of the fibular head. Halfway between these points, and a distance 1.5 cm below the joint line, a 1.5-mm longitudinal incision is made. There normally is a palpable depression here with overlying periosteum that, when incised, nicely exposes the anatomical ALL tibial attachment. A 2.4-mm pin is drilled here parallel to the joint line.

The next step is isometry determination with my goal for a nonisometric graft that tightens 2 to 3 mm in extension and loosens in flexion. A #2 FiberWire suture is looped around the femoral pin and passed deep to the ITB to the tibial pin where a hemostat is placed on both sutures (▶ Fig. 39.4). The knee is

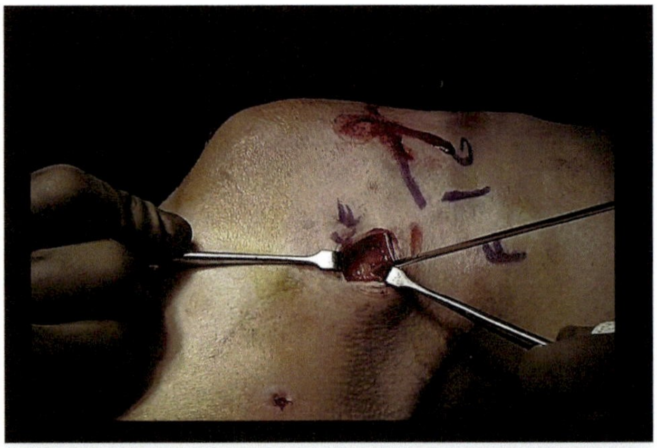

Fig. 39.3 Left knee: Femoral guide pin drilled at anatomical landmark of lateral gastrocnemius tubercle.

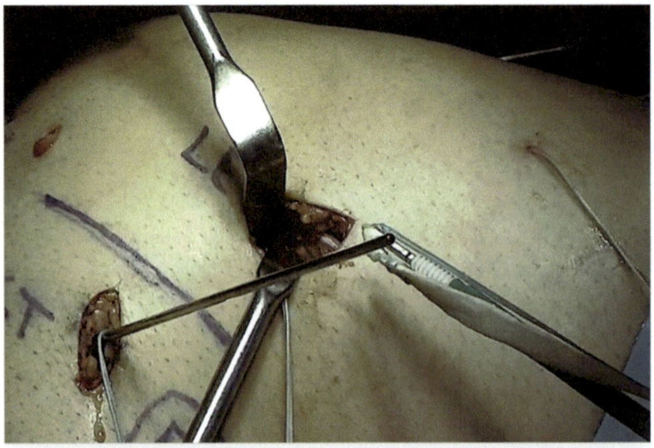

Fig. 39.5 Left knee: Graft fixation at the femur is done with 4.5-mm Biocomposite SwiveLock anchor. Key is making sure the sutures holding the graft stay tight at the tip of the anchor as it is inserted into the hole to ensure sutured part of graft is completely in hole as screw is tightened down.

then taken from 100 degrees of flexion to full extension to gauge the suture excursion. Generally, if this lengthening pattern is not achieved, the femoral pin needs to be moved posteriorly and isometric testing repeated.

Having determined appropriate pin position on the femur and tibia, attention is directed toward graft fixation. The femoral pin is overreamed with a 5.0-mm reamer to a depth of 20 mm. Fixation of the sutured end of the graft is done here with a 4.75-mm Biocomposite SwiveLock anchor. Be sure the sutured end of the graft fully inserts into the socket before the anchor itself is screwed into position. The #2 FiberWire suture in this anchor is left in place to be used later to reattach the important capsulo-osseous fibers back to the femur (▶ Fig. 39.5). On the tibia, the pin is overreamed with a 7.0-mm reamer to a depth of 20 mm. The graft is shuttled from the femoral incision deep to the ITB and holding the graft taut, the knee is cycled several times to eliminate any graft laxity. Then with the leg on the table in normal resting extension (or hyperextension if present), and *neutral* tibial rotation, tibial fixation

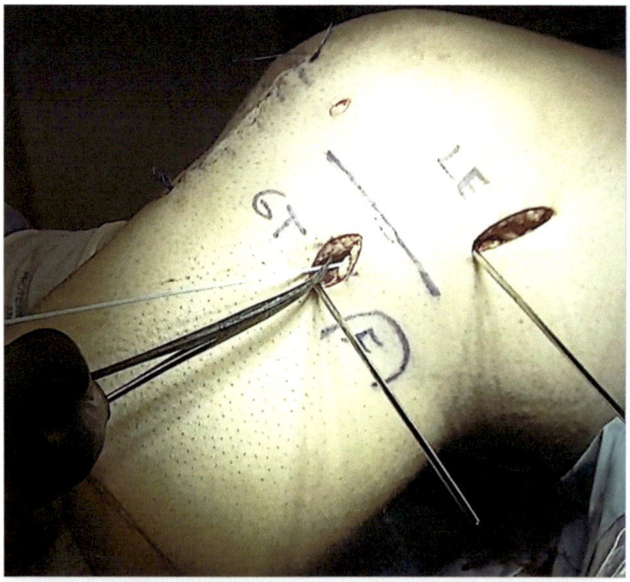

Fig. 39.4 Left knee: #2 FiberWire suture passed around the femoral guide pin beneath iliotibial band and held with hemostat at tibial pin. Desired is lengthening pattern taking the knee into full extension, meaning hemostat with suture travels 2 to 3 mm proximally.

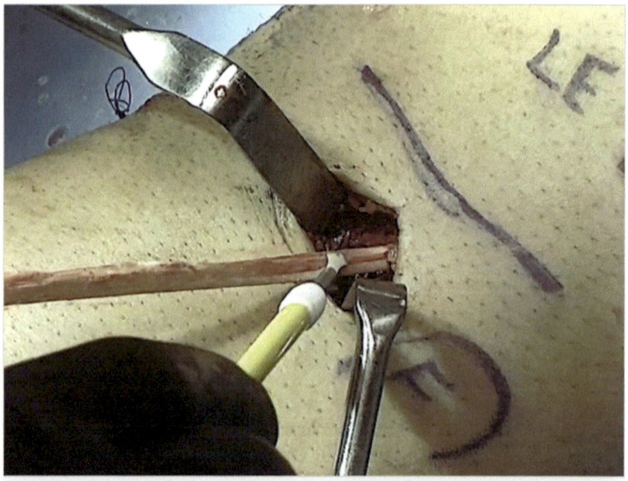

Fig. 39.6 Left knee: Fixation of graft on the tibial side. Knee is held in full extension (or hyperextension) with neutral rotation of the foot. 7-mm Biocomposite forked SwiveLock anchor is used to fixate the graft here. Key point is allowing some slack in graft before inserting anchor to ensure screw can be completely inserted in hole.

is done using a 7.0-mm forked Biocomposite SwiveLock anchor (▶ Fig. 39.6). With this fixation technique, the free end of the graft is held over the tibial socket leaving slight laxity in the graft itself; the graft is captured by the forked device so it can be inserted in this 20-mm socket eliminating any laxity as the SwiveLock anchor is screwed down flush to the cortex. Excess graft is then cut off (▶ Fig. 39.7). The capsulo-osseous fibers of the deep ITB are then reattached by using the retained #2 FiberWire suture in the femoral SwiveLock anchor (▶ Fig. 39.8). The incision in the ITB is then closed.

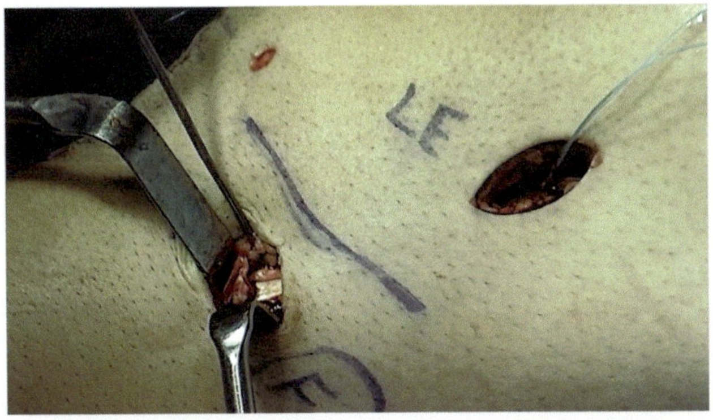

Fig. 39.7 Final anterolateral graft seen on tibia after final fixation.

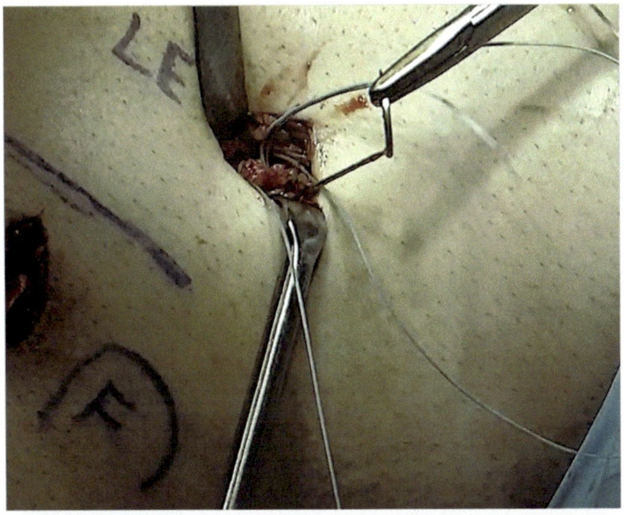

Fig. 39.8 Use of #2 FiberWire suture from femoral SwiveLock anchor to reattach capsulo-osseous fibers to femur here with a mattress-type suture.

39.11 Bailout, Rescue, and Salvage Procedures

On the femoral side, one potential salvage scenario occurs if one utilizes suspensory fixation for the ACL graft and creates a more central "down-the-wall" ACL femoral socket. This ACL fixation may then be close to the femoral ALL graft placement socket. If in drilling for the ALL femoral socket there is any inadvertent compromise to the ACL suspensory fixation device via cutting of the sutures, the bailout is to immediately go back in the joint and place an interference screw over the graft in the femoral socket to avoid the risk of losing graft stability. On the tibial side, if loss of fixation occurs with use of the forked SwiveLock device, the bailout is to cut the graft length down and suture the end of the graft with a FiberWire whipstitch. Next drill a Beath pin from the lateral tibial socket out the skin medially and use this pin to pull the graft into the tibial socket and maintain tension while the graft is then fixed with a standard interference screw usually 1 mm less in diameter than the socket itself.

39.12 Pitfalls

First, a major potential pitfall with any extra-articular reconstruction is the risk of iatrogenic injury to the lateral collateral ligament attachment on the femur related to femoral drilling and fixation. It is important to be proximal and posterior to the lateral epicondyle when drilling the femoral socket to avoid this complication. An advantage of this described ALR procedure is that the landmark of the lateral gastrocnemius tubercle for femoral graft position provides an inherent "safe zone" well away from the lateral collateral ligament. A second pitfall with extra-articular reconstruction relates to the knee angle for final graft fixation. I believe it is critical to fix the ALR graft in full knee extension or hyperextension, otherwise fixing the graft in flexion could lead to joint overconstraint by limiting normal joint internal rotation present in knee flexion. Furthermore, by placing the graft nonisometrically so it lengthens in extension, I believe the resultant graft tightening helps control internal rotation of the tibia toward extension which is when the pivot shift tends to occur.

Section III

Adult Reconstruction

III

40 Opening Wedge High Tibia Osteotomy—Varus Knee

Philipp Lobenhoffer

40.1 Description

The medial open wedge biplanar high tibia osteotomy (OWHTO) is a well-established and relatively safe procedure to correct a varus deformity of the tibia. Fixation with a stable angle plate allows for early weight-bearing and avoids bone grafts or substitutes.

40.2 Key Principles

Varus frontal plane malalignment will cause overload in the medial compartment of the knee. Chronic overload is likely to damage the cartilage. Osteotomy may correct frontal plane malalignment and has been proven to normalize cartilage loading. Varus deformity usually results from a disproportional growth of the proximal tibial epiphysis with relative inhibition of the medial side's growth. As a result, the medial metaphyseal aspect of the tibia is shorter than usual. The open wedge tibial osteotomy is the most logical treatment to address this deformity. The anterior cruciate ligament (ACL) or posterior cruciate ligament (PCL) deficiencies are not contraindications to this procedure. The correction of the malalignment may be associated with a planned modification of the tibial slope, which ultimately may improve knee stability.

40.3 Expectations

In general, the activity level after HTO is significantly higher than after any arthroplasty procedure. High tibia osteotomy has reported 87 to 99% survival rates after 5 years and 66 to 84% after 10 years. A recent meta-analysis including 46 peer-reviewed papers demonstrated a survival rate of tibia osteotomies of 82% after 8 to 12 years. The latest Cochrane review indicates silver evidence that osteotomy improves clinical outcomes in 70% of the patients for 10 years.

40.4 Indications

Osteotomies around the knee are indicated for active individuals, presenting constitutional deformities over 3 degrees in the coronal plane, and with unilateral osteoarthritis grade Kellgren Lawrence II and III. Age above 65 years is not an exclusion criterion for an osteotomy. Our multicenter study demonstrated that high tibia osteotomy was also successful in patients with osteoarthritis grade IV in the involved compartment (bone-on-bone) as long as we followed the other indication criteria. Obesity and nicotine use are not exclusion criteria for an osteotomy around the knee.

The valgus producing high tibia osteotomy should be considered in individuals with proximal metaphyseal tibial deformity undergoing medial compartment cartilage reconstruction or meniscus transplantation.

40.5 Contraindications

Patients with a typical bone configuration of the tibia, which means a normal mechanical proximal tibial angle (MPTA), should not receive OWHTO since the procedure would lead to an abnormal design of the proximal tibia and an oblique joint line. Deformities of the shaft and the distal tibia are usually not suitable for OWHTO because the center of correction is not at the site of deformity. OWHTO is indicated for frontal plane deformities. Simultaneous sagittal plane as well as torsional corrections is possible but only to a limited degree. A healthy and intact soft tissue envelope is mandatory for performing an OWHTO. Any skin defects, skin infections, or soft tissue alterations of the tibia are exclusion criteria for this type of procedure.

40.6 Special Considerations

Weight-bearing radiographs, including a long-leg radiograph, should be obtained. The long-leg film is crucial for analysis and planning and must be performed in a two-leg stance and with correct torsion of the leg. A detailed deformity analysis is mandatory. The main parameters are the Mikulicz line, the distal femur (mLDFA), and proximal tibia joint angles (MPTA), and the joint convergence angle (JLCA). In the preoperative radiograph, the Mikulicz line must be shifted to the medial compartment, corroborating an indication for an HTO. The normal range for the medial proximal tibia angle is 85 to 90 degrees. Patients for HTO will usually have MPTA values at the lower normal range or below (86 degrees or less). The lateral distal femur angle should be normal (85 to 90 degrees) in patients suitable for HTO. The JLCA may be abnormal (over 2 degrees), reflecting lateral joint opening in a standing position. The abnormal JLCA must be considered when planning the correction, which may be performed following the established techniques. The postoperative rehabilitation is critical. The patient may mobilize the joint according to pain tolerance and following the surgeon's guidelines. No immobilization or protection is necessary. Weight-bearing is allowed but is dependent on pain tolerance. Studies have proven that this type of osteotomy and fixation allows for early weight-bearing without loss of correction. We usually expect our patients to walk short distances without crutches after 4 weeks. Manual lymph drainage is helpful; physical therapy is usually not necessary. Radiographic controls are performed after the surgery and after 4 weeks. If the hinge is intact at this stage and the patient has no problems, we do not implement more controls. We know that healing of the gap takes 8 to 12 months, but under the protection of the plate, the patient can perform all activities. We also inform the patient that plate removal is only necessary if local problems occur.

40.7 Special Instructions, Position, and Anesthesia

40.7.1 Patient Positioning and Preliminary Steps

The patient is positioned on a straight radiolucent operative table, allowing for fluoroscopy of the hip, knee, and ankle. A foot stop and a side post are helpful to stabilize the leg in the extended and at 90-degree flexed position. The entire leg, including the pelvic crest, is draped. A tourniquet is not necessary for this type of surgery. An arthroscopy is carried out on the same day of the osteotomy only if the patient presents with locking mechanical symptoms, or any other intra-articular derangement that the surgeon should address.

40.8 Tips, Pearls, and Lessons Learned

40.8.1 Lateral Hinge

Placement of the lateral hinge is critical in this procedure. The optimum location of the hinge is at the upper end of the proximal tibiofibular joint aiming for the tip of the proximal fibula.

40.8.2 Overcorrection

A common source of overcorrection is preoperative joint line opening on the noninvolved side. The joint line will close to normal values after realignment of the leg, resulting in a final overcorrection when the patient stands up. If the surgeon has not considered this aspect in his planning (pathological joint line convergence angle), gross valgus deformity may be the result. There are mathematical ways to solve this problem as well as digital planning solutions. The easiest way is to use the planning software to create a virtual closing wedge osteotomy at the level of the joint space with a lateral base as the first step. When the lateral joint line has normal width, the planning process is continued, and the opening wedge is then calculated based on the corrected joint space. During surgery, closure of the lateral joint line can be simulated by axial compression and valgus stress. The postoperative loading situation can be reproduced, and an alignment rod and fluoroscopy can be used to check the correct postoperative mechanical axis.

40.8.3 Unintended Increase of Tibial Slope

For geometrical reasons, the osteotomy must be opened one-third more in the posterior aspect than in the anterior aspect if the tibial slope should stay unchanged. We recommend using a spreader in the posteromedial corner of the tibia and rechecking the distal medial collateral ligament (MCL) release after the osteotomy is opened. When the leg hangs free and full extension is achieved, the gap is automatically opened more in the posterior aspect of the tibia. The fixator should be fixed in this position.

40.9 Difficulties Encountered

High tibia osteotomies may be associated with some difficulties, which should be overcome in case the surgical technique is perfectly executed.

We list the most typical difficulties that may be associated with poorer outcomes.

- Perfect placement of the hinge.
- Fracture of the hinge.
- Overcorrection or undercorrection in the coronal plane.
- Unintended change in the tibial slope.

40.10 Key Procedural Steps

40.10.1 Surgical Exposure

It is important to understand that the fixation of the osteotomy relies on the minimal invasive plate osteosynthesis (MIPO) technique. The implant is placed under intact soft tissues, and the distal screws are inserted percutaneously via a stab incision. It is not recommended to expose the entire area where the implant will be placed. We use a longitudinal medial incision of 4 to 5 cm length starting around 1 cm below the joint line and ending at the upper border of the pes anserinus. The incision is placed in the middle portion of the medial tibial plateau and can be extended as necessary.

40.10.2 MCL Release

The medial retinaculum, the pes anserinus, and the MCL are exposed. The interval between the patella tendon and the tibia is palpated. A line is drawn starting posterior to the patella tendon insertion and aiming distally parallel to the tibial crest. This line reflects the second osteotomy line in the biplanar technique. The bursa between pes anserinus and the MCL is opened. By retraction of the pes tendons, the distal part of the MCL below the pes tendons comes into view. This part of the MCL is now stripped off the tibia by sharp dissection. This maneuver exposes the posteromedial tibia shaft. It is essential to restrict this MCL release to the distal part of the ligament and not progress more proximal than the sartorius aponeurosis. The space between the posterior tibia and the popliteus muscle is opened with a blunt rasp. A retractor is inserted into this window, protecting the popliteus muscle and the neurovascular structures during the next steps of the surgery. The distal MCL should also be retracted either by the retractor or by a separate small Hohmann retractor to avoid damage by the saw cut.

40.10.3 Guidewire Placement

The leg is now placed in the extended position. The C-arm is adjusted over the knee so that the entire lateral tibial joint line is oriented precisely in the anteroposterior plane. The surgeon now places two wires in the tibia, from medial to lateral, defining the plane of the first osteotomy line. We recommend placing the tips of the wires at the superior end of the proximal tibiofibular joint. It is crucial to notice that we only use wires 2.5 mm with drill tips because they allow for exact placement. These two wires will guide the saw cut in the next step (▸ Fig. 40.1). The length of the osteotomy cut is now defined.

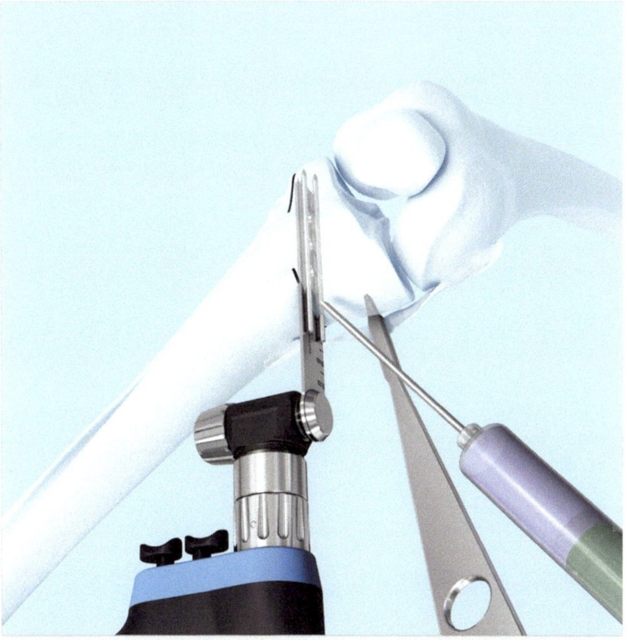

Fig. 40.1 The first osteotomy cut is performed guided by two wires. The osteotomy is limited to the posterior two-thirds of the tibia and ends 5 to 10 mm from the lateral cortex.

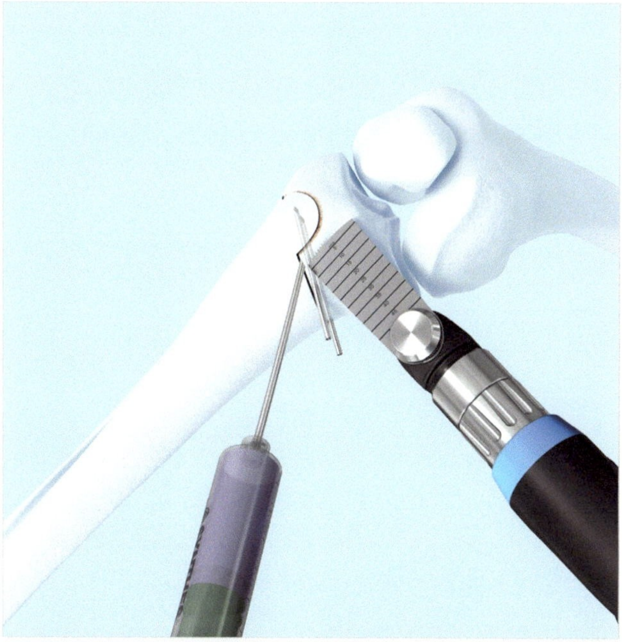

Fig. 40.2 The second osteotomy cut is performed with an angle of 100 degrees to the first cut behind the tibial tuberosity. This is a complete cut to the opposite side.

A third wire of the same length is placed on the cortex adjacent to the guidewires. The length difference of the wires is measured with a ruler. This measurement reflects the entire width of the tibia at the level of the osteotomy. We usually subtract 10 mm from this value in very hard bone 5 mm and mark this value on the sawblade.

40.10.4 Osteotomy

We recommend using specific saw blades for this procedure. We use either two special blades designed for biplanar tibia osteotomy or a special front-cutting blade with a rigid shaft. The osteotomies can be done either in the extended or the flexed position. The saw is inserted under the two wires on the anteromedial aspect of the tibia. The surgeon first makes a window in the cortex of the tibia. From this window, he can direct the saw against the posterior cortex and gradually cut the cortex. By gently tapping the saw against the cortex, he can feel clearly when the bone is cut (loss of resistance). Thus, the surgeon can cut the middle and posterior section of the tibia as planned by advancing the saw in an oscillating mode. The last step is to complete the osteotomy in the anterior section up to the marking line for the ascending cut drawn under the patellar tendon. We recommend irrigation during the procedure, and the pace of the saw should be as slow as possible. The saw blade should have a length of at least 90 mm and a width of 25 mm. Hyperaggressive saw blades like those used in arthroplasty are not recommended for this procedure. The next step is the ascending osteotomy behind the anterior tibial tubercle. We recommend using a small blade for this osteotomy to avoid too much bone loss (▶ Fig. 40.2).

40.10.5 Opening of the Osteotomy

A first chisel is now inserted below the two wires. We prefer specific chisels with length markings. The chisel is inserted in the posterior aspect of the osteotomy and as deep as the saw cut was performed. A second chisel is now inserted between the wires and the first chisel. The insertion may need very careful small blows with a hammer, and the insertion depth is 15 mm less than the first chisel. Two more chisels are inserted between the first chisels. The osteotomy gap in front of the chisels is monitored during this step: the gap should open gradually, and the ascending cut should not translate or open. When 6 mm opening is achieved, a metal wedge is inserted in the anterior gap and blocked with small hammer blows. The chisels are removed one by one and the wires are removed. A bone spreader is inserted on the posteromedial crest of the tibia. The spreader is opened until resistance and the anterior wedge is now removed. This spreader is used to achieve the planned opening of the osteotomy gap. Our planning gives us the opening of the gap in millimeters, and we use a caliper to measure the actual gap opening during the surgery. This measurement should be done in front of the spreader (posteromedial) since this is the area reflecting the valgus correction. For geometrical reasons, the gap during the surgery should be one-third smaller in the anterior area of the osteotomy if the slope should be unchanged. One millimeter should be subtracted from the measured value because of the bone loss by the saw blade. The leg is placed in the extended position. A forceps is used to palpate the MCL between the branches of the spreader. If the MCL is still tight (bowstring), trepanation of these specific areas of the ligament should be performed with a scalpel number 11 until there is no residual tightness (▶ Fig. 40.3).

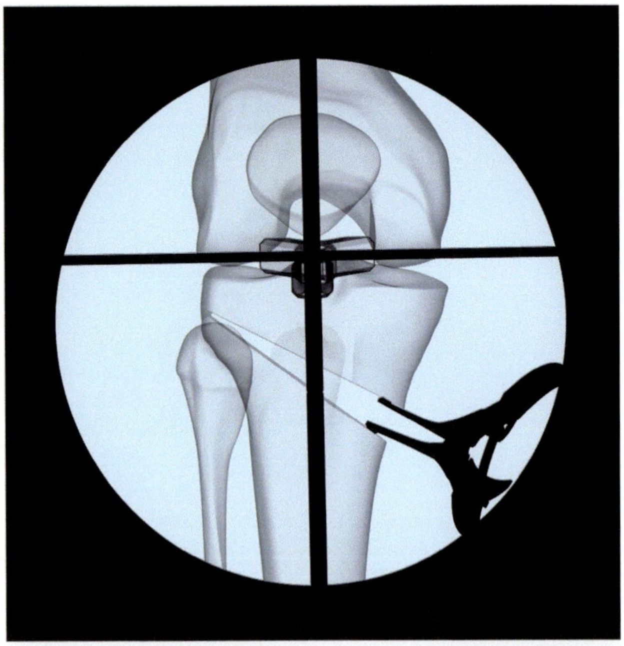

Fig. 40.3 The osteotomy is opened, and the correction is fine-tuned with the aid of an alignment rod placed between the center of hip and the center of ankle under fluoroscopy.

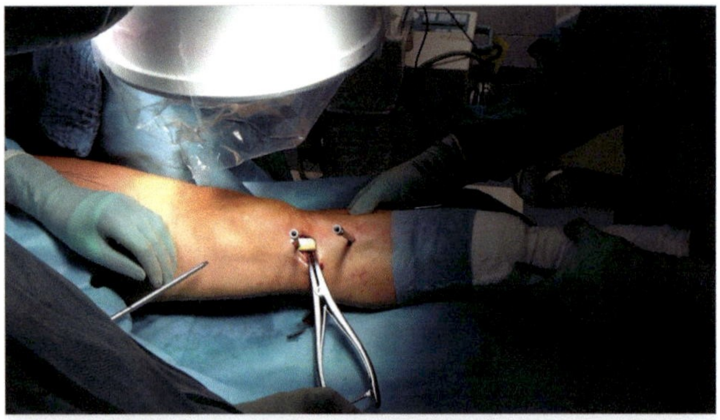

Fig. 40.4 Intraoperative view of the osteotomy with the spreader on the posterior cortex. The plate is already inserted in the subcutaneous plane. The distal fixation is achieved by a stab incision over the shaft section of the plate.

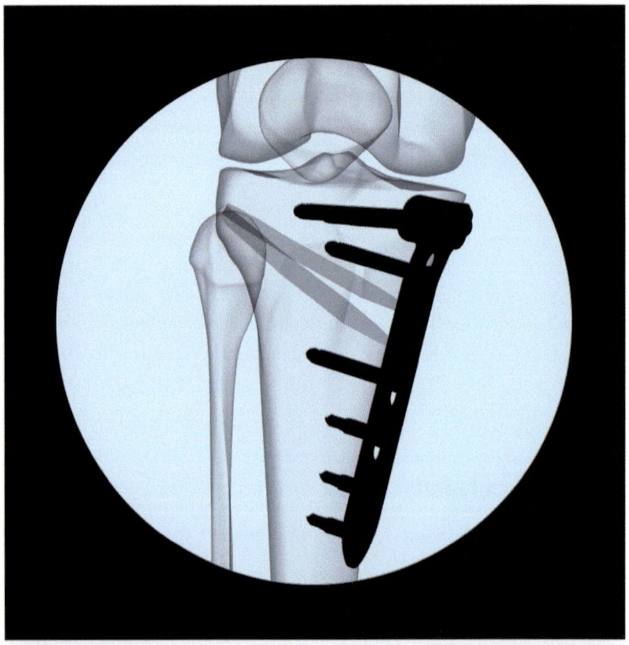

Fig. 40.5 Final view of the open wedge osteotomy with the plate fixator. Unicortical locking screws are used in the shaft area.

40.10.6 "Fine-tuning" the Correction

The final step is the fine adjustment of the correction. The leg is brought into full extension by pressure on the anterior aspect of the tibia. The knee must be hanging free with the heel on the foot support. A long metal rod is placed over the leg. The center of the hip is identified fluoroscopically and the rod is placed there. The assistant fixes the rod over the hip. The distal aspect of the rod is now placed over the center of the ankle by the aid of the fluoroscopy and held in place. Axial load on the leg is simulated by the assistant who leans against the foot with his body weight. The fluoroscope is now shifted to the knee. The metal rod should project at the planned crossing point of the Mikulicz line with the knee joint line. There is a special alignment rod available which incorporates a stand that allows inserting a second wire simulating the joint line. This wire is helpful to check the correction of the MPTA angle because it shows an MPTA of 90 degrees and the actual medial joint line can be referred to this line. If joint convergence angle is pathological before the correction, a valgus stress should be introduced by the assistant to normalize the lateral joint opening. The new Mikulicz line should only be accepted if this normalization is achieved. Otherwise, the correction can easily be increased or decreased by opening or closing the spreader (▶ Fig. 40.4).

40.10.7 Fixation of the Osteotomy

When optimum correction is achieved, fixation of the osteotomy can be performed. The Tomofix ® implant is mounted with drill sleeves. The implant is pushed into the layer under subcutaneous tissue and aligned distally with the shaft by palpation. Proximally, it is placed as far posteriorly as possible and adjusted under fluoroscopy so that all screws are placed safely. A reduction sleeve is inserted into the proximal drill guide, and a 2-mm wire is drilled into the tibia plateau. This wire reflects the direction of the proximal screws, which should be parallel to the joint line and at least 10 mm below the cartilage layer. The three proximal screws are now inserted and locked (▶ Fig. 40.5).

Distal to the osteotomy gap, the combination hole is identified, and a cortical 4.5-mm screw is placed in the dynamic compression section of this hole, aiming distally and anteriorly. This screw is tightened very carefully with a manual screwdriver. The effect of this screw is a prebending of the implant and a compression of the lateral hinge of the osteotomy, improving the biomechanics of the construct significantly. Fluoroscopic control of this step is recommended to avoid overtightening of the standard screw. A stab incision is made at the level of the third screw hole of the plate on the shaft. Drill sleeves are attached to the plate, and unicortical locking screws are inserted. The conventional cortical screw is removed, and a bicortical locking screw is inserted into the combination hole. A locking screw is placed in the second proximal row of screws. Due to the screw direction, this screw will be shorter than the first three proximal screws. The fixation is now completed and documented with the fluoroscope. A drain is inserted from proximal and placed very far distally parallel to the plate. The MCL fibers are reduced over the osteotomy gap. The anterior gap may be covered with periosteum or sealed with collagen fleece. The incision is closed meticulously with subcutaneous sutures and skin sutures. A padded compression bandage is applied.

40.11 Bailout, Rescue, and Salvage Procedures

40.11.1 Hinge Fractures

To avoid fractures of the lateral hinge of the osteotomy, the horizontal osteotomy must end at a point 5 to 10 mm to the lateral cortex, especially in the posterolateral aspect of the tibia. Fluoroscopy is used to control the osteotomy depth.

Fractures can occur in the line of the osteotomy (type 1) or an ascending (type 3) or descending direction (type 2). Type 1 fractures may be compressed by using a lag screw in the plate and do not interfere with the stability and the rehabilitation. Type 3 intra-articular fractures should first be reduced and stabilized. The spreader should be closed, which usually results in a reduction of any fracture gap. One or two small-fragment screws should be placed directly under the joint surface from lateral to medial. Then the osteotomy can be opened again and the Tomofix ℬ plate placed as planned. Type 2 fractures decrease the stability of the lateral aspect of the osteotomy and the hinge significantly. The patient has to be informed that the rehabilitation time will be prolonged. In extreme cases, a small-fragment plate can be placed on the lateral side to restore the lateral cortex and stabilize the hinge.

40.11.2 Arterial Bleeding

Severe bleeding may occur when the posterolateral cortex is addressed by saw or chisel. Since the popliteus muscle protects the popliteal artery at the level the biplanar osteotomy is performed, in our experience the reason in most cases is a variation of the arterial supply to the tibia with a high division of the truncus tibiofibularis, thus placing the tibialis anterior artery directly on the periosteum of the posterior tibia. This variation occurs in at least 1% of all humans and can be identified in the routine preop magnetic resonance (MR) scans. We recommend as the first step to use manual compression of the thigh or a sterile tourniquet to control the bleeding. The osteotomies should then be completed and opened as much as possible, at least 20 mm. The posterior tibia area can now be visualized through the osteotomy gap. By the careful release of compression on the thigh, the artery is identified. We could achieve direct control of bleeding by coagulation and hemostatic agents in all cases in our practice. The gap can then be closed to the planned width, and the procedure is completed as usual.

40.11.3 Pseudarthrosis

Delayed healing results in pain with weight-bearing. In these cases, the pain is usually on the lateral side of the knee. Delayed healing is correlated with type 2 fractures of the lateral hinge in most cases. We recommend a minimal invasive bone graft if the patient cannot load the leg pain-free after 8 weeks. Cancellous bone is harvested from the iliac crest and inserted into the gap without modifications of the osteosynthesis. We observed bony healing after this procedure within 4 to 6 weeks.

40.12 Pitfalls

40.12.1 Lateral Hinge

Placement of the lateral hinge is critical in this procedure. The optimum location of the hinge is at the upper end of the proximal tibiofibular joint aiming for the tip of the proximal fibula.

40.12.2 Overcorrection

A common source of overcorrection is preoperative joint line opening on the noninvolved side. The joint line will close to normal values after realignment of the leg, resulting in a final overcorrection when the patient stands up. If the surgeon has not considered this aspect in his planning (pathological joint line convergence angle), gross valgus deformity may be the result. There are mathematical ways to solve this problem as well as digital planning solutions. The easiest way is to use the planning software to create a virtual closing wedge osteotomy at the level of the joint space with a lateral base as the first step. When the lateral joint line has normal width, the planning process is continued, and the opening wedge is then calculated based on the corrected joint space. During surgery, closure of the lateral joint line can be simulated by axial compression and valgus stress. The postoperative loading situation can be reproduced, and an alignment rod and fluoroscopy can be used to check the correct postoperative mechanical axis.

40.12.3 Unintended Increase of Tibial Slope

For geometrical reasons, the osteotomy must be opened one-third more in the posterior aspect than in the anterior aspect if the tibial slope should stay unchanged. We recommend using a spreader in the posteromedial corner of the tibia and rechecking the distal MCL release after the osteotomy is opened. When the leg hangs free and full extension is achieved, the gap is automatically opened more in the posterior aspect of the tibia. The fixator should be fixed in this position.

41 Lateral Closing-Wedge High Tibia Osteotomy (LCW HTO) in Varus Knee

Jörg Harrer, Felix Hüttner, and Wolf Strecker

41.1 Description

The authors describe a technique to correct varus deformities around the knee by performing a proximal tibia lateral closing-wedge valgus-producing osteotomy. The method is also used to correct inwardly pointing knees, where the goals are to address not just the varus but the external torsion of the proximal tibia. In this clinical scenario, we obtain realignment in the coronal and axial planes by producing valgus and internal torsion of the tibia, which improves the patellofemoral tracking.

41.2 Key Principles

The main goal of a valgus-producing osteotomy around the knee is shifting the mechanical load from a symptomatic and overloaded medial knee compartment to the lateral compartment of the joint. The resulting biomechanical changes are expected to reduce pain, slowing down the progression of degenerative changes in the medial compartment of the knee. Specifically, the lateral closing wedge aims to increase the surface area at the osteotomy site, promoting early bone healing without producing a patella baja.

41.3 Expectations

Tibial valgus-producing osteotomies may be performed by either opening a wedge on the medial metaphyseal aspect of the bone or closing a wedge on its lateral aspect. Medial opening wedge techniques gained popularity after the advent of angle stable implants. Lateral closing-wedge techniques require a precise preoperative planning, as there will be no options for progressive intraoperative adjustments as observed in cases of medial closing-wedge osteotomies. Lateral closing-wedge osteotomies are inherently stable, have a broader surface area, and do not require angle stable implants.

41.4 Indications

A high tibial valgus-producing osteotomy should be considered in very active individuals, with a varus alignment of the knee caused by a metaphyseal tibial deformity. The varus of the proximal tibia results from an abnormal mechanical proximal tibial angle inferior to 87 degrees. The valgus-producing osteotomy is indicated if the patient has medial knee pain, clinical and radiographic evidences of degenerative changes in the medial compartment of the joint, and a range of motion of at least 100 degrees of flexion, with a maximum lack of extension of 10 degrees.

Lateral closing-wedge techniques should be particularly considered in cases where the affected limb is longer than the opposite one, and/or the patient already has patella baja. Lateral closing-wedge tibial osteotomies allow correction of the alignment without increasing the overall leg length.

Another indication for a lateral closing-wedge proximal tibia osteotomy is a clinical situation described by Cooke in 1990, the so-called inwardly pointing knee. This deformity is characterized by an abnormal increased external tibial torsion, excess varus angulation of the tibial plateau, and varus knee. The congenital increased external torsion is located in the most proximal portion of the tibia, generating an increased Tibial Tubercle–Trochlear Groove (TT-TG) distance. This deformity is associated with abnormal patellar tracking. At the time of the lateral closing wedge, it is possible to rotate the distal part of the tibia internally. The osteotomy site is proximal to the anterior tibial tuberosity, and the internal torsion of the tibia will shift the anterior tuberosity medially. As a result, there will be a reduction of the TT-TG and improved patellofemoral tracking.

The potential advantages of utilizing lateral closing-wedge valgus-producing osteotomy are:

- No increase in leg length.
- Possibility of correction in three dimensions: coronal, sagittal, and axial planes.
- Minimal or no impact to patellar height.
- No tendency to increase the posterior tibial slope.
- No additional tension to the soft tissues and therefore lesser likelihood of wound healing problems when compared with medial opening techniques.
- No need to perform a fibular osteotomy, if the desired correction in the frontal plane is inferior to 10 degrees.
- Easier access to the peroneal nerve, especially in cases where a neurolysis is planned.

41.5 Contraindications

A lateral closing-wedge valgus-producing osteotomy is contraindicated in the presence of.

- Advanced signs of degeneration in the lateral tibial-femoral compartment of the knee (Outerbridge IV; insufficient or extruded lateral meniscus).
- Flexion contracture superior to 10 degrees, which may not be corrected with arthroscopic notchplasty, resection of the tibial eminences' osteophytes, and/or an additional simultaneous slope correction (extension osteotomy).
- Severe ligament laxity, with joint subluxation.
- Clinical comorbidities associated with impending bone healing (e.g., rheumatoid arthritis, use of immunosuppressants).
- Varus deformity, which is not originated from a metaphyseal tibial deformity, but from the metaphyseal femoral deformity (normal mechanical proximal tibial angle, and abnormal mechanical lateral distal femoral angle). Advanced tricompartimental knee arthritis.

These are the potential disadvantages of utilizing lateral closing-wedge valgus-producing osteotomy when compared with a medial open-wedge technique.

- Need for a fibular osteotomy, for corrections superior to 10 degrees.
- Increased risk of peroneal nerve injury.
- Increased surgical time.
- Increased bone loss (wedge resection).
- Potential risk of a translational deformity of the proximal tibia (shaft medialization in relationship to the epiphyseal segment).

41.6 Special Considerations

A detailed medical history and physical exam should be obtained.

In the physical exam we should document the range of motion of the hip, knee, and ankle. The torsional profiles of the tibia and of the femur are documented by measuring the foot/thigh angle, the progression foot angle along the gait, and hip range of motion with the patient lying supine and prone. We document the patellofemoral tracking assessing it for presence of instability and/or apprehension. A comprehensive knee exam is then performed, documenting the integrity status of the main ligaments of the knee.

The following image studies are requested.

- Knee radiographs: anteroposterior, lateral, patellar axial, and Rosenberg.
- Extremity alignment study (full weight-bearing standing long-leg radiographs).
- Magnetic resonance: for cases of suspected associated soft tissues injuries (cartilage, ligaments, and menisci).

Based on these studies, the following measurements are obtained.

- Joint orientation angles (mechanical proximal tibial, mechanical lateral distal femoral, joint convergence).
- Femorotibial angle.
- Patellar height (Blackburn-Peal or Insall-Salvati-Index).
- Tibial slope.

The preoperative planning should be based on the principles described by Paley (CORA: Center of rotation of angulation) and Strecker. The planning calculates a lateral closing wedge that will correct the mechanical proximal tibial angle and bring the mechanical femorotibial angle (mFTA) to a value of 0 to 2 degrees of valgus, depending on the degree of cartilage loss in the medial compartment. It is important to consider that if the preoperative planning determines that the only way to correct the mechanical femorotibial angle is by increasing the mechanical proximal tibial angle to a value superior to 93 degrees, a new planning should be carried out considering a double-level osteotomy (distal femur and proximal tibia). A mechanical proximal tibial angle superior to 93 degrees may have adverse effects to knee ligament balance in case of a future conversion to a total knee replacement.

41.7 Special Instructions, Position, and Anesthesia

The patient should be positioned supine on a radiolucent operative table.

General anesthesia and regional anesthesia are both appropriate.

We leave a tourniquet on the most proximal aspect of the thigh, but we rarely use it. We consider important to be prepared in case an unexpected bleeding takes place.

A single antibiotics dose is provided at the time of anesthesia induction.

The legs are not leveled on the table, and this facilitates intraoperative fluoroscopic images on multiple projections.

41.8 Tips, Pearls, and Lessons Learned

- Fibula osteotomy is not necessary for corrections in the coronal plane varying from 8 to 10 degrees of valgization. For corrections superior to 10 degrees, an oblique osteotomy performed at the midshaft of the fibula will facilitate the closing of the tibial wedge.
- A subperiosteal dissection is needed at the level of the osteotomy. A blunt, curved, periosteal elevator should elevate the popliteus muscles on the posterior edge of the tibia. A blunt Hohmann retractor should be placed in front of the popliteus muscle and on the posterior tibial cortical. This retractor will protect the neurovascular bundle along the osteotomy procedure.
- In case of a pure coronal plane correction, two oblique Kirschner wires are inserted from lateral to medial, converging on the epiphyseal medial cortical. The oscillating saw will cut the bone following the direction of the wires. It is important that we preserve the hinge intact, which increases the stability of the final construct.
- If an associated torsional correction is planned, the most proximal Kirschner wire is inserted perpendicular to the axis of the tibia, and the second wire is inserted from distal lateral to proximal medial, converging to the perpendicular wire on the medial tibial cortical. In this case, the hinge will not be preserved, as the perpendicular cut will allow for the torsional correction, followed by the coronal plane realignment, after the resection of the lateral-based bone wedge.
- Nonlocking implants provide enough stability to a tibial lateral closing-wedge osteotomy. We recommend the use of a large fragment 4.5-mm five-hole dynamic compression plate (DCP). The plate is contoured to match the curvature of the proximal tibia. The osteotomy site is located between the second and the third holes of this plate.
- The most distal screw of the plate should be inserted from proximal lateral to distal medial. The orientation of this screw is critical as it will push the plate against the bone, compress the osteotomy site, and secure the correction of the alignment.

41.9 Difficulties Encountered

- The fibula may prevent the reduction of the osteotomy gap, and in this case a fibula osteotomy is needed: It is important to perform an oblique osteotomy, which allows for displacement of the fibula favoring the closure of the tibial osteotomy.

- Variations of anatomy may occur in the proximal tibia and significant bleeding may occur if the dissection is not performed subperiosteally.
- Fractures of the medial tibial cortical may occur if the wedge was not completely removed and the surgeon pushes very hard to close the osteotomy. The removal of the wedge may be difficult due to adhesions of soft tissues on the posterior tibial cortical.
- Significant hematoma and compartment syndrome may develop and require prompt recognition and urgent treatment, especially when a lateral closing wedge is associated with torsional correction of the proximal tibia.

41.10 Key Procedural Steps

- The surgical procedure starts with a diagnostic/therapeutic knee arthroscopy. The purpose of the arthroscopy is to document the extent of cartilage/meniscus damage and, moreover, to confirm the integrity of the lateral compartment of the joint. During the arthroscopy, cartilage and meniscal flaps may be excised. We have performed a concomitant anterior cruciate ligament reconstruction in a few cases, especially in individuals who had varus knee in association with anterior knee instability.
- An anterolateral incision measuring approximately 8 cm is performed. The subcuticular and superficialis fascia are opened in line with the skin. The fascia of the tibialis anterior is opened leaving a stripe of 5 mm parallel to the anterior tibial crest. A subperiosteal elevation of the tibialis anterior is carried out. Hemostasis is performed with electrocautery. Once the anterolateral quadrant of the tibia is exposed, we perform a blunt dissection of the popliteus muscle, on the posterior cortical of the tibia. It is critical to keep the periosteal elevator on bone and in front of the popliteus muscle. The anterolateral and posterolateral quadrants of the tibia are then freed up from soft tissues. A Hohmann elevator is placed anteriorly under the patellar tendon. A second Hohmann is placed posteriorly in front of the popliteus muscle (▶ Fig. 41.1a,b).
- Two Kirschner wires are inserted to determine the wedge of the osteotomy. The level of the osteotomy will coincide with the interval between the second and third holes of the plate. The wires will be inserted in an oblique fashion from distal lateral converging to the medial cortical on the proximal tibia. The distances between the wires on the lateral cortical should match the preoperative planning. This distance represents the lateral base of the closing wedge and has to correlate with the desired angle of correction.
- The osteotomy is performed with an oscillating saw, under protection of Hohmann retractors. Special attention should be given to protect the patellar tendon anteriorly and the neurovascular structures posteriorly (▶ Fig. 41.1c,d).
- The osteotomy is performed above the level of the anterior tibial tubercle. In case the anterior tibial tubercle is too proximal, and the epiphyseal segment is relatively short, we perform a biplanar cut as described in the technique of medial open-wedge tibial osteotomy. Having a cut behind and parallel to the anterior tibial tubercle allows us to perform the transverse cut posterior to this initial cut, and when we rotate the leg internally the tibial tubercle will follow the tibial shaft.
- The wedge is removed, and the osteotomy is gradually closed.
- A prebent narrow 4.5-mm DCP plate is applied to the proximal tibia. The first screw is a 6.5-mm cancellous fully threaded screw, which is applied parallel to the joint, at the most proximal hole of the plate. The second screw is a 4.5-mm cortical screw which is inserted in an oblique fashion, from proximal lateral to distal medial, at the most distal hole of the plate. This screw will compress the osteotomy laterally and push the plate distally against the tibia. The two following

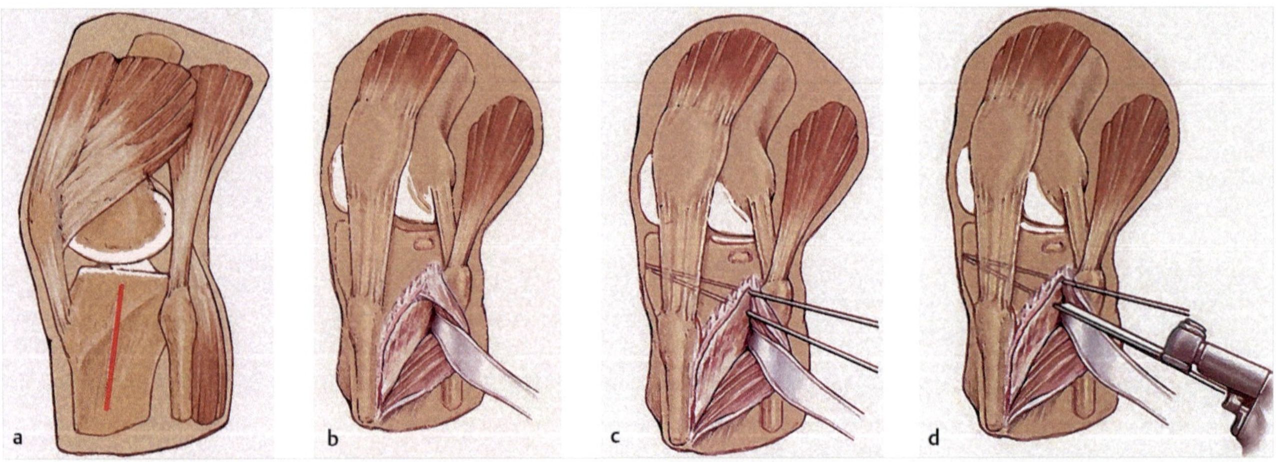

Fig. 41.1 Key Steps of the surgical procedure. **(a)** Anterolateral approach to the proximal tibia; **(b)** a blunt Hohmann retractor is placed on the posterior cortical of the proximal tibia, in front of the popliteus muscle; **(c)** two Kirschner wires, determining the angle of the wedge to be resected are inserted from lateral to medial, converging on the medial cortical of the proximal tibia; **(d)** an oscillating saw is used to resect a proximal tibial wedge, using the Kirschner wires to guide the resection.

screws are applied through the second and third holes of the plate, respectively. The screw inserted through the second proximal hole of the plate is directed from proximal lateral to distal medial, compressing the medial cortical. The screw inserted in the third hole of the plate is angled from distal lateral to proximal medial, crossing the osteotomy site complementing the compression and improving the stability of the bone-implant construct. The final screw is inserted through the hole number four of the plate, with the purpose of neutralization (▶ Fig. 41.2).

- If the intact fibula blocks the complete closure of the tibial osteotomy, a fibular osteotomy is necessary. This is the typical outcome for osteotomies aimed to correct deformities superior to 10 degrees of varus. We prefer a midshaft fibular osteotomy, which is performed through a small longitudinal incision just proximal to the distal third of the fibula. After a blunt preparation at the osteotomy site, Hohmann retractors are placed around the fibula, protecting the surrounding soft tissues. A delicate oscillating saw is used to perform a short oblique fibular osteotomy. It is critical to irrigate the fibula along with the use of the oscillating saw. It is also mandatory to protect the entire surface of the osteotomy with retractors, preventing iatrogenic soft tissues damage.
- It is possible to add up to about 18 degrees of torsional correction in addition to the correction of the varus deformity in the coronal plane, but in these cases a prophylactic fasciotomy and neurolysis of the peroneal nerve in the technique described by Paley must be done. To correct the axial plan, the most proximal osteotomy line should be perpendicular to the tibial axis, and parallel to the joint line. A 5.0-mm Schanz pin is inserted proximal and distal to the osteotomy line. The Schanz pins should be inserted with an inclination that reproduces the amount of desired correction. For example, if 10 degrees of internal torsional correction of the distal segment is desired, the most proximal Schanz pin is inserted perpendicular to the axis, while the distal Schanz pin is inserted with 10 degrees of external torsion in relationship to the proximal pin. Once the osteotomy is completed, the

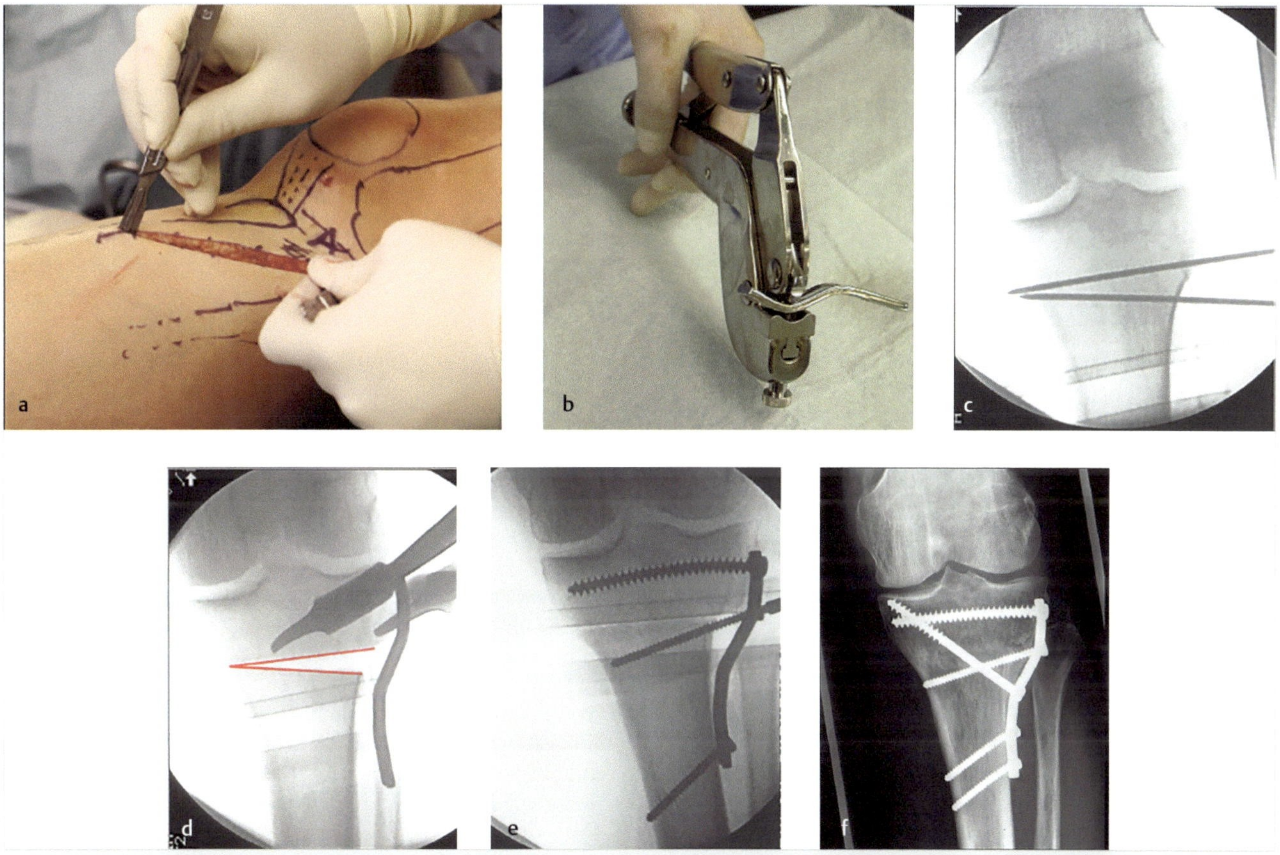

Fig. 41.2 Surgical steps of a lateral tibia closing-wedge valgus-producing osteotomy. **(a)** Anterolateral approach to the lateral tibial head; **(b)** precontouring a 5-hole 4.5-mm dynamic compression plate (DCP) plate; **(c)** two K-wires are placed in the proximal tibia determining the angle of the desired correction; **(d)** after performing the saw cuts and removal of the wedge, the plate is contoured to match the offset of the anterolateral aspect of the proximal tibia taking into consideration the amount of correction; **(e)** the first screw is inserted in the proximal aspect of the tibia and parallel to the joint. It is a fully threaded 6.5-mm cancellous screw. The second screw is a 4.5-mm cortical screw inserted distally and obliquely to promote compression at the lateral osteotomy site. We insert the third screw (4.5-mm cortical) into the second proximal hole of the plate. **(f)** Final construct depicting alignment correction and a technique of absolute stability, which may allow for early weight-bearing. Observe that we insert a partially threaded 6.5-mm cancellous screw in hole number 3 of the plate, from distal to proximal, crossing the osteotomy site and, therefore, promoting compression on the medial column of the tibia.

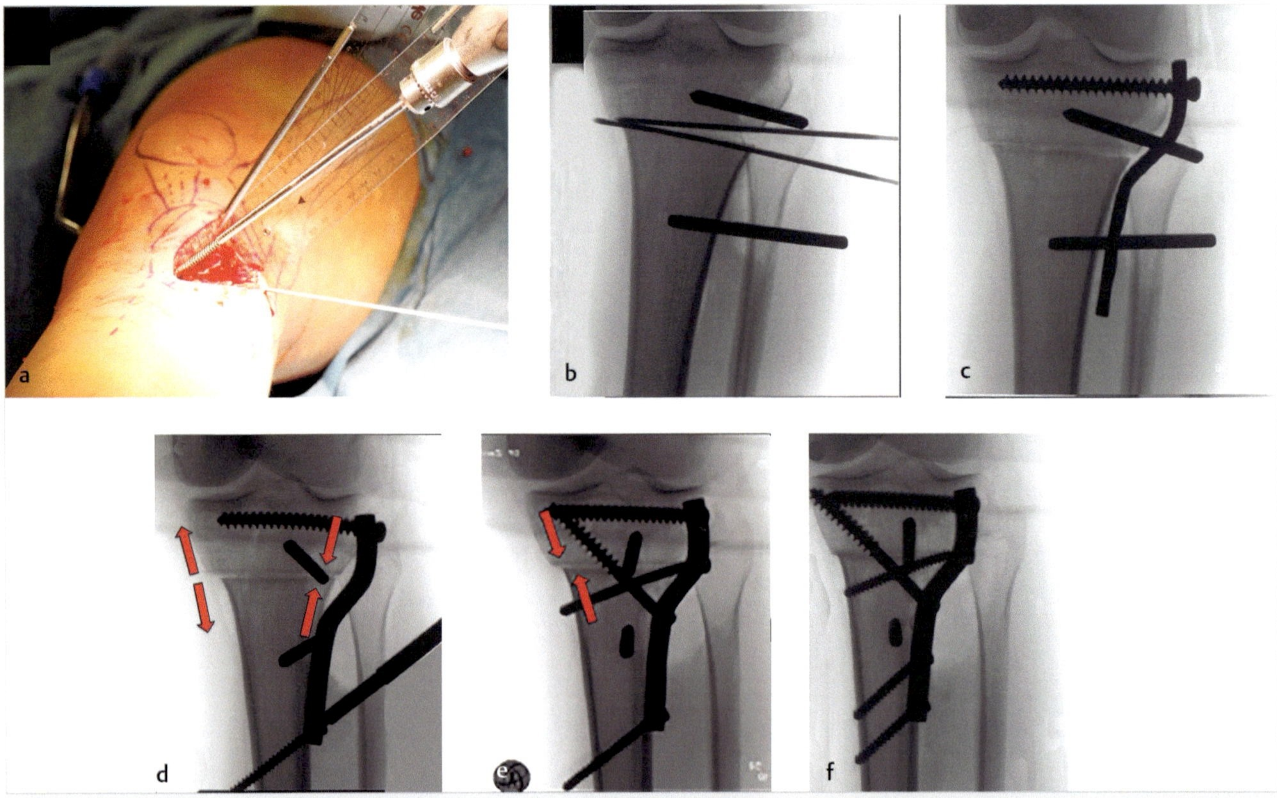

Fig. 41.3 Clinical intraoperatives illustrating a torsional correction in association with a lateral proximal tibial valgus-producing closing-wedge osteotomy. **(a)** Strategic placement of 5.0 Schanz pins to the proximal tibia, determining the angle of torsional correction; **(b)** illustration of the osteotomy site after resected wedge; **(c)** aspect of the osteotomy after complete lateral gap closure; **(d)** the application of the distal oblique screw promotes compression at the lateral osteotomy site, but may add gap in the medial cortical; **(e)** the two following screws cross the osteotomy and promote compression at the medial cortical of the tibia; **(f)** final construct illustrating that the Schanz pins are parallel to each other in the axial plane, and the osteotomy is fixed with absolute stability. The Schanz pins are removed at the end of the procedure.

two pins are lined up and this will generate 10 degrees of internal torsion of the distal fragment. The Schanz pins should be used as guiding pointers—they must not be used as levers. An additional external fixator bar may provide mechanical control and hold the pins in line if needed. Next, an ascending oblique osteotomy, directed from distal lateral to proximal medial is performed. This second osteotomy line should determine an angle with the first osteotomy line, which will determine the amount of correction in the coronal plane (▶ Fig. 41.3).

41.11 Bailout, Rescue, and Salvage Procedures

- It is critical to protect the neurovascular bundle with a Hohmann retractor placed in front of the popliteus muscle and on the posterior cortical of the proximal tibia. A tourniquet should be left on the most proximal aspect of the thigh and in case significant bleeding takes place, a vascular repair may be necessary. The surgeon should be prepared for this unexpected outcome.
- The fracture of the medial hinge does not have the same impact and outcomes as observed in open-wedge osteotomies. A closing-wedge osteotomy has a broader surface area and is fixed under axial compression. This reduces the importance of an additional hinge fixation.
- In cases of associated torsional correction, one should consider a maximum of about 18 degrees of internal torsional correction of the distal fragment. The greater the correction the higher the likelihood of compartment syndrome and peroneal nerve compromise. In those cases, a preventive release of the peroneal nerve should be performed in addition to an oblique fasciotomy of the tibialis anterior muscle.
- Postoperative hematoma should be promptly identified and drained avoiding compression to neurovascular structures and compartment syndrome.
- Nonunion cases are rare but should be addressed following protocols for long bones nonunion emphasizing the improvement of biomechanics and biology at the osteotomy site.

41.12 Pitfalls

- Preoperative planning should include not just the analysis of the coronal plane but also the sagittal and axial plane.
- Under- or overcorrection is possible while performing corrective osteotomies. It is important to stick to a detailed preoperative planning and to confirm it intraoperatively with

fluoroscopy and usage of an alignment rod. The patient should also be informed that the postoperative correction may not match the exact preoperative planning and in case this is only noticed postoperatively, a revision procedure may be considered to optimize the lower limb alignment.

- A closing-wedge osteotomy is more demanding than a proximal tibial open-wedge technique. The closing wedge requires a precise execution of the wedge resection, and sometimes an additional fibular osteotomy. If the osteotomies are not complete and the wedge is not completely removed, the tibial gap will not be completely closable. Consequently, undercorrection and delayed union may take place.
- Patients should be advised to stop smoking prior to surgery and should not be using nonsteroid anti-inflammatory drugs after surgery aiming to optimize their chances of a faster and uneventful bone healing.

42 Opening Wedge Distal Femur Osteotomy—Valgus Knee

Mitchell I. Kennedy, Zachary S. Aman, Connor Ziegler, Robert F. LaPrade, and Lars Engebretsen

42.1 Description

Varus-producing lateral opening-wedge distal femoral osteotomy (DFO) is a well-documented treatment option for genu valgum deformity with associated lateral compartment overload and isolated lateral compartment osteoarthritis (OA) in the young adult patient and for patients with chronic medial collateral ligament (MCL) injuries with genu valgus alignment.

42.2 Key Principles

When a DFO is combined with a cartilage repair procedure, the aim of the correction is neutral alignment of the limb. The amount of correction is calculated by the offset of the mechanical axis, which represents a straight line from the center of the femoral head to the center of the talar dome. The percentage across the tibial plateau is designated by the medial edge representing 0% and the lateral edge 100%. Valgus malalignment is thereby determined from a mechanical axis falling at or further than the apex of the lateral tibial eminence, or > 56% across the tibial plateau in the coronal plane. If there is mild degenerative disease in the lateral compartment, the mechanical axis should be adjusted a few degrees beyond neutral alignment, with overcorrection to the apex of the medial tibial eminence. With advanced degenerative disease, overcorrecting the axis to unload the degenerated compartment may be desired.

The osteotomy correction angle aims to restore the mechanical axis through the apex of the medial tibial eminence, or 41% of the width along the tibial plateau from medial to lateral. The intersection of two lines drawn through the apex of the medial tibial eminence, one originating from the femoral head and the other from the center of the talar dome, creates the necessary osteotomy correction angle. This angle is then transposed to the distal femur creating a triangle (apex medial pointed toward adductor tubercle) with the angle measured in degrees correlating to the height in mm of the osteotomy cut required for the alignment correction (▶ Fig. 42.1).

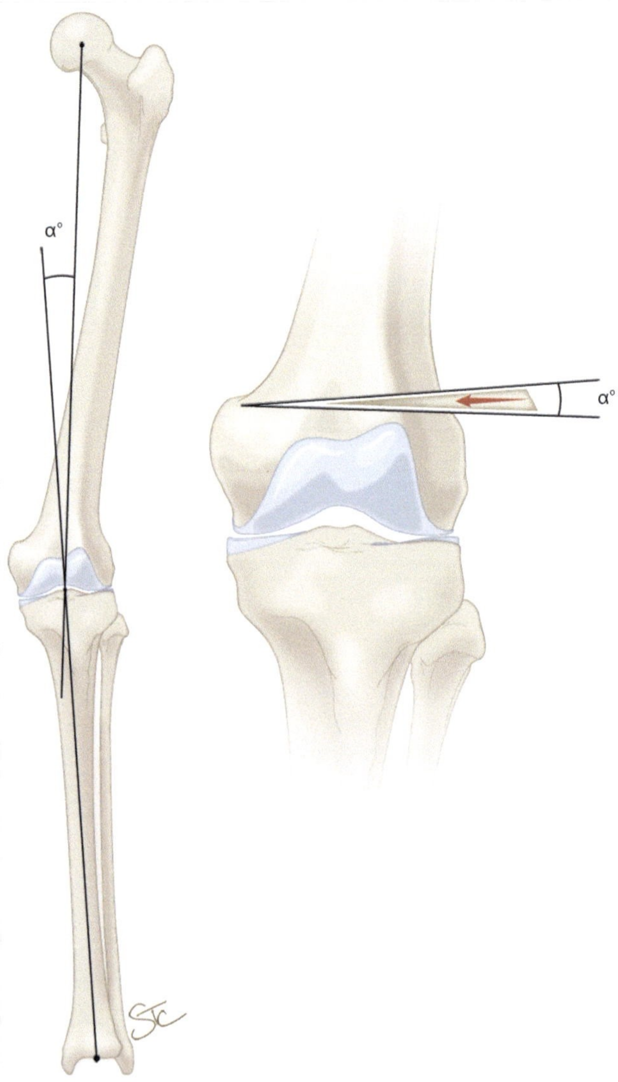

Fig. 42.1 Preoperative planning. The angular difference between the mechanical axes of the femur and tibia is transposed to the site of the planned osteotomy and represents the magnitude of correction needed to restore limb alignment (neutral mechanical axis).

42.3 Expectations

High survival rates, improved knee scores, and correction of valgus deformity to a near-neutral tibiofemoral angle or mechanical axis have been consistently reported following DFOs, which is especially vital for postponing the requirement for a total knee replacement. At 10 years follow-up, 80% survival rates have been reported. At a mean follow-up of 78 months, DFO has an approximately 10% reported complication rate and a 35 to 40% reported reoperation rate with the most common reasons cited as the removal of hardware or conversion to arthroplasty. If the patient requires a TKA in the future following a DFO, the procedure can be more challenging and associated with greater complications. Reports have correlated a decrease in clinical outcomes for TKA following both opening- and closing-wedge DFO procedures.

42.4 Indications

Patients of young age who have unicompartmental chondral pathology and malalignment may undergo an osteotomy procedure to allow preservation of the native knee joint; neutral alignment of the limb is the primary goal. Valgus malalignment can result from trauma, lateral meniscectomy, or metabolic diseases. The initial approach for treatment of isolated lateral compartment OA and valgus malalignment is conservative management, but failure leads to possible treatment options of osteotomy or arthroplasty. Specific indications are:

- Genu valgus deformity with concurrent isolated lateral compartment OA in young active patients or symptomatic MCL incompetence.
- Valgus tibiofemoral angulation of ≥ 12 degrees with narrowing of the lateral joint space.
- Valgus malalignment of > 10 degrees in a patient with a biological age of < 65 years.

42.5 Contraindications

- Patellofemoral or medial compartment joint pain.
- Osteoarthritis or meniscal deficiency in the compartment intended for weightbearing.
- Active smoking.
- Knee range of motion less than 90 degrees.
- Severe medial compartment arthritis.
- Severe tricompartmental osteoarthritis.
- Tibiofemoral subluxation.

42.6 Special Considerations

In the setting of an abnormally steep sagittal-plane slope with ACL insufficiency or an abnormally flat sagittal-plane with posterior cruciate ligament insufficiency, an anterolateral or lateral opening wedge tibial osteotomy may be more effective as opposed to a DFO because a DFO does not change the joint slope.

42.7 Special Instructions, Position, and Anesthesia

- The patient should be placed in the supine positioning on the operating table with a well-padded high-thigh tourniquet on the operative leg, and a bump to secure the knee at 30 degrees of flexion.
- General endotracheal anesthesia is typical; epidural or spinal anesthesia can also be used.
- To prevent venous thrombosis, the contralateral knee is positioned in extension with a pneumatic compression device.
- Examination under anesthesia is performed to evaluate the cruciate and collateral ligaments, as well as to assess range of motion and the presence of recurvatum.
- Postoperatively, the patient remains non-weightbearing with full knee motion allowed and an immobilizer for 8 weeks.

42.8 Tips, Pearls, and Lessons Learned

- Patients with chronic central and/or medial ligamentous laxity and concurrent genu valgum deformity should be managed with a varus-producing DFO in addition to ligamentous reconstruction/repair.
- Preoperative templating via full-leg standing alignment radiographs permit a reproducible approach for determining the amount of correction necessary using the osteotomy correction angle.
- During the procedure, the following tips will guide the surgeon in avoiding undesired surgical outcomes:
- Slow and meticulous progression will contribute to avoiding fracture propagation of the medial cortex.
- Ensuring the complete release of both the anterior and posterior femoral cortices allows for expansion of the osteotomy site.
- Leaving 1 cm of medial cortex creates a sufficient hinge to prevent medial cortex fracture.
- Following the placement of hardware for the osteotomy, malleable bone graft should be used for complete filling of the void.
- Lastly, for the purposes of improving postoperative range of motion and reducing risk of arthrofibrosis, an early rehabilitation program should be instigated immediately postsurgery.

42.9 Difficulties Encountered

- Major complications can occur when blunt retractors are not used to effectively protect the posterior neurovascular bundle.
- When creating the osteotomy too quickly, a medial sided fracture can occur, necessitating fracture management of the medial femoral cortex and increased operative time.
- Plate and screw placement must be meticulously performed to assure no penetration of hardware into the knee joint and to prevent ITB irritation.
- Plates should be contoured around the lateral femoral cortex to prevent hardware prominence.
- To determine the proper correction angle and osteotomy trajectory aimed at achieving a neutral axis; long-leg weightbearing mechanical axis radiograph is imperative.

42.10 Key Procedural Steps

- A 4- to 6-cm skin incision is made along the axis of the distal ITB (▶ Fig. 42.2). The ITB is incised in the direction of its fibers to expose the vastus lateralis muscle, which is subsequently separated from the posterior aspect of the ITB gently with a Cobb elevator.
- Next, careful subperiosteal dissection is performed, and the vastus lateralis is elevated until the femoral diaphysis and metadiaphyseal flare are identified.
- At this point, neurovascular structures must be protected using a blunt retractor placed anteriorly underneath the quadriceps tendon and another placed posteriorly above the hamstrings. In addition, a radiolucent retractor should be used to visualize the posterior femoral cortex under fluoroscopy for further protection of the neurovascular structures.
- Intraoperative fluoroscopy should be utilized while creating the osteotomy. Once a guide pin is inserted into the lateral femoral cortex, an osteotomy guide is placed over the pin and adjusted until fixed at the desired angle with a second guide pin.
- After assurance that retractors are adequately protecting the neurovascular structures, a reciprocating saw is used to penetrate the lateral femoral cortex for a depth of 3 to 4 mm

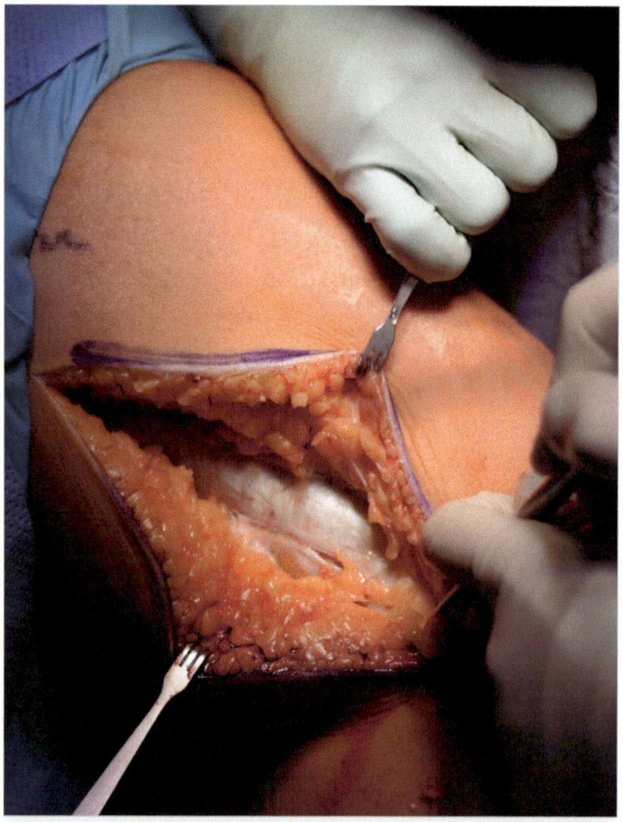

Fig. 42.2 An initial hockey-stick incision of 4 to 6 cm along the axis of the distal ITB is made, followed by an incision of the distal ITB in the direction of its fibers exposing the VLM. ITB, iliotibial band; VLM, vastus laterals muscle.

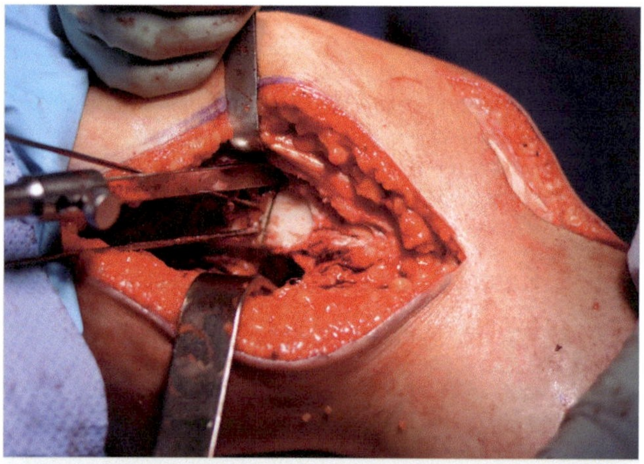

Fig. 42.3 Following the use of a reciprocating saw along the osteotomy guide to a depth of 3 to 4 mm, a series of osteotomes from lateral to medial and progressing from small-medium-small in size are utilized for penetrating the anterior cortex through the posterior cortex; live fluoroscopy aids in ensuring protection of the posterior neurovascular structures.

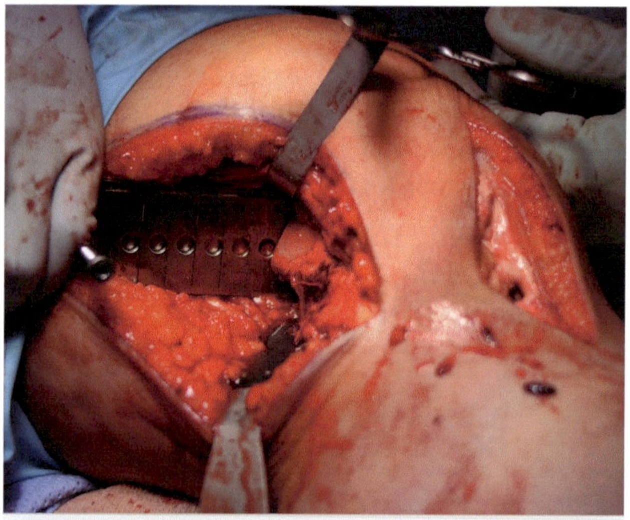

Fig. 42.4 Angular correction is obtained by a spreading device that consists of two blunt angled tines and a handled compactor, which is slowly inserted into the path created by the series of osteotomes and expanded to the degree of varus correction desired.

while following the osteotomy guide border to ensure proper directionality.

- Once this is achieved, the saw and guidewires are removed.
- The completion of the osteotomy is performed by advancing a series of osteotomes from lateral to medial (▶ Fig. 42.3). A small osteotome is first used to penetrate the anterior cortex, a medium osteotome is used for the midcortex, and finally a small osteotome is used to complete the posterior cortex cut while using both live fluoroscopy and direct palpation posteriorly to ensure protection of the posterior neurovascular structures. A medial cortical hinge of 1 to 2 cm is necessary to prevent iatrogenic fracture of the medial cortex.
- Angular correction begins with a spreading device, which is inserted into the path created by the osteotomy and slowly expanded to the desired degree of varus correction (▶ Fig. 42.4).
- The angle of correction is then stabilized by two blunt angled tines assembled with a handled compactor slowly inserted into the defect. It is essential that this step be taken in a slow, controlled fashion to avoid iatrogenic fracture of the medial cortex.
- Final confirmation of angular correction and overall fixation is performed under fluoroscopy.
- Fixation of the osteotomy site begins with the removal of the handled compactor and subsequent placement of the osteotomy plate into the defect.
- The plate is then fixed proximally using 4.5-mm fully threaded bicortical nonlocking screws. In addition, 6.5-mm fully threaded cancellous screws are inserted distally (▶ Fig. 42.5). The choice of plate varies according to surgeon preference; however, Tomofix (Synthes, West Chester, PA) and Puddu plates (Arthrex, Naples, FL) are the most commonly used.
- Once the plate is confirmed to be secured and the fixation hardware in the desired position, demineralized bone matrix allograft is then compacted into the osteotomy defect (▶ Fig. 42.6 and ▶ Fig. 42.7). It is imperative that care be taken to assure soft tissue, muscle fibers, and neurovascular structures are carefully protected.

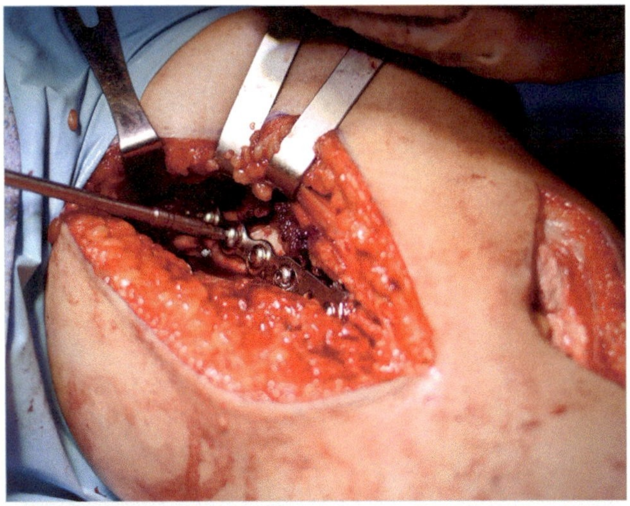

Fig. 42.5 The osteotomy site fixation is secured by a plate that is fixed proximally with a 4.5-mm fully threaded bicortical nonlocking screws, and distally by 6.5-mm fully threaded cancellous screws.

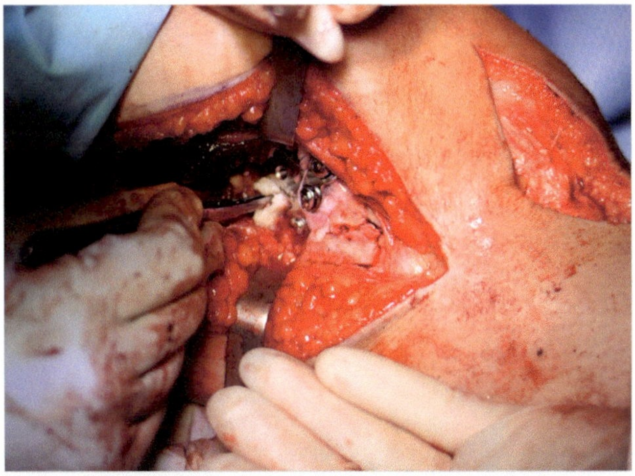

Fig. 42.6 Following plate fixation and confirmation of its positioning, demineralized bone matrix allograft is then compacted into the osteotomy defect, filling the void created by the osteotomy procedure.

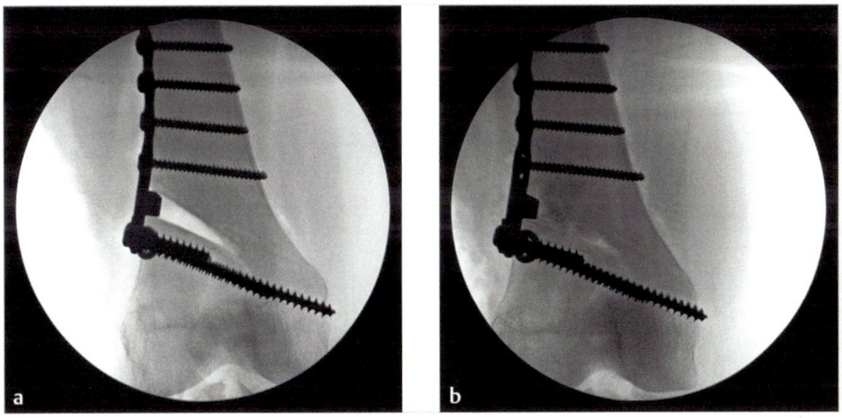

Fig. 42.7 Intraoperative fluoroscopy confirming plate positioning and length of fully threaded screws **(a)** and following insertion of demineralized bone matrix allograft into the osteotomy void **(b)**.

42.11 Bailout, Rescue, and Salvage Procedures

If the osteotomy is progressed too aggressively, the medial femoral cortex may fracture and result in instability of the distal femur. In this case, the medial side of the distal femur must undergo an open reduction and internal fixation. Additional hardware can lead to higher risk of complications and possible compromise of the desired osteotomy correction angle. Also, rehabilitation protocols must be slowed to allow more time for sufficient bony healing after a rescue procedure.

42.12 Pitfalls

- Improper directionality of guide pins or failure to utilize imaging can result in undercorrection or residual malalignment (▶ Fig. 42.7).
- Neurovascular structures must be protected throughout the entirety of the procedure; failure to use proper posterior retractors can lead to iatrogenic neurovascular injury.
- Aggressive use of an osteotome can result in medial femoral cortex fracture or instability leaving little medial cortex for adequate hinging.
- Improper screw placement can lead to diminished outcomes particularly with intra-articular penetration.
- The lateral distal femoral plate may cause ITB irritation.
- Failure to adhere to rehabilitative protocols can lead to poor motion or compromise of the osteotomy correction as a result of early weightbearing before bony healing.
- Failure to allow sufficient time for bone graft incorporation prior to initiation of weightbearing can potentially lead to loss of reduction and undercorrection of the valgus deformity; more secure fixation may make this less of an issue.
- Full range of motion (ROM) must be achieved within 4 to 6 weeks of surgery otherwise knee stiffness can result and limit overall functionality and restoration of normal knee kinematics.

43 Closing Wedge Femur Osteotomy—Valgus Knee

Philipp Lobenhoffer

43.1 Description

The medial distal femur closing wedge varus-producing osteotomy (MDFCWO) is a procedure indicated to correct frontal plane deformities around the knee, offloading the lateral compartment of the joint. A biplanar technique and fixation with a specific plate fixator allow for fast healing.

43.2 Key Principles

The wedge resection is performed only in the posterior two-thirds of the femur. An ascending osteotomy is created in the anterior third of femur which exits the bone 3 cm proximal to the horizontal osteotomy line. After gradual closure of the osteotomy gap, a plate fixator with specific configuration is used for fixation.

43.3 Expectations

No large patient series exist on distal femur osteotomies. Survival rates of 80% at 10 years are reported for a lateral open wedge as well as for medial closing wedge procedures. A series of 107 MDFCWO performed in our institution from 2014 to 2015 revealed only four cases with delayed healing which needed revision with bone graft and a supplemental small-fragment plate on the opposite cortex. We found one plate breakage in a female obese patient. This case required a revision fixation with a lateral locking plate and bone graft. Overall, the series showed free knee range of motion in all patients, since we used a muscle-sparing surgical technique.

43.4 Indications

Constitutional and posttraumatic frontal plane valgus deformities of the distal femur of more than 3 degrees in symptomatic patients.

43.5 Contraindications

- Osteoarthritis of the medial compartment (Outerbridge grade 3 or 4).
- Total loss of the medial meniscus.
- Acute or chronic infections.
- Significant deficit of range of motion (this type of extra-articular osteotomy does not improve range of motion).
- Poor soft tissue conditions on the surgical site.
- Degeneration of the patellofemoral joint is not a contraindication, since the realignment in the coronal plane will improve patellofemoral tracking.

43.6 Special Considerations

A detailed deformity analysis and planning using a high-quality long-leg radiograph is mandatory. The wedge resection is defined using established planning routines. In valgus deformity, the target of correction is neutral alignment of the leg. This implicates that the Mikulicz line crosses the tibial plateau at 44% of the entire width medial to lateral after the operation. Formal overcorrection should not be aimed for in valgus cases. Technically, software planning allows for calculation of the wedge base width. This parameter is easy to control during surgery. After closure of the osteotomy gap, the alignment can be rechecked under fluoroscopy by use of an alignment rod oriented between center of the hip and center of the ankle joint.

43.7 Special Instructions, Position, and Anesthesia

The procedure can be performed with general or regional anesthesia. The patient is placed supine on a radiolucent table. The hip, knee, and ankle must be accessible for fluoroscopy. The opposite leg should be lowered at the level of the hip around 20 degrees. This allows access to the medial distal femur of the operated leg. Alternatively, the involved leg can be raised by placing flat bolsters under the femur. The entire leg including the iliac crest is prepared and draped. A tourniquet is not necessary in this procedure. The fluoroscope is placed on the ipsilateral side.

43.8 Tips, Pearls, and Lessons Learned

This procedure may be performed with a formal medial subvastus approach elevating the vastus medialis from the distal femur. This approach allows the surgeon the control of the anatomy at the medial side of the femur directly. With more practice the surgeon may reduce the incision length and the exposure to the metaphyseal area of the femur. In case of small skin incisions, the use of a particular saw (Precision saw), which oscillates only at the tip, helps to avoid skin damage. The fixation of the plate is then performed with an additional stab incision over the shaft area of the femur.

The osteotomy of the posterior cortex of the distal femur in its central and lateral aspect has inherent risks of vascular injuries due to the small distance of the saw to the femoral artery and vein. This saw cut should only be performed with protection of the posterior area. We use the special Tomofix retractor, alternatively a flat Hohmann retractor (preferable radiolucent), which we place under fluoroscopy in line with the osteotomy. When using the Precision saw, the surgeon may place one finger of his nondominant hand behind the bone to protect the vessels. This special saw has minimal oscillations and does not cause collateral injuries.

The wedge resection should be marked with Kirschner wires. The hinge point is placed 5 mm medial of the lateral cortex as low as possible in the distal femur condyle. The osteotomy should be placed just above the posterior chondral border of the lateral femur condyle which can be identified in the fluoroscope.

The osteotomy should be closed gradually by axial compression from the foot. All bone remnants have to be removed from the gap allowing for precise closure.

The position of the plate should be checked with the fluoroscope in anteroposterior and lateral projections before final fixation. The plate should be aligned with the shaft and have no overhang anteriorly or posteriorly.

43.9 Difficulties Encountered

The three-dimensional anatomy of the distal femur is not easy to understand. The surgeon should train this procedure on models and pass a cadaver training ahead of the surgery.

The hinge point of this osteotomy should be very low in the lateral femur condyle, with a distance of 5 mm to the lateral cortex. The wedge resection must be defined precisely with two or four K-wires. The amount of resection on the medial cortex must be calculated by the planning program ahead of the surgery. A caliper can be used during the procedure to define the right distance of the K-wires.

The saw should be advanced inside of the space created by the K-wires ("cage").

The ascending osteotomy should start 10 mm posterior to the anterior border of the distal femur at the level of the osteotomy. This osteotomy aims to leave the femur cortex 30 mm proximal to the horizontal cut. This osteotomy line is roughly parallel to the posterior cortex of the femur shaft, ascending with an angle of 10 degrees. The anterior cortex must be divided completely to allow the osteotomy to close.

43.10 Key Procedural Steps

A medial skin incision starting at medial epicondyle and extending 3 to 5 cm proximal. Incision of the fascia of the vastus medialis muscle. The intermuscular septum is exposed and incised parallel near to the posterior edge of the femur. The posterior soft tissues are gently separated from the posterior cortex of the femur. The planned wedge osteotomy is marked with K-wires. Osteotomy of the posterior two-thirds of the femur is guided by the K-wires. The posterior saw cut must be protected by a retractor. Anterior ascending osteotomy. Removal of the wedge (▶ Fig. 43.1). Gradual closing of the osteotomy. Correct alignment is checked by fluoroscopy and an alignment rod. Fixation with a specific plate fixator for the medial femur (Tomofix Medial Distal Femur, Depuy Synthes). Submuscular (MIPO) insertion of the plate. Distal screw placement, compression screw, and proximal screw placement by stab incision and transmuscular screw insertion (▶ Fig. 43.2 and ▶ Fig. 43.3).

43.11 Bailout, Rescue, and Salvage Procedures

Closure of the osteotomy may be blocked by residual cortical bone areas which have not been addressed by the saw. We use a thin metal liner to palpate the osteotomy line under fluoroscopic control. Remaining cortical bone (usually in the posterolateral condyle area) is then cut under fluoroscopy. The lateral

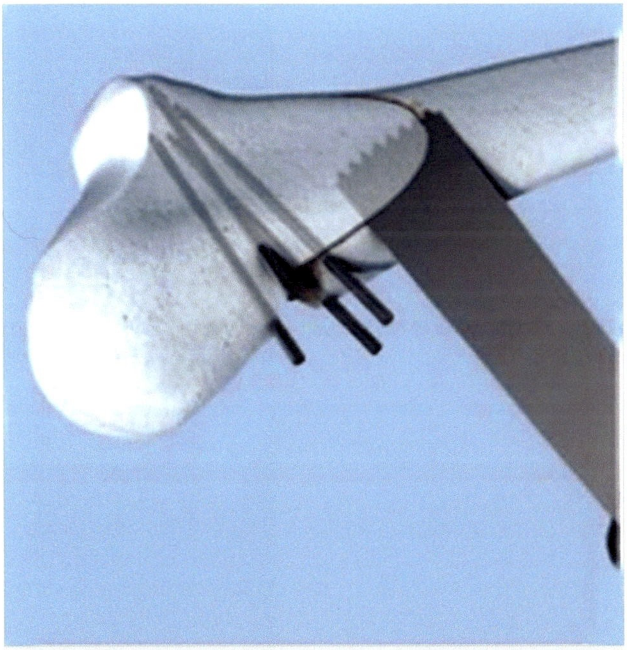

Fig. 43.1 Principle of closed wedge biplanar osteotomy to treat valgus deformity. A wedge of suitable size is removed from the posterior two-third of the medial femur metaphysis. The hinge point is placed 5 mm medial to the lateral cortex as inferior as possible, avoiding damage to the cartilage of the lateral femur condyle. A second osteotomy plane is created in the frontal plane. This bone cut exits the femur cortex around 3 cm proximal.

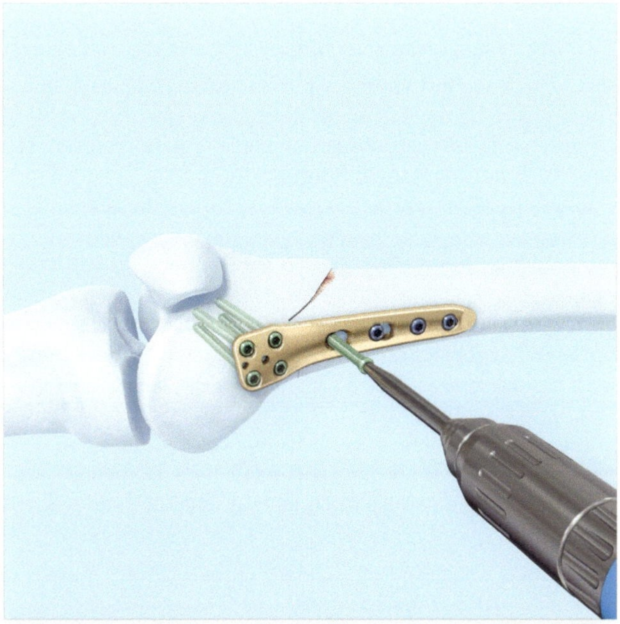

Fig. 43.2 The osteotomy is closed gradually by axial compression. A specific plate fixator is placed on the bone. The distal locking screws are inserted. Compression of the osteotomy gap can be achieved by inserting a cortical screw in the combination hole proximal to the osteotomy gap. The screw is replaced by a locking screw after placement of the other screws. The proximal screws can be inserted either via the incision or by a separate stab incision placed over the second plate shaft hole.

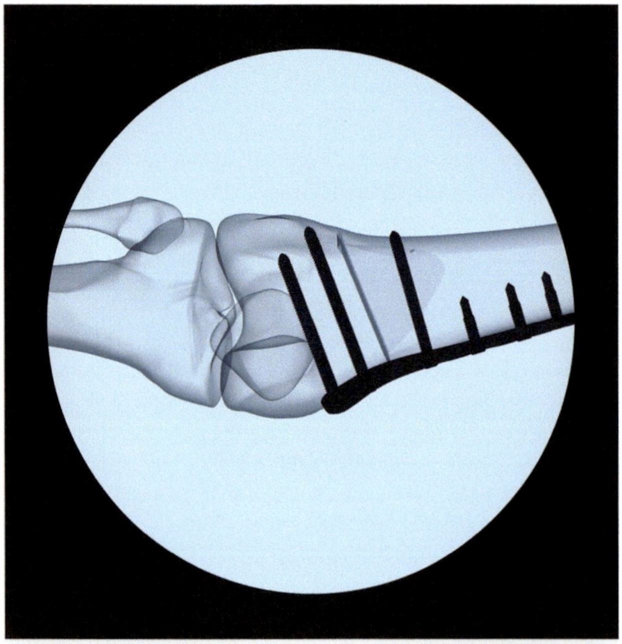

Fig. 43.3 Picture illustrating an intraoperative fluoroscopic control, which reveals proper placement of the hardware and an intact contralateral hinge.

hinge can also be weakened carefully with the oscillating saw under fluoroscopy. Complete bone-on-bone closure may be hindered by small fragments in the gap. We gradually close the osteotomy with the saw inserted. The two osteotomy planes now act as a slotted guide block for the saw. The saw is carefully moved back and forth in the gap, thus cleaning out all obstacles. The pressure on the foot is increased and finally the saw blade is captured in the gap. When the blade is then removed, the osteotomy should close completely.

Instability of the osteotomy may occur when the lateral hinge is disrupted. Usually, translation of the fragments will be recognized in the fluoroscope. Due to the biplanar configuration, manual reduction is normally possible. The hinge can be stabilized by a K-wire starting in the lateral condyle and passing into the lateral femur shaft. The plate fixator should be fixed distally with locking screws. Then a lag screw is inserted into the proximal fragment. Tightening of the screw results in compression of the osteotomy planes and reduction of any translation. Further locking screws are inserted and at the end the lag screw can be exchanged to a bicortical locking screw. If there is doubt on the stability, we recommend placing an additional small fragment plate on the lateral side bridging the osteotomy hinge. This plate reproduces the hinge and increases the stability dramatically. Dislocation of the osteotomy in the sagittal plane is very uncommon because of the second osteotomy plane on the anterior cortex. The surgeon has to ensure that the proximal and distal part of the femur is supported by bolsters during the procedure. If the osteotomy area is not supported, a posterior gap may occur causing an extension deformity of the distal fragment.

Distal femur osteotomy has a significant risk for vascular injury due to the close anatomical relationship of femoral artery and vein. When an oscillating saw is used, a special long and narrow saw blade is mandatory due to the throw of the saw tip (width 15 mm, length 90–110 mm). The design of the tip is crucial. Aggressive tooth as used for arthroplasty is dangerous in this procedure and should not be used. We prefer a specific saw design where only the tip of the saw moves (Precision Saw). If significant bleeding occurs during the procedure, injury to the femoral artery and vein must be anticipated and treated following the standards of vascular surgery.

Delayed healing may occur after femur osteotomy. If the patient cannot load his leg after 6 weeks and radiographs show signs of instability (gap formation, hypertrophic callus formation around the osteotomy), a computed tomography (CT) scan is performed. We recommend autologous bone grafting plus an additional small plate on the lateral side in these cases to speed healing.

43.12 Pitfalls

- Overcorrection or undercorrection: exact planning is mandatory because intraoperative adjustments are difficult to achieve once the wedge is resected.
- Hinge disruption: the osteotomy should only be closed by axial compression from the foot. The use of varus stress will break to hinge and cause instability.
- Instability of the fixation: varus stress after final fixation of the plate should not result in opening of the lateral hinge area of the osteotomy. If instability is observed, an additional lateral small-fragment plate should be used to support the lateral hinge.
- Misplacement of the plate: the position of the plate should always be checked with the fluoroscope in both planes before final fixation. Misplacement may compromise screw insertion due to the uniaxial locking mechanism and cause pain.

44 Unicompartmental Knee Replacement—Medial Compartment

Douglas D.R. Naudie

44.1 Description

Medial unicompartmental knee arthroplasty (UKA) is an attractive alternative to total knee arthroplasty (TKA) or osteotomy for selected patients with pain and degenerative disease confined to the medial compartment of the knee.

44.2 Key Principles

- UKA can provide excellent patient satisfaction, function, and long-term survivorship in carefully selected patients.
- In joint replacement registries, UKA demonstrates a lower risk of infection than TKA, but an inferior survivorship to TKA with higher revision rates.
- In interpreting registry data, we need to consider that many different models of UKAs have been performed.
- UKA has been shown to a cost-effective alternative to TKA.
- UKA is less tolerant for limb malalignment or component malposition than TKA.

44.3 Expectations

Patients undergoing medial UKA can experience a faster recovery and return to work and recreational activity than TKA. Excellent second-decade survivorship can be achieved in properly selected patients using UKA implants that have demonstrated a successful clinical performance. Patients aged 60 years or younger can expect to return to their regular physical activities after medial UKA, with approximately two-thirds of the patients achieving a high level of activity.

44.4 Indications

- Specific indications for UKA are highly variable among surgeons.
- Medial UKA is traditionally reserved for older (> 60 years), thin (< 82 kg), and low demand patients.
- Traditional indications for medial UKA also included patients with good preoperative flexion (> 90 degrees), a flexion contracture less than 5 degrees, angular deformity less than 10 degrees of varus (that is passively correctable), and intact cruciate ligaments.
- However, indications have since expanded to include younger, heavier patients and patients with anterior cruciate ligament (ACL) deficiency.
- Some recent studies have reported simultaneous or staged ACL reconstruction in addition to medial UKA in younger patients with higher functional demands, but further studies are required to validate these recommendations.

44.5 Contraindications

- Tricompartmental arthritis (with diffuse pain), inflammatory arthritis, and severe flexion contractures (> 10 degrees) are strong contraindications to medial UKA.
- Global pain symptom distribution or patellofemoral pain in the absence of radiographic patellofemoral disease should also be considered contraindications to medial UKA.
- Fixed, noncorrectable varus deformities should be considered a relative contraindication to medial UKA. Preoperative stress radiographs can assist in determining correctability of coronal plane deformity.
- ACL deficiency should be considered a contraindication for mobile-bearing UKA and lateral UKA.
- Surgeons should be wary of recommending medial UKA in patients who have undergone previous meniscectomy or who have severe chondrocalcinosis in the lateral compartment.
- Young age and obesity are not absolute contraindications to medial UKA, but UKA should be used with caution in young patients with high activity levels and morbid obesity.
- Intraoperatively, surgeons should consider conversion to TKA if they identify exposed subchondral bone beneath the patella, particularly under the lateral patellar facet, or in the lateral compartment.

44.6 Special Considerations

Progression of disease (sometimes secondary to overcorrection of mechanical alignment) and aseptic loosening are the two most common reasons for early revision of UKA. These reasons emphasize the need for proper patient selection and meticulous surgical technique. The overall complication and reoperation rates and implant survivorship are comparable for mobile-bearing and fixed-bearing UKA designs.

44.7 Special Instructions, Position, and Anesthesia

Unicompartmental knee arthroplasty is always performed with the patient in the supine position. The use of a thigh support or commercially available footrests and/or lateral bolsters, as well as the use of an upper thigh tourniquet, is up to the individual surgeon's discretion. The contralateral leg should always be well padded, especially under the heel. We shave the hair around the area of the planned incision just prior to sterile preparation of the leg. The nurses scrub the leg with an iodine or chlorhexidine solution as the surgical team scrubs. The entire leg is then prepared with an iodine or chlorhexidine solution, based on surgeon preference. A limb extremity sheet with a rubberized central portion having a hole is placed over the

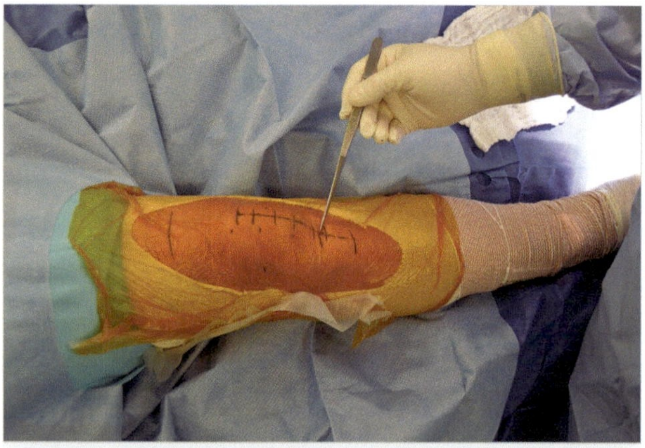

Fig. 44.1 In this case, a small parapatellar incision is marked in preparation for a medial unicompartmental knee arthroplasty. As can be seen in the picture, the skin marking extends distally in the event that a total knee arthroplasty is deemed more appropriate intraoperatively.

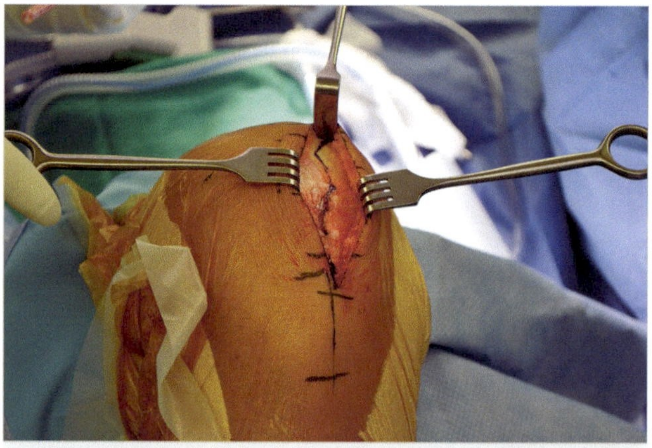

Fig. 44.2 The proximal midvastus extension of the medial parapatellar arthrotomy is marked with a sterile marking pen in this muscular male patient.

stockinet and pulled proximally to the tourniquet level. The foot and ankle are wrapped with an elastocrepe bandage or flannel roll to prevent the stockinet from sliding during manipulation of the foot during the procedure. As an alternative, a sterile surgical glove can be placed over the foot. A window is cut in front of the stockinet on the anterior aspect of the knee, and the appropriate landmarks about the knee are palpated and marked with a sterile pen. The incision is drawn to include a distal extension in the event conversion to TKA is required, and transverse lines are made to assist with wound alignment at the time of closure (▶ Fig. 44.1). If a tourniquet is employed, it is usually inflated to 300 mm Hg, so as to have the tourniquet at least 100 mm Hg above the systolic blood pressure. The pressure can be elevated as high as 350 mm Hg in hypertensive or obese patients. Intravenous prophylactic antibiotics and tranexamic acid are given within 20 minutes of tourniquet inflation.

44.8 Tips, Pearls, and Lessons Learned

We have found that a systematic approach to exposure has allowed us to rapidly and safely expose even the most complex patients and deformities. Our preference is to bring the leg into a figure-four position and apply a thyroid grasper to the medial soft tissue sleeve. This aids in the exposure of the medial side of the joint by subperiosteal dissection of the medial collateral ligament. The medial collateral ligament is dissected in a continuous flap using electrocautery with vertical strokes for a variable distance depending on the type and degree of preoperative deformity. It is very important not to inadvertently over-release the medial collateral ligament. A limited proximal midvastus release can also be employed and allows the patella to slide out of the way in stiff, muscular knees (▶ Fig. 44.2). After resection of the proximal tibia, we have found it useful to inspect the bone cut to evaluate the pattern and distribution of arthritis, and to ensure that the resected fragment is appropriate and matches the patient's native tibia slope (▶ Fig. 44.3). Using conventional instrumentation, it is also very helpful to check the alignment using an extramedullary reference.

44.9 Difficulties Encountered

The most common complications of minimally invasive medial parapatellar arthrotomies are those associated with wound healing. Unless adequate soft tissue closure is achieved, areas of wound separation or drainage can occur. Therefore, careful management of the soft tissue and meticulous deep and superficial wound closure is important. Overzealous retraction of the patella during flexion of the knee can result in damage to the patellar cartilage or avulsion of the patellar tendon from the tibial tubercle. This can be an extremely disabling problem and every effort should be made to avoid it. Problems with insufficient or aggressive tibial resection can also occur. It is usually best to begin with a conservative tibial resection, as it is easy to take additional bone if required. Tibial malrotation can also occur if there is poor exposure or if there are retained intercondylar notch osteophytes that can push the reciprocating vertical saw cut into excessive internal or external rotation. Finally, careful attention must be made to implant trials to ensure there is no overhanging or edge loading of the tibial or femoral components.

44.10 Key Procedural Steps

44.10.1 Exposure

A short medial arthrotomy incision is generally employed for medial UKA. The incision is made from the superomedial pole of the patella to the top of the tibial tubercle. It is taken through the skin and subcutaneous tissue and down through the deep fascia. The skin can be gently undermined with Metzenbaum scissors to create a mobile window to work through. The arthrotomy is taken through the medial capsule and synovium approximately 5 mm from the medial border of the patella. The quadriceps can be spared or for wider exposure a "mini" midvastus incision can be performed (▶ Fig. 44.2). This minimally invasive incision gives

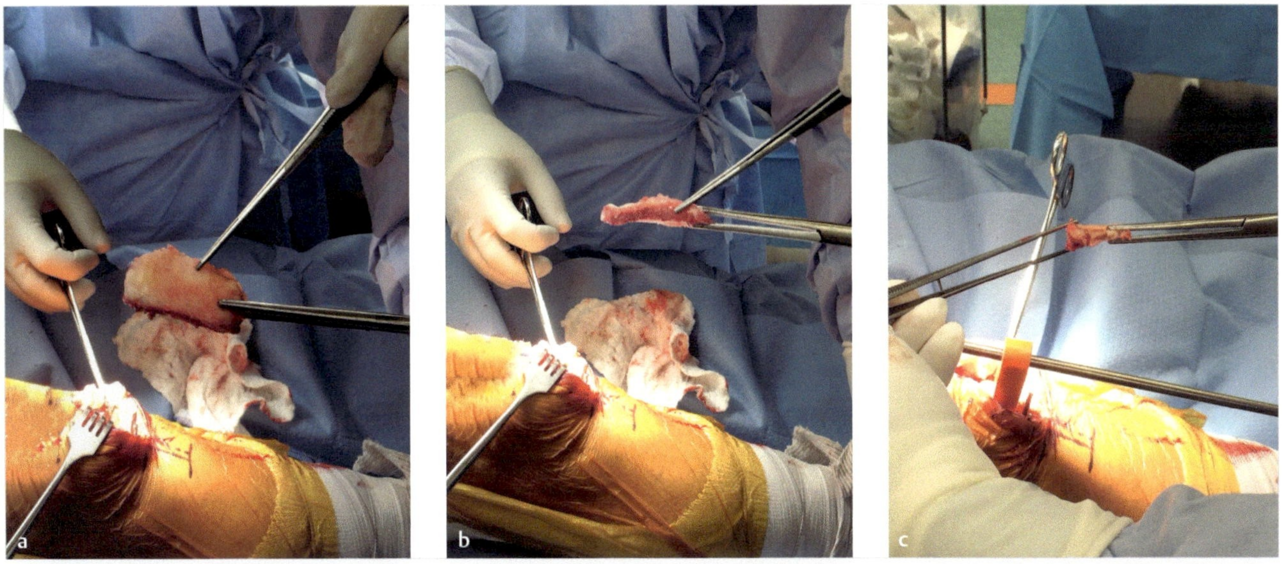

Fig. 44.3 The resected fragment of proximal tibia is evaluated to assess **(a)** the disease pattern, **(b)** the resected tibial slope, and **(c)** the varus-valgus resection. In this patient, the resected tibial slope matches the patient's anatomy and is slightly thicker mesially (held by the forceps) than medially (as is the desired case in medial unicompartmental knee arthroplasty [UKA]).

excellent visualization of the medial condyle and medial proximal tibia without patellar eversion.

After the initial exposure is performed, it is important to inspect the patellofemoral joint, the ACL, and the lateral compartment to decide whether to proceed with UKA or whether conversion to TKA is indicated. It is also important to remove intercondylar notch osteophytes as these may push the vertical tibial cut into excessive internal or external rotation. Removal of medial patellar osteophytes and distal femoral medial osteophytes also facilitates retraction of the patella and helps with sagittal and coronal plane balancing. Removal of the medial meniscus is typically performed after proximal tibial resection and/or distal femoral resection, as the extension space is especially well visualized.

44.10.2 Tibial Preparation

The sequence of bone cuts performed will depend on the specific UKA system used, but most begin with the proximal tibia cut. The tibial cut is typically done with an extramedullary (EM) referencing technique, which is familiar to most surgeons. The EM guide is aligned with the tibial crest and/or the base of the second metatarsal. It is very important to ensure proper varus/valgus positioning, tibial slope, and depth of resection. Too much tibial resection exposes weaker tibial bone, can result in fracture, and can make any future revision surgery very difficult. The vertical tibial cut is made along the lateral margin of the medial femoral condyle at the medial edge of ACL insertion. It is important to limit the distal extent of this resection, as this can create a stress riser for medial plateau fracture, but it is typically limited by the tibial cutting block. It is important to try and remove the proximal tibial fragment in one piece, as the resected fragment can be inspected to ensure it matches the patient's native tibia slope (▶ Fig. 44.3). The bone fragment can also assist with implant sizing; the appropriate size can be measured off the inferior aspect of the resected fragment using the opposite-side trial for comparison.

44.10.3 Femoral Preparation

The sequence of femoral bone cuts performed will again depend on the UKA system used, and specifically whether the femur is referenced using an intramedullary (IM) technique (and somewhat independent of the tibial cut) or using an EM technique based off the proximal tibial resection. Intramedullary systems require the use of an IM femoral guide rod, to which the posterior and/or distal femoral resection guides attach. The insertion position of the IM rod is important and is typically located 1.0 cm anterior and 0.5 cm medial to the intercondylar notch aiming toward the femoral head. The advantages of IM guides are that they can assist with retraction of the patella and help determine flexion/extension of the femoral component as well as rotation. Extramedullary UKA systems typically proceed with resection of the distal femur after tibial resection to create a rectangular extension space. Distal femoral resection guides are inserted into the knee in extension and are aligned off the initial tibial cut. These are pinned in place and resection of the distal femur is completed in extension (▶ Fig. 44.4). Once distal resection has been performed, sizing and rotation of the posterior femoral resection is accomplished with the knee in flexion (▶ Fig. 44.5).

44.10.4 Balance, Trialing, and Insertion

Balancing the UKA to the appropriate tension also depends on the specific UKA system employed. Those systems that resect the posterior femur using IM alignment guides calculate the amount of distal resection required to balance the knee, often using feeler gauges and milling techniques. Those systems that resect the distal femur using EM alignment typically employ

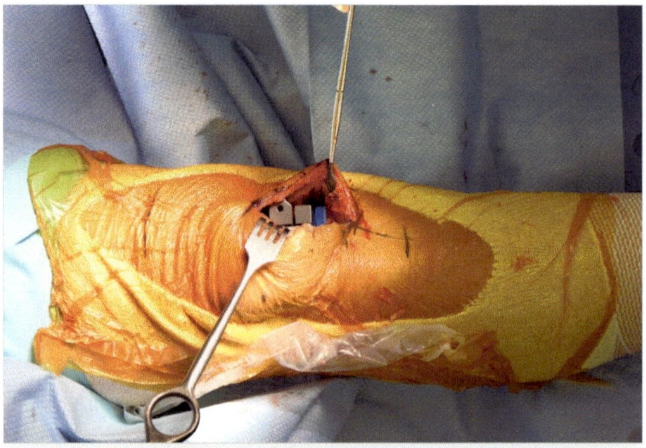

Fig. 44.4 In this extramedullary technique, the distal femoral cutting block is linked to the cut surface of the tibia and pinned in place to allow resection of the distal femur in extension.

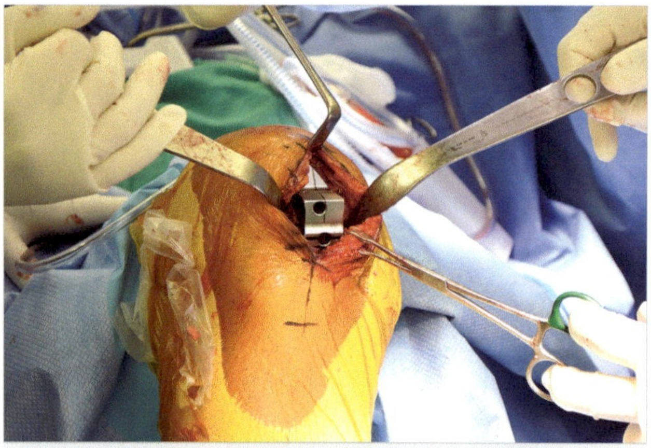

Fig. 44.5 In this extramedullary technique, femoral sizing and rotation of the posterior femoral resection is accomplished with the knee in flexion.

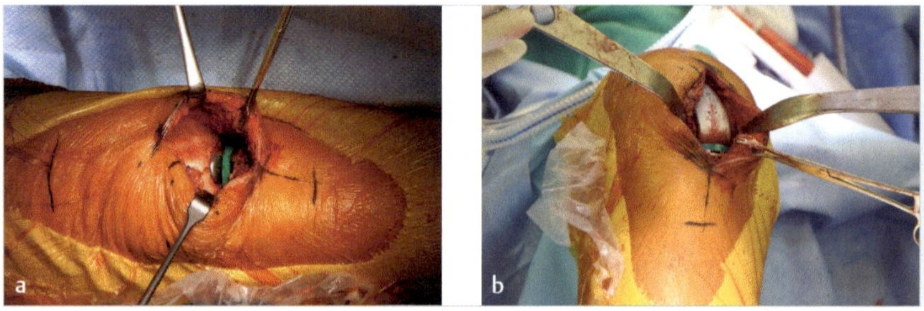

Fig. 44.6 These fixed-bearing implant trials demonstrate excellent sizing and component-to-component orientation in **(a)** extension and **(b)** flexion.

spacer blocks and recutting jigs to ensure symmetrical extension and flexion spaces.

All UKA techniques require implant trialing to ensure proper soft tissue balance (which is especially important in mobile-bearing implants), alignment, and component-to-component orientation (▶ Fig. 44.6). Great care should be taken to avoid overhang of the tibial component anteromedially or of the femoral component anteriorly (as this may cause patellofemoral impingement). Polyethylene trials are necessary to determine the correct polyethylene thickness to optimize soft tissue balance and mechanical axis alignment.

Once trialing is completed and the surgeon is pleased with the selected implants, the femur and tibial are prepared for final implantation. The individual UKA system employed will determine whether this involves lugs, pegs, or keel preparation. During tibial preparation, it is very important to avoid penetration of the anterior or posterior tibial cortex. During cementation, it is best to try and extrude any cement out anteriorly to avoid any retained cement on the posterior aspects of the femur or tibia.

44.10.5 Postoperative Management

The postoperative recovery of the medial UKA performed through a short medial incision is very brief. Most procedures can be performed on an outpatient basis with limited need for postoperative narcotics. Local infiltration of long-acting anesthetic agents into the posterior capsule and periarticular soft tissues can greatly assist with pain management. Patients can expect to return to usual activities within 6 weeks.

44.11 Bailout, Rescue, and Salvage Procedures

The surgeon should always be prepared to convert to a TKA, should intraoperative findings dictate that a UKA is not appropriate, or in the case of intraoperative fracture, ligament injury, or inability to correctly balance the knee. If conversion to TKA is required, adequate exposure is essential. Fortunately, with a systematic approach, even the most complex problems can be exposed without the need for any major extensile exposure. Stemmed implants may be needed if an intraoperative fracture occurs.

44.12 Pitfalls

- Impingement of the femoral component on the patella can occur and result in progression of patellofemoral arthrosis leading to need for revision.
- When performing medial UKA with a mobile-bearing design, impingement of the mobile bearing on the lateral wall of the tibial tray in UKA must be avoided or bearing dislocation may occur.
- A deep vertical cut of the tibial should be avoided to prevent fracture of the medial tibial plateau.

45 Unicompartmental Arthroplasty—Lateral Compartment

Eli Kamara and Stefano A. Bini

45.1 Description

This procedure addresses symptomatic unicompartmental arthrosis of the lateral compartment of the knee.

45.2 Key Principles

Lateral unicompartmental knee arthroplasty (UKA) is a resurfacing procedure that can replace a painful articulation due to loss of articular cartilage. It cannot correct severe deformity, ligamentous injury and imbalance, severe bone loss, or significant knee flexion contracture.

45.3 Expectations

Compared to total knee arthroplasty (TKA), UKA patients feel that their knee is closer to a physiologic knee. Knee pain should be nearly absent, with improved coronal-plane alignment and nearly normal knee range-of-motion. UKA is associated with fewer complications and a more rapid recovery than total knee arthroplasty.

45.4 Indications

Patients are evaluated using a combination of clinical and radiographic criteria. On physical examination, symptoms should be localized to the lateral compartment only. The cruciate and collateral ligaments should be intact without any signs of instability or incompetency. Range of motion must be close to full extension with a minimum of 100 degrees of flexion. Valgus angulation should be less than ten degrees and correctable to neutral or at the very least to their native, nonarthritic alignment (if this can be assessed using the contralateral limb). Restoration of physiologic valgus can be confirmed with stress radiographs. On X-ray, the arthritis should be localized to the lateral compartment. The medial and patellofemoral compartments should ideally be free of osteophytes and subchondral sclerosis. The medial knee joint space should be normal; the patellofemoral compartment may have minor joint space narrowing. Asymptomatic mild patellofemoral disease can generally be accepted but should be addressed with the patient as a potential source of early failure. Magnetic resonance imaging (MRI) may be helpful to visualize the medial meniscus and anterior cruciate ligament (ACL). It is the practice of the authors to avoid lateral compartment UKA in the context of an ACL injury or medial meniscal tears. The former can lead to failure due to instability and the latter has a moderately high incidence of progression to osteoarthritis requiring TKA. Patients with posttraumatic arthritis from a healed lateral tibial plateau fracture may be candidates.

45.5 Contraindications

Patients less than 40 years of age may have a higher failure rate for UKA. However, for some patients, the idea of undergoing a procedure that bridges them to the fifth or sixth decade before their first TKA is an acceptable compromise. Obesity (body mass index [BMI] > 40) is not currently considered a specific contraindication for UKA. Patients with inflammatory arthritis, calcium pyrophosphate disease, less than 90 degrees of flexion, symptomatic medial meniscal tears, or ligamentous deficiency should not be offered this procedure. An adequate amount of bone stock is necessary for fixation; patients with severe bone loss or advanced osteonecrosis should not be treated with lateral UKA.

45.6 Special Considerations

In normal knee kinematics, femoral rollback occurs laterally, while the medial contact point is mostly stationary. The lateral collateral and posterior cruciate ligaments facilitate this rollback by keeping the lateral compartment relatively taught in full extension but loose in flexion. To allow for physiologic rollback, the surgeon must be mindful of recreating this relationship—a tight extension gap but a looser lateral flexion gap and ensure that the tibial component extends to the back of the tibial plateau, fully covering it. To achieve this relationship, careful consideration must be given to matching the patient's native tibial slope. In addition, due to the extent of the anteroposterior movement in the lateral compartment during flexion and the differential in the flexion and extension space, lateral UKAs do not tolerate mobile bearings as these have a high risk of "spinning out" and dislocating. Unconstrained mobile bearings are contraindicated in this procedure.

45.7 Special Instructions, Position, and Anesthesia

An adductor canal block is performed in the preoperative area and spinal or general anesthesia is administered in the operating room. The patient is positioned supine on a standard operating room table with a tourniquet placed on the proximal thigh. The leg can be held with a combination of sandbags taped to the bed, positioning posts, a side kidney post, or a leg holder depending on surgeon preference. Some surgeons prefer placing the leg in an arthroscopy-style leg holder to allow greater joint distraction.

45.8 Tips, Pearls, and Lessons Learned

- The lateral compartment of a normal knee has inherent laxity in flexion to allow for rollback of the knee to occur. In extension, the screw home mechanism tightens the lateral compartment for maximum stability at heel strike. Therefore, balancing the lateral compartment differs from balancing a medial UKA in which the gaps are evenly tensioned in flexion and extension. There should be 0 to 1 mm of tibiofemoral

gapping in extension (to avoid overloading the medial compartment), and 2 to 3 mm of gapping in flexion.
- UKA is very sensitive to cement technique. The authors prefer careful hand packing of cement into a dry bone bed along with cement coating of the implants.

45.9 Difficulties Encountered

It is the authors' preference to expose the knee through a medial parapatellar arthrotomy; exposure of the lateral compartment requires a standard arthrotomy, almost identical to that of a TKA. Patients with severe patella baja may require a more extensile exposure. Patients with a severe valgus deformity and laterally tracking patella may benefit from a lateral arthrotomy but generally are not candidates for a lateral UKA due to advanced patello-femoral arthritis.

45.10 Key Procedural Steps

45.10.1 Surgical Approach

- The knee is placed in 110 degrees of flexion.
- A midline incision is made centered over the superior pole of the patella and extended distally to the medial aspect of the tibial tubercle. It must be sufficiently proximal to allow exposure of the anterior femur and proximal femoral condyle; it is slightly smaller than the standard incision for a total knee replacement.
- A medial parapatellar arthrotomy is performed; the arthrotomy extends approximately 1–3 cm above the superior pole of the patella into the quadriceps tendon. The arthrotomy is carefully performed to avoid damage to the underlying medial and patellofemoral compartments. Care must be taken to not damage the anterior horn of the medial meniscus at the time of the arthrotomy.
- The ACL, medial compartment, and patellofemoral compartments are examined for pathology prior to proceeding.
- The anterior half of the lateral meniscus is removed, and the rim of the lateral tibial plateau is exposed (▶ Fig. 45.1).
- The weight-bearing center of the lateral compartment is marked with electrocautery on the tibia; the knee is brought to full extension and a corresponding mark is made on the femur (▶ Fig. 45.2). This mark will be used to set femoral component rotation and ensure that weight-bearing loads are transferred to the center of the tibial tray throughout the arc of motion.
- The knee is brought into 90 to 100 degrees of flexion and the patella is mobilized laterally; if the patella cannot be subluxated laterally at this point, extend the arthrotomy proximally an additional 1 to 2 cm into the quadriceps tendon. The suprapatellar synovium should be visible prior to proceeding and the patella subluxated sufficiently with a 90-degree angled retractor to access the lateral compartment.

45.10.2 Femoral Preparation

- The surgical technique guide for the selected UKA device should now be followed. It is our preference to perform the distal femoral cut first. Next the tibia is extended, and a mark made on the femur at the point where the center of the longitudinal axis of the tibia meets the femur in extension. The rotation of the femoral component should be set to match the mark made on the femoral condyle. This ensures that as the knee "screws home" and the tibia externally rotates in extension, the femoral component does not load the tibial tray at its outer rim, a common cause for early aseptic loosening and wear. Furthermore, the femoral component should be positioned as medially as necessary so that the center of the component contacts the center of the tibial tray at 90 degrees of flexion. Setting the rotation and medial to lateral position of the femoral component using this technique will ensure that the contact point between the two implants is always centered throughout the arc of motion. This frequently requires more medial translation than would seem appropriate. The tibial tray positioning should be in neutral coronal alignment or slight varus relative to the

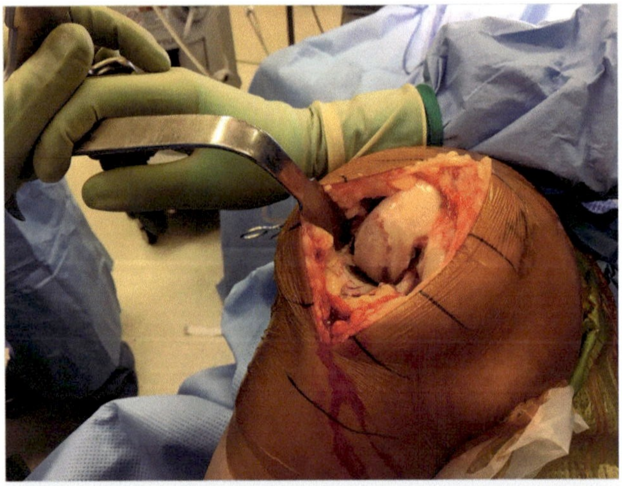

Fig. 45.1 Complete exposure of the lateral compartment is made using a midline incision and medial parapatellar arthrotomy.

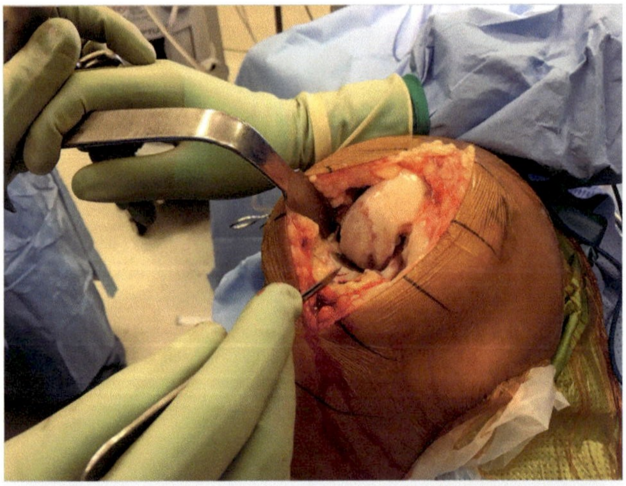

Fig. 45.2 The weight-bearing center of the lateral compartment is marked on the anterior edge of the tibia.

anatomic axis of the tibia and match the patient's anatomic slope; it should be sized to cover the tibia completely in the anterior-posterior plane and not overhang over the lateral cortical margin of the tibia.

- The author's preference is to use an intramedullary guide for the distal femoral cut if available. The medullary canal is entered using a drill and the marrow contents irrigated and suctioned to reduce the risk of a fat embolism. As most distal femoral cutting guides for UKAs assume that the medial joint cartilage has been worn through, any residual cartilage left on the femoral condyle is removed with a knife, saw, or burr until the subchondral bone is exposed. The guide is set in 4 degrees of valgus and pinned to the femur (▶ Fig. 45.3). The cut is performed with careful attention to not damage the patella or trochlea. The cut bone is measured with a caliper and confirmed to match the thickness of the implant minus the width of the saw and no adjustment is usually necessary for lost cartilage as wear in valgus arthritis is usually on the posterior, not distal condyle. If the resection is not deemed sufficient it is critical that more bone be resected at this point by advancing the cutting block and removing the necessary bone. It is very difficult to recut the femur at later stages of the procedure and under-resection at this stage could lead to a permanent flexion contracture following surgery.
- At this point the author's preference is to complete the femoral preparation. The femur is sized, and rotation is set using the resection guide. The guide is placed flat on the distal femoral cut and centered over the previously made rotational guide marks (▶ Fig. 45.4a, b). Hyperflexing the knee frequently helps position the guide correctly. A properly sized femur will have 1 to 2 mm of exposed bone above the anterior aspect of the guide to avoid impingement between the femoral component and the patella. The chamfer and posterior condyle cuts are performed paying attention to not cut the popliteus tendon in the process. The posterior condyle is measured to ensure a resection equal to that of the implant's posterior femoral condyle's thickness. It is important to understand the resection height built into the cutting jig for the posterior condyle in the system being used because the lateral compartment is particularly sensitive to over-resection of the posterior chamfer. Frequently, the posterior condylar cartilage is already worn down to subchondral bone and no cartilage needs to be removed. If the posterior chamfer bone resection is too thick, consideration should be given to moving the cutting block down by 1 or 2 mm prior to drilling the peg holes. No bone graft is required if this is done.

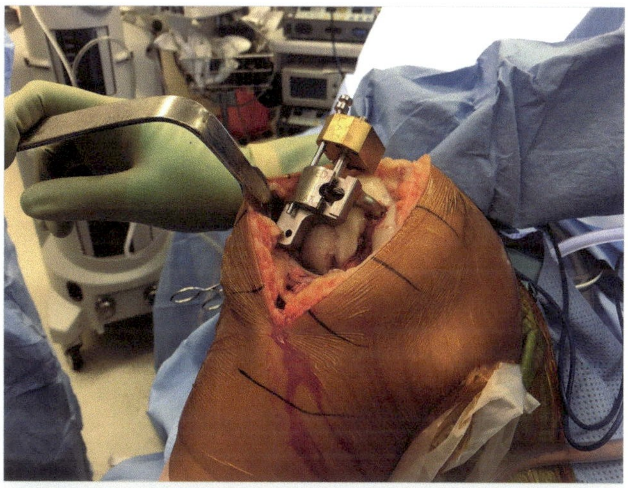

Fig. 45.3 The intramedullary femoral guide is shown pinned in correct position to the distal femur.

45.10.3 Tibial Preparation

- The tibia is then exposed by hyperflexing the knee and placing a 90-degree bent Homan retractor laterally to protect the lateral structures.
- An extramedullary guide is used for the tibia cut. In a fixed-bearing UKA, the tibial cut should follow the resection height recommended in the technique guide, often 4–6 mm in depth, in neutral mechanical alignment and aimed to recreate the patient's native slope (▶ Fig. 45.5a, b). The vertical tibial cut is performed first using a reciprocating saw. The rotation of the cutting block should match that of the tibial spine or the second metatarsal ray when looking from the top of the tibia (a drop rod is frequently used in this situation) to ensure appropriate positioning of the tibial tray as the knee "screws home" in extension. Further, the cut should not be so medial as to jeopardize the cruciate ligaments. If the angle for the vertical, coronal cut is difficult with the exposure, it can be made through a small vertical incision in the patellar ligament in line with its fibers (▶ Fig. 45.6a, b).
- The horizontal tibial cut is then made while protecting the patellar ligament and popliteus tendon with a curved Homan retractor purposefully placed by the surgeon at the level of the intended cut and behind the femoral condyle. Protecting the popliteus tendon is absolutely critical to the integrity of the lateral flexion gap. The cutting block will have already been positioned and pinned in place in order to replicate the

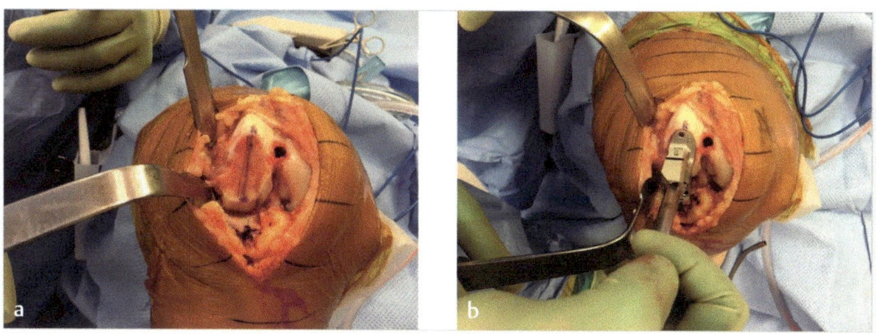

Fig. 45.4 After the distal femoral cut is made, the knee is extended, and the previous mark made in the center of the tibia is used to mark femoral rotation (**a**). The cutting-block for the anterior and posterior chamfers is then pinned in correct rotation (**b**).

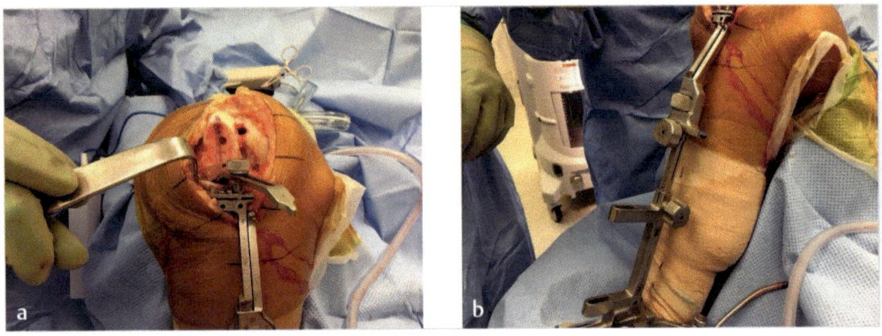

Fig. 45.5 An extramedullary guide is placed on the tibia and a stylus used to set the correct depth of resection (**a**). The extramedullary guide is shown set to reproduce the patient's anatomic tibial axis and posterior tibial slope (**b**).

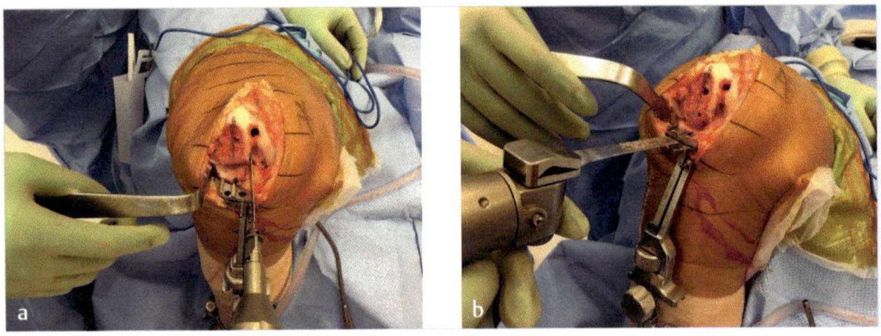

Fig. 45.6 A reciprocating saw is used to perform the vertical (**a**) and horizontal (**b**) tibial resections.

patient's native posterior slope adjusting for any posterior-lateral tibial bone loss. The height of the block should be positioned so that the resected bone and lost cartilage plus the thickness of the saw should equal the thickness of the tibial tray plus the thinnest available insert, generally 9 mm. Care should be taken to not undermine the tibial spine with the tibial saw. The resected bone is loosened using an osteotome, removed with a rongeur, ideally in one piece and measured for thickness with a caliper. Examining the resected tibial bone's sagittal profile from the side of the tibial spine shows the accuracy of the slope of the tibial cut.

45.10.4 Soft Tissue Balancing and Trialing

- At this point, any residual meniscal tissue and peripheral osteophytes are removed. Spacer blocks are used to perform a gross check of the gaps. The thickest spacer block should be selected that allows the knee to come into full extension with no more than 1 mm of slack. With the same block, the flexion gap should be 2 to 3 mm and not symmetric.
- The authors prefer to inject the periarticular injection cocktail at this time to give the epinephrine time to act and prevent postoperative bleeding.
- The tibial sizing jig is then used to size the tibia in the anterior-posterior and medial-lateral planes. Occasionally, a 1 to 2 mm sliver of bone needs to be resected from the tibial spine to accommodate the appropriate size tibial tray in the medial to lateral plane.
- Any peg holes or keel slots are then prepared for the tibial tray as needed for the implant being used.
- All the trial components are now inserted. With the trials in place, the flexion and extension gaps are checked; as previously stated, unlike a medial UKA 2 to 3 mm more laxity is preferred in flexion compared to extension to allow for unimpaired femoral rollback and to restore native joint laxity. In extension, there should be a 1 mm increased lateral laxity to avoid overstressing the medial joint.
- Minor adjustments can still be made at this point by varying the slope of the cut on the tibial side. If the knee does not come into full extension, the tibial slope can be decreased by 1 to 2 degrees (achieved by resecting 1–2 mm of bone from the front of the tibia but not the back) using the extramedullary cutting jig appropriately repositioned on the tibia to guide the saw. Similarly, if the knee is too loose in flexion the slope can again be decreased and a thicker insert inserted. If the knee hyperextends, the tibia and femur should be cemented separately, and the femoral component allowed to cure 1 to 2 mm proud of the subadjacent bone cuts. This can be achieved by placing the tip of the "wing" (or any flat instrument 2 mm thick) between the implant and the bone while seating it.

45.10.5 Component Insertion

- To prepare for cementation, the bony surfaces are irrigated with normal saline and then carefully dried. A sponge is packed into the back of the knee to catch any excess cement and prevent extrusion thereof into the back of the knee. The cement is hand pressurized diligently into the tibial cancellous bone as well as carefully placed on the back of the tibial tray component. The tray is inserted and impacted. The sponge is removed while applying manual pressure on the tibial component and any excess cement is removed. Cement is then hand pressurized into the femoral bone and the component is impacted in an identical fashion. After the liner is inserted the knee is taken through a range of motion to allow the cement to pressurize. Any excess cement is removed and the rest is allowed to set with the knee in extension.

- After releasing the tourniquet and checking for any bleeding, the arthrotomy is closed with #2 barbed suture, subcutaneous tissue is closed with a 2–0 barbed suture, and the skin is closed with 3–0 resorbable barbed suture, and skin glue. The senior author has stopped using steri strips for the closure without any undue complications. A thin, two-layer gauze dressing is now applied along with a thin occlusive dressing (Tegaderm, 3 M, St. Paul, MN). These are placed with the knee in full flexion to avoid blistering.

45.10.6 Postoperative Care

- The dressings are generally not removed until day 5 (unless soiled) and patients may wash at will immediately and after the dressing is removed.
- Patients are allowed to weight bear as tolerated and discharged home the same day with self-directed physical therapy for the first month; the authors' have seldom had any issues with poor range of motion or slow recovery after UKA and prefer to let the knee rest and rehabilitate at its own pace.
- When necessary to regain lost lower extremity musculature, formal strengthening exercises are begun after 4 to 6 weeks following surgery assuming normal recovery.

45.11 Bailout, Rescue, and Salvage Procedures

The authors always consent patients for a possible TKA; if the patient is an inappropriate candidate for a lateral UKA due to previously undiagnosed medial knee arthritis, focal articular lesions > 0.5 cm^2, or advanced lateral facet arthropathy, a TKA is performed. It is also possible to over-resect the lateral tibial plateau and find it difficult to balance the knee. In such a case a TKA is an excellent option.

45.12 Pitfalls

The success of a lateral UKA is dependent upon rigorous patient selection and careful balancing of the knee allowing for femoral rollback. With current patient selection guidelines and modern implants, 10-year survivorship is over 90% for lateral UKA and higher than medial UKA.

46 Unicompartmental Knee Replacement—Patellofemoral Compartment

Patrick Horst and Elizabeth A. Arendt

46.1 Description

Patellofemoral arthroplasty (PFA) is a surgical option that can lead to long-term pain relief and improved functional outcomes for patients with severe anterior knee pain and isolated patellofemoral (PF) osteoarthritis (OA).

46.2 Key Principles

Preoperative clinical symptoms, examination findings, and radiographic appearance of PF OA are important preoperative considerations for patient selection. Implant positioning and proper surgical technique are crucial to functional improvement, pain relief, and long-term implant survival. Complications and poor outcomes can be minimized with appropriate indications and surgical technique.

46.3 Expectations

Newer implant designs are shown to have excellent functional outcomes and long-term implant survivorship when strict indications and contraindications are followed. Most studies demonstrate a revision rate of less than 10 to 20% at 10 to 15 years.

The most common short-term complications following the procedure include synovitis, swelling, pain, and PF subluxation; these are largely due to lack of restoration of PF tracking mechanics. Longer term "complications" are revisions associated with progression of tibiofemoral (TF) arthritis. Implant loosening and polyethylene wear are uncommon occurrences; reports are sparse in our literature. Prosthetic joint infection is a rare complication following PFA.

46.4 Indications

PFA is considered in patients who have anterior knee pain with bent knee activities (walking up and down a hill, up and down stairs, and sit to stand activities) that are of sufficient severity to affect quality of life, and who have not had resolution of symptoms after nonoperative management. Severe clinical symptoms should correlate with severe PF arthrosis on imaging studies. The typical progression of isolated PF arthritis is one of narrowing of the lateral PF joint space, leading to (relative) lateral tilt and/or lateral translation of the patella. ▶ Fig. 46.1 demonstrates the Iwano Classification for staging of PF OA. PFA performed for patients with high-grade PF OA (Iwano III/IV) has better clinical and patient-reported outcomes than when performed for patients with low-grade PF OA (Iwano I/II). Cartilage loss based on magnetic imaging alone, without radiographic correlation, is not an indication for PF arthroplasty.

46.5 Contraindications

Important contraindications to PFA include pain localized to or radiographic degeneration of the medial or lateral TF joint, PF chondromalacia without complete joint space loss or patients with Iwano Stage I/II disease, fixed loss of knee range of motion greater than 10 degrees of extension loss or less than 110 degrees of knee flexion, and distal femoral or global knee osteopenia. Relative contraindications include a history of systemic inflammatory arthritis, uncorrected lower extremity malalignment greater than 5 degrees of valgus or 3 degrees of varus, and body mass index greater than 30.

46.6 Special Considerations

The ideal use of PFA is in a patient in which the implant is expected to last a lifetime. However, the revision of a PFA to a total knee arthroplasty (TKA) is less onerous than a revision of TKA, or a conversion of medial or lateral partial replacement to TKA. Its use in the younger age group (age 40–55) may acceptably carry with it the expectation of revision to a TKA in their lifetime.

Alternative surgical techniques include.

- Partial lateral facetectomy with lateral retinacular lengthening/release: ideal in early lateral-sided PF wear associated with lateral tightness associated with a positive clinical response to lateral to medial McConnell taping.
- Anteriomedialization (AMZ) of the tibial tubercle: ideal in unipolar patellar arthritis based inferior and lateral, with an elevated quadricep vector (increased Q-angle or increased TT-TG).
- Cartilage restoration procedures including osteochondral allografts, and cell-based therapies (i.e., autologous

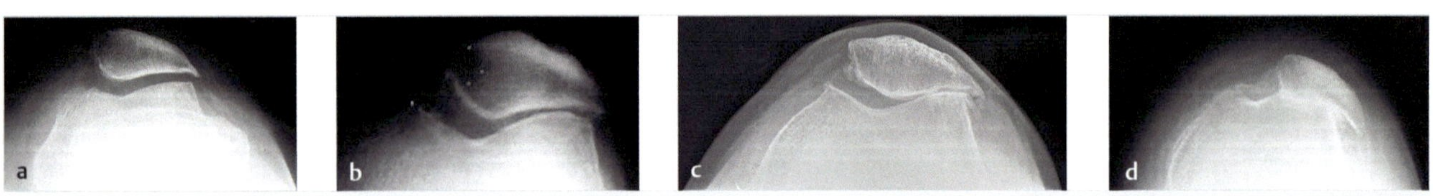

Fig. 46.1 Iwano classification for patellofemoral (PF) osteoarthritis. **(a)** Stage I: mild osteoarthritis with joint space at least 3 mm; **(b)** Stage II: moderate osteoarthritis with joint space < 3 mm but no bony contact; **(c)** Stage III: severe osteoarthritis with bony contact less than one quarter of the joint surface; **(d)** Stage IV: very severe osteoarthritis with joint surfaces entirely touching each other, often accompanied by a large lateral patellar osteophyte, and bone loss of the lateral patellar facet.

osteochondral chondrocyte implantation). Ideal in focal unipolar patella or femoral groove lesions.

- TKA has long been shown to be a viable treatment option for isolated PF OA and should be discussed with patients as TF joint wear is the leading reason for conversion of PFA to TKA. A recent randomized controlled trial has shown that functional patient reported outcomes, knee range of motion, and recovery time following PFA for isolated PF arthritis are superior to TKA.

46.7 Special Instructions, Position, and Anesthesia

The procedure is performed with the patient in the supine position, similar to TKA. A nonsterile tourniquet is routinely used to minimize blood loss during the procedure and during implant cementation. Positioning aids such as a bump under the operative hip, De Mayo or Alvarado leg positioners, or a sterile bump under the knee can aid in limb positioning for successful completion of the procedure. Placement of a Foley catheter is not routinely necessary.

Short-acting spinal and regional anesthesia techniques are preferred to general or endotracheal tube intubation and helps aid in early mobilization. If regional anesthesia is used as an adjunct for postoperative pain control, intraoperative periarticular joint infiltration or adductor canal block is preferable to femoral nerve block as femoral nerve block results in quadriceps weakness, risk for falls, and a delay in mobilization. Early mobilization and multimodal postoperative pain control is imperative to improving recovery time, limiting early postoperative complications, and if considering performing PFA in the short-stay or outpatient setting.

46.8 Tips, Pearls, and Lessons Learned

- Patients with radiographic evidence of arthritis have superior outcomes over arthritis diagnosed by MR imaging alone.
- Isolated PF OA is associated with high grade trochlear dysplasia, with PF joint forces concentrated laterally.
- Medial PF arthritis (▶ Fig. 46.2a) can be associated with previous (overmedialized) patella realignment surgeries, or with a genu varum. It is important to note that early medial-sided PF OA is a prognostic factor for future medial-sided tibiofemoral arthritis and possible need for conversion to TKA.
- Patients with central groove defects, which are often identified on MR sagittal imaging or arthroscopy, are often considered for inlay methods of PF resurfacing.
- Onlay prostheses have greater utility with high-grade trochlear dysplasia as the anterior femoral cut eliminates the dysplastic portion of the trochlear. However, they have greater potential of PF overstuffing. With end-stage PF OA, there is often bone loss on the lateral trochlea and/or lateral patellar facet. At a minimum, one is expanding the height of the lateral patella facet and lateral trochlear height, as well as recentering the patella, all of which can lead to increased height of the PF joint and possible overstuffing. Lateral lengthening of the soft tissues and minimizing the patellar button thickness are strategies to avoid this problem.
- Inlay designs, which has no anterior femoral cut, offer more technical challenges trying to accommodate dysplastic PF elements when used in association with high-grade trochlea dysplasia.
- Global PF arthritis (▶ Fig. 46.2b) can be related to previous fracture or severe blunt knee trauma. However, the absence of an identifiable cause is a harbinger of global knee arthritis.
- Valgus knee alignment associated with hypoplastic lateral femoral condyle can present intraoperative challenges to achieve correct femoral component positioning as well as acceptable interface between component and cartilage surface.
- Patella alta vs. patella baja.
  - Engagement of metal femoral flange and prosthetic button:
    - Patella alta has concerns for catching in extension to flexion.
    - 1. Solutions: patellar component positioning more caudad, choosing a prosthesis with a longer proximal flange, distalizing proximal tibial tubercle osteotomy (TTO).
    - Patella baja has concerns for plastic on cartilage interface in flexion with potential for pain and further cartilage wear distal to the femoral prosthesis.
    - 1. Solutions: patellar component positioning more cephalad, choosing a prosthesis with a wider distal nose, proximal TTO.

46.9 Difficulties Encountered

Early implant failure typically results from implant or technique-related problems such as component malposition that can result in maltracking, patellar instability, or patellar catching. Patellar catching in early flexion can be caused by lack of patella/groove engagement due to patella alta, knee hyperextension, and/or a too short *femoral* component anterior flange (▶ Fig. 46.3). An iatrogenic "J-sign," with the patella jumping into the groove from a lateralized position, is typically due to varus positioning of the femoral prosthesis (▶ Fig. 46.4). Patella catching in deep flexion is caused by lack of congruency of the distal femoral prosthesis

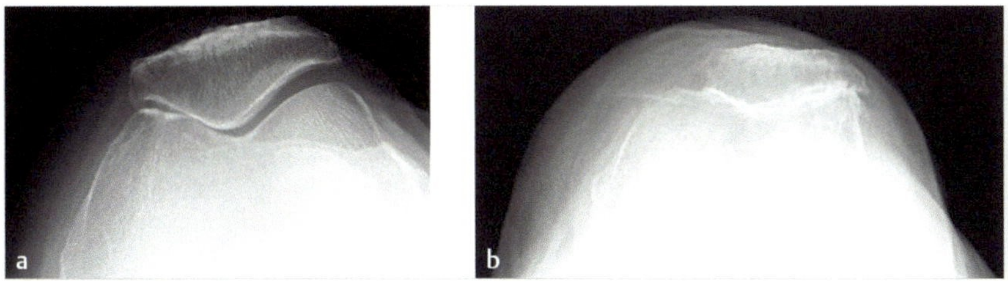

Fig. 46.2 **(a)** Axial radiograph of a patient with medial patellofemoral (PF) osteoarthritis (OA); **(b)** Axial radiograph of a patient with global PF OA.

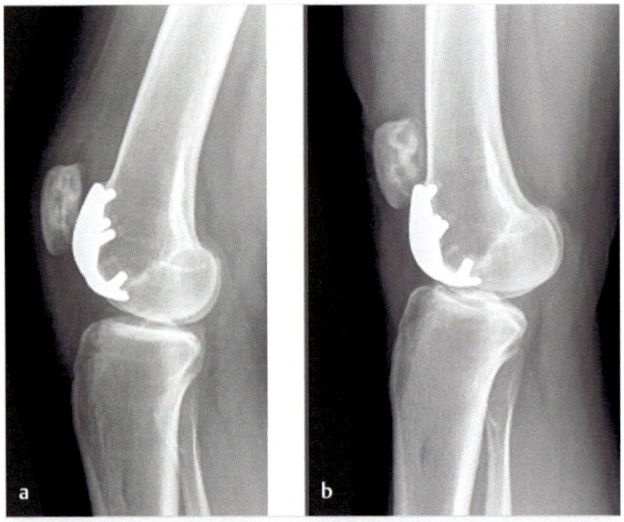

Fig. 46.3 **(a)** Sagittal knee image with acceptable engagement between patellofemoral arthroplasty. **(b)** A sagittal of this same knee in hyperextension, which clinically demonstrated a clinic when flexion was attempted from a hyperextended position.

with cartilage surface and is more common in femoral designs with wider proximal femoral coverage and a narrow distal component. Postoperative knee stiffness and arthrofibrosis are reported in approximately 5 to 10% of patients and can be treated with manipulation in the early (< 3 mo) postoperative period. Difficulty in regaining quad strength: due to preexisting weakness combined with surgical trauma. This can be minimized with focused physical therapy, mid-vastus splitting approach, and therapy-related strategies to re-engage quad activation. In the presence of normal patella alignment, continued swelling/synovitis can indicate overstuffing of the PF joint, or lack of concentric tracking. Long-term failure of PFA most commonly results from progression of TF arthritis. The conversion rate to TKA over 10 to 15 years is approximately 10 to 20%, depending on the series reviewed.

46.10 Key Procedural Steps

46.10.1 Choosing a Prosthesis

- Onlay prosthetic design ideal for patients with high-grade trochlear dysplasia, as the initial anterior femoral cut eliminates most if not all of the trochlear bony dysplastic elements.
- Patella alta should be measured and matched against the length of the femoral flange, as individual design lengths vary considerably.
- The option for a thinner patella button (7.5–8 mm) is optimal for those patellae with significant wear, as adding 9 to 10 mm of patella height can add to overstuffing.

46.10.2 Operative Approach

- A standard medial parapatellar or mid-vastus arthrotomy is used for surgical exposure.

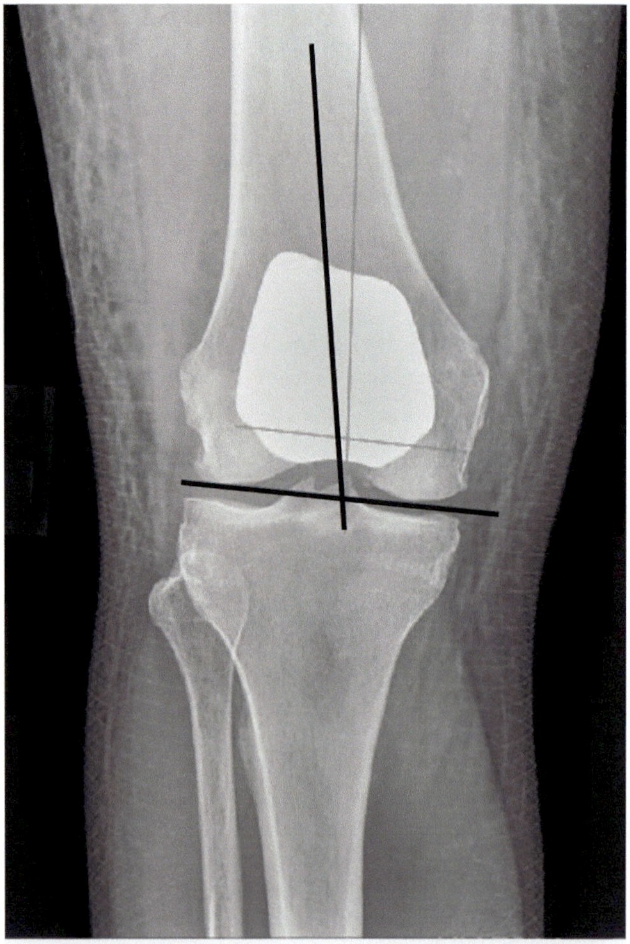

Fig. 46.4 Anteroposterior knee radiograph showing femoral valgus (*black line*) and femoral component varus (*grey line*). Placing the component aligned with the distal femur in a patient with hypoplastic lateral femoral condyle risks patellar maltracking to a medialized proximal groove entry.

- Preservation of the meniscus and anterior intrameniscal ligament is important during the surgical approach.
- Careful intraoperative examination for wear of the medial and lateral TF joints is important and if noted may necessitate consideration of TKA.

46.10.3 Femoral Component Positioning

- Each operative system has unique instrumentation to aid in implant positioning and bone resection. Knowledge of this instrumentation and characteristics of each system are important to understand for successful completion of the procedure.
- The majority of the systems (onlay type systems) utilize anterior trochlear femoral resection guide, similar to that used for the anterior distal femoral cut in TKA.
- Proper medial to lateral coverage of the femoral component is important and any medial or lateral overhang of the component should be avoided. Undersize if necessary.

- The transition from the medial and lateral femoral cartilage to the medial and lateral aspects of the trochlear component should be smooth to help limit impingement of patellar tracking against prominent osteochondral anatomy or the implant. However, this cannot always be achieved, while maintaining proper femoral component valgus. Recession of the medial aspect of the femoral component is favored over protrusion of the lateral aspect of the component. Flexion of the component is also a strategy than can be used to obtain a flush surface distally but can lead to catching in extension to flexion if patella alta and/or a short femoral flange is present.
- Each implant design and company has specific instrumentation to ensure proper rotation and coronal alignment of the femoral component. Femoral component positioning in these planes is important for patellar tracking and implant longevity. However, it is more important to set rotation of the femoral component to the anatomy of the femur (than to align the femoral component with the tibia).

46.10.4 Patellar Resection and Positioning

Prior to patellar resection, the native patellar thickness should be measured with a caliper. Significant bone loss can create a very thin bony patella, primarily lateral. This can be managed by doing a partial lateral facetectomy and removing the lateral 10 to 12 mm which is often the thinnest portion. Residual patellar thickness after resection should exceed 10 mm to minimize the risk of patellar fracture.

- Patellar resection should be performed carefully and the proper resection plane may be difficult to determine as a result of lateral patellar facet bone loss, as well as patellar dysplasia resulting in a vertical medial facet (Wiberg type IV patella) (▶ Fig. 46.5).
- The patellar button should be medialized to aid in patellar tracking, similar to TKA.
- In cases of mild alta, a smaller patella button placed distal on the bony patella surface may aid in patellar tracking without catching.

46.10.5 Trial Component Evaluation

- Implant position should be carefully evaluated with trial components.
- Partial closure of the arthrotomy with suture or clamps, and checking passive knee range of motion, can aid in evaluation of patellar tracking and implant position. Important to look at early extension to flexion, and deep flexion to extension.
- With the trial components in place, the patella should track smoothly throughout range of motion. There should be full fluid tracking of the patella from full extension to flexion greater than 120 degrees, based on the patient's preoperative range of motion.
- If a problem with trial component position is noted or patellar tracking is noted, the implants should be reassessed and repositioned as necessary.
- Lateral release/lengthening may be considered to aid in patellar tilt or tracking issues. Lateral release should not be relied upon to correct lateral patellar subluxation if noted when trialing implants. In this case, component positioning should be further assessed.

46.10.6 Cementation and Closure

- Once satisfied with position of the implants, the trial components are removed and the knee is irrigated with pulsatile lavage. The bony ends are then dried.
- A tourniquet should be used during cementation to ensure proper interdigitation of the cement into the cancellous bone.
- The implants should be carefully impacted to avoid fracture and to ensure proper implant position.
- All excess cement should be removed. Any retained cement will result in third body wear and can lead to cartilage injury and progression of TF arthritis.
- After cementation, the tourniquet is released and hemostasis is obtained. A deep drain is not routinely used.
- The subcutaneous and skin layer is closed according to the surgeon's preference.

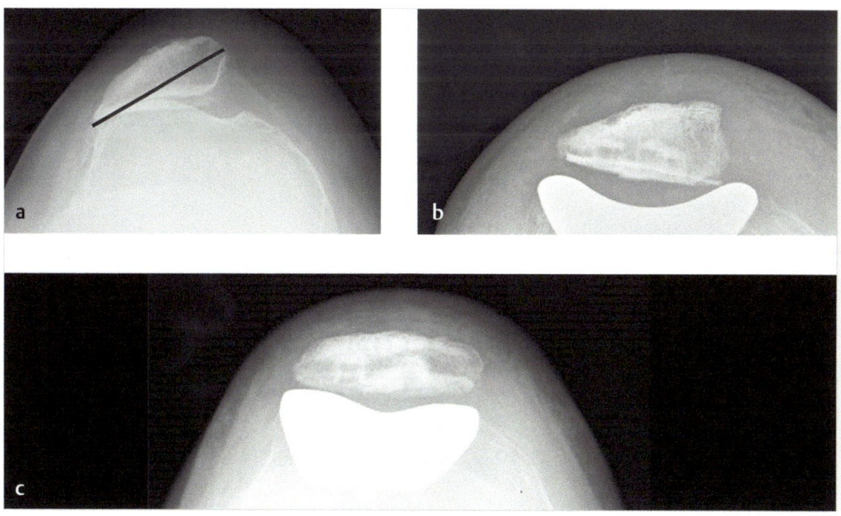

Fig. 46.5 **(a)** Lateral patellar facet wear; **(b)** a commonly made error is to assume that the lateral facet is the surface of the patella. In this case, when the patellar resection is made, too much medial bone remains and the patellar component is improperly positioned; **(c)** proper patellar resection where the residual medial and lateral bone is similar.

46.11 Bailout, Rescue, and Salvage Procedures

TF joint wear and patellar maltracking are the most common reasons for failure of PFA. TF joint pain that is nonresponsive to conservative treatments can be treated with conversion of the PFA to TKA. The results from conversion to TKA are often successful with durable pain relief and implant longevity. The patellar component can typically be retained for use with the TKA implants.

In patellar maltracking or mechanical symptoms, it is important to understand the etiology of the problem. If the problem is component positioning of the PFA implants, revision PFA or soft tissue realignment/releases may be considered if there is adequate bone stock. However, conversion to TKA may be a more reliable and definitive treatment. In general, the outcomes of TKA are generally not compromised by prior PFA.

46.12 Pitfalls

Poor outcomes and a high rate of implant failure are noted when the indications and contraindications for PFA are not closely followed. Proper use of implant-specific instrumentation is imperative to allow for accurate implant positioning, patellar tracking, and implant longevity.

47 Cruciate-Retaining Total Knee Arthroplasty

James Keeney

47.1 Description

Total knee arthroplasty (TKA) using cruciate-retaining components addresses end-stage osteoarthritis occurring in a knee that has a competent posterior cruciate ligament (PCL).

47.2 Key Principles

There are several key principles to keep in mind when performing a cruciate-retaining (CR) knee replacement. The first principle is to define which patients are suitable candidates for the CR technique and which patients will be better managed with another type of implant constraint. Successful PCL retention during TKA requires a near-symmetric flexion and extension space. Patients with increased tibial slope or with anterior tibial translation on preoperative lateral X-rays will likely need PCL release and increased implant constraint (highly conforming polyethylene or a cam-post articulation). The second principle is to understand whether you are using an anterior referencing or posterior referencing implant system. Anterior referencing systems may introduce flexion-extension imbalance in cases where femoral anatomy falls between available implant sizes. The third principle is to properly execute the operative plan during surgery, with careful assessment to the amount of bone resected from each of the bone surfaces, rotational component alignment, and selection tibial component thickness that is appropriate for TKA balance. Under-resection of bone during initial tibial and femoral osteotomies may impact component placement and soft tissue balance.

47.3 Expectations

Posterior-referenced, cruciate-retaining knee replacement provides most patients with a successful knee reconstruction. Patients should expect substantial improvement in pain (70–90%) with moderate improvement in function after surgery. Individual patient physical characteristics—preoperative range of motion, postoperative range of motion, body weight, and lower extremity functional strength—can all affect the loading of soft tissues around the knee and can contribute to pain with higher activity levels. Because knee replacements have mechanical components and surgery stimulates intra-articular scar tissue formation, some patients may also note mechanical symptoms (e.g., clicking, grinding) or a feeling of tightness even with well-performing knee replacements.

47.4 Indications

Cruciate-retaining TKA can be performed for most patients with knee osteoarthritis, as long as there is absence of major deformity, cruciate ligament imbalance, and structural bone loss.

47.5 Contraindications

There are several potential contraindications to cruciate-retaining total knee replacement including preoperative cruciate ligament imbalance, excessive tibial slope, excessive proximal tibial bone resection, and preoperative collateral ligament instability. These conditions can generally be identified on routine preoperative plain radiographs.

A careful review of preoperative lateral knee radiographs can be helpful to anticipate whether a PCL release may be required during TKA and whether standard bone preparation may be expected to release enough of the PCL from the tibia to create flexion instability. If the cruciate ligaments are unbalanced before surgery, a PCL release may be predictably required, and this may favor selection of a PCL sacrificing/substituting approach during TKA (▶ Fig. 47.1). If significant posterior tibial slope is noted on the lateral X-ray, reversal of this slope may be necessary to optimize femorotibial loading. The combination of tibial slope reversal and PCL retention may result in increased PCL tension, the need for a release, and the use of an implant system that will better accommodate a released PCL (▶ Fig. 47.2). For patients who do not have a significant coronal plane deformity, a more substantial tibial bone resection may be performed and may result in decreased tension in the PCL (▶ Fig. 47.3a, b).

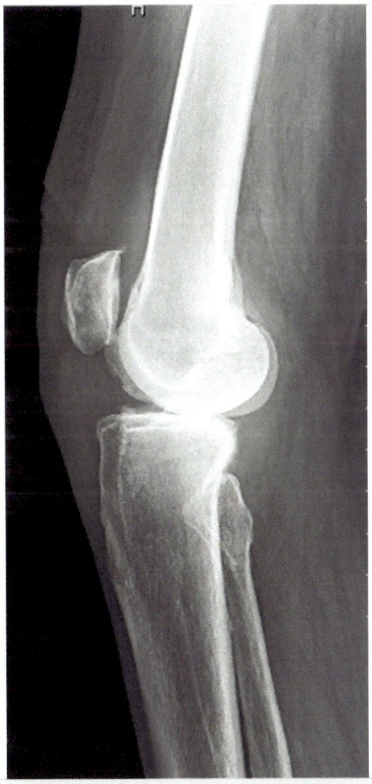

Fig. 47.1 Anterior tibial translation demonstrating anterior cruciate ligament-posterior cruciate ligament (ACL-PCL) imbalance.

The considerations for knee instability may be magnified among patients with a smaller native PCL or with generalized soft tissue laxity, which may be more common among female than among male patients. Finally, there are cases with significant collateral ligament instability or structural bone loss that require implant systems that may provide a higher degree of constraint (► Fig. 47.4).

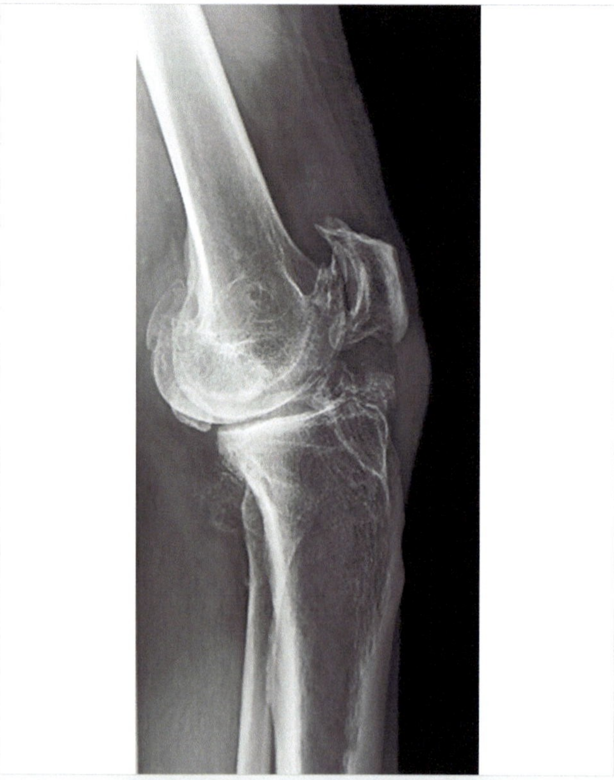

Fig. 47.2 Increased tibial slope with anterior cruciate ligament-posterior cruciate ligament (ACL-PCL) imbalance.

47.6 Special Considerations

Some implant systems may have highly conformed or ultra-congruent tibial-bearing articular surfaces that may allow cruciate-retaining implant systems to still be used even when there is some laxity created in the PCL. If a cruciate-retaining system is used that does not have a highly conformed articular surface option, it is appropriate to have a posterior-stabilized system available as a back-up option for an uncommon occurrence where a PCL deficiency is created intraoperatively by either intentional or inadvertent PCL release.

Whether or not to routinely perform patellofemoral resurfacing during TKA remains a point of controversy. The author's preference is to retain the native patella for patients less than 50 years old, a body mass index > 40 kg/m^2, or patellar thickness ≤ 21 mm. Resurfacing is generally performed for patients ≥ 65 years old, patients of all ages with severe patellar cartilage loss, or for surgeries performed for patients with radiographic patellofemoral arthritis.

The descriptions used in this chapter are based on mechanical instrumentation systems that are used in most conventional TKA surgeries. Patient-specific instrumentation systems exist that do not require consideration of femoral component sizing using anterior cortical or posterior condylar referencing. Careful performance of technique with resections as outlined by the PSI system remains important, but consideration of these approaches is outside the scope of this chapter.

47.7 Special Instructions, Position, and Anesthesia

Standard TKA positioning and techniques are utilized. Surgery can be accomplished using either regional or general anesthetic techniques. Perioperative analgesia can be added using pericapsular injection, intra-articular injection, or adductor canal injection.

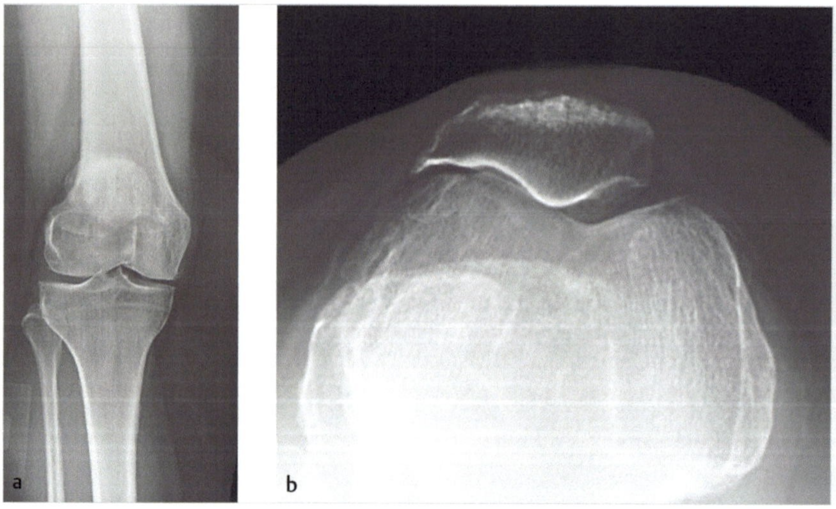

Fig. 47.3 (a,b) Neutral tibiofemoral alignment in total knee arthroplasty (TKA) performed for patellofemoral arthritis.

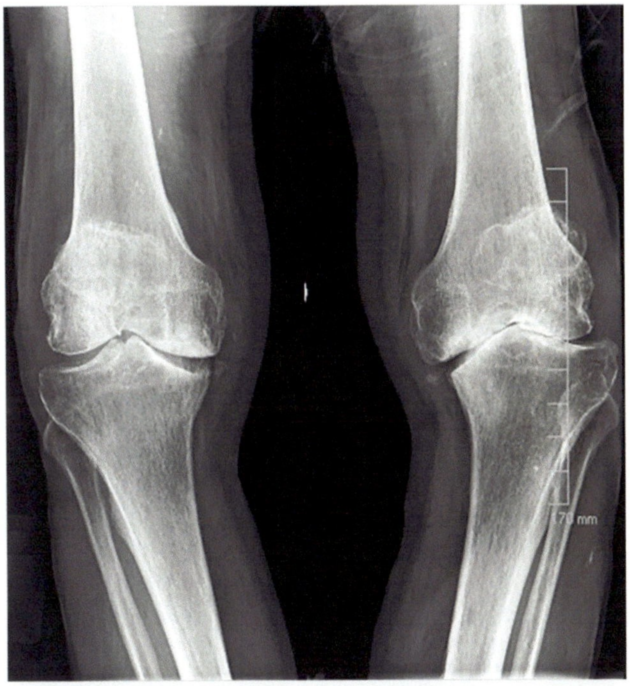

Fig. 47.4 Patient with major limb deformity and structural bone loss requiring augmentation.

47.8 Tips, Pearls, and Lessons Learned

- Correct bone resection is needed to avoid instability or stiffness following TKA; therefore, the surgeon must carefully assess all bone resections performed during TKA.
- The use of reduced profile instrumentation and flexible saw blades can result in under-resection of bone from sclerotic areas of bone. If bone resection from the distal medial and posteromedial femoral condyle is not symmetric, this can result in difficulty gaining full knee extension (if a thicker tibial insert is used to stabilize the knee in flexion) or in flexion instability (if a smaller insert is used to allow the knee to fully extend).
- The first step in successful CR-TKA is to define and select the instrument referencing system that will be used. Most conventional instrumentation systems will accommodate either an anterior or a posterior referencing approach. Both referencing systems should be able to accommodate knees where the anteroposterior dimensions of the patients' femur—measured from the anterior femoral cortex to the posterior femoral condyles—matches available implant sizes. If an anterior referencing knee system is used and a patient's femoral bone is "in between" component sizes, use of a downsized femoral component results in a looser flexion gap and this can cause either flexion instability (if a thinner insert is placed to balance the knee appropriately in extension) or an inability to fully extend the knee (if a thicker insert is used to balance the knee in flexion). If an anterior referencing system is used for "in between" cases and a larger femoral component size is selected, this can result in either extension instability (if a thinner insert is utilized) or difficulty gaining knee flexion (if a thicker insert is used to avoid extension instability).
- If tibial slope is reversed, this can result in a tight PCL and restriction in knee flexion requiring PCL release. Over extended periods, this tightness in flexion can result in anterior tibial translation, posterior tibial loading in flexion, anterior tibial component lift off, and component loosening. Increased tibial slope can result in flexion instability, and over extended periods of time can produce increased loading on the posterior tibial baseplate, anterior tibial component lift off, and component loosening.
- For patients (approximately 10–15% from my experience) whose anatomic femoral size falls in between implant sizes, proceeding with femoral bone resections without making an adjustment in technique may result in flexion-extension gap asymmetry and instability (anterior referencing) or patellofemoral (PF) compartment asymmetry (posterior referencing) with either femoral cortex notching or PF joint overstuffing. My preference is to use a posterior femoral referencing system for both CR and PS reconstructions. This allows flexion and extension spaces to be maintained in a consistent relationship during femoral bone preparation. For the minority of cases with "in between" femoral sizing, my preference is to select the smaller size, resect an additional 2 mm from the distal femur, and to shift the femoral cutting block 2 mm anteriorly. This maintains knee flexion and extension balance while avoiding PF compartment asymmetry.

47.9 Difficulties Encountered

47.9.1 Intramedullary Alignment Guides

Tibial bone resection can be accomplished using either an intramedullary or extramedullary alignment guide. The authors prefer to use an extramedullary alignment guide during primary TKA to allow compensation for diaphyseal and metaphyseal deformity and to reduce total marrow embolization during the procedure. While intramedullary alignment is almost always used for femoral preparation in primary TKA, there are some cases where retained hardware, previous distal femoral osteotomy, or distal femoral fracture healing may limit the ability to utilize femoral IM alignment guides. In these cases, the author's preference is to either use a patient-specific instrumentation or surgical navigation platform for the distal femoral resection. Axial plane (external rotation) femoral implant preparation can be performed in most cases using conventional instrumentation using traditional landmarks—posterior condylar axis, Whiteside line, and the transepicondylar axis.

47.9.2 Visualization

Smaller surgical exposures can affect the ability to see and appropriately size implants used during primary TKA. It is important to adequately mobilize soft tissues to expose the posterolateral tibia. The lateral meniscus resection should be performed adequately to fully expose the lateral tibial plateau with visualization of the popliteus tendon. Anterior cruciate ligament release generally affords adequate anterior tibial translation, but some patients may have less compliant soft tissues and this may not be readily attained. The author will occasionally perform a partial release of the PCL from the roof of the intercondylar notch—preserving the medial femoral PCL attachment—in extreme cases.

47.9.3 Patellar Maltracking

Patellar maltracking can be minimized with careful attention to surgical technique. When bone resections and component placement is appropriate, patellar malalignment should not be present after most cases. Correction of preoperative valgus deformity may increase tension in the lateral retinacular tissue. The author routinely performs a lateral release in valgus TKA even when tracking appears to be appropriate. If maltracking is otherwise noted with trial components in place, it is appropriate to undergo a stepwise assessment of technical considerations that may contribute to maltracking.

Tibial Rotation

In the author's experience, the tibia will be one size smaller than the femur in female patients and same size or one size larger than the femur in male patients. The author prefers to establish tibial rotation by aligning the baseplate on the anteromedial and posterolateral tibial plateau, leaving a portion of the posteromedial plateau uncovered. The center of the baseplate viewed from the front should be aligned with the dorsiflexion plane of the ankle joint and should fall along or slightly external to the medial border of the tibial tubercle.

Femoral Rotation

Femoral component rotational malalignment is generally noted when assessing the knee in flexion. An externally rotated femoral component will have increased medial (valgus) knee laxity. An internally rotated femoral component will typically have increased medial compartment tightness or lateral (varus) laxity. With an appropriately sized insert placed with the knee in extension, medial compartment flexion tightness can produce anteromedial tibial translation.

Patellar Implant

If the patella has been resurfaced, the component should be placed in a position where the high spot of the insert is in a similar position as the central ridge of the native patella. Medial placement of the patellar implant will help to maintain patellofemoral relationships.

Lateral Patellar Facetectomy

Removing of a small amount of exposed bone from the lateral facet along with partial lateral retinacular release from the edge of the resected bone may help reduce lateral patellar tilt.

Surgical Approach

If a median parapatellar approach was used during the TKA procedure, VMO and medial capsule releases may result in preferential pull from the vastus lateralis and *pseudo-maltracking*. If reapproximation of the medial soft tissues with a towel clip restores normal patellar tracking, the maltracking is expected to be managed with standard wound closure.

Tourniquet

Before making a final determination of patellar tracking concerns, a tourniquet—if used—should be released.

47.9.4 Flexion-Extension Imbalance

Managing knees that are "tight in flexion" or "tight in extension" is an important consideration in finishing the TKA procedure with a balanced knee. (Refer to Tips, Pearls, and Lessons Learned—#2–5.) It is important to recognize that these are relative terms. Knees with symmetric tightness or laxity in both flexion and extension are managed from the tibial reconstruction. Knees that are too tight require additional bone resection. Knees that are too loose require a thicker tibial insert.

Flexion-extension imbalance exists with two general patterns: (1) knees that are tighter in flexion than in extension (flexion tightness-extension laxity); (2) knees that are looser in flexion than in extension (extension tightness-flexion laxity). In addition, the asymmetric flexion-extension relationships can result from errors with the tibial reconstruction (tibial slope), with the femoral relationships (asymmetric distal medial/posteromedial bone resection) or a combination of both.

47.9.5 Tibial Slope

If tibial slope is decreased, the flexion space will be decreased (tight in flexion) and the extension space will be relatively increased (loose in extension). If tibial slope is increased, the flexion space will be increased (loose in flexion) and the extension space will be relatively decreased (tight in extension).

47.9.6 Asymmetric Femoral Bone Resection

Posterior Referencing

For a posterior-referenced TKA, flexion and extension relationships should be symmetric if bone resections from the proximal tibia and distal femur have been made correctly. If a knee is tight in flexion, carefully assess tibial slope first. Second, consider whether excessive bone had been resected from the distal femur. If the knee is not substantially tight, bone resection relationships are appropriate, and a mild flexion tightness remains, a partial recession of the PCL from the intercondylar roof may be considered. The release should be performed while applying posterior translation force to the anterior tibia with the release stopped as soon as the tibial returns to a neutral translation position. If the knee is tight in extension, and bone resection relationships appear to be appropriate, consider whether the patient may have had a preoperative flexion contracture and removing an additional 1 to 2 mm to facilitate gaining balanced extension-flexion motion.

Anterior Referencing

In an anterior-referenced total knee replacement, it is possible for flexion-extension imbalance to exist for patients with native femoral anatomy falling between component sizes—if compensating adjustments in femoral component placement are not made. Selection of a smaller implant during anterior-referenced TKA results in flexion laxity (extension tightness). Selection of a larger implant during anterior-referenced TKA results in extension laxity (flexion tightness). For knees that fall in between sizes, consider selecting the smaller knee component size, but removing a balanced amount of distal femur so the distal medial bone removal matches the posteromedial bone removed during the component downsizing.

47.9.7 Varus-Valgus Laxity

Coronal plane imbalance can be present prior to a surgical procedure, or may be produced during the operative procedure if either the distal femoral bone resection or the proximal tibial bone resection remove bone asymmetrically from the medial (valgus laxity) or lateral (varus laxity) side of the joint.

Cases without Significant Preoperative Malalignment or Ligament Attenuation

Patients who do not have substantial varus-valgus laxity instability relationships before surgery should have a balanced knee if bone resections have been performed correctly. If an instability pattern is noted after surgery, it is important to carefully evaluate the tibial bone resection and competence of the medial and lateral collateral ligament structures.

Tibial Bone Resection

A varus proximal tibial resection will result in a relatively tighter lateral joint space and relatively looser medial compartment (valgus instability). A valgus proximal tibial resection can result in a relatively tighter medial joint space (varus instability). Before performing lateral soft tissue releases to balance this valgus laxity, it is important to reassess the tibial bone resection and to reaccomplish the osteotomy if a varus cut is confirmed.

Soft Tissue Competence

Loss of soft tissue support during primary TKA is uncommon in primary TKA. Medial laxity in extension can occur with intentional or unintentional release of the superficial medial collateral ligament (MCL). Medial laxity in flexion can occur with intentional or unintentional release of the deep MCL and posteromedial capsule. Lateral laxity in extension can occur with intentional or unintentional release of the iliotibial band and lateral collateral ligament. Lateral laxity in flexion can occur with intentional or unintentional release of the popliteus tendon and posterolateral capsule. The magnitude of collateral ligament-related instabilities is attenuated when the PCL is retained. Simple repair of injured ligament structures and postoperative bracing is generally adequate to manage minor instabilities. Care must be taken to not excessively increase tibial insert thickness, as this may alter isometric relationships for collateral ligament balance.

Cases with Significant Preoperative Malalignment or Ligament Attenuation

Patients with major pre-existing coronal plane deformity and ligament attenuation may have balancing considerations driven by the integrity of the collateral ligaments. This is more frequently a concern for severe valgus deformity (attenuated MCL), although there may be some considerations for patients with severe varus deformity and chronic medial ligament and PCL contracture. The author does not perform cruciate-retaining TKA for most patients with severe malalignment or ligament attenuation, as these cases are more likely to require substantial release and consideration for implants with increased varus-valgus constraint.

47.10 Key Procedural Steps

- A midline incision is used for superficial exposure. The incision length should be guided based on surgeon experience and patient physical characteristics (size, soft tissue compliance).
- Deep surgical exposure is performed using a medial parapatellar approach, midvastus approach, or subvastus approach. The deep exposure should be based on the surgeon's experience and patient physical characteristics (bone size, arthritis severity). Medial parapatellar approach affords better visibility. Midvastus and subvastus exposures may allow earlier quadriceps function, but decrease visibility.
- Medial soft tissue release is performed based on the patient's preoperative alignment and medial soft tissue laxity. For patients with valgus deformity or lax medial soft tissues, the medial soft tissue release should be limited to the joint line (1 cm). An elevator or thin (1/2 inch) osteotome may be used to elevate the posteromedial capsule and deep MCL.
- The patella is displaced laterally and synovial tissues are elevated from the distal femur.
- With the knee in flexion, deep retractors are placed around the tibia for exposure.
- A portion of the retropatellar fat pad is removed as needed to visualize the lateral femoral condyle.
- Anterior cruciate ligament is released from its tibial insertion.
- Anterior horn of the lateral meniscus is released.
- Anteromedial tibial osteophytes are removed.
- Extramedullary alignment guide is oriented and fixed to the proximal medial tibia for adequate bone resection for varus (9–10 mm from the lateral tibia) or valgus (4–8 mm from the medial tibia) deformities. Tibial slope is set at either 5 to 7 degrees to most appropriately match the patient's native slope on lateral X-rays.
- Proximal tibial osteotomy is initiated with an oscillating saw straight posterior through the tibia in line with the medial femoral condyle and obliquely toward the posterolateral tibia.
- The extramedullary guide and tibial cutting block are removed. Tibial bone resection is completed through the visualized anteromedial and anterolateral tibia.
- The femur is entered with a chamfered drill. Bone marrow is suctioned from the femoral canal.
- Intramedullary alignment rod is fully inserted into the femoral canal. The distal femoral cutting guide is placed against the distal medial femoral surface. Depending on the

patient's native distal femoral valgus, the lateral side of the cutting block may/may not touch against the lateral distal femur.

- The distal femoral cutting block is secured. Distal osteotomy is performed. Distal bone resections are measured. Additional bone is resected through the cutting block (without resetting it) if the initial cut did not adequately remove bone. The distal femoral and proximal tibial resections should result in a reasonably symmetric joint space with the knee in extension (▶ Fig. 47.5).
- Femoral rotation and sizing guide is placed on the resected surface. Three-degree drill markings are made. For patients with a hypoplastic lateral condyle, a pin is placed into the medial drill guide hole and the femoral guide is rotated to place it in a parallel relationship with the resected tibial surface.
- A four-in-one femoral cutting guide is placed against the distal femur. A size larger than the measured femoral size is selected initially to ensure that femoral notching is avoided. A provisional anterior femoral resection is performed. The anterior resection is assessed and decision is made to completely downsize, or to adjust for femur that is "in between" sizes.
  - If the femoral cutting block size is appropriate, it is secured in position.
  - If the femur sizes "in between" the larger and smaller sizes, consider removal of an additional 2 mm from both the distal and posterior femur.
    - The distal femoral guide is placed against the resected surface while placing a resection guide and free saw blade through the bone resection slot.
    - Pins are placed and the femur is advanced 2 mm proximally and secured into a + 2-mm resection position. The block is secured and distal bone resection is performed.
    - The final femoral guide is advanced 2 mm anterior (+ 2 mm posterior resection) and secured in position.
- After the final femoral cutting guide is secured in place, final anterior, posterior, and chamfer resections are performed. Evaluate the posterior femoral condyle width. If it is narrower than the saw blade being used, change the saw blade to a smaller size to decrease the risk of iatrogenic injury to intercondylar structures or collateral ligaments. The distal femoral and proximal tibial resections should result in a reasonably symmetric joint space with the knee in flexion (▶ Fig. 47.6).
- Perform trochlear recess osteotomy using cutting guide (if appropriate).
- Re-expose the tibia. Excise meniscus tissues to facilitate exposure of the entire tibial plateau.
- With deep retractors in place, reposition the extramedullary tibial cutting guide to remove no additional bone from the deepest area of resection (usually the medial plateau). Secure the cutting guide and leave the extramedullary guide in place.

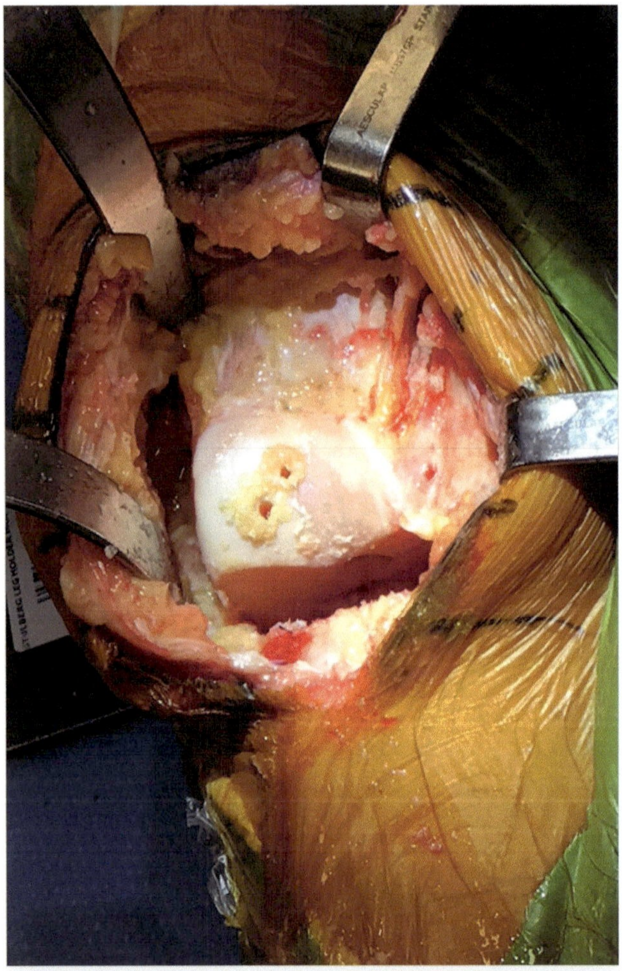

Fig. 47.5 Symmetric extension space after initial bone resections.

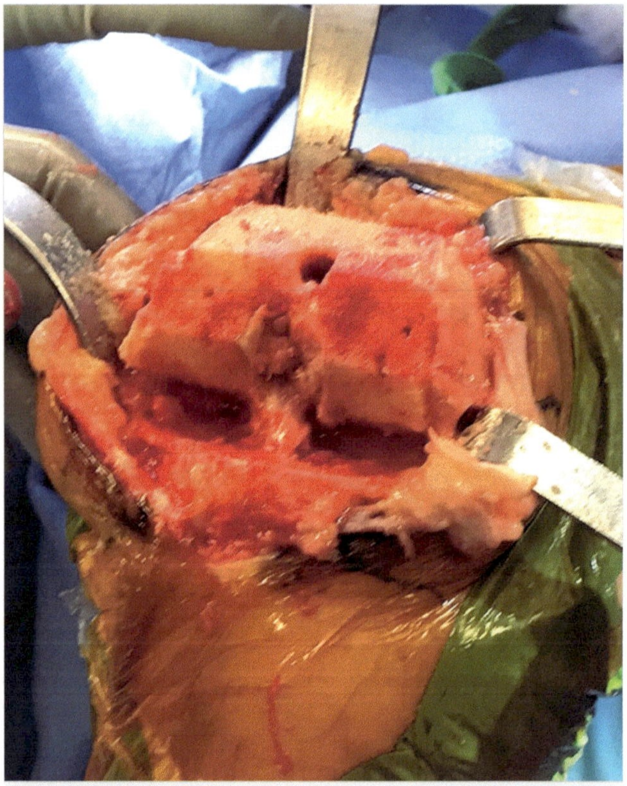

Fig. 47.6 Symmetric flexion space with intact posterior cruciate ligament (PCL).

- Recut the tibial bone under direct visualization through the cutting guide.
- Remove the extramedullary guide and tibial cutting block. Finalize bone and soft tissue removal from the tibial surface.
- Place the trial tibial baseplate. Select a size that allows contact against the anteromedial tibia and the posterolateral tibial cortex. A portion of the posteromedial cortex will be uncovered (▶ Fig. 47.7).
- Secure the tibial baseplate in position. Prepare the tibia using manufacturer-approved technique.
- Place the trial femoral component. Ensure appropriate medial-lateral sizing. The femoral component should not overhang the lateral cortex or the PCL.
- Select a trial insert appropriate for the amount of bone resection performed. Evaluate the knee stability in flexion and extension. Adjust the tibial insert thickness as appropriate based on soft tissue balance.
- Evert the patella and assess the patellar articular surface (▶ Fig. 47.8). Measure the maximum thickness of the patella using a caliper.
- If retaining the patella without resurfacing, consider performing a lateral facetectomy.
- If resurfacing the patella, place the knee in a position of slight flexion. Remove 8 to 10 mm of patellar bone as appropriate for patellar implant thickness (▶ Fig. 47.9).
- Assess the residual patellar thickness and symmetry of the bone resection. Adjust patellar bone resection as appropriate to create an even, resected surface at the desired thickness.
- Prepare for patellar implant placement, favoring placement of the implant along the medial patellar border.
- Assess patellar tracking (▶ Fig. 47.10). Consider causes of maltracking if this is noted during the procedure.
- Place final components (▶ Fig. 47.11) and perform wound closure in standard fashion.

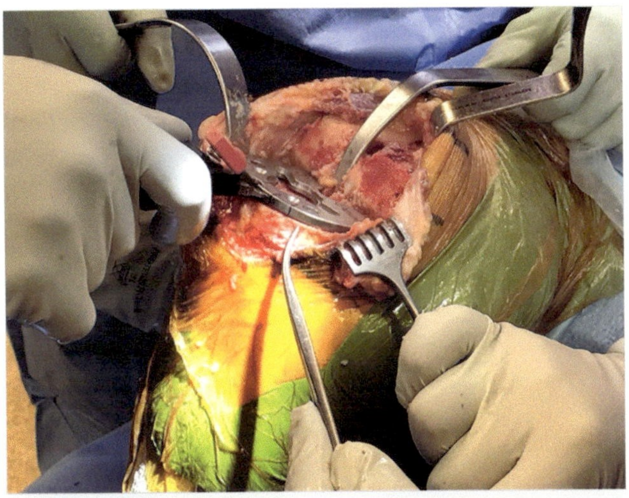

Fig. 47.7 Establishing tibial component rotation and positioning.

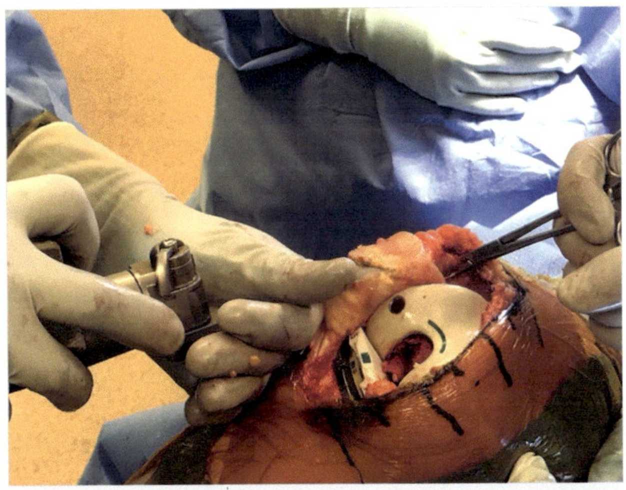

Fig. 47.9 Patellar bone measurement.

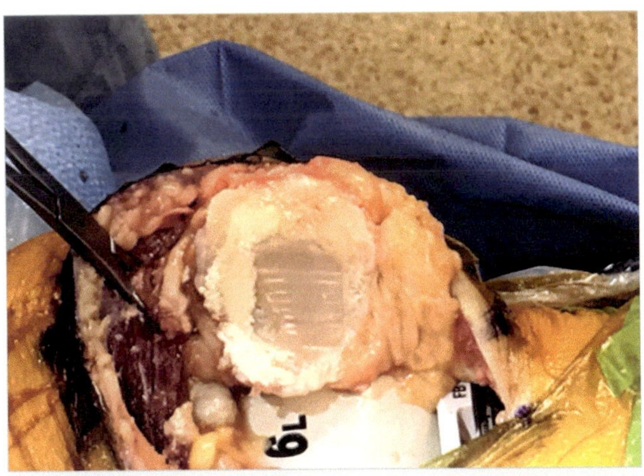

Fig. 47.8 Patellar bone and cartilage assessment.

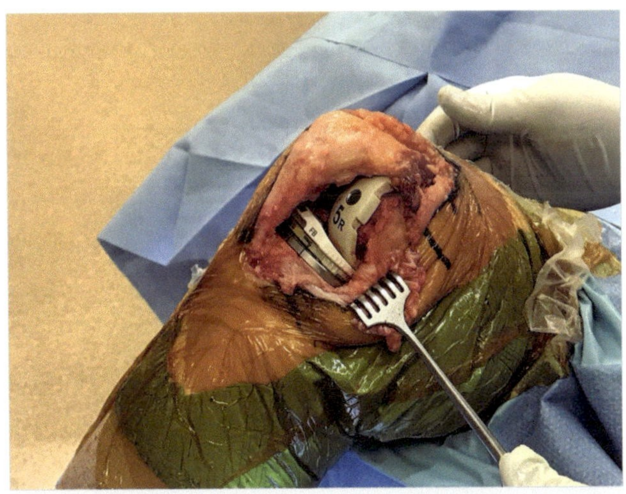

Fig. 47.10 Patellar bone resection.

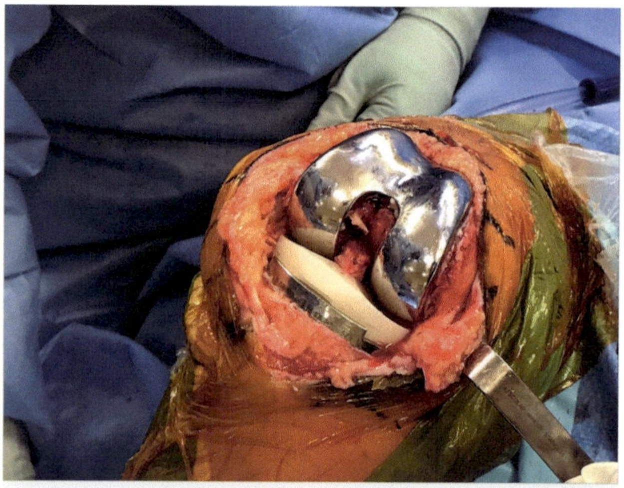

Fig. 47.11 Final balanced cruciate-retaining total knee arthroplasty (CR-TKA) with sized tibial insert.

47.11 Bailout, Rescue, and Salvage Procedures

With attention to surgical technique, bailout, rescue, and salvage procedures should not be necessary. Inadvertent injury to the deep or superficial MCL or PCL may require an increase in implant constraint. Intended release of the posterolateral soft tissues during valgus knee deformity correction may increase instability to varus or external rotation forces and may also require conversion to a revision knee replacement component system with either a semiconstrained (constrained condylar) or a constrained (hinge) reconstruction system.

47.12 Pitfalls

There are generally no significant pitfalls associated with the cruciate-retaining technique. But, the technique cannot be performed uniformly for all knee replacement procedures. For surgeons who prefer to use a single technique for all surgeries, a posterior-stabilized implant system may provide a more predictable and consistent technique. With limited differences in clinical and functional outcomes following CR- or PS-TKA, it is reasonable to use either system during primary TKA. The author's experience with both cruciate-retaining and posterior-stabilized knee replacements has suggested that PS-TKA is associated with a higher rate of mechanical symptoms (clicking) resulting from the engagement of femoral cam and tibial insert post. CR-TKA is selected for patients with higher expected activity demands. PS-TKA may be utilized for lower demand patients who are less likely to engage their knee in ways that will increase their risk for mechanical symptoms.

48 Primary Total Knee Replacement: Posterior Stabilized

Ajay Aggarwal

48.1 Description

Total knee arthroplasty (TKA) using posterior-stabilized components addresses end-stage osteoarthritis occurring in a knee that has an incompetent posterior cruciate ligament (PCL), whether due to preoperative pathology or intraoperative release.

48.2 Key Principles

Although being debated for many years, the superiority of posterior cruciate-retaining (CR) total knee arthroplasty (TKA) and posterior-stabilized (PS) TKA still remains controversial. The choice of CR or PS knee design should be based on the surgeon's preference and condition of the PCL.

Posterior-stabilized implants compensate for the absence of the PCL with a polyethylene post and femoral cam that interact to prevent anterior translation of the femur on the tibia, while allowing femoral rollback during flexion. Potential advantages of these designs include a less technically demanding procedure, easier correction of deformity, decreased polyethylene wear, a more stable component interface, and increased range of motion. Disadvantages include the potential for increased risk of loosening, reduced proprioception, and more bone loss due to incorporation of intercondylar cam-and-post mechanism.

Although the PCL is often attenuated in arthritic knees, it is usually present. The PCL causes the femoral condyles to glide and roll back on the tibial plateau as the knee is flexed, which is defined as the femoral rollback phenomenon. In a normal knee, the shape of the plateau does not restrain this motion and the laxity of the meniscal attachments allows the menisci to move posteriorly with the femur. This femoral rollback is crucial in prosthetic design to achieve optimal functional outcome. If the cruciate ligaments are excised, a more conforming tibial polyethylene component can be used to provide some degree of anterior and posterior stability. However, without a functional PCL, femoral rollback will not occur, which theoretically limits the ultimate flexion that can be obtained. If the PCL is retained, the tibial surface must be flat or even sloped posteriorly to allow the roll back to occur. If a more conforming component is used in these circumstances, posterior impingement will occur. Substitution of the PCL with a cam-and-post mechanism not only recreates femoral rollback, but also allows a conforming articulation to be used without risk of posterior impingement.

In the physiological knee, the PCL has different kinematic functions. During flexion, it guides rollback of the femoral condyles on the tibial plateau, prevents posterior subluxation of the tibia on the femur in flexion, and plays a decisive secondary role in varus/valgus stability. Resection of PCL tends to reduce flexion moment on the knee, which is compensated by leaning the body forward. It also causes transfer of shear forces that are normally absorbed by PCL to the interface between the bone and cement; greater stress is also transferred to the patella, and patellar fractures are more frequent.

48.3 Expectations

Since the PS knee has been designed on the principle of substituting the function of PCL with the presence of a cam-and-post mechanism, this provides the advantage of preventing anterior translation by facilitating femoral rollback phenomenon leading to increased range of motion in flexion. PS knee provides more predictable restoration of knee kinematics, improved range of motion, decreased polyethylene wear because of more conforming articular surfaces, easier correction of severe deformities, and easier ligament balancing.

48.4 Indications

PS TKA can be done on all patients with symptomatic end-stage knee arthritis. However, there are a few special circumstances when the use of a PS knee implant is preferred over a CR knee, which includes severe preoperative deformity, knees with flexion contracture > 40 degrees, insufficient or ruptured PCL, ankylosed knee, post-patellectomy TKA, and previous osteotomies of distal femur or proximal tibia and revision surgeries.

48.5 Contraindications

Infection and neuropathic joint disease are contraindications for any TKA. Specifically, PS knee is contraindicated when one or both collateral ligaments are significantly lax or disrupted and it necessitates the conversion to a valgus-varus constrained implant or the use of hinged prosthesis.

48.6 Special Considerations

Before deciding whether a PS or CR knee has to be used in a specific patient, a history of prior trauma (that might affect the integrity of PCL), patellectomy, or inflammatory arthritis should be elicited, as these patients become a better candidate for a PS design.

48.7 Special Instructions, Position, and Anesthesia

The patient is positioned supine. A foot-holding device is used to keep the knee in alternate flexion and extension during the procedure. A tourniquet is placed over the upper thigh and elevated after exsanguination of the limb. Standard preparation and draping are used with leg draped free for hyperflexion during the procedure.

Anesthesia options are epidural anesthesia with intravenous (IV) sedation as needed and postoperative epidural patient-controlled analgesia (PCA), or general anesthesia with postoperative IV PCA.

48.8 Tips, Pearls, and Lessons Learned

1. Consider the conversion of CR to PS when PCL or the popliteus tendon is accidently cut or when the PCL has not sufficient tension to preserve it.
2. Femoral component, if aligned in flexion, will lead to cam-and-post impingement as it brings roof of the box closer to the position of the post in extension. While using an anterior referencing system in PS knee, since the PCL resection causes asymmetrical opening of the flexion gap, the intermediate size of the femur should be rounded up to a larger size to tighten up the flexion. In PS design, care must be taken to minimize the box cut, as this may lead to stress riser causing medial or lateral femoral condyle fractures. Typically, no posterior slope is used in a PS design as resection of the PCL has already loosened up the flexion gap.

48.9 Difficulties Encountered

In a small femur (less mediolateral dimension), it is sometimes difficult to incorporate box cut in the intercondylar notch to accommodate cam-and-post mechanism without increasing the risk of causing iatrogenic fracture. In such cases, narrow femoral component or the use of cruciate-substituting (CS) prosthesis should be considered. CS designs have deep-dished, highly congruent, anterior-lipped polyethylene for femoral roll-back instead of cam-and-post mechanism. Similarly, in osteoporotic bone, due caution should be taken during box cut to avoid risk of femoral condyle fracture.

48.10 Key Procedural Steps

- Make the anterior midline incision with the knee flexed. I prefer the classical medial parapatellar approach. Transverse markings made at the proximal and distal poles of the patella before arthrotomy make for easier closure. While doing the arthrotomy, I prefer to leave ~0.5-cm cuff of retinaculum on the medial border of the patella.
- The periosteum of the proximal medial tibia is elevated. It is sometimes necessary to release structures off the posteromedial tibia up to the semimembranosus bursa for better anterior tibial subluxation.
- Avoid excessive medial release in a valgus knee. Resect the anterior cruciate ligament (ACL) from the tibial articular surface.
- Whether to cut the distal femur or the proximal tibia first is the surgeon's preference. I prefer to perform the distal femoral resection first with five-degree valgus resection in a varus knee and 3- to 4-degree cut in a valgus knee. Draw Whiteside's line and a second horizontal line on the medial femoral condyle over the meniscal impression. The intersection of these lines is the preferred starting-hole location for the intramedullary rod (▶ Fig. 48.1).
- The sequence of cuts to achieve predictable balancing in a primary TKA: patellar resection, distal femoral resection, proximal tibial resection, balance the knee in extension, choose femoral rotation and sizing for rectangular flexion space, femoral anterior-posterior chamfer cuts, balance knee for equal flexion and extension space (▶ Fig. 48.2 and ▶ Fig. 48.3).
- Measure all bony cuts with a caliper. (Tip: In most varus and valgus knees, the posteromedial femoral cut is around 9 mm to 9.5 mm thick. This will ensure you have 3-degree external rotation on your femoral component.)

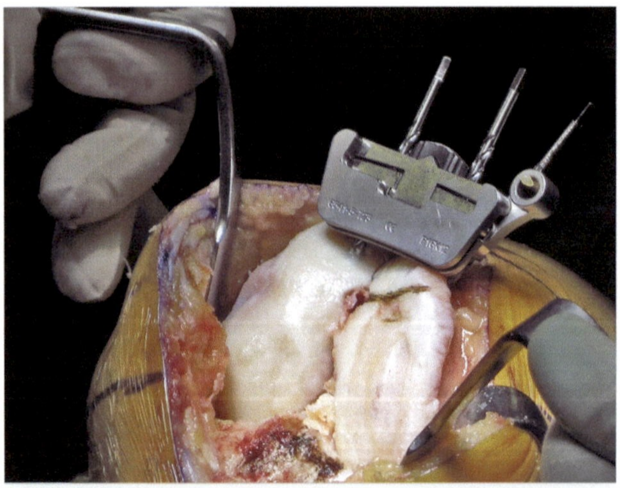

Fig. 48.1 A distal femoral cutting jig with Whiteside's line and a horizontal line on the medial femoral condyle from meniscal impression. The intersection represents the starting point for the intramedullary guide.

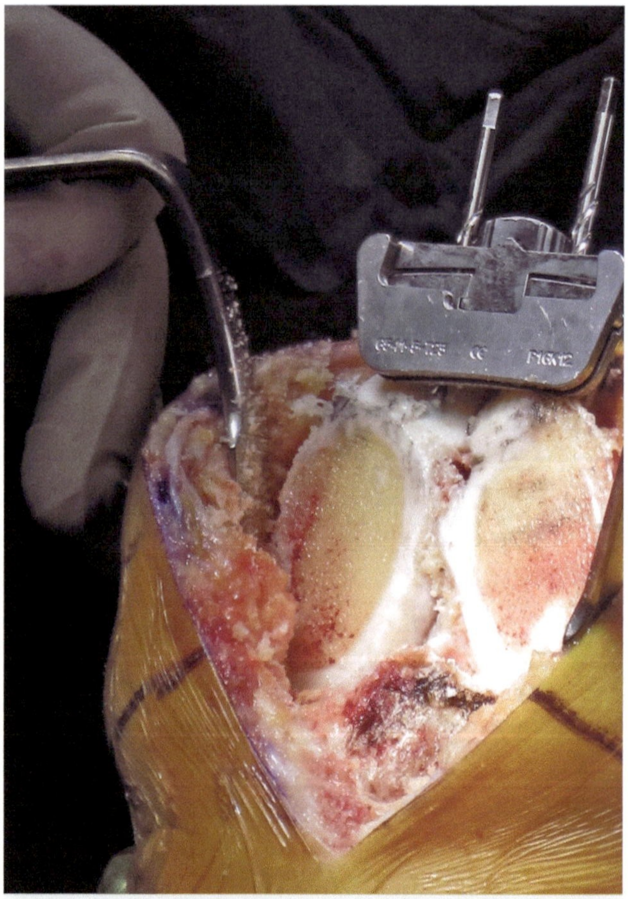

Fig. 48.2 A flat distal femoral cut.

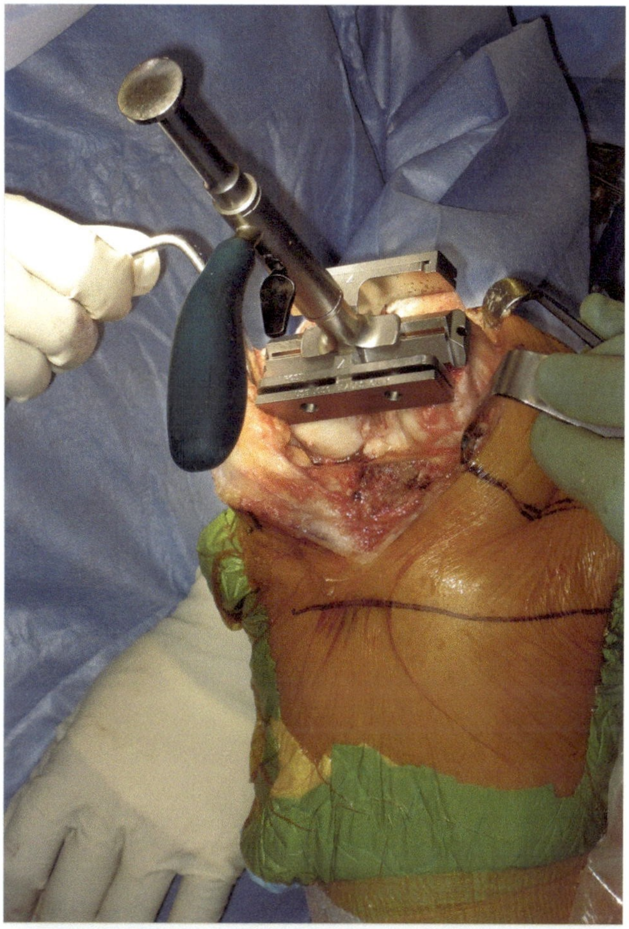

Fig. 48.3 A femoral "4-in-1" cutting jig.

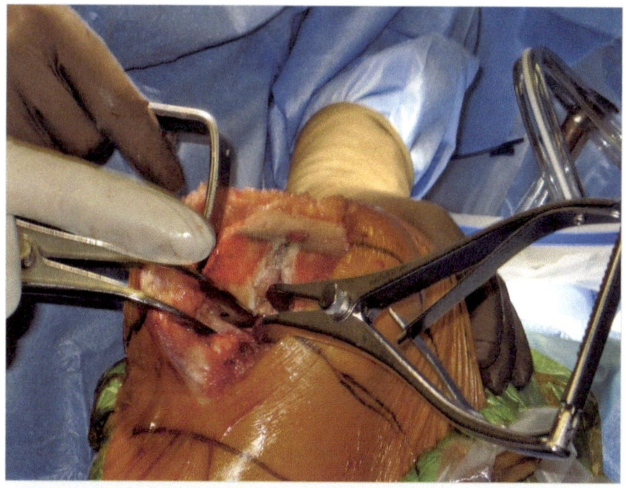

Fig. 48.4 Lamina spreaders are used to place tension on the soft tissues medially and laterally. The bone resection gap should be rectangular with both sides tensioned.

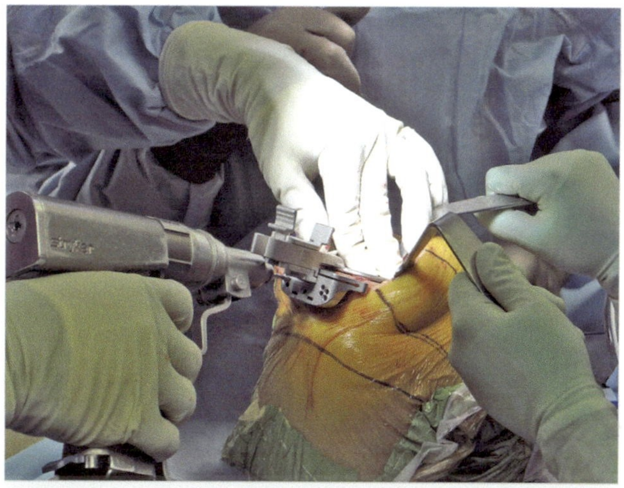

Fig. 48.5 A varus-cutting block is used for revising the tibial cut.

- The bone resections are made in a standard fashion. The tibial resection is made perpendicular to the mechanical axis of the tibia with no posterior slope. With distraction from a laminar spreader, the PCL is excised. It is important to remain on bone rather than soft tissues (▶ Fig. 48.4). The medial meniscus is excised with careful preservation of the peripheral rim of the meniscus and the medial collateral ligament (MCL), while the lateral meniscus is resected with preservation of the popliteus tendon. (Tip: If the tibial cut is in varus or valgus, one can use a varus- or valgus-cutting block for revising the cut and balancing the knee rather than using whole jig again (▶ Fig. 48.5.)
- Place the notch guide laterally to decrease the chance of intraoperative fracture of the medial femoral condyle and to enhance patellar tracking.
- The intramedullary guide hole is filled with bone graft.
- Posterior capsular subperiosteal elevation is done, and posterior condyle osteophyte removal is performed to eliminate flexion contractures and to prevent impingement in high flexion.
- The size of the tibial base plate is assessed based on the anteromedial and posterolateral edges. To achieve correct rotational alignment of the tibial tray, the center of the tibial component is set over the medial one-third of the tibial tubercle. Keep the cam and post in correct alignment. Rotation of tibial tray is confirmed based on a line passing through anterior third of the tibial tubercle and notch of femur, which must pass through the center of the tibia plate. An alignment rod, if used, should point toward the second ray of the ipsilateral foot.
- Creation of a composite resurfaced patellar that is 1 to 2 mm thinner than the native patella helps tracking and avoids overstuffing of the joint.
- Check for impingement—do a full-extension check for impingement of the femur on post. This can be due to excess slope or flexed femur component.

48.11 Bailout, Rescue, and Salvage Procedures

In case of severe collateral insufficiency or perioperative femoral condyle fracture, keep the constrained implant (hinged or tumor prosthesis) ready as a part of armamentarium.

48.12 Pitfalls

Increased bone loss, patellar clunk syndrome, cam-and-post dislocation, and rare post breakage are the pitfalls associated with the PS knee. Increased bone loss due to the femoral box cut may cause femoral fracture or can make revision surgery more challenging.

Patellar clunk syndrome—this is a phenomenon exclusive to PS knees where a collection of scar tissue located just proximal to the proximal pole of the patella on the underside of the quadriceps tendon becomes entrapped in the box as the knee goes into extension from flexion.

Cam-and-post dislocation—if the flexion gap is too loose, the post can come disengaged from the cam and fall posterior to it.

49 Primary Total Knee Replacement using Navigation

Dominique Saragaglia

49.1 Description

We describe using a navigation system in the set of a primary total knee replacement (TKR). We have adopted this technology since 1997, aiming to reduce the revision surgery rate due to either implant malalignment or joint instability.

49.2 Key Principles

Navigation in orthopaedic surgery is a concept that uses computer technology for surgical planning and guidance during a surgical procedure. Therefore, it is essential to have a precise three-dimensional model that reproduces the anatomical area of interest used as a map for intraoperative guidance. Computer tomography, fluoroscopy, and other technologies (i.e., image-free) provide the surgeon the desired model for navigation. We describe the use of one navigation platform, the Orthopilot (BBraun-Aesculap, Tuttlingen, Germany), an image-free navigation system based on intraoperative data acquisition. The equipment includes a navigation station (▶ Fig. 49.1), which allows the system to locate the surgical area of interest. The navigation station comprises a personal computer, an infrared Spectra localizer (Northern Digital Inc.), and a dual-command foot pedal. The knee is connected to markers, the so-called "rigid bodies," which are a collection of four reflective spheres rigidly held together (▶ Fig. 49.2). The navigation system locates the markers spatially in real time using infrared technology. The markers are rigidly attached to the bone using special bicortical screws. The surgeon uses ancillary devices, like metallic pointers, wireless markers containing detectable spheres, locating specific anatomic areas around the knee as the computer registers their three-dimensional location. The computer determines a protocol for capturing specific areas of reference, which will allow for the construction of a three-dimensional model of the knee. The surgeon uses a foot pedal and a dedicated graphic interface to provide information to the navigation system. Therefore, each marker's attitude (position and orientation) is computed from spheres positions and the marker's shape.

The cutting guides are equipped with markers that are firmly attached to the bone by four threaded pins. Therefore, the navigation system's cutting guides are spatially detected and guide the tibial cut (height of cut, valgus varus, tibial slope) and the femoral cut (height of cut, valgus varus, procurvatum, recurvatum). In addition, we use a distractor to guide the ligament balance in flexion and extension.

49.3 Expectations

Navigation-assisted primary TKR should allow for.

- Implantation of the hardware at a hip knee angle (HKA) of 180 + /- 3 degrees.
- Improved ligament balance.
- Improved patellofemoral tracking.
- Surgical implantation of components without opening the medullary canal.

49.4 Indications

Computer-assisted TKR is a technology applicable to patients who have a formal indication for a TKR. It is particularly advantageous in cases of extra-articular deformities, in cases where the medullary canal is obliterated/occupied by hardware (▶ Fig. 49.3a,b), or if the removal of hardware would increase the risks of periprosthetic fracture (▶ Fig. 49.4).

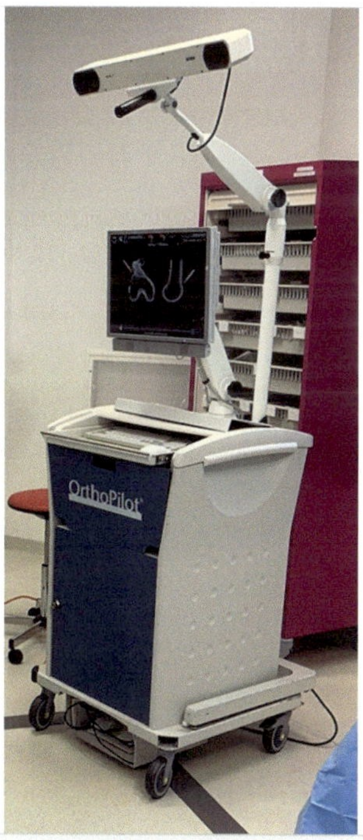

Fig. 49.1 The Orthopilot device.

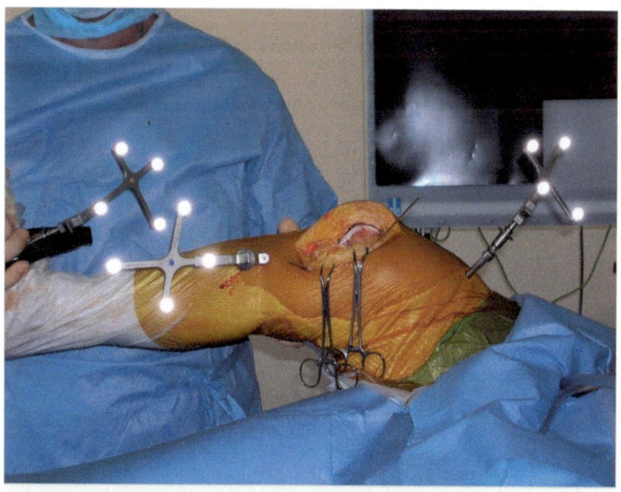

Fig. 49.2 Marker with four reflecting balls (passive marker).

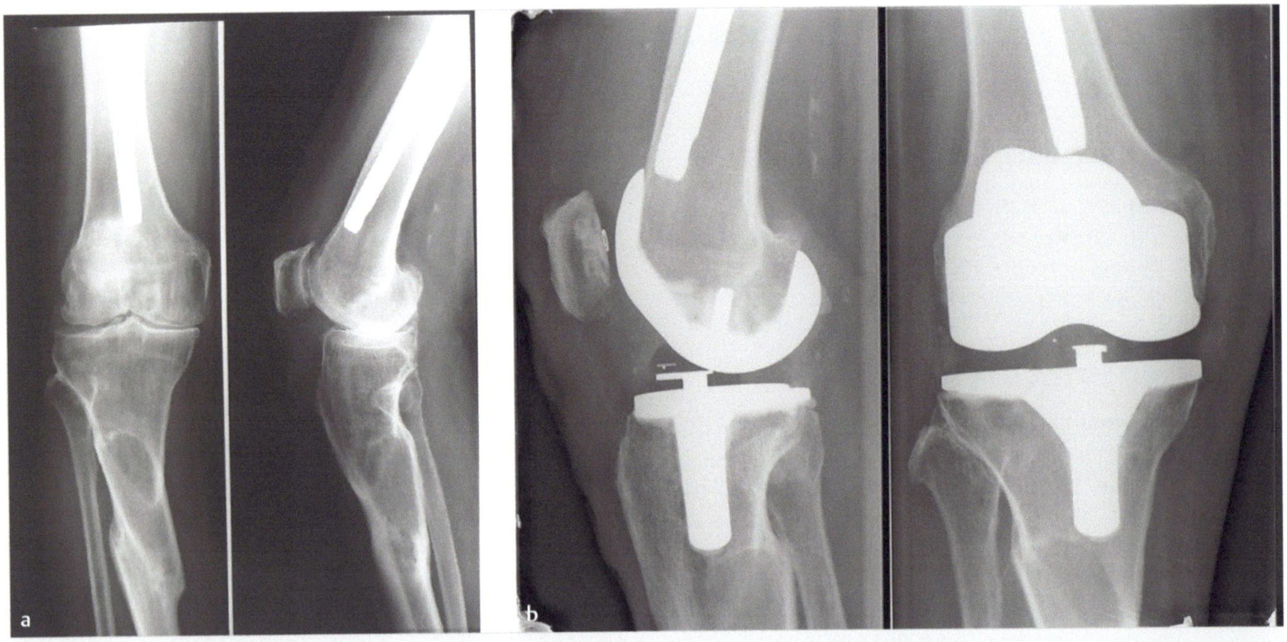

Fig. 49.3 (a) Osteoarthritis of the knee with a retained nail in the femoral medullary canal. (b) Total knee arthroplasty (TKA) implanted using navigation.

49.5 Contraindications

Navigation systems that use a kinematic model (capture of multiple images of reference in association with the mobilization of the hip and knee) cannot be used when there is ankylosis or arthrodesis of the hip or the knee.

49.6 Special Considerations

Navigation is an evolving technology that also requires a learning curve. It is critical to be well trained in standard total knee arthroplasty so that the surgeon may question the guidance provided by the system during the surgery. It also adds extra equipment to the operation theater, which requires training for the staff.

49.7 Special Instructions, Positioning, and Anesthesia

General or regional anesthesia is used in our primary TKR surgeries. The patient is placed supine on the operation table. We leave a tourniquet on the proximal aspect of the thigh. The navigation system should ideally detect the markers applied to the knee. The computer navigation system is placed 1.8 to 2.2 meters away from the knee on the contralateral side, closer to the patient's head (▶ Fig. 49.5). Members of the surgical staff should not obstruct the navigation camera and the markers applied to the knee during the procedure. When the navigated HKA angle matches with the radiographs, the operating procedure will run smoothly. It is essential not to change the position of the rigid bodies from the beginning of the surgery until the arthrotomy closure.

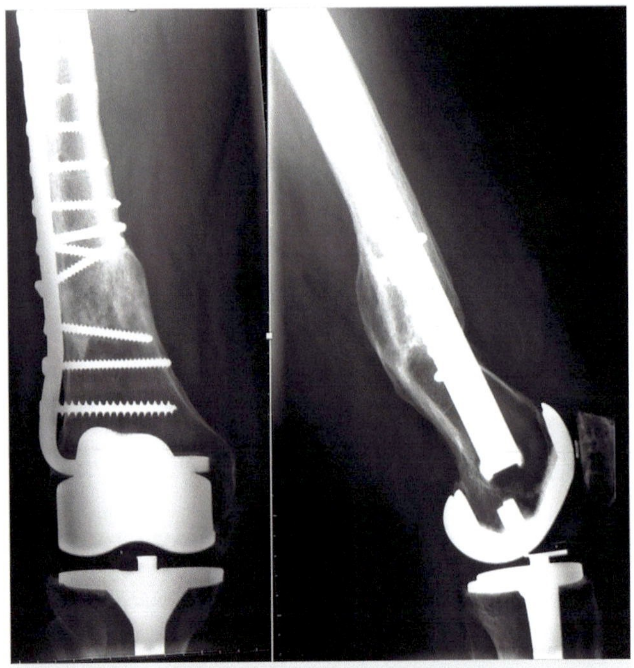

Fig. 49.4 Computer-assisted total knee arthroplasty (TKA) with a retained plate and an extra-articular recurvatum malunion: 5-year follow-up.

Checking the reducibility of the deformity (see below) is essential in determining whether soft tissue release is necessary. The analysis of the stability to valgus and varus stress in combination with the alignment of the femur in the coronal plane (valgus/varus) is critical to determine how we manage the rotation of the femoral component.

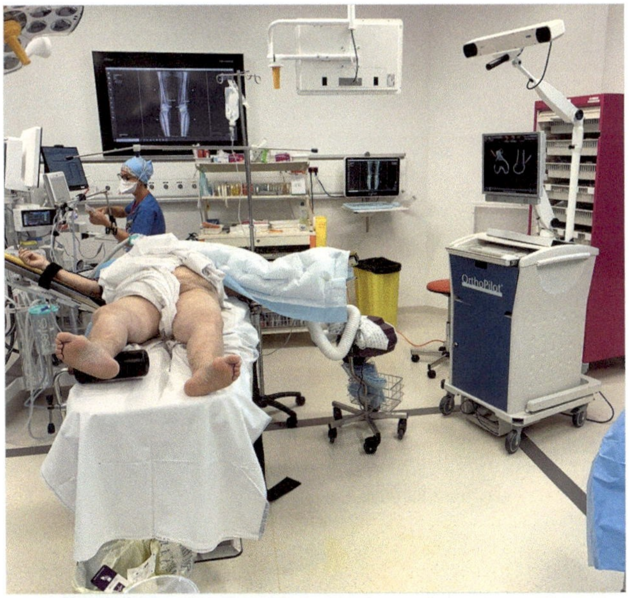

Fig. 49.5 Position of the navigation device in the operative room.

Flexion deformity inferior to 15 degrees is easily corrected by the bone cuts and by removing the osteophytes, especially when there are substantial posterior osteophytes of the medial femoral condyle. In rare cases, it is necessary to cut more at the level of the distal femur by moving the femoral cutting guide proximally, as we can do with a conventional technique.

In the case of preoperative excessive recurvatum (more than 10 degrees, which is measured with navigation), it is straightforward to move the femoral cutting guide distally and resect less bone than the thickness of the femoral implant.

49.8 Tips, Pearls, and Lessons Learned

- Before beginning the surgical procedure, it is essential to check that the localizer is in the correct position to avoid changing its spatial location during the operation.
- No assistant or nurse must be between the camera (localizer) and the markers. The field must be accessible for the camera to locate the markers.
- It is necessary to have an alternative plan with conventional instruments, in case rare problems may occur (for instead, computer crash or impossible fixation of the rigid bodies due to severe osteoporosis).
- We should avoid multiple drilling holes at the site of the implantation of the rigid bodies, as it increases the risk of fractures on those sites.
- Preoperative radiographs are always helpful (anteroposterior [AP], lateral, skyline views, and long-leg + + +) to check if the deformities match the navigation data. If it does not match, we advise making a new acquisition of the lower leg axis. In case the discrepancy persists, we follow the guidance of the navigation system.
- We avoid any soft tissue release before removing all osteophytes and verifying how much of the deformity we may reduce by stressing the joint. Thus, we perform significant releases in less than 10% of cases.

49.9 Difficulties Encountered

Sometimes, markers are not seen by the localizer after the bone cuts, which is usually related to drops of blood on the sensor balls. A good cleaning of the balls with gauze pads solves the problem.

Rarely, the navigated HKA angle does not match the radiographic angle. When it happens, it may be related to either inadequate preoperative radiographs or an intraoperative bad acquisition of the anatomical landmarks. A mismatch between preoperative radiographs and intraoperative navigation measurements requires that the surgeon verify the adequacy of the radiographs and the intraoperative data collection.

If the mismatch persists, after data collection has been repeated once again, we follow the navigation measurements.

49.10 Key Procedural Steps

We prefer a medial parapatellar approach for the majority of the cases. We evert the patella and expose the joint. We insert the femoral and tibial markers percutaneously (▸ Fig. 49.2), reducing the surgical incision length. The markers should be accessible to the navigation system during the entire procedure without moving the navigation localizer. The femoral marker is placed 15 centimeters above the joint line in an oblique position to the frontal plane, and the tibial marker is placed 10 centimeters below the joint, parallel to the frontal plane.

49.10.1 Navigation of the Femorotibial Mechanical Angle

The navigation begins with the collection of anatomical landmarks on the patient's knee. We use a wireless metallic pointer to capture points predetermined by a software protocol. The following points of reference are registered:.

- The anterior cortex of the femur just above the upper margin of the trochlea.
- The posterior aspect of the medial and lateral condyles.
- The point in the middle of tibial spines.
- The center of either the medial or the lateral tibial plateau. When the tibial mechanical axis is in varus, the lateral plateau is used as a reference. When the tibial mechanical axis is in valgus, the medial tibial plateau is used. The idea is to reference the higher point of the tibial plateau and plan for minor bone resection.
- At the end of this step, the center of the knee is determined, and the femoral implant size is registered on the computer.
- The acquisition of the center of the ankle is obtained by informing the system where the medial and lateral malleoli are located and the center of the tibiotalar joint.
- Finally, the femoral head center is located by moving the leg in a small circular motion, slowly and progressively, with the knee in extension or in flexion.
- At this step of the procedure, we know the HKA angle, which is compared to the preoperative radiographic measurements. Before applying the cutting jigs, it is essential to check the reducibility of the deformity, above all in extension (10 degrees

of flexion) predicting any soft tissue release. In the genu varum, we stress the knee in valgus and check the HKA angle informed by the computer. In case of hyperreducibility (varus going into valgus) or hyporeducibility less than 3 degrees, there is no need to release the medial collateral ligament (MCL). If there is a varus contracture determining that we cannot reduce the varus and persist with 3 to 6 degrees, a release of the MCL is needed (pie-crusting). If the lack of reducibility is above 6 degrees, a significant release is required (release of the MCL at its femoral insertion). If these adjustments are not performed, the balance will not be symmetric, and the side of the knee, which was convex before surgery, will be lax.

49.10.2 Navigation of the Bone Cuts

The tibial cutting guide is mounted on a support, which allows the valgus varus, the height of the cut, and the posterior tibial slope to be measured (▶ Fig. 49.6). We currently prefer to position this cutting guide freehand without any external support, which means smaller incisions. The tibial cutting guide is equipped with its rigid body. We fix the tibial cutting guide with four threaded pins when the computer shows a valgus-varus angle of 0 degree, a posterior tibial slope from 0 to 2 degrees, and a cutting height of 8 or 10 mm, which corresponds to the thickness of the tibial plateau implant (▶ Fig. 49.7). The tibia is then cut with an oscillating saw. The femoral cutting guide equipped with its "rigid body" is then placed against the anterior cortical of the distal end of the femur, with the knee flexed at 90 degrees. Any additional trochlear overhang on the anterior cortical is resected before placing the femoral cutting guide. The femoral mechanical axis is determined and compared with the radiological preoperative measurements (▶ Fig. 49.8). The surgeon then adjusts the valgus varus of the distal femoral cutting guide (0 degree for us), the posterior slope (between 0 and 2 degrees of flexion avoiding the notching of the anterior cortex), and the height of the resection corresponding to the thickness of the implant. We try to do a minimal resection on the side of the preoperative deformity convexity. Once the two initial cuts are performed, proximal tibia and distal femur, the extension gap is known, and the subsequent femoral cuts will follow the classic technique for a primary TKR.

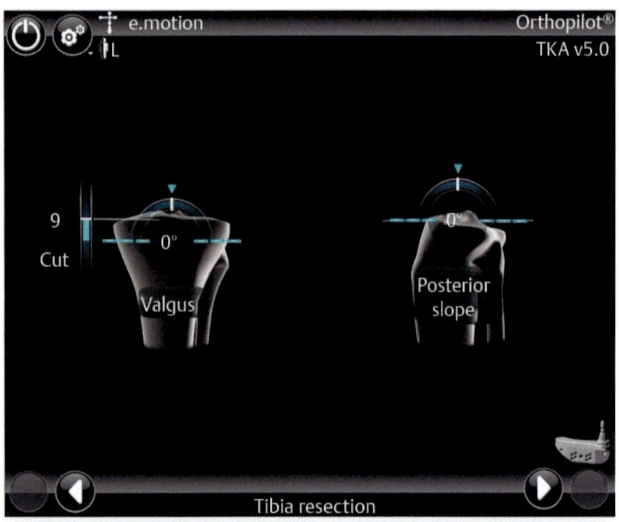

Fig. 49.6 Intraoperative measurements: resection height of the tibial plateau, varus-valgus alignment, and posterior slope.

49.10.3 Implanting the Prosthetic Trial

The implantation of the trial prosthesis uses computer assistance to check the mechanical leg axis in extension. Ligament balance is also controlled by performing valgus or varus stress measurements and assessing any medial or lateral gaping. We also check the mechanical axis of the leg with the permanent implants. This measurement allows double-checking if the implants were properly cemented. For every 1 mm of cement in excess, there is 1 degree of impact to the mechanical axis.

49.10.4 Rotation of the Femoral Implant

We do not systematically apply external rotation to the femoral implant, at least in genu varum. The femoral component rotation depends on pre- and intraoperative measurements of the mechanical axis of the femur (▶ Fig. 49.9). We use the following algorithm.

- The knee is in varus, but the femur has 3 or more degrees of valgus: In this case, it is expected to have more distal femur resection from the medial femoral condyle. Therefore, to obtain a proportional cut in flexion, one has to rotate the distal femur cutting guide externally.

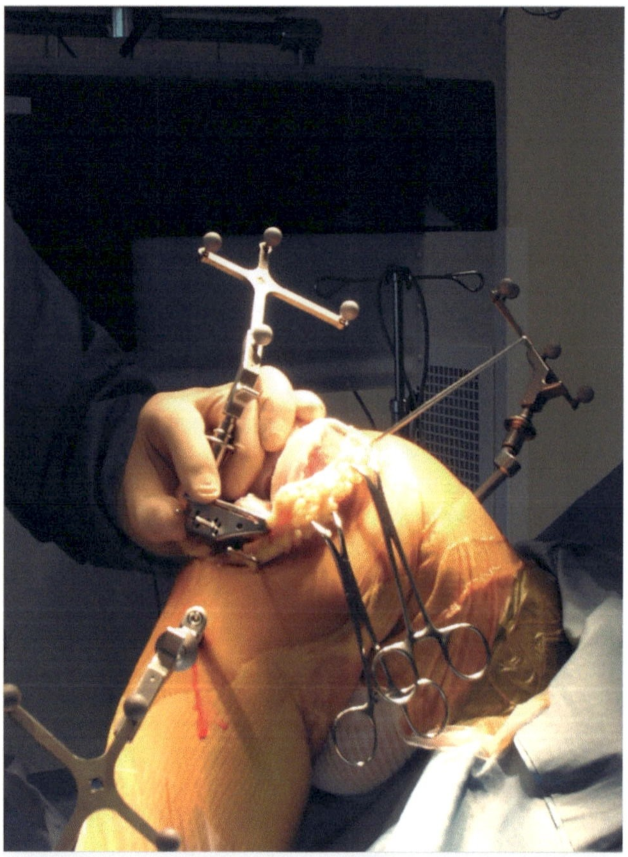

Fig. 49.7 Implanting freehand the tibial cutting guide.

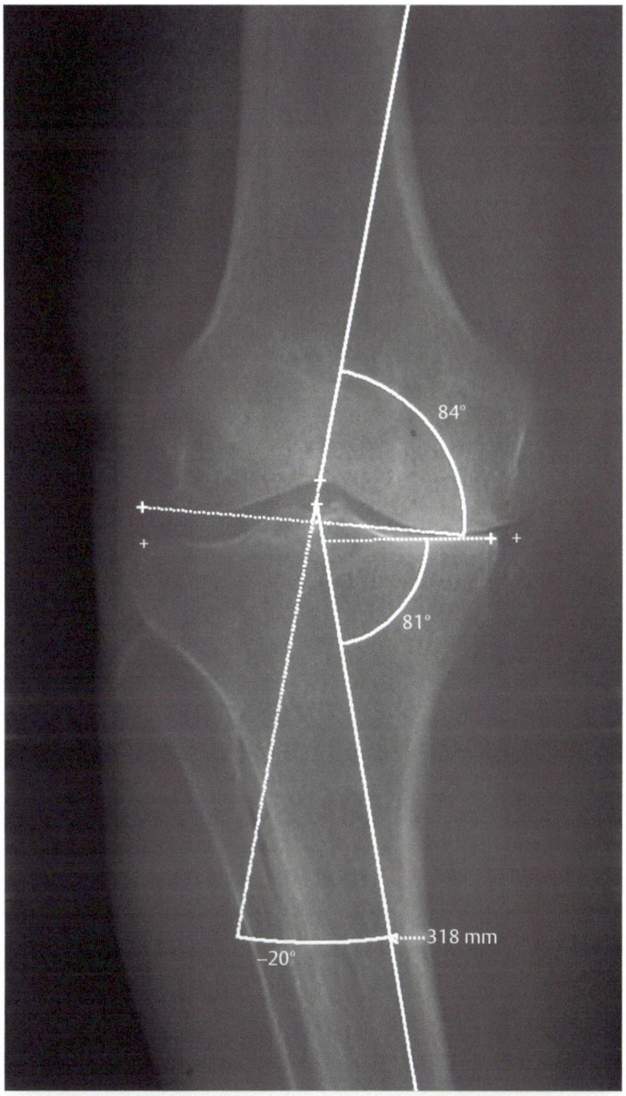

Fig. 49.8 Radiological measurement of the varus deformity: hip knee angle (HKA), medial femoral mechanical angle, medial tibial mechanical angle.

- The knee is in varus, and the femur is varus: In this case, if the knee is overreducible under stress, we foresee a less distal femur cut. Thus, to cut less posteromedial femur, it is appropriate to rotate the distal femur cutting guide internally.
- In the case of genu valgum: External rotation is systematically applied to the distal femur. We usually use 1 degree of external rotation for every 1 degree of femoral valgus and do not exceed 5 to 6 degrees of rotation, limiting the cut in the anterolateral cortex of the femur.

49.10.5 Ligament Balance

There are two ways to proceed: either by working from reducibility of the deformity tests (valgus and varus stress near extension) or by following ligament balance management software. We prefer to use the first method (software TKA smart 1.0), which allows the surgeon to consider and remain master of his/her decisions.

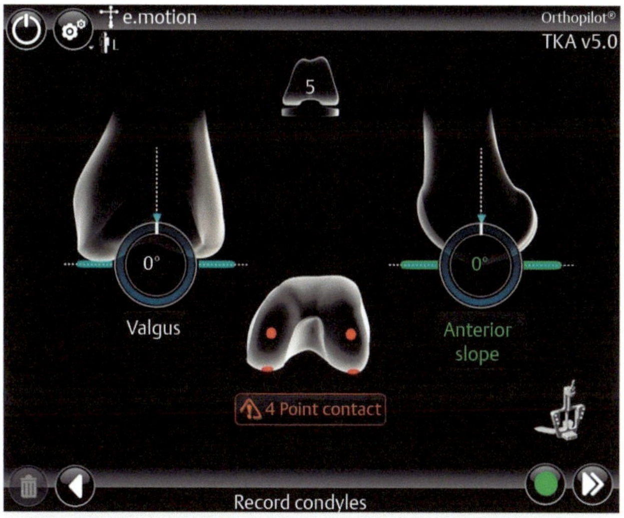

Fig. 49.9 Measurement of the femoral mechanical angle with the computer.

We proceed in the following way: when the mechanical leg axis appears on the computer screen, before any ablation of osteophytes, a manual force is applied in varus and valgus, with the knee at 5 to 10 degrees of flexion, to assess the reducibility of the deformity and the gap in convexity. If the deformity is entirely reducible or even hyperreducible, we are confident that we will achieve ligament balance, and no soft tissue release is needed in the concavity. The same is true if reducibility gives a hypocorrection of 2 to 3 degrees. If hypocorrection is more significant than this, it will be necessary to allow for the progressive release of soft tissue with trial implants after removing the osteophytes. However, a perfect balance does not necessarily mean a symmetrical gap between the medial and the lateral sides since it is known that the lateral compartment is laxer than the medial compartment in a normal knee. We therefore readily accept, in genu varum, a difference of 3 or 4 degrees more for the lateral compartment of the knee.

As far as the management of gaps between extension and flexion is concerned, we never have an imbalance since, on the one hand, we commonly use a PCL-retaining prosthesis which is a good "keeper" of the gaps, and on the other hand, the bone resection thickness is identical to the thickness of the implants. Thus, we maintain the balance in flexion as it was preoperatively.

Finally, we control the medial-lateral balance in flexion without using any distractor. We believe that using lamina spreaders is an artificial procedure that does not guarantee an adequate balance. Creating tension between the two compartments of the knee is subjective and challenging to reproduce among surgeons. To check this balance, it is sufficient, once the cutting guide for the chamfers has been applied at the distal femur level, to raise the thigh through the use of this supporting point, to manually pull into the axis of the knee flexed at 90 degrees, and to check the parallelism of the cutting guide with the cut of the tibial plateau (▶ Fig. 49.10). In genu varum, parallelism is perfect in most cases, and it is unnecessary to release soft tissue. Otherwise, especially in genu valgum, it is necessary to release the medial or lateral collateral

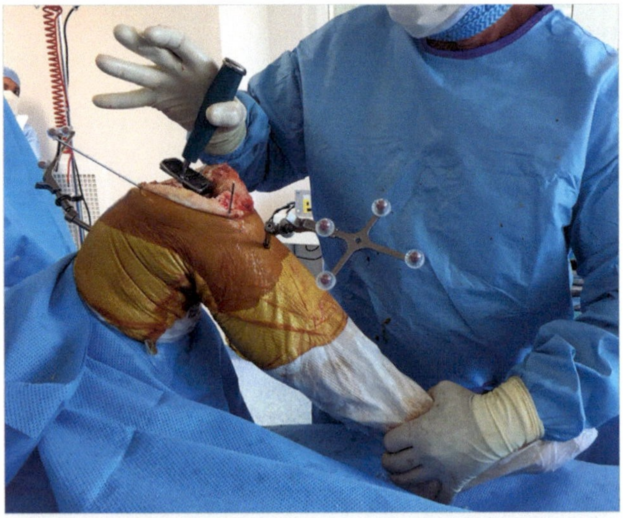

Fig. 49.10 Verification of ligament balance in flexion at 90 degrees.

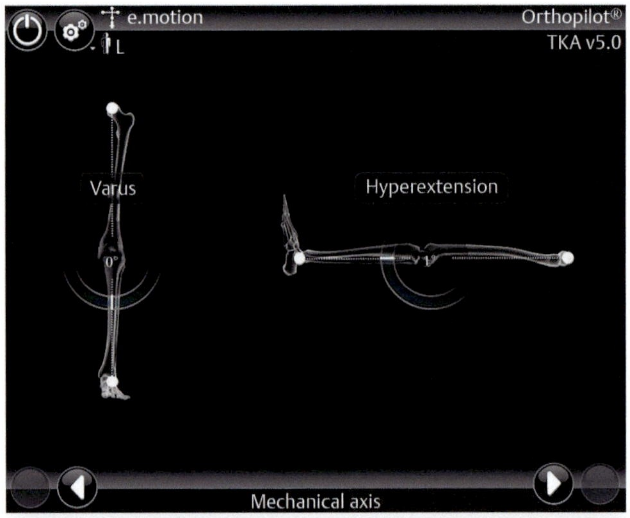

Fig. 49.11 Final hip knee angle (HKA) displayed on the computer's screen.

ligaments (LCL) progressively (fascia lata first, then LCL, and last the popliteus tendon and the capsule).

49.10.6 Implanting the Final Prosthesis

The final prosthesis is cemented (or not, in the case of cementless prostheses) when the HKA angle is at 180+/-3 degrees (▶ Fig. 49.11), the ligaments are well balanced and the tracking of the patella is optimal as well as the range of motion. The knee is closed in a standard fashion.

49.11 Bailout, Rescue, and Salvage Procedures

The main problem is when the rigid bodies move intraoperatively. At the beginning of the procedure, one can change the position of the rigid bodies and start the operation again. We don't advise it because, at the femur level, to do two or three drillings is at risk of fracture. The best is to move to a conventional TKR. If the rigid bodies move after the alignment with the trials has been checked, one may proceed to the final steps of the procedure without implanting the rigid bodies again.

49.12 Pitfalls

Important aspects to consider:

- The procedure is smoother when the radiographic preoperative HKA angle matches the navigated angle.
- The rigid bodies have to be perfectly fixed to the bones, or the system's accuracy is lost.
- The cutting guides should be well fixed. Otherwise, it may introduce a malalignment to the implants.
- Fail to plan is planning to fail. The procedure should follow all the pre-established steps.

50 Revision Total Knee Arthroplasty: Femoral and Tibial Components

Steven F. Harwin and Julio César Palacio-Villegas

50.1 Description

This chapter describes revision of the femoral and/or tibial components of a total knee arthroplasty (TKA), which may be done as part of a complete total knee revision, such as in cases of prosthetic joint infection (PJI), or to address problems specific to the femoral or tibial component itself, such as malposition (including malrotation), incorrect sizing, subsidence, stiffness, instability, and/or loosening. Isolated polyethylene liner replacement is sometimes performed in cases of acute infection to facilitate thorough knee debridement, for management of polyethylene wear, and in some cases of knee instability that require addition of a dished insert or a change of polyethylene thickness.

50.2 Key Principles

It is best to approach all surgical procedures in a systematic fashion.

The prime principle of revision surgery is to first establish the cause of failure. The most common causes of revision TKA are instability, infection, aseptic loosening, extensor mechanism dysfunction, arthrofibrosis, and osteolysis. While we commonly see a knee that "looks bad and feels bad," it is not uncommon to also see a knee that "looks good and feels bad." Knees that look good and feel bad will often be found to have subtle causes of failure such as unsuspected infection, mechanical loosening which is not readily evident (debonding), instability especially in flexion (seen in cruciate-substituting as well as cruciate-retaining knees), impingement, malrotation, or unrealistic expectations on the part of the patient. Complete knee arthroplasty revision is most often needed to successfully address most of these issues, but occasionally a problem isolated to the femoral or tibial component may present itself, such as use of a component that is too large or small, bone resections that were made incorrectly causing sagittal or coronal-plane malalignment, or loosening.

Occasionally isolated tibial polyethylene liner exchange is considered. A patient with mild anterior or posterior instability may have improved knee function if a dished liner is used to provide more constraint. A patient with a similar degree of coronal plane instability in extension and flexion may be more stable with a thicker tibial insert. However, most painful and/or unstable TKAs are not treated successfully with simple tibial polyethylene exchange because the underlying cause is not addressed (such as femoral and/or tibial malrotation, femoral over- or undersizing, or extensor mechanism problems).

50.3 Expectations

In general, revision TKA is an effective procedure. Over 80% of patients that undergo revision TKA for conditions not associated with PJI have a good-excellent outcome. The clinical outcomes associated with revision of knees affected by PJI are not as good, but patient satisfaction is nearly equal in both types of revisions. Patients must be counseled when discussing revision surgery that there cannot be certainty that every one of their symptoms will be cured and they will have "normal" knee. The outcomes of revision surgery are not as good and predictable as primary surgery.

50.4 Indications

Revision surgery is indicated when a verifiable objective failure of a primary arthroplasty can be documented. Exploratory surgery for a dissatisfied patient with no objective evidence of pathology often results in continued dissatisfaction. The timing of revision surgery should be a decision made by the treating physician who is acquainted with the situation and the problems that may arise if revision surgery is delayed, especially with respect to the risk of progression of the primary pathology that the revision surgery would address.

50.5 Contraindications

An absolute contraindication is a patient that is too frail for major surgery. Relative contraindications are lack of adequate home health resources/support for a successful recovery, or patients with pain who have no identifiable problem. Revision surgery should not be performed without a clear diagnosis.

50.6 Special Considerations

50.6.1 Diagnosis

To increase the likelihood of success, it is important to establish the correct diagnosis before recommending TKA revision. There should be no "exploratory surgery." The most frequent technical errors that may need to be corrected during revision surgery are malposition of components, alteration of the joint line, joint instability, failure to reproduce the correct limb axis, and poor fixation of the components. If planning to replace only one or two of the total knee components, one should try to obtain the previous operation note to be certain of the manufacturer and sizes of the implants in place.

A thorough history must be obtained, and a detailed physical examination done. The character, pattern, onset, and intensity of the patient's pain must be understood and the presence of a positive response to provocative physical signs noted. Flexion instability can be demonstrated by having the patient dangle the limb from the examination table and testing varus and valgus stress as well as anterior and posterior stability. The gait pattern should be observed, and the skin should be assessed especially as it relates to old or poorly placed incisions or poor soft-tissue coverage. The neurovascular status should be assessed. Patients with unexplained pain, swelling, and skin sensitivity should be evaluated for regional complex pain syndrome. PJI should be considered in a knee arthroplasty that is painful and swollen. Finally, the preoperative assessment should include a review of all available prior radiographs.

If no clear evidence of common causes for failure is apparent, such as infection, loosening, instability, extensor mechanism dysfunction, malposition, osteolysis, arthrofibrosis, and component failure, then remote causes of knee pain should be ruled out including problems in the spine, hip disease, vascular disease, or emotional or psychological issues and unrealistic expectations. Other less common causes of knee pain after surgery include soft tissue and bony impingement (including the popliteus tendon), pain from an unresurfaced patella, patella clunk syndrome, polyethylene-induced synovitis from wear, osteonecrosis of the resurfaced patella, and incisional neuroma.

An appropriate work-up for the painful total knee includes complete blood count (CBC), sedimentation rate, C-reactive protein, bone scans (technetium, indium, sulfa colloid marrow), computed tomography (CT) scan with 3D reconstruction, and magnetic resonance imaging (MRI) with metal suppression software. The gold standard to rule out PJI is aspiration of the knee for aerobic and anaerobic cultures and cytochemical evaluation. There are an increasing number of available serum and synovial fluid biomarkers that may be useful in the diagnosis of PJI such as leukocyte esterase and alpha-defensin; the authors recommend that surgeons be familiar with the latest guidelines and what is available at their institution.

50.7 Special Instructions, Position, Anesthesia

We perform virtually all joint replacements using regional anesthesia. We use spinal or epidural anesthesia and use nerve blocks postoperatively for pain control.

50.8 Tips, Pearls, and Lessons Learned

To ensure success, preoperative planning should include the following.

- Establish the best approach.
- Have a plan for implant removal.
- Determine the implants and instruments required, considering potential bone defects and ligament condition.
- Establish the need for a bone graft.
- Always be prepared for the worst-case scenario.
- Be aware of PJI. Consider obtaining cytochemical samples and aerobic and anaerobic cultures and delay the reimplantation until there is certainty regarding whether infection is present and the organism(s) responsible.

50.8.1 Have all Prosthetic Options Available

While some revisions require only a simple change of polyethylene, most will require removal of implants, debridement, and soft tissue balancing. One might also encounter unexpected ligament collateral ligament insufficiency. Therefore, one should have all prosthetic options available including posteriorly stabilized implants, totally stabilized implants, and on rare occasions a rotating hinge or even a modular tumor-type distal femoral or proximal tibial replacement implant. The importance of having the prior operation report cannot be overemphasized. One should not have to remove solidly fixed, well-positioned unaffected components simply because the accompanying revision implant was not available.

50.8.2 Consider the Possibility of Infection in All Revisions

If there is any suspicion of PJI, there are intraoperative investigations available to the surgeon that provide additional information, although none have perfect sensitivity and specificity. One such option is to use a leucocyte esterase urine test strip, which has been shown to be sensitive and is simple and inexpensive. More traditionally, multiple specimens (at least five) are taken and sent for frozen sections, although results are clearly subject to sampling error as well as the availability of a pathologist with appropriate experience. If histopathologic findings are consistent with acute inflammation (greater than 10 white blood cells per high-powered field) or positive leucocyte esterase, then one should consider removing the implants. In such cases, it is the author's preference to insert a spacer consisting of a new "loosely cemented" femoral component and all-polyethylene tibial component that can be easily removed after the infection is eradicated, or antibiotic-impregnated articulating cement spacer or also static spacer with antibiotics depending on the surgeon's preferences or the severity of the case. Antibiotic-loaded cement fashioned into "cigars" or "chains" and placed in the femoral and tibial canals can be an option.

50.9 Difficulties Encountered

Adequate exposure of the knee is mandatory for avoiding complications and can be very difficult in revision TKA situations. If adequate exposure cannot be obtained even with the quadriceps snip, then thought should be given to performing a tibial tubercle osteotomy. An extended osteotomy allows visualization of the canal and later reattachment using cerclage wires. We suggest detaching the tubercle proximally to provide a buttress for reattachment and extending the tibial osteotomy along the medial aspect of the tibial tubercle distally for a distance of 8 to 10 cm, leaving the lateral soft tissue sleeve intact. Drill holes are made laterally and the bone flap is "cracked" laterally in situ. In some cases in which the extensor mechanism is severely contracted, it may be necessary to perform a lateral retinacular release early in the procedure to allow for satisfactory visualization and mobilization of the patella, including its eversion when necessary. When removing a well-cemented implant that already has stems in place, it may also be necessary to perform an osteotomy or "window" of the anterolateral femur in order to gain access to the femoral canal.

50.10 Key Procedural Steps

50.10.1 Obtain Adequate Exposure

The surgical exposure must be wide enough to allow for proper visualization and assessment of the entire knee. A tourniquet is used in all cases and regional anesthesia is preferred, using tranexamic acid either intravenously, topically, or both. In general, the previous incision can be utilized, extending proximally and distally as needed. The cutaneous vasculature of the anterior aspect of the knee primarily arises from the medial genicular arteries, placing laterally based skin flaps at risk. If several incisions are present, one should utilize the most lateral incision that allows adequate exposure for the planned surgery (▶ Fig. 50.1). There should be no tension on the skin edges during surgery. If the previous procedure was performed with a poorly placed incision, or if prior surgery had been performed with an incision that would preclude a standard midline approach, then plastic surgical consultation should be considered to avoid wound problems postoperatively. Once the fascia is exposed, it can be determined if there is adequate mobilization of the patella and extensor mechanism. A medial parapatellar incision is made initially to open the joint, leaving a cuff of soft tissue on the patella for later capsular closure. Any fluid within the joint is noted and sent for Gram stain, aerobic and anaerobic culture and sensitivity, and cytochemical studies. If the patella cannot be adequately mobilized with the knee flexed 90 degrees, consider performing a quadriceps snip by crossing the lateral aspect of the proximal quadriceps tendon at a 45-degree angle approximately 5 cm above the patella. Both sides of the extensor mechanism are elevated with tenaculae. The suprapatellar pouch, medial and lateral gutters, and anterior chamber are debrided and debulked. One should ensure that there is adequate patellar and patellar tendon mobility, and the posterior capsule should be released to be able to mobilize the tibia anteriorly.

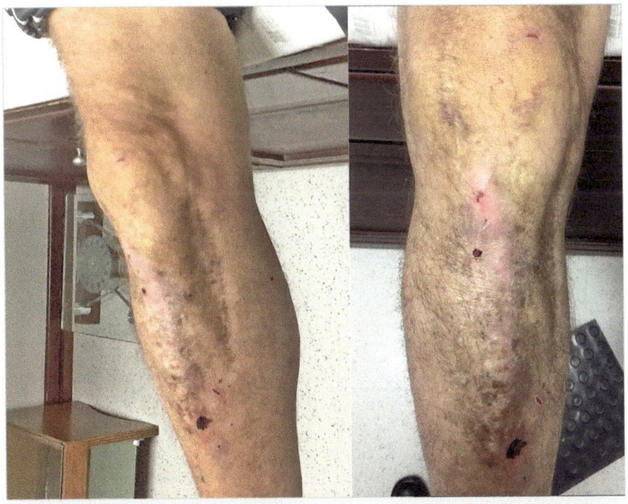

Fig. 50.1 Example of a patient with multiple knee incisions. The most lateral incision should be used for revision arthroplasty.

50.10.2 Remove the Implants Carefully with Minimal Bone Loss

Once the source of pathology is confirmed and it is determined that the implant must be changed, then atraumatic removal of the existing implant must be undertaken. The procedure must be done with care and patience. One starts by assessing the patella component first. If it is in satisfactory condition and well cemented, it may be left in place even though it may be from a different manufacturer. Most patella components are simple domes that are compatible with all revision femoral components. Removing a well-cemented patella component runs the risk of fracture or being left with too thin a bony remnant on which to place a new component. If the patellar component is to be removed sharp thin osteotomes can be used at the prosthesis–cement interface dislodging the component. Alternatively, in the case of a well-fixed patellar component, one may use a sharp oscillating saw just beneath the polyethylene and then remove the pegs with a drill. Once the patellar button has been removed, any residual cement is then removed by performing a skim cut with a thin rigid oscillating saw and then removing the residual cement by hand with small rongeurs and small curettes. If the patella component is loose and the remnant is less than 12 mm thick, then a "salvage patelloplasty" is performed by trimming the residual bone and centralizing it for proper tracking. See Chapter XX for further discussion of patellar component revision.

50.10.3 Femoral Component Removal

Typically, the femoral component is addressed next, since doing so will improve exposure for the tibia. The tibial polyethylene is removed to further improve exposure and "loosen" the knee. The surgeon should understand the locking mechanism of the specific implant used; a locking pin or screw may be present and need to be removed first. The tibial insert can be removed easily by drilling a 3.2-mm hole in the plateau and then inserting a large cancellous screw that lifts up the poly, or prying the polyethylene out using an osteotome or sharp Homan between the insert and the metal tibial component. A short, thin oscillating saw can be used to carefully disrupt the cement–component interface of the femoral component. Manual instruments typically suffice to complete the removal. A thin osteotome may be used to disrupt the cement-prosthesis interval, moving circumferentially around the implant freeing up all fixation, including the intercondylar notch. A Gigli saw is ideal for freeing up the anterior bone–cement interface. These steps should be done carefully with preservation of bone stock as the goal. Once that is performed, a lipped instrument is slipped beneath the anterior flange of the femoral component and is gently tapped to dislodge it. Using this method, bone loss is minimal. All residual cement is removed, and osteolytic areas are debrided.

50.10.4 Tibial Component Removal

The next step is to assess the tibial component. If it needs to be replaced, the tibial tray and cement are removed in a similar fashion to the femur. A thin osteotome is placed between the implant and cement, starting anteromedially and progressing

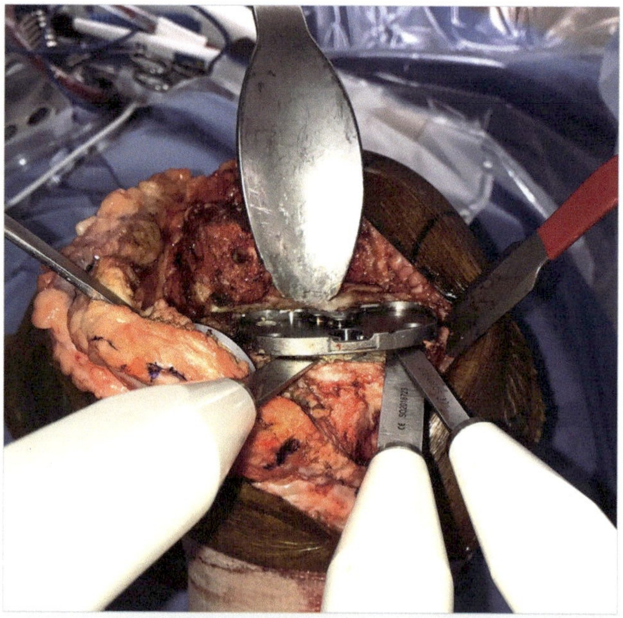

Fig. 50.2 Stacked osteotomes are used to gently pry out the tibial component. This technique minimizes damage to the proximal tibia that can occur by levering out the tibial tray from a single fulcrum.

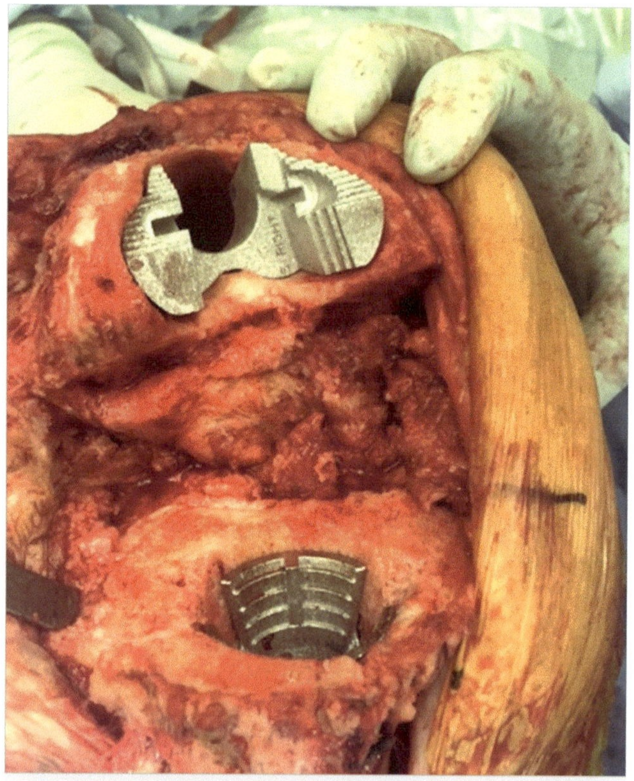

Fig. 50.3 An intraoperative photograph showing the placement of metaphyseal cone trials in both the femur and tibia.

posteriorly and then laterally and posteriorly. The posterolateral corner and the areas near the cutout for the posterior cruciate ligament (PCL) can be troublesome and exposure is key. Once the interface is disrupted, the stacked osteotome technique is used (▶ Fig. 50.2). If needed, a small notch can be made in the anterior aspect of the tibia directly below the center of implant to allow for a punch to elevate the implant without applying torque. Commercial extractor instruments can be helpful, but patience and meticulous technique is essential. If needed, a thin, rigid oscillating saw may be used to disrupt stubborn areas. Attempting to remove an implant without disrupting the entire interface can result in significant loss of bone.

50.10.5 Debride the Knee, Assess Residual Defects, and Determine the Management Strategy

Once all implants are removed, the residual bone and soft tissues are debrided, especially the posterior portion to recreate the flexion space. The bone is examined for defects and the need for bone graft or augments. Very small defects can be filled with cement, but bone graft or augments are preferred for larger defects. Commonly, there is a central defect in the tibia and bone loss medially and/or laterally. For medial and lateral tibial plateau defects, either 5- or 10-mm thick augments are typically available. For central defects, multiple sizes of cone augments are available for the tibia and femur (▶ Fig. 50.3). Uncontained defects can be effectively treated with a bilobed augment. The exact size and shape of the augments will be dictated by the configuration of the defects, the distance from the femoral and tibial joint lines, and the size of the flexion and extension gaps (▶ Fig. 50.4).

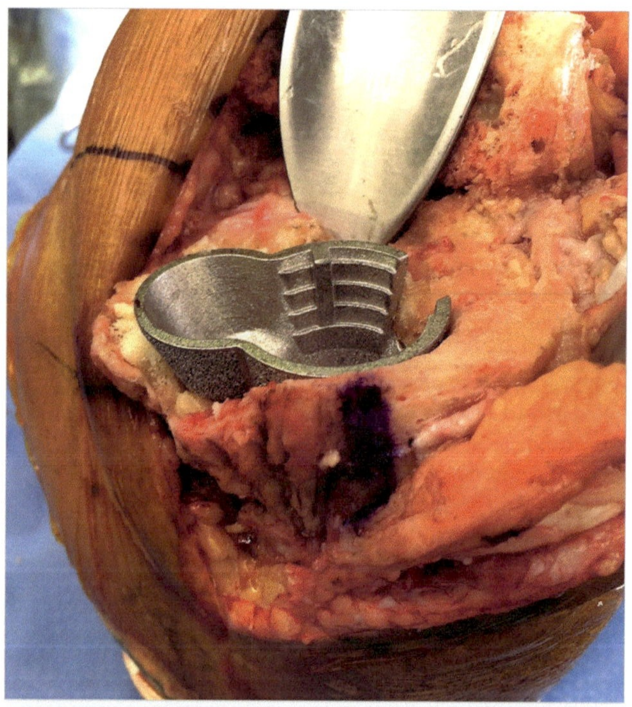

Fig. 50.4 An example of a "bi-lobed" tibial metaphyseal cone used in a patient with extensive loss of bone from the medial aspect of the tibial plateau.

50.10.6 Preparation of the Femur and Tibia

The femur is prepared for the revision implant, with the goal of reproducing the original joint line. Stems are nearly always used in the revision setting, and the surgeon will have to choose the length, diameter, and mode of fixation of the stem (cemented or uncemented). There are advantages and disadvantages to the use of short vs. long and cemented vs. uncemented stems. If bone stock is adequate, use of a short stem avoids the need to use an offset adapter. Longer stems that engage the diaphysis provide increased biomechanical stability, but unfortunately dictate the final position of the component and typically necessitate use of an offset coupler so that the position of the femoral component on the metaphysis is optimized. Short stems are simpler, maintain bone stock, and are typically adequate except in cases of severe bone loss or osteopenia. Since the specific technique of total knee revision is dependent on instrumentation, for purposes of illustration, the procedure of preparing the femur for a Triathlon TS (Stryker Orthopaedics, Mahwah, New Jersey, USA) revision component with a short-cemented stem is shown (▶ Fig. 50.8). Revision using other knee systems will utilize similar steps as shown in ▶ Fig. 50.3 and ▶ Fig. 50.4. Large central metaphyseal defects of the femur or tibia are treated with the Triathlon Tritanium Metaphyseal Cone Augment System; other systems will have similar cone options and steps. Ensuring appropriate construct support and stability in the metaphyseal zone is critical to long-term success of the reconstruction.

After debridement and removal of all cement, the first step is to open up the medullary canals and curette the contents. If infection is suspected, specimens are sent from the canal. A trial implant is assembled with the stem length chosen and the length measured to determine the depth of reaming. Medullary reaming is carried out to the previously determined depth until consistent cortical chatter is heard and felt. Power or hand reamer can be used according to surgeon's preferences. Once the reamer is stable in the canal, the size of the component to be used is determined with a sizer, taking into account the width of the femur and the anterior-posterior distance. Once this is determined, the appropriate-size distal femoral cutting guide is applied with distal and posterior augments, if necessary. We are then able to go up or down one size on the tibia. The epicondyles are located and the cutting guide, with the epicondylar line referenced, is positioned to reproduce the joint line, usually 2 to 2.5 cm distal to the epicondylar axis. The distal femoral cutting guide is set at the angle of the stem on the femoral component (typically 6 degrees). Excess flexion and extension of the implant should be avoided. The guide with its augment trials is rotated to match the epicondylar axis and placed against the distal femur. If the epicondyle reference for the femoral rotation is identifiable, the tibial base can be used as a reference for the femoral rotation (▶ Fig. 50.5). A blade runner is used to assure that the implant sits properly on the anterior femur. Then determination can be made as to the necessity for posterior augments. Once the proper anterior/posterior position and the proper rotation of the implant are determined, the jig is pinned in place securely. Correct rotation of the femoral component is assessed using the transepicondylar axis, as well as making sure that medial and lateral flexion gaps are symmetric (the latter is easily checked after the tibial trial is in place.

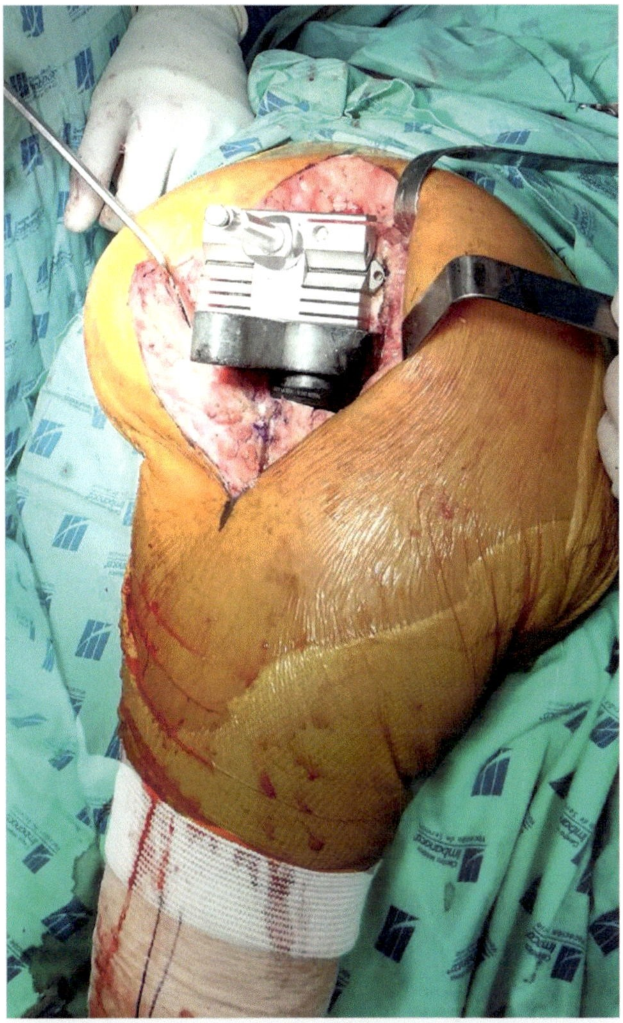

Fig. 50.5 With the knee in flexion, the rotation of the femoral component should match that of the tibial trial, with equal flexion gaps medially and laterally.

The cuts are made in the following order: anterior femur, anterior chamfer, posterior femur, and then posterior chamfer. The posterior cut can accommodate a 5- or 10-mm augment if needed. The distal femoral augments on the medial and lateral side have already been determined based upon the distance from the epicondylar line. At this point, an accessory guide is applied to the jig anteriorly and the intercondylar notch is fashioned. Once this is accomplished, the jigs and intramedullary reamer are removed. If there is a large central defect, the femur must be prepared for the use of a femoral metaphyseal augment. The femur is prepared by a machining process: first with medullary reaming and then metaphyseal reaming to the proper size implant (▶ Fig. 50.6).

Attention is then turned to the tibia. Previously, we removed the implant and any loose or retained cement. We assess the residual bone for the need of an augment medially or laterally or for a metaphyseal cone augment. Similarly to the femur, the medullary canal is reamed to the distance determined by the length of the base plate, augment, and stem. The size of the tibial component has already been measured preliminarily by applying a template to the surface prior to final preparation.

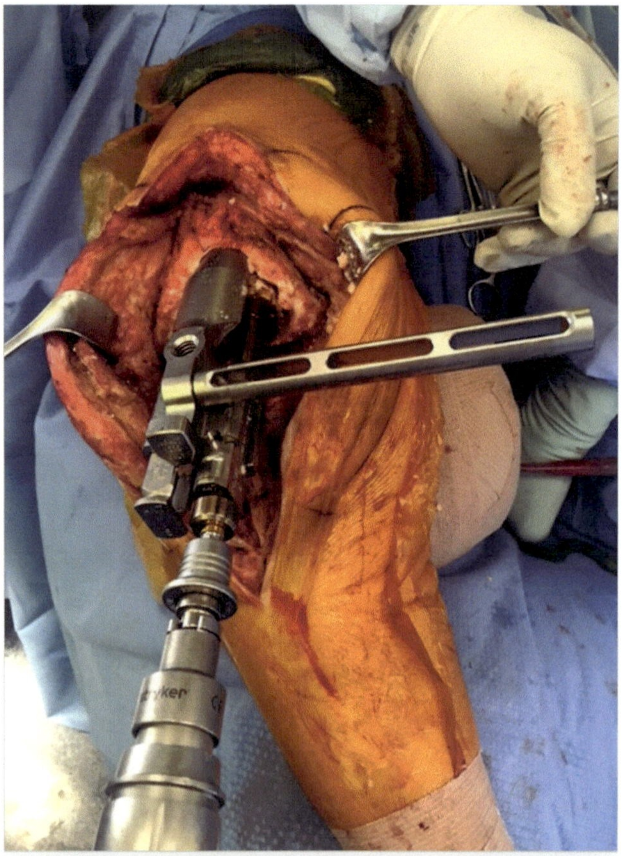

Fig. 50.6 Intraoperative photograph showing the instrumentation used to prepare the distal femur for a stemmed revision component with a metaphyseal augment.

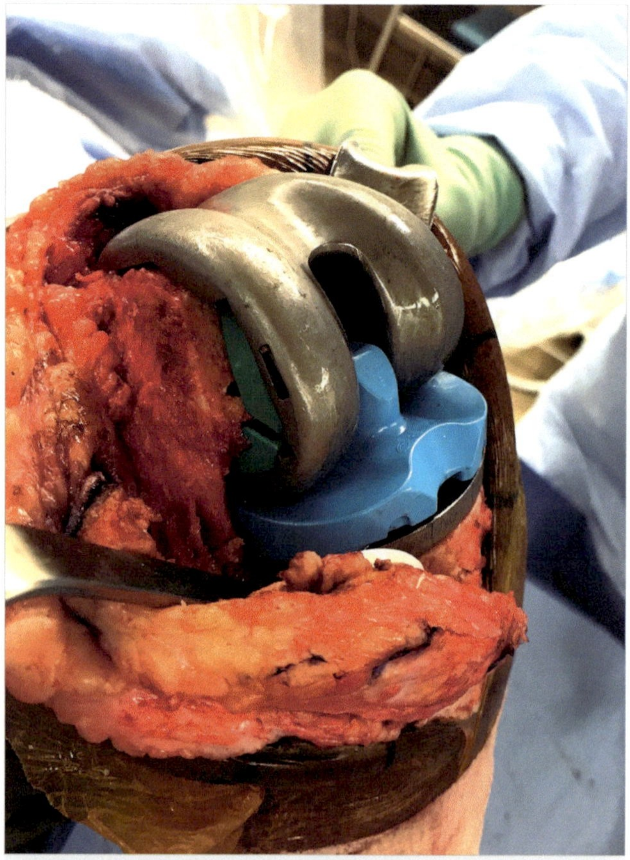

Fig. 50.7 Intraoperative photograph showing trial reduction of the knee.

The medullary canal is opened and curetted and specimens are taken for culture and pathology, if necessary. Sequential reaming is carried out similarly to that on the femur. A preliminary construct of a baseplate with its possible augments and stem is measured before beginning the reaming process. Once the reamer is stable in the canal, the tibial cutting guide is applied. Adjustments in the cut are made based upon the need for augmentation medially or laterally. It is preferable to use an augment if there is a bone deficiency rather than to remove more bone. The tibial cutting guide accounts for step cuts and a 5- or 10-mm augment can be utilized medially and laterally independently. These can also be used with a metaphyseal cone augment if needed. The fibular head can be used as a landmark to judge the original tibial joint line. The tibial component template is applied covering cortex to cortex and pinned in place in the proper rotation, just medial to the center of the tibial tubercle. Internal rotation must be avoided. If a metaphyseal cone augment is needed, the metaphysis is machined using first a medullary reamer, then a central and/or lobe reamer for use either medially or laterally (▶ Fig. 50.4).

50.10.7 Apply the Trials and Assess Stability and Kinematics

Once the bones are cut, cleaned, and prepared for augmentation, the flexion and extension gaps are evaluated and appropriate releases are performed to balance the gaps. The trials are assembled and placed. The trial tibial metaphyseal cone is placed and the trial tibial component with its augments is inserted. Again, final adjustments in position of the tibial are made, if needed. The femoral trial with its stem extension and any distal and posterior augments is applied to the distal femur after inserting the metaphyseal cone trial, if needed. Adjustments in fit and final position of the femur are made, if needed. Finally, sequential trial tibial polyethylene inserts are used, and the size is chosen that gives full extension and maximal flexion, with adequate medial/lateral and anterior/posterior stability. Trialing should be done with standard cruciate retaining (CR) and posteriorly stabilized (PS) implants in order to assess the true stability (▶ Fig. 50.7). A totally stabilized or constrained insert with a wider post can be used if adequate coronal stability cannot be achieved. The knee is taken through a full range of motion, checking the kinematics and patella tracking. If not already done, a lateral retinacular release is performed if necessary. However, before performing, the implants should be checked for proper position and rotation. It is important to put the quadriceps mechanism under direct proximal tension before doing a release. It is not uncommon for the patella to appear subluxed without proper tension restored. This is done by putting a tenaculum on the edge of the lateral flap and pulling proximally, not medially.

50.10.8 Deflate the Tourniquet, Achieve Hemostasis, Prepare the Bone Ends, and Cement the Implants

Most full revisions will include a wide debridement and debulking of scar tissue, especially in the back of the knee to recreate the flexion space. Therefore, it is best to pack the knee, deflate the tourniquet if used, and achieve hemostasis prior to proceeding. Once done, the limb is elevated, exsanguinated, and the tourniquet reapplied. If cemented stems are used, cement or biodegradable plugs are placed in the proximal femur and distal tibia, about one centimeter from the tip of the stem. A "baby bottle brush" is used to thoroughly remove any loose bone or debris. The bone ends and canals are prepared by using pulsating lavage, dry sponges, hydrogen peroxide-soaked sponges (to remove blood from the interface), and dry sponges again. The tibial component is usually placed first. For relatively short stems (100 mm) that are intended to be cemented, two batches of methyl methacrylate cement with tobramycin are mixed in a vacuum mixer and inserted in a retrograde fashion in a slightly more liquid, than doughy, state and pressurized. Alternatively, if the surgeon prefers uncemented stems, the medullary canals are plugged with a finger or lap sponge while the cement is applied to the bone surface. The component is coated with cement and inserted with an impactor flush with the bone. The position is checked with the template and alignment rod. Excess cement is trimmed away. The femoral component is inserted in a similar way. Once the cement is doughy, the knee can be reduced with the trial poly insert in place and the knee extended for cement pressurization. Care must be taken not to change the component position. Once the cement is hard, the trial is removed and the back of the joint is checked for any excess cement or debris. A periarticular injection with Marcaine, epinephrine, morphine, Toradol, and Depo-Medrol is given. The real poly insert is impacted and the knee reduced and checked for alignment, stability, range of motion, kinematics, and patella tracking (▶ Fig. 50.8).

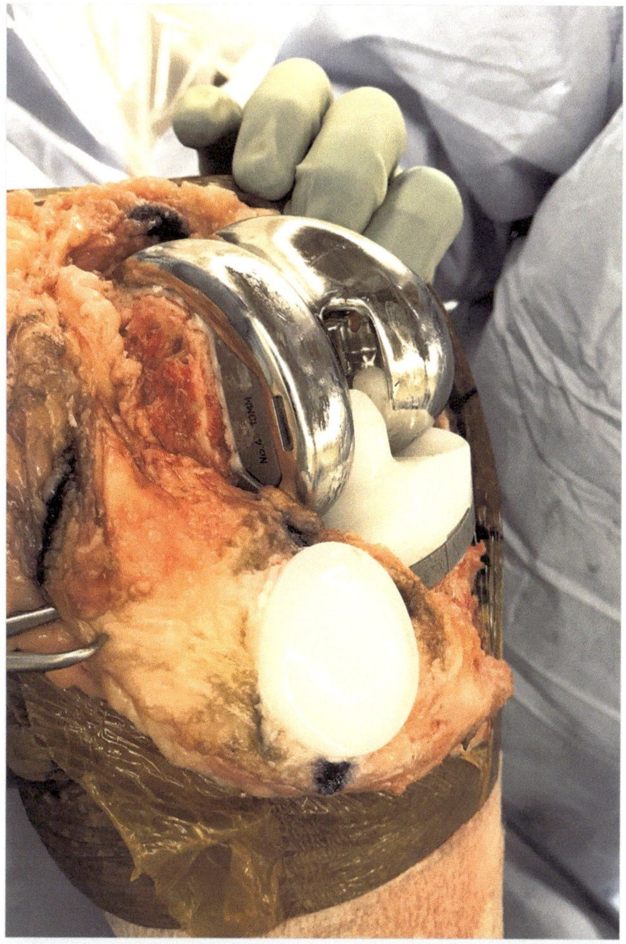

Fig. 50.8 Intraoperative photograph showing the final revision knee components in place.

50.10.9 Close the Wound Securely

Once the implants are in, the wound is soaked in a dilute solution of Betadine (0.35%) for 3 minutes and then thoroughly and completely washed away with a pulsating lavage. A deep and superficial suction recovery drain is placed in most cases of full revision. The quadriceps mechanism and snip are closed with #1 Maxon suture, the subcutaneous tissue is closed with #2–0 Vicryl, and the skin is closed with a subcuticular Monocryl suture or staples. The wound is coated with the dilute Betadine solution and an Aquacel dressing is applied, as well as a large, bulky dressing. The tourniquet is then deflated and the circulatory return is checked.

50.10.10 Wound Healing Must Supersede Rehabilitation

We would all agree that postoperative rehabilitation is very important to achieving satisfactory outcomes. Most revisions can undergo a standard rehab program with immediate range of motion exercises and full weight bearing as tolerated. However, if the wound does not heal properly, with drainage, bleeding, redness, or disruption, then all rehab should be held until the wound improves and seals. An elegant reconstruction is cancelled out by postoperative wound problems or infection. Persistent wound drainage or significant necrosis should be addressed by early rather than later surgical intervention.

50.11 Bailout, Rescue, and Salvage Procedures

For extreme ligament loss with instability, a rotating hinge component should be considered. For extreme bone loss, a tumor-type distal femoral replacement implant is utilized.

50.12 Pitfalls

Inadequate release of the extensor mechanism can lead to inadvertent disruption of the patellar tendon insertion on the anterior aspect of the proximal tibia. Patellar tendon injury must be avoided. If that possibility exists and/or patellar tendon mobility is not as expected, the first option should be to realize a vastus snip, and if that is not enough, then an expanded anterior tibial tuberosity osteotomy should be performed.

Inadequate exposure of the implants before removing them can lead to fractures and more bone loss.

Stemmed femoral and tibial components are often used during revision TKA. If any doubt with the position of the stem, consider using image intensification during surgery to ensure proper positioning of the stems and to avoid inadvertent canal penetration or malposition.

51 Revision Total Knee Replacement—Patellar Component

Benjamin Hansen

51.1 Description

Revision of the patellar component can be done in isolation or as part of a complete knee revision or reimplantation. This procedure can address isolated loosening of the patellar component or can be combined with more extensive procedures to correct patellofemoral symptoms associated with malpositioning, specifically due to malrotation or immproper sizing/positioning of the femoral and/or tibial components.

51.2 Key Principles

A key principle in revision of the patellar component is to be aware of the thickness of the remaining patella, especially the amount of bone available to support a revision patellar component. The risk of patellar fracture and subsequent extensor mechanism deficiency increases as the patellar bone stock decreases. If the remaining patellar bone thickness is 10 mm or less, it is not advisable to remove further bone in order to place another patellar component. In this case, the patella should be left without resurfacing. In many knee revisions, the end result of the patellar revision is an unresurfaced patella. A new patellar component should not be cemented to the remaining thin, sclerotic bone. Revision to a new patellar component should only be done when there is a healthy bone for cement fixation. Cementing into sclerotic bone is likely to fail due to loosening of the patellar component. On the other hand, overstuffing the patellofemoral compartment of the knee with a femoral component that is placed too anterior, oversized, or final patellar construct (patella + patellar component) that is too thick can lead to anterior knee pain and/or reduced knee flexion.

A second important principle when considering a revision of the patellar component is that it is essential to evaluate the alignment and rotation and positioning of the femoral and tibial components. Failure to address malrotation and/or malalignment/postitioning of the femoral and tibial components.

51.3 Expectations

The main goal after revision of the patellar component is to maintain the integrity of the extensor mechanism. This is paramount to keep in mind when considering revision of the patellar component. Patients can have an acceptable outcome after revision surgery even if the patellar bone stock was not adequate to resurface. When patellar revision is done, either as an isolated revision or when associated with tibial and/or femoral component revision, 2-year survivorship is approximately 95%. Revision of the patellar component for patellofemoral pain without evidence of component malposition, infection, or loosening will be less successful.

51.4 Indications

Once the patella resurfaces during the initial arthroplasty procedure, the indications for revision of the patellar component are loosening, infection, or extensor mechanism dysfunction This dysfunction may be due to associated overstuffing of the patellofemoral compartment, malalignment of the knee or malrotation of the femoral and/or tibial components. In cases of malalignment or instability of the patella, revision of the femoral and/or tibial components is often necessary. In these cases, the primary patellar component can be preserved if it is well fixed. In the case of loosening of the patellar component, often there is adequate bone stock to place a new polyethylene liner. The underlying sclerotic bone and old cement should be removed in order to get to healthy bone for new cementation of the polyethylene patellar component. A new patellar component should not be placed on sclerotic bone. This will lead to poor cement contact with bone and early loosening of the patellar component. In the case of infection, all hardware in the knee should be removed, including the patellar component. Many times, the patellar component is well fixed, and care should be taken to remove the patellar component with as little bone loss as possible. Revision for malpositioning of the patellar component may be necessary if the patellar component is grossly malpositioned. This is possible if the component is positioned too far inferior or medial on the patella. This can lead to patellar maltracking problems and pain. The patella may also need to be revised if it is found that the total patellar thickness (patellar bone plus patellar component) is too large, leading to anterior knee pain and/or knee stiffness.

51.5 Contraindications

Revision of the patellar component is contraindicated if there is a well fixed, appropriately sized patellar component. If the patellar component has to be removed secondary to infection, loosening, or gross malposition then a new patellar component should only be reimplanted if there is greater than 10 mm of native patellar bone remaining. It is not advisable to cement a new patellar component to sclerotic bone or old cement as this leads to early loosening and failure. Although it has been proposed that trabecular metal patellar implants can be sewn into soft tissue in the absence of any residual patellar bone stock, this technique is associated with early loosening. I retain the original patellar component in the the majority of the knee revisions that I perform.

51.6 Special Considerations

In the setting of infection, do not place a "cement spacer" on the patella. It is more advisable to place antibiotic-loaded cement on the anterior aspect of the femur in order to fill the patellofemoral joint space. Later removal of an adherent patellar spacer can lead to further bone loss and increased risk of fracture and subsequent extensor mechanism disruption (▶ Fig. 51.1, ▶ Fig. 51.2, ▶ Fig. 51.3).

Revision of the patellar component for malpositioning is rarely indicated. More commonly, there are times when a patellar revision is indicated if the patella is medialized appropriately but

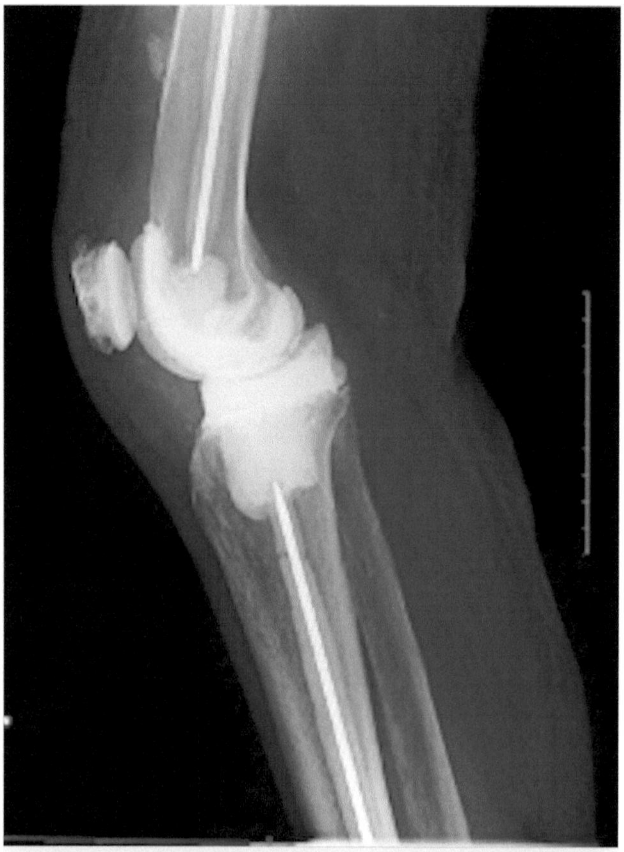

Fig. 51.1 Lateral radiograph of a knee after resection of an infected total knee replacement and placement of an articulating antibiotic spacer. Note the cement that has been placed on the patella. This cement was firmly attached to the patella and during removal further patellar bone was lost.

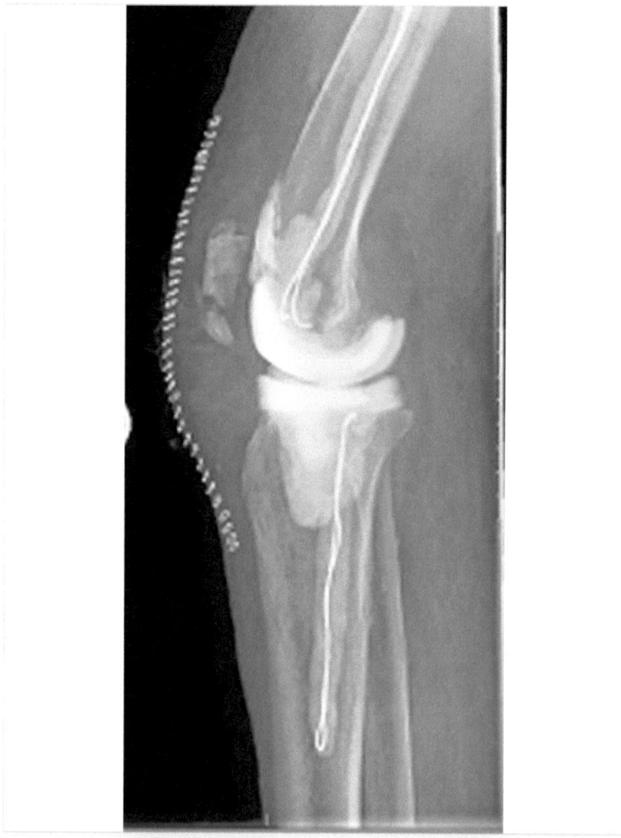

Fig. 51.2 Lateral radiograph of the same patient. She did not clear the infection after the first spacer and another spacer was placed. She had a fall postoperatively and sustained a fracture of the patella, resulting in loss of the function of the extensor mechanism. The patient went on to an above-knee amputation.

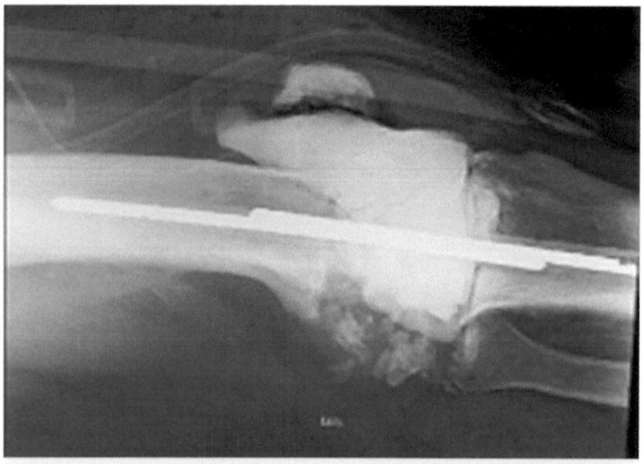

Fig. 51.3 Lateral radiograph of a knee after resection of an infected knee replacement and placement of a static antibiotic spacer. Note the cement filling the patellofemoral compartment. Adequate fill of the patellofemoral compartment is essential for a successful static spacer. No cement was directly placed on the remaining patella which maintains patellar bone stock.

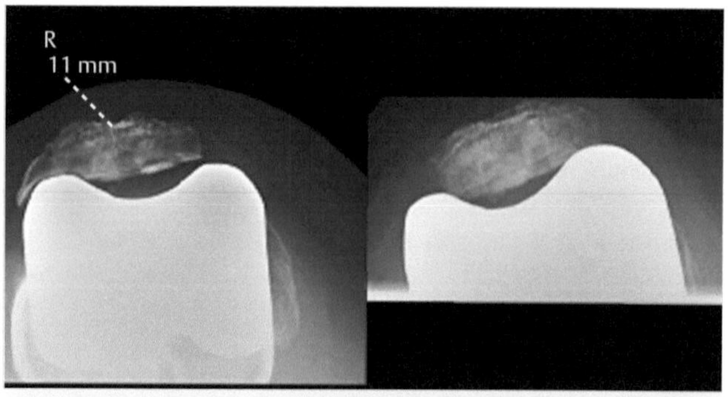

Fig. 51.4 Pre- and postoperative Merchant views of the knee showing uncovered lateral bone with contact of the lateral aspect of the patella with the lateral trochlea of the femoral component. This was removed during revision of the patellar component. The patellar polyethylene button was loose and adequate bone stock was available for a new polyethylene button. Postoperatively the patient had better function and no pain.

there is uncovered bone laterally. This uncovered patellar bone can contact the lateral aspect of the femoral component in the trochlea with flexion and lead to pain (▶ Fig. 51.4). In this case, during revision surgery, the stability of the patellar component should be checked. This can be done by trying to place an osteotome by hand under the patellar component and manually trying to lift the patellar component from the patella. If it is stable, then it is left in place. At this point, all of the remaining bone laterally should be removed until the bone is flush with the patellar component. This is easily done with a saw and/or rongeur.

51.7 Special Instructions, Position, and Anesthesia

Spinal or general anesthesia may be used. When revising the patellar component, the knee is in full extension. Full revision instrumentation and components should be available, as well as a wide array of straight and angled curettes, curved and flat osteotomes in many widths, and a pencil-tipped burr.

51.8 Tips, Pearls, and Lessons Learned

Preoperative planning is important. Tibial and femoral malrotation and total patellar thickness (bone plus patellar component) should always be considered as factors contributing to patellofemoral problems after total knee arthroplasty. The surgeon should be prepared to perform a complete total knee revision if such problems are noted intraoperatively. Preop computed tomography (CT) comparing the posterior condylar axis to the femoral neck axis can sometimes provide clues to femoral component rotation.

51.9 Difficulties Encountered

Adequate surgical exposure is mandatory. In the case of isolated patellar revision, simply extending the incision farther proximally and releasing adhesions is usually sufficient to evert the patella. A quad snip may be needed on rare occasions.

Removing a well-fixed patella, such as in the setting of infection, can be difficult. An oscillating saw can be used to cut just under the polyethylene. Be careful not to cut through the bone with the saw. It is preferable to either cut through the polyethylene or the cement. After that, a pencil tip burr or drill bit is used in order to meticulously remove the remaining cement and polyethylene from both the flat surface of the patella and from the lug holes in the central aspect of the patella. There is better bone preservation when the pencil tip burr is used.

Persistent patellar maltracking may signify an underlying problem with femoral or tibial component rotation. Options to correct maltracking include complete knee revision or tibial tubercle osteotomy.

51.10 Key Procedural Steps

- Expose the knee using the same incision used for the prior arthroplasty. The proximal incision may need to be longer, and releases should be performed as needed to be able to evert the patella. A sharp towel clamp is placed just inferior and superior to the patella as close to the bone as possible in order to evert the patella for adequate exposure. The soft tissue from the lateral edge of the patella will need to be removed just enough to delineate the true border of the patella for adequate exposure. If this is not done, excessive tension can be placed on the patellar tendon.
- After the patella is everted, the entire patellar component–bone interface should be exposed.
- The patella component may be grasped with a pointed towel clip while small osteotomes can be inserted parallel to the undersurface of the patella in order to loosen it. If the patella is well fixed, it may be cut off with a saw, aiming for a resection level that is just beneath the patella, cutting across any prongs or lugs. Remaining cement is then carefully removed. The surface should be recut if not done already. Small drill holes may be placed in any sclerotic bone areas.
- The patella is sized according to the specific implant used, and the undersurface of the patella prepared using the appropriate instrumentation.
- A trial component is placed, and patellar tracking evaluated.
- The patellar undersurface is debrided with pulsatile jet-lavage, the bone is dried, and the definitive patellar component cemented in place.
- The wound is closed according to the surgeon's preference.
- Postop rehabilitation will depend on the nature of the revision. If a standard arthrotomy is done, there are typically few restrictions. If a quad snip or tibial tubercle osteotomy is done, protection of the quad mechanism may be needed.

51.11 Bailout, Rescue, and Salvage Procedures

In cases where the patient has significant patellar bone loss without enough remaining bone (< 10 mm) to cement a new standard polyethylene liner in place, then salvage procedures can be used. These salvage procedures are only advisable if the patient has pain from the unresurfaced patella, or poor function due to maltracking. In the case of inadequate bone stock, the usual scenario is a central defect with an intact cortical rim. The preferred treatment is to restore bone stock. This can be done by packing cancellous bone graft into the central defect and then using a synovial flap from the adjacent synovium to contain the bone graft in the defect. This synovium is elevated, rotated, and sown over the bone graft. This has the advantage of restoring bone stock without further metal implants. Trabecular metal patellar implants are also available to use if there is inadequate bone stock available for a revision to a polyethylene component. These trabecular metal implants rely on bony ingrowth for long-term stability. They do require bony contact for a successful outcome and should not be placed in soft tissue alone as a substitute for the patella entirely. When faced with poor bone stock, my initial approach is to leave the patella alone, especially if there has been a history of infection. If there is not a history of infection and the patient requires restoration of the function of the fulcrum that the patella provides, then my initial approach would be to restore the bone stock with bone grafting procedure. I prefer this approach over a trabecular metal implant. At this stage, if a metal implant has to be removed again, further bone will be lost and the extensor mechanism function will be at higher risk for failure.

51.12 Pitfalls

- Pain associated with the patella after knee replacement can be unrelated to the actual patella implant itself.
- Beware of unrecognized component malposition or the presence of an oversized femoral component as a cause of patellofemoral problems.

52 Extensor Mechanism Reconstruction—Synthetic Mesh

Kevin I. Perry and Arlen D. Hanssen

52.1 Description

This procedure addresses extensor mechanism disruption after primary or revision total knee arthroplasty (TKA). Previously treated with isolated suture fixation, allograft tendon, or whole extensor mechanism allograft, synthetic mesh reconstruction of the extensor mechanism provides a favorable, inexpensive alternative. This reconstruction utilizes a knitted monofilament polypropylene graft folded onto itself and secured with heavy nonabsorbable suture. The graft is then secured to the anterior tibia either in an extramedullary position through a bone trough or through intramedullary position prior to cementation of the tibial component in the setting of tibial component revision. Following mobilization of the vastus lateralis and vastus medialis, the mesh is brought over the patella through an inferolateral portal and secured proximally with a combination of nonabsorbable and absorbable suture. The mesh is covered with a pants-over-vest technique ensuring complete coverage of the mesh graft. Utilization of this technique has demonstrated improved clinical outcomes with increased Knee Society scores for pain and function, maintained knee flexion, improved extensor lag, cost-effectiveness, and reproducibility.

52.2 Key Principles

- A 10 × 14 in (25–35.5 cm) sheet of knitted monofilament polypropylene mesh (Bard Mesh, Davol, Inc., Warwick, RI) is folded upon itself and secured with heavy nonabsorbable suture.
- The mesh is secured to the anterior tibia either via extramedullary fixation (usually through a bone trough) or intramedullary fixation with poylmethylmethacrylate and nonabsorbable suture.
- The vastus lateralis and vastus medialis oblique (VMO) are mobilized distally, while the mesh is tensioned proximally and secured with nonabsorbable suture in a pants-over-vest fashion.

52.3 Expectations

Historically, extensor mechanism disruption has been treated with isolated suture fixation (in the acute setting), Achilles tendon allograft, or whole extensor mechanism allograft. These modalities have offered modest results with substantial expense. Specific complications with allograft have included increased mid- and long-term extensor lag, immune reaction and disease transmission, tissue availability, and cost. An inexpensive alternative involves reconstruction of the extensor mechanism with a knitted monofilament polypropylene mesh. Initial series utilizing this technique have demonstrated that a specific synthetic mesh can provide a cost-effective, favorable alternative.

Patients treated with synthetic mesh for extensor mechanism disruption have demonstrated improved Knee Society score for both pain and function. The mean Knee Society pain score for aseptic reconstruction improved from 36 points preoperatively to 75 points postoperatively. The mean Knee Society function score for aseptic reconstruction improved from 20 points preoperatively to 50 points postoperatively. Utilization of synthetic mesh improved extensor lag at midterm follow-up without progressive extensor lag over time and maintained knee flexion throughout. There have been no direct correlations of synthetic mesh-related infection and overall survivorship in both the aseptic and septic settings has been quite favorable.

52.4 Indications and Contraindications

While primary repair of the extensor mechanism is often reserved for acute disruptions, utilization of synthetic mesh is indicated for reconstruction of acute, subacute, and chronic extensor mechanism disruption after TKA in both the aseptic and septic settings. Contraindications to performing synthetic mesh reconstruction include medical comorbidities that preclude the patient safely undergoing the operative intervention, ongoing infection, or soft-tissue complications preventing wound closure. While not a contraindication, comorbid association of diabetes mellitus has been demonstrated as a risk factor for reconstruction, given abnormal physical and vascular properties inhibiting successful healing following reconstruction of extensor mechanism.

52.5 Special Instructions, Position, and Anesthesia

All patients being evaluated for extensor mechanism reconstruction should obtain plain radiographs of the knee (anteroposterior [AP], lateral, and patellar views) as well as an erythrocyte sedimentation rate (ESR) and C-reactive protein (CRP) to rule out concurrent joint infection. If concurrent periprosthetic joint infection (PJI) is confirmed, two-stage exchange with extensor mechanism reconstruction is preferred.

The patient is placed in the supine position in the operating suite. A sterile tourniquet is typically placed after preparation and draping of the affected extremity. Preparation of the sterile synthetic mesh is completed on the back table. A 10 × 14 in (25–35.5 cm) sheet of knitted monofilament polypropylene mesh is folded upon itself approximately 8 to 10 times to a width of 2 to 2.5 cm wide and secured with heavy nonabsorbable suture.

52.6 Tips, Pearls, and Lessons Learned

While synthetic mesh has been demonstrated to retain tensile strength, it is crucial to ensure incorporation of mesh with host tissue. Fixation of mesh through avascular allograft tissue not previously excised at the time of initial reconstruction leads to failure of incorporation. Therefore, in the setting of previous reconstruction, it is vital to ensure appropriate excision and debridement of avascular tissue surrounding mesh graft.

Intramedullary fixation has been found to be superior to extramedullary fixation, primarily in the setting of tibial component revision. Intramedullary fixation avoids risk of tibial tubercle nonunion, proximal tibial fracture at the site of allograft bone fixation, and bone-block avulsion.

Reconstruction should be performed with the knee in extension to ensure maximal VMO advancement. Typical flexion ranges from 40 to 60 degrees after closure.

52.7 Difficulties Encountered

- Failure to properly mobilize the vastus medialis and vastus lateralis will lead to significant extensor lag and/or failure of the reconstruction. Often these structures have retracted considerably into the proximal thigh and the incision must be extended proximally to find and mobilize them down to the knee.
- Failure to properly excise avascular tissue will inhibit incorporation of mesh and lead to mechanism failure.
- Failure to ensure complete coverage of the mesh can allow joint fluid to wick through into the soft tissues and cause a subcutaneous seroma. Every effort should be made to provide complete coverage of the mesh graft.

52.8 Key Procedural Steps

- Sterile synthetic mesh is prepared on the back table and secured with heavy nonabsorbable suture (▶ Fig. 52.1).
- An incision is made through patient's previous skin incision, utilizing the most lateral incision that can safely access the knee, thus preserving blood supply over the anterior aspect of the knee. Sharp dissection is carried down through the skin and subcutaneous tissue down to the capsule. A standard median parapatellar arthrotomy is made.
- The mesh is secured to the anterior tibia either through a bone trough or in an intramedullary fashion if the tibial component is being revised at the time of surgery.
  a) If tibial component revision is not required, a burr is used to make a trough through the anteromedial tibial cortex anterior and distal to the tibial component tray. The mesh is inserted and secured with poylmethylmethacrylate and transfixation lag screw to ensure fixation (▶ Figs. 52.2a, b and 52.4).
  b) In the setting of tibial component revision, the mesh graft should be inserted prior to cementation anterior to the component stem and exiting the intramedullary canal of the tibia in an anteromedial location just medial to the anterior tibial crest (▶ Figs. 52.3 and 52.4). The tibial stem should extend 4 to 6 cm beyond the mesh graft in order to ensure appropriate tibial component fixation. Methylmethacrylate cement is used to obtain fixation.
- After tibial fixation, a laterally based flap of fibrinous tissue or retinaculum is mobilized and interposed between the mesh and the tibial polyethylene insert to prevent abrasive irritation from the polyethylene.
- A small incision should be made through the level of the patellar tendon remnant fibrinous tissue or retinaculum. The mesh graft is then advanced through the remnant patellar tendon scar tissue or retinaculum and secured medially with nonabsorbable suture. The mesh is then advanced deep to

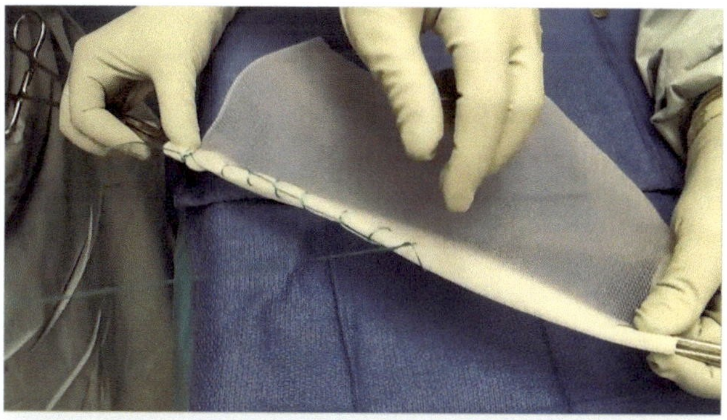

Fig. 52.1 Preparation of the mesh on the back table with nonabsorbable suture.

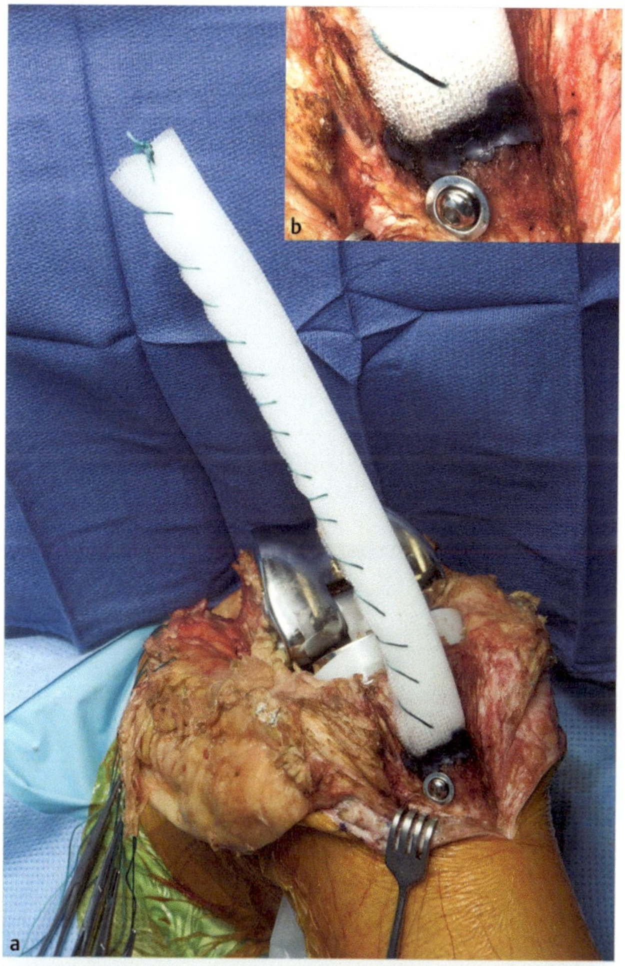

Fig. 52.2 (a) Mesh secured through bone trough with screw fixation. (b) Close-up of the mesh, cement, bone interface with screw fixation. Typically, the trough for the mesh is 2 cm × 2 cm and the most distal aspect of the mesh is cemented into the trough.

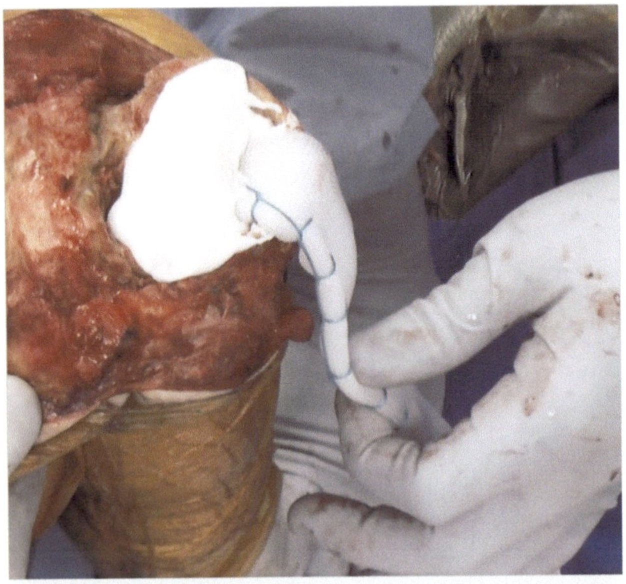

Fig. 52.3 Placement of the mesh into intramedullary canal during tibial component revision.

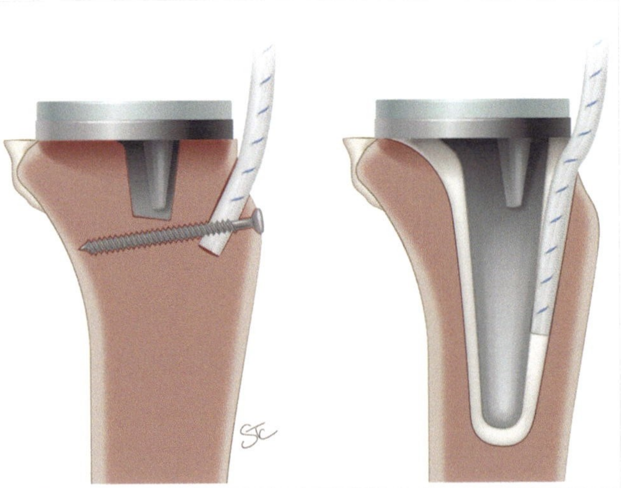

Fig. 52.4 The left panel demonstrates how the mesh is placed into a trough in the tibia if the tibial component is being retained. The right panel demonstrates how the mesh is placed anterior to the tibial component during cementing if the tibial component is being revised.

superficial to lie anterior to the patella. Patellectomy is not routine, but can be performed if soft tissue is sparse in order to make room for the mesh graft.

- With the knee in extension, mobilization of the VMO and vastus lateralis with use of blunt dissection is performed to release any adhesions. The skin incision should be extended proximally as needed for appropriate visualization. VMO and vastus lateralis are advanced distally to restore appropriate tension and patellar height. Nonabsorbable sutures are utilized to assist with distal traction of the vastus lateralis and VMO. Synthetic mesh is simultaneously tensioned proximally. The graft is secured with nonabsorbable suture to the lateral retinaculum, vastus lateralis, and quadriceps tendon. Redundant mesh is excised proximally. Mesh is secured superficially to the vastus lateralis and deep to the vastus medialis in a pants-over-vest fashion. Mesh should be completely enveloped by host soft tissue.
- Capsule closure is then performed in standard fashion.
- Postoperative management includes long leg cast for 12 weeks. After cast removal, patient flexion is advanced by 30 degrees every 4 weeks to achieve a total range of motion of 90 degrees by 12 weeks out of the cast.

52.9 Bailout, Rescue, and Salvage Procedures

In the setting of a failed mesh reconstruction of the extensor mechanism, bailout options include repeat mesh reconstruction, complete extensor mechanism reconstruction using allograft, above-knee amputation, or knee arthrodesis.

52.10 Pitfalls

- Failure to excise avascular tissue can lead to failure of mesh incorporation. This is most commonly encountered in patients who have had prior failed attempts at extensor mechanism reconstruction with allografts.
- Failure to mobilize the vastus medialis and vastus lateralis and bring them distal can lead to failure or significant extensor mechanism lag. To mobilize them in the chronic setting, the incision must often be carried quite proximal to localize the muscle and bring them down distally.
- Failure to immobilize the patients for an extended period of time can lead to failure of the mesh to fully incorporate and early failure. The authors recommend a period of immobilization in a cast for 12 weeks followed by stepwise progressive flexion in a brace for an additional 12 weeks.

53 Unipolar Osteochondral Femoral Replacement

Luis Eduardo Passarelli Tirico and William D. Bugbee

53.1 Description

Unipolar osteochondral femoral replacement using fresh osteochondral allograft (OCA) transplantation addresses full-thickness articular cartilage lesions of the femoral condyle. OCA has over a century of clinical history. Many clinical and basic scientific studies have been performed with the result that allografting is now part of the cartilage repair paradigm for the treatment of chondral or osteochondral lesions. Surgical technique of allografting of the femoral condyle can be performed utilizing a dowel osteochondral plug (dowel technique) or small fragment grafts (shell technique) in order to restore the osteochondral unit (bone and cartilage) of the femoral condyle with mature, hyaline articular cartilage.

53.2 Key Principles

- Limb malalignment and ligament instability must be addressed prior or simultaneously to the allograft procedure.
- Allografts are obtained from an organ/tissue donor and are preserved fresh in positive temperatures until transplantation.
- Transplantation is usually performed between 2 and 6 weeks of tissue recovery, typically in an average of 20 days.
- Chondrocyte viability decreases over time with storage. New medium of tissue culture is being investigated in order to increase storage time with high cell viability.
- Fresh OCAs are usually indicated for osteochondral lesions larger than 2 cm^2 or as a salvage procedure in cases of failure of previous cartilage repair procedures.
- Advantages include a single stage procedure, with no donor site morbidity, restoring mature, hyaline articular cartilage to the affected area.
- Disadvantages of OCA include limited allograft tissue availability and the potential for transmission of infectious disease from the graft or immunologic response by the recipient.
- Surgical techniques can be performed using specific instrumentation (dowel technique) or small fragment grafts (shell technique) in order to restore the osteochondral unit.

Regardless of the technique used, the following general principles should be followed.

- Matching donor and recipient within 2 mm difference.
- Resection of recipient area to be grafted must be kept to a minimum.
- Harvest graft from donor at the same location as the lesion on the recipient.
- Prepare donor graft with the same depth as measured at the recipient site, beveling the edges and trimming with a rasp.
- Very gentle tamping is performed to fully seat the graft when needed.

53.3 Expectations

Good and excellent results with OCA for the femoral condyle have been published, and ongoing investigations with modern surgical techniques continue to clarify the indications and clinical outcomes of osteochondral allografting on the knee joint.

53.4 Indications

Indications for fresh OCAs include a broad range of pathology, such as cartilage repair procedures and complex osteochondral reconstruction.

53.4.1 Cartilage Repair

- Chondral or osteochondral defects larger than 2 cm^2.
- Osteochondritis dissecans.
- Revision of previous failed cartilage repair surgery.
- Subchondral bone lesions without full-thickness cartilage defect.

53.4.2 Complex Reconstruction

- Posttraumatic periarticular fracture malunion.
- Selected cases of single compartment arthritis or multifocal degenerative lesions.
- Massive type III or IV osteochondritis dissecans.
- Osteonecrosis of the femoral condyle.

53.5 Contraindications

Fresh OCAs should not be used in some pathology, due to increased risk of complications. Some of these situations are:

- Generalized osteoarthritis.
- Use of tobacco containing nicotine.
- Active inflammatory joint disease.
- Ongoing joint infection.

53.6 Special Considerations

When considering using OCA for cartilage repair, the surgeon needs to understand that a compatible donor must be found in order to match the recipient defect characteristics with donor morphology, and a scheduled surgical procedure with a specific date and time is not always possible. Often the patient receives notice that a donor is available less than 7 to 10 days before the surgical procedure, in order to perform transplantation of graft with high cell viability. Matching of donor and recipient is usually performed by size of the proximal tibia, using plain anteroposterior knee radiographs. A standard anteroposterior radiograph of the recipient corrected for magnification is measured and matched with a direct caliper measurement of the tibial width for the donor. A size match is considered acceptable when donor and recipient are within 2 to 3 mm, although matching by donor sex, height, and weight is often adequate. When performing the dowel technique, the size of the donor tibial width should be equal or larger than the recipient, in order to have the convexity of the donor femoral condyle similar or flatter in shape compared with the recipient.

The two commonly used techniques for preparation and implantation of OCAs include the press-fit plug technique and the shell graft technique. Each technique has advantages and disadvantages. The press-fit plug technique is similar in principle to autologous osteochondral transfer (OATS). A number of commercially available instruments can be used for this procedure. This technique is optimal for contained condylar lesions between 15 and 30 mm in diameter. Fixation is generally not required due to the stability achieved with the press fit. Disadvantages include the fact that very posterior femoral condyle and tibial plateau lesions are not conducive to the use of a circular coring system (which requires a perpendicular approach to the joint surface) and may be more amenable to shell allografts. In addition, the more ovoid or elongated a lesion is in shape, the more normal cartilage needs to be sacrificed at the recipient site in order to accommodate the circular donor plug. Shell grafts are technically more difficult to perform and typically require fixation. However, depending on the technique employed, less normal cartilage may need to be sacrificed.

53.7 Special Instructions, Position, and Anesthesia

The surgical procedure is performed with the patient in a supine position, with a tourniquet on the proximal ipsilateral thigh under spinal anesthesia or general anesthesia and femoral nerve block. An anteromedial or anterolateral 5 cm arthrotomy is executed, depending where the lesion is located. The size of the lesion is recorded.

53.8 Tips, Pearls, and Lessons Learned

- OCA may be used for primary cartilage repair of large osteochondral lesions or as a salvage procedure following a failed previous cartilage repair. OCA can anatomically restore large or complex lesions of any anatomic surface and is particularly useful in dealing with disorders of subchondral bone.
- OCA has the advantage of restoring both the osseous and chondral components caused by osteochondritis dissecans (OCD) lesion.
- The guidewire for OCA dowel technique must be placed perpendicular to the articular surface when preparing the host area. This is of paramount importance particularly in cases of classic OCD on the lateral wall of the medial femoral condyle, once the center of the lesion is usually situated oblique to the weight-bearing central area of the condyle.
- The depth of resection of the area to be grafted must be kept to a minimum, until healthy subchondral bone is found.
- Pulsatile lavage of the osseous surface is used to remove marrow elements in order to decrease immunogenicity of the graft.
- Medial condyle lesions are usually long and narrow and two grafts might be needed in cases of larger lesions. When using two grafts, they can be placed adjacent to one another ("snowman") or overlapping a small part in its interface ("MasterCard").
- When using more than one plug, the direction of the plugs must be convergent to one another, in order to restore the curved articular surface of the femoral condyle.
- For simple dowel plugs, adjunct fixation is rarely necessary.

53.9 Difficulties Encountered

Early complications unique to the allografting procedure are few. There does not appear to be any increased risk of surgical site infection with the use of allografts as compared with other procedures. The use of a miniarthrotomy in the knee decreases the risk of postoperative stiffness. Occasionally, one sees a persistent effusion, which is typically a sign of overuse, but which may indicate an immune-mediated synovitis. Delayed union or nonunion of the fresh allograft is the most common early finding. This is evidenced by persistent discomfort and/or visible graft–host interface on serial radiographic evaluation. Delayed union or nonunion is more common in larger grafts, such as those used in the tibial plateau, or in the setting of compromised bone, such as in the treatment of osteonecrosis. In this setting, patience is essential and complete healing or recovery may take an extended period.

Decreasing activities, the institution of weight-bearing precautions, or use of braces may be helpful in the early management of a delayed healing. In this setting, careful evaluation of serial radiographs can provide insight into the healing process. Magnetic resonance imaging (MRI) scans are rarely diagnostic, particularly prior to 6 months postoperatively, as they typically show extensive signal abnormality that is difficult to interpret. The natural history of the graft that fails to osseointegrate is unpredictable. Clinical symptoms may be minimal, or there may be progressive clinical deterioration and radiographic evidence of fragmentation, fracture, or collapse.

53.10 Key Procedural Steps

53.10.1 Dowel Technique

- When performing the dowel OCA technique, a 2.5-mm Kirschner guidewire is drilled in the center of the lesion and 15- to 30-mm cylindrical templates are used to measure the appropriate size of the repair.
- The recipient site is debrided and prepared with circular reamers. The depth of the debridement is determined when healthy bleeding subchondral bone is encountered and is usually no more than 3 to 7 mm of subchondral bone, yielding a total prepared recipient site depth of 5 to 11 mm (▶ Fig. 53.1a–d).
- Donor grafts are typically cored out at the exact same (orthotopic) location as the lesion on the recipient, and then trimmed to the same thickness. Pulsatile lavage (1–2 L) is used on the donor graft, in order to wash out potentially immunogenic marrow elements from the osseous portion of the graft and to reduce overall allograft bioburden (▶ Fig. 53.2a–f).
- The graft is then inserted by hand in the appropriate rotation and is gently pressed into place manually and with manually

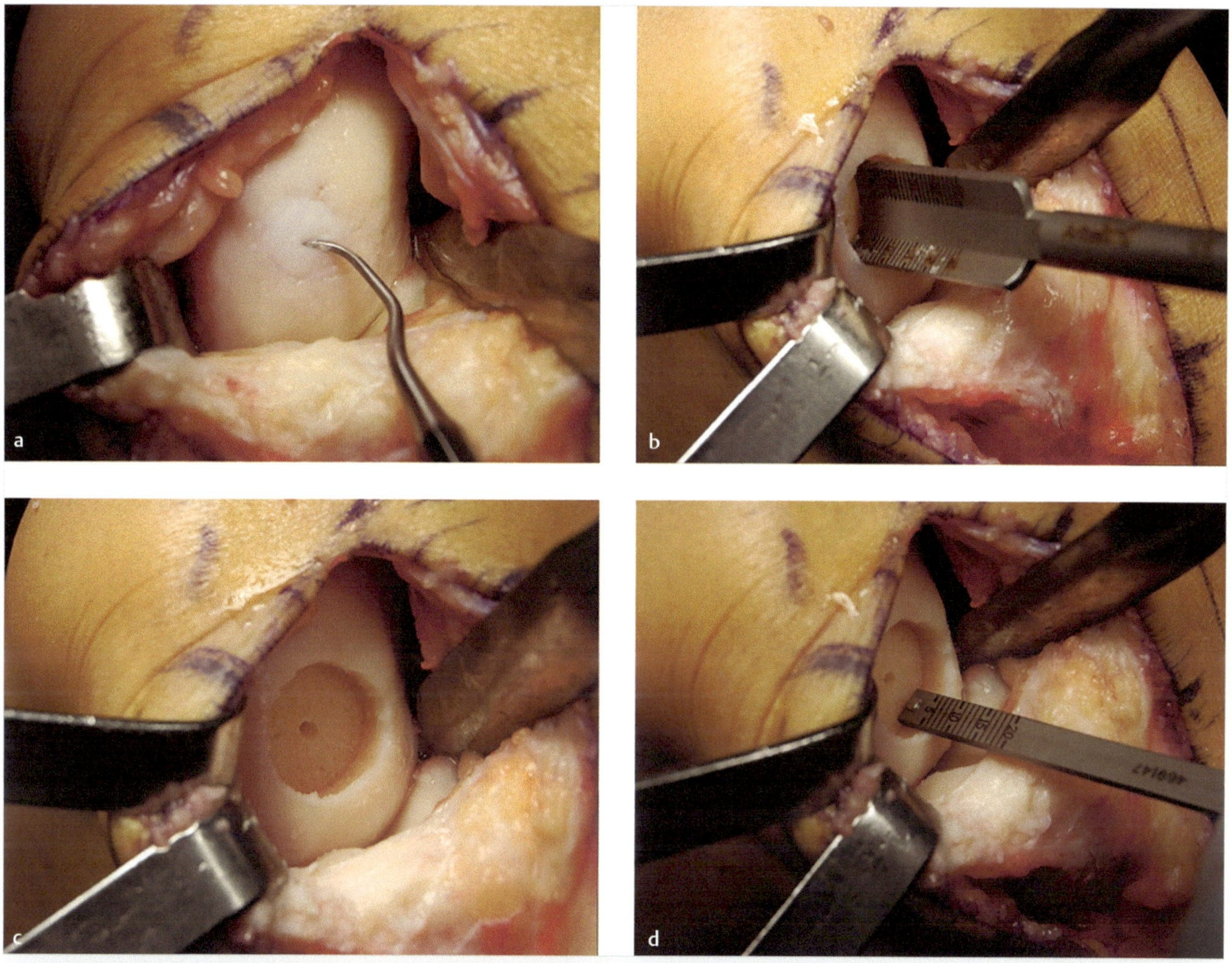

Fig. 53.1 **(a)** Failed autologous osteochondral transplantation graft of the medial femoral condyle. **(b)** Reamer to prepare the recipient defect and remove damaged articular cartilage and subchondral bone. **(c)** View of the lesion site after preparation. Note the shallow bed. **(d)** Depth measurement of the lesion after preparation in four quadrants.

cycling the joint. Finally, very gentle tamping is performed to fully seat the graft when needed (▶ Fig. 53.3a,b). Fixation is achieved by a press-fit technique in the majority of cases with supplemental fixation using absorbable internal fixation devices in a minority of cases.

- Postoperatively, full range of motion is implemented as tolerated immediately after surgery. No immunosuppressive therapy is used. Patients are allowed 25% weight bearing for 4 to 6 weeks after surgery. After 6 weeks, progressive weight bearing is implemented as tolerated. Patients are allowed to return to recreational and sports activities between 4 and 6 months.

53.10.2 Shell Technique

Although the dowel or plug allograft method is generally preferred for most lesions, the surgeon should be prepared to perform a shell graft if the lesion size or location do not allow for proper placement of the dowel graft instruments.

- For the shell graft technique, the defect is identified through the previously described arthrotomy, and the dimensions of the lesion are marked with a surgical pen.
- Using motorized burrs, sharp curettes, and osteotomes, the subchondral bone is removed down to a depth of 4 to 5 mm.
- The shape is transferred to the graft, using length, width, and depth measurements or a foil template. A saw is used to cut the basic graft shape from the donor condyle, initially slightly oversizing the graft by a few millimeters. Excess bone and cartilage is removed as necessary through multiple trial fittings.
- The graft and host bed are then copiously irrigated, and the graft placed flush with the articular surface.
- The need for fixation is based on the degree of inherent stability. Bioabsorbable pins are typically used when fixation is required, but countersunk compression screws may be used as an alternative (▶ Fig. 53.4a–h).
- After cycling the knee through a full range of motion to ensure graft stability, standard closure is performed.
- Initial postoperative management includes attention to control of pain, swelling, and restoration of limb control and range of motion. Patients generally are maintained on touch-down weight bearing for 4 to 6 weeks, depending on the size of the graft and stability of fixation. Patients with

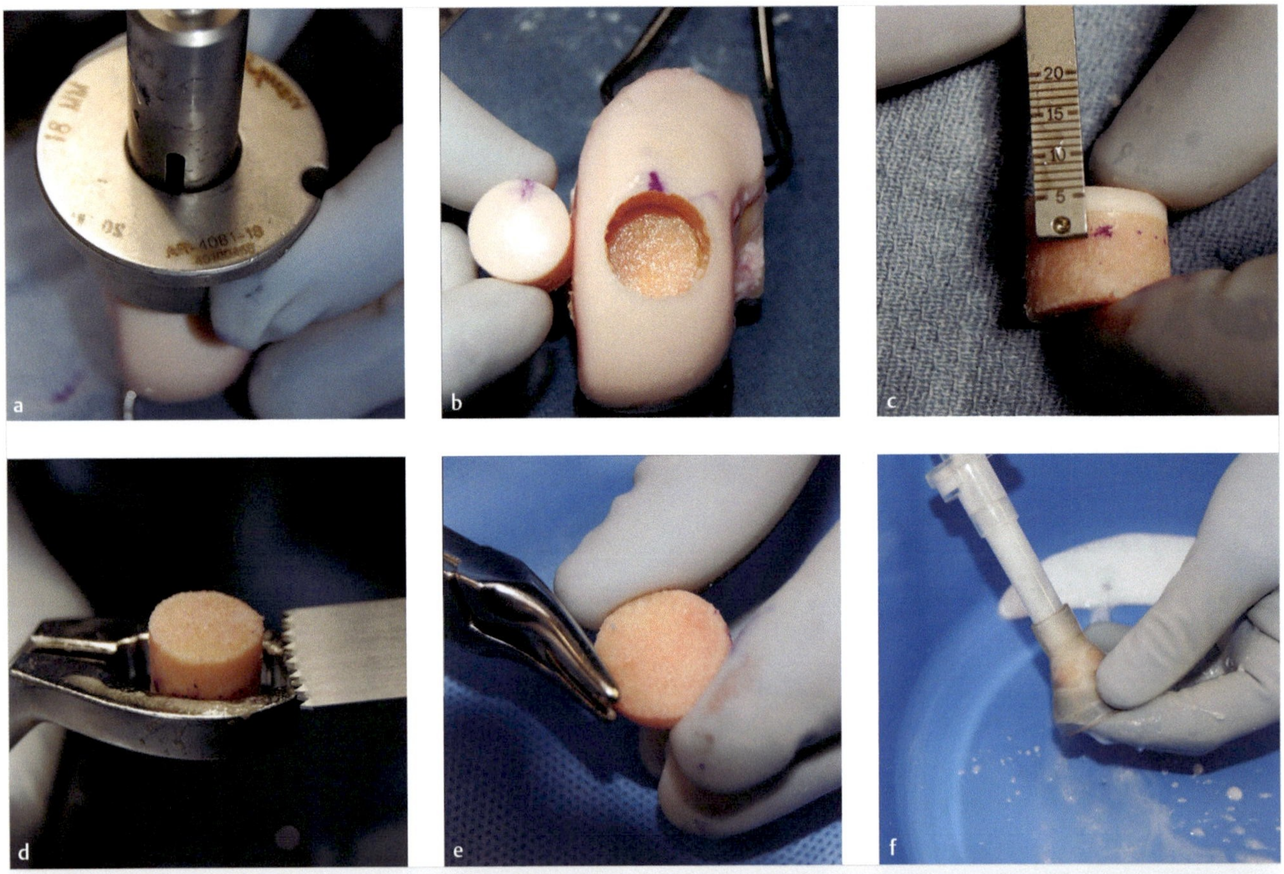

Fig. 53.2 (a) Graft harvesting guide and saw placed in the appropriate position, perpendicular to the articular surface. **(b)** Allograft after harvesting of plug with donor femoral condyle. **(c)** Recipient depth map to be used to trim graft to proper thickness. **(d)** Graft mounted on the graft holder, serving as a cutting guide and cut with an oscillating saw. **(e)** Beveling the edges of the graft to facilitate insertion at the recipient defect. **(f)** Irrigation with a high-pressure lavage to remove marrow elements from the bone.

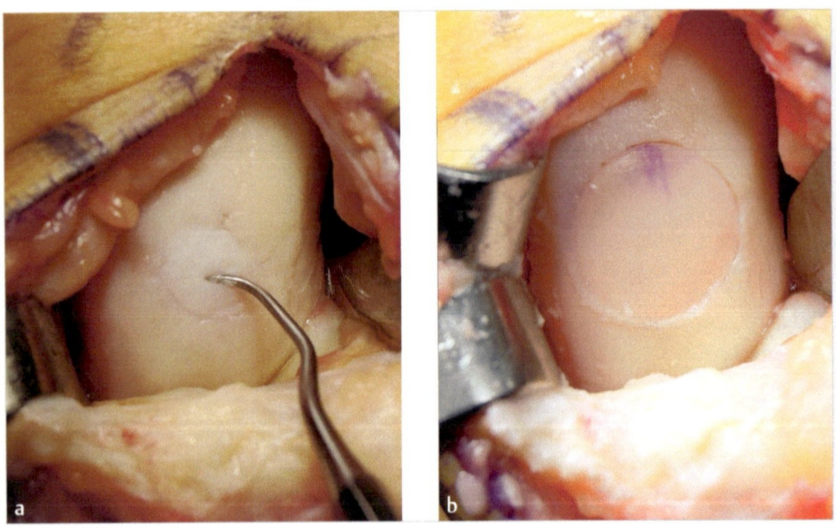

Fig. 53.3 (a) Macroscopic aspect of the lesion prior to transplantation. **(b)** Final macroscopic aspect of the graft, addressing the osteochondral defect.

patellofemoral grafts are allowed weight bearing as tolerated in extension, and generally are limited to 45 degrees of flexion for the first 4 weeks, utilizing an immobilizer or range-of-motion brace. Closed-chain exercise such as cycling is introduced between weeks 2 and 4. Weight bearing is progressed slowly between the second and fourth month, with full weight bearing utilizing a cane or crutch. Full weight bearing and normal gait pattern are generally tolerated between the third and fourth month. Recreation and sports are not reintroduced until joint rehabilitation is complete and

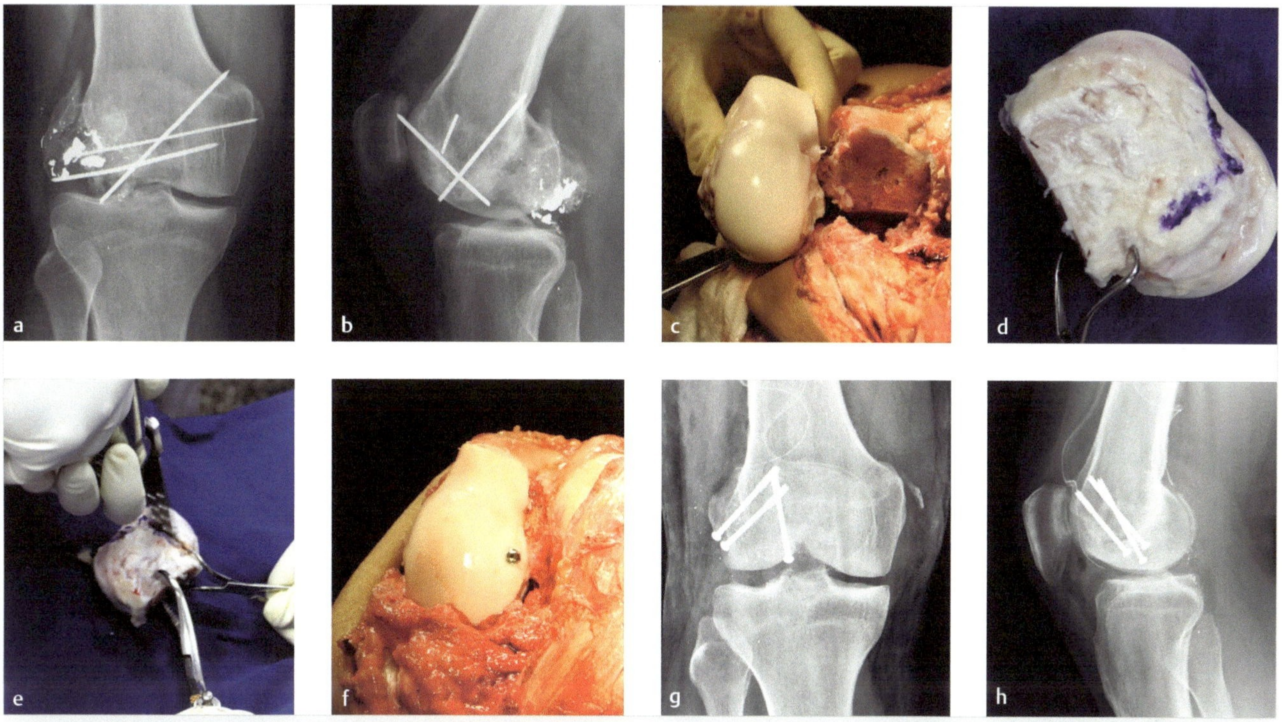

Fig. 53.4 **(a)** Anteroposterior radiograph of the right knee showing a blowout of the lateral femoral condyle following a gunshot wound and a failed attempt of fixation. **(b)** Lateral radiographic view of the right knee showing a displaced fracture of the distal and posterior parts of the lateral femoral condyle. **(c)** Lateral femoral condyle prepared for transplantation using a freehand technique with a saw blade and the donor graft. **(d)** Matching recipient anatomic measurements at the donor graft with a surgical pen. **(e)** Cutting the donor graft to match the recipient defect with a saw blade. **(f)** Final macroscopic aspect of the donor lateral femoral condyle fixed in place with three cannulated screws. **(g)** Postoperative anteroposterior radiograph showing restoration of the lateral femoral condyle after transplantation. **(h)** Postoperative lateral radiographic view showing restoration of the contour of the femoral condyle, similar in size as the medial femoral condyle, restoring knee range of motion.

radiographic healing has been demonstrated, which generally occurs no earlier than 6 months postoperatively.

53.11 Bailout, Rescue, and Salvage Procedures

Treatment options for failed allografts include observation if the patient is minimally symptomatic and the joint is thought to be at low risk for further progression of disease. Arthroscopic evaluation and debridement also may be utilized in many cases. Lastly, revision allografting can be performed with success rates approaching those of primary allografting. This appears to be one of the particular advantages to fresh osteochondral allografting, in that fresh allografting does not preclude a revision allograft as a salvage procedure for failure of the initial allograft. In cases of more extensive joint disease, particularly in older individuals, conversion to prosthetic arthroplasty is appropriate.

53.12 Pitfalls

- Malalignment and ligament instability increase the risk of cartilage repair failure if not properly addressed.
- Matching donor and recipient is extremely important, especially when using shell technique.
- Depth of the graft must be equal to the recipient. Tamping hard on the graft in order to impact it in place might lead to chondrocyte death and graft failure
- Healing of the graft is achieved by creeping substitution. Larger grafts take longer to heal.

54 Patellofemoral Osteochondral Replacement

James P. Stannard

54.1 Description

This procedure addresses large full-thickness articular cartilage defects of the patella and/or the trochlea.

54.2 Key Principles

Successful transplant surgery with fresh osteochondral allografts (OA) requires adherence to a number of key principles. First, the grafts must have at least 70% chondrocyte viability at the time of transplant for long-term success. This can be assured by using grafts preserved using MOPS (Missouri Osteochondral Preservation System) technology. A series that evaluated chondrocyte viability using conventional storage techniques found only 27% of grafts were above the 70% threshold, and all of those grafts were between 17 and 20 days old. All MOPS grafts were remarkably above the 70% threshold and were a mean of 44 days old.

The second key principle for patellofemoral OCAs is to replace the entire patella or entire trochlea in most situations. The topography of both the trochlea and patella makes them poorly suited for replacement with an osteochondral dowel. The third key principle is to cut the grafts thin, with a thickness of approximately 7 mm total of articular cartilage and bone. The fourth key principle is to soak the cancellous bone of the allograft in bone marrow aspirate concentrate harvested from the recipient.

54.3 Expectations

This technique is very new and long-term follow-up data is not available yet. Early published results are encouraging once grafts are fully incorporated. The process of creeping substitution and graft incorporation is thought to take approximately a year. Patients should avoid impact activities and shear forces for one year from the time of grafting.

54.4 Indications

Fresh OCA transplantation is indicated for active patients with large (> 2.5 cm^2) full-thickness articular cartilage loss and functional disability secondary to pain. In most cases patients should be no more than 55 years of age with a high level of activity. Active patients more than 55 years old may also be appropriate surgical candidates. The patient should have failed treatment with rest, anti-inflammatory medications, and physical therapy prior to resorting to OCA transplant surgery.

54.5 Contraindications

Sedentary patients are not good candidates for OCA transplantation. Patients with an underlying disease (example: rheumatoid arthritis) that led to the joint degeneration are not candidates unless it can be demonstrated that the underlying disease is well controlled and not likely to cause premature degeneration of the graft. Patients with a Body Mass Index (BMI) greater than 35 and smokers are also relative contraindications for large transplants.

54.6 Special Considerations

As a general statement, active patients are the best candidates for OCA transplants. Patients under the age of 40 years who are not active may also be considered. Patients must have a stable knee and normal alignment to have success with OCA transplants. Patellar alignment and patellar or trochlea dysplasia are also considerations that must be addressed. All of these issues must either be normal, or the patient must undergo a concomitant or staged procedure (such as tibial tubercle osteotomy) to address the abnormality.

Marked trochlea dysplasia with normal articular cartilage is a challenge that must be addressed. We have had outstanding success with transplantation of a new trochlea with normal morphology that matches the patella that is being transplanted. A second option that can be considered is a trochleoplasty. There is inadequate data available at this time to give a clear evidence-based recommendation between the two procedures.

54.7 Special Instructions, Position, and Anesthesia

Patients are placed in the supine position with a Stulberg leg holder attached to the table. General anesthesia is normally used, with a preoperative peripheral nerve block to help control postoperative pain.

54.8 Tips, Pearls, and Lessons Learned

- Reaming circular grafts from the patella and trochlea have not been associated with good outcomes in the literature. This is likely due to the shape of the structures and difficulty matching the graft and patient morphology.
- If the patella requires replacement, we strongly recommend replacing the entire articular surface.
- The parapatellar arthrotomy must be carried up into the quadriceps tendon so that the entire patella can be everted during the procedure.
- A distal bone block and a proximal bone trough provide three-dimensional stability to the patella graft to allow early knee motion (▶ Fig. 54.1).
- Occasionally, only one facet of the patella or trochlea is damaged. When that is the case, consideration can be

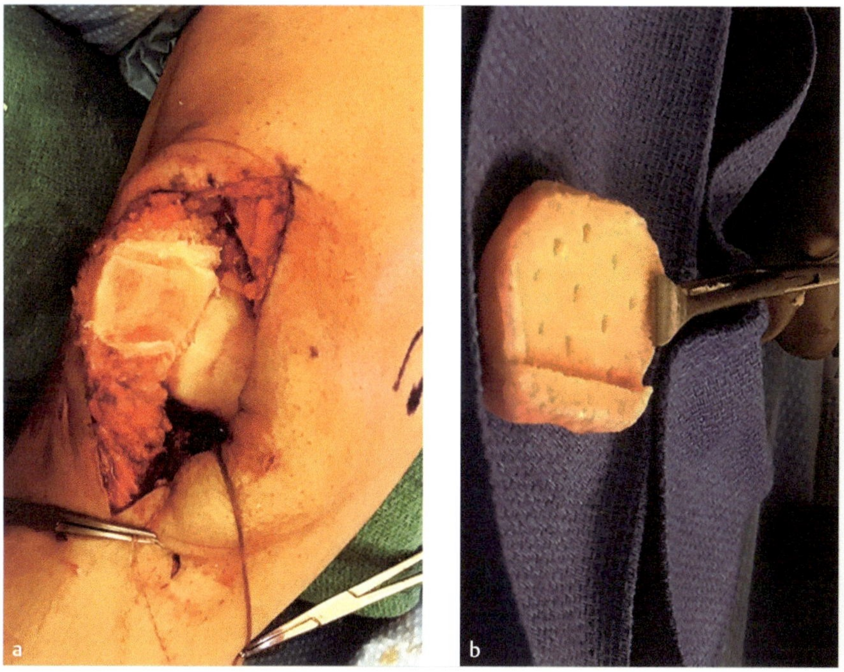

Fig. 54.1 Preparation for the patellar allograft implantation. **(a)** The recipient site is cut with an oscillating saw. We resect the articular surface and we create an offset to it, with a positive tab on the superior pole, and a negative tab on the inferior pole. **(b)** The allograft has the cartilage facing down. The docking area has the offset that matches the recipient bone.

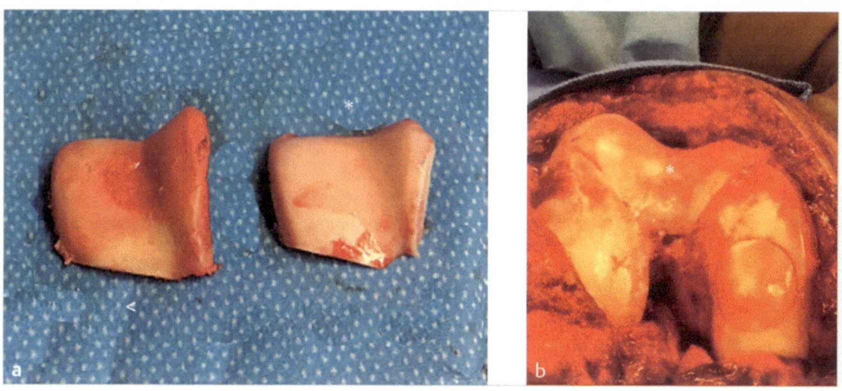

Fig. 54.2 Trochlear allograft. **(a)** Resected damaged osteochondral surface of the trochlear (<) and the matched fresh osteochondral allograft (*); **(b)** trochlear allograft implanted (*).

given to replacing only the damaged facet. In many ways, this is more difficult than replacing the entire articular surface.

- The cancellous bone side of the grafts should be washed out with pulsatile lavage and then soaked in the recipient patients bone marrow aspirate concentrate (BMAC). This remarkably improves both the speed and degree of graft incorporation. We harvest the bone marrow aspirate from the distal femur as the first step of the procedure.
- Fixation of the patella is achieved by cutting the graft and patient as described in ▶ Fig. 54.1 and then pinning it with four bioabsorbable pins.
- Trochlear stabilization is achieved by a combination of the three-dimensional anatomy, two or three bioabsorbable implants that can achieve compression (Smart Nail, Convatech) and bioabsorbable pins if needed (▶ Fig. 54.2).
- Initial knee motion is from 0 to 60 degrees after patellofemoral replacement. If the patient is doing well, we advance to 90 degrees of flexion after 2 to 4 weeks. Full range of motion is allowed after 6 weeks of rehabilitation.

54.9 Difficulties Encountered

In many cases the patellar width is correct, but the length of the graft is shorter than the original patella. This works well as long as the width is a good match.

Cutting the trochlea to get a perfect surface match with the recipient's trochlea is difficult. It is very common to have some small spaces between part of the trochlea graft and the recipient patient. Bone grafting these small spaces with a mixture of autograft bone (harvested from the excised patella and trochlea) and BMAC works well. The graft should be cut into small pieces and soaked in the BMAC. That combination should then be packed into the small spaces between the trochlear graft and the recipient patient.

54.10 Key Procedural Steps

54.10.1 Trochlea

- Make an anterior midline surgical incision to the knee.

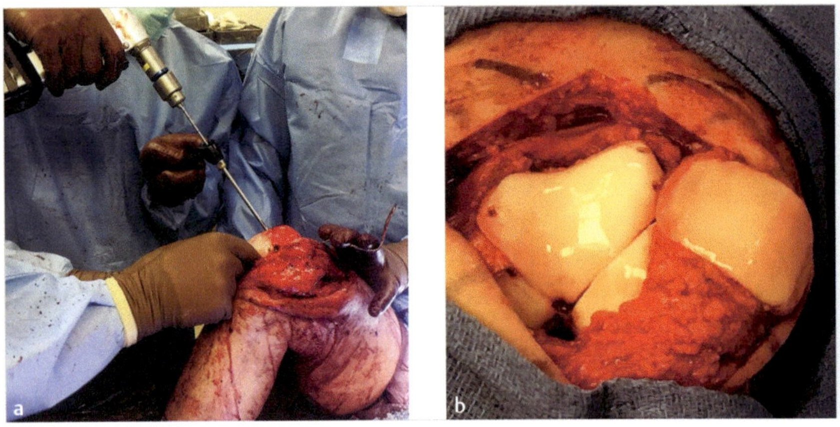

Fig. 54.3 Fixation of the graft with resorbable pins. **(a)** Drilling of the drill holes on the periphery of the graft. **(b)** Final aspect of the graft with the resorbable pins buried under the cartilage (*dark dots* on the periphery of the graft).

- A Jamshidi needle is used to harvest 60 to 120 mL of bone marrow aspirate which is concentrated for use later in the case.
- Medial or lateral parapatellar arthrotomy are both acceptable approaches. We routinely perform a medial parapatellar arthrotomy unless the patient has concomitant injuries on the lateral side that dictate a lateral parapatellar arthrotomy as the appropriate choice.
- The trochlea is excised to a depth of 7 millimeters (bone and cartilage) using an oscillating saw. In most cases the entire trochlea is removed. If all cartilage damage is located on either the medial or the lateral side, consideration can be given to excising only the damaged portion of the trochlea. Cutting guides are being developed but currently these cuts are made using a free-hand technique.
- The excised portion is taken to the back table and used as a template for cutting the allograft trochlea.
- Following the initial cut of the allograft, it is taken to the patient and fine-tuning finishing cuts are performed with the oscillating saw to get the best fit possible. This step often involves multiple small refinements of the initial cut to achieve the best possible fit.
- Once the ideal fit is obtained, the allograft is taken to the back table and the cancellous bone side is washed out with pulse lavage.
- BMAC from the recipient is then soaked onto the cancellous surface of the allograft.
- The graft is temporarily pinned in place with one or two Kirschner wires 1.25 mm in diameter.
- Compression fixation is achieved by drilling and placing two bioabsorbable compression nails (Convatech, NJ). These implants are generally placed through the nonarticular surfaces on the medial and lateral surface of the trochlea (▸ Fig. 54.3).
- Two additional bioabsorbable pins (Arthrex, Naples, FL or Convatech, NJ) are placed through the proximal portion of the graft.
- Bone graft mixed with BMAC is packed into any open spaces between the graft and the patient. Attention is now turned to the patella.

54.10.2 Patella

- The native patella is everted and held in that position using sharp towel clamps through the quadriceps and patellar tendons.
- A caliper is used to measure the thickness of the patella, taking into account the missing articular cartilage. This measurement will be used to assess the appropriate thickness of the graft and avoid making a graft that is either too thick or too thin. It is important to avoid "overstuffing" the patella.
- In most cases the entire articular surface is resected at a depth of 7 millimeters. If all damage is limited to either the medial or lateral facet, consideration can be given to excising and replacing only the involved facet. The cut portion is taken to the back table and used as a template for cutting the allograft.
- A distal bone block is left on the native patella and a proximal bone trough is cut into the patella. Similarly, a boney tab is left on the proximal end of the graft so that it fits into the boney cuts on the patella and provides three-dimensional stability.
- After the initial cut, the graft is taken to the patient and finishing cuts to perfect the fit are performed with the sagittal saw. The thickness of the graft and native bone should be assessed with the caliper to match the original patellofemoral joint. When a good fit has been achieved, the graft is taken to the back table.
- The cancellous bone side of the graft is washed out using pulsatile lavage.
- The bone is then soaked in the recipients BMAC.
- The graft is placed back on the patient and fixed in place with four bioabsorbable pins. Two are generally placed from the proximal end and two from the distal end (▸ Fig. 54.4).

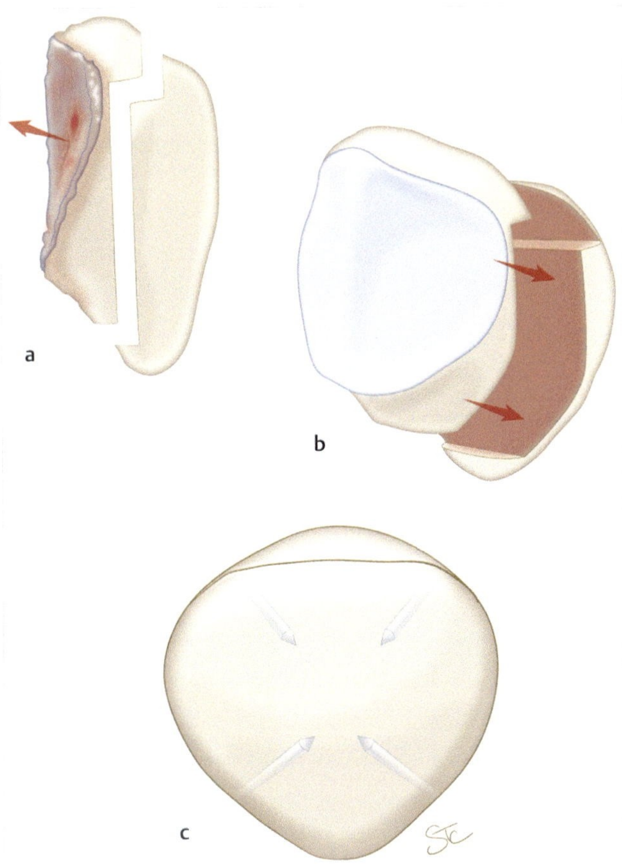

Fig. 54.4 Patellar allograft. **(a)** Resected damaged osteochondral surface (>), and matched fresh osteochondral allograft (*); **(b)** the osteochondral allograft is soaked with autologous bone marrow aspirate concentrate obtained from the recipient's distal femur. **(c)** Final aspect of the osteochondral graft after implantation.

- The graft is then returned to its normal anatomic position and tracking of the patella is assessed either through observation with knee motion or arthroscopy or both.
- The parapatellar arthrotomy is closed and adjustments can be made to address eventual mild maltracking issues. Major issues may require a tibial tubercle osteotomy. The need for an osteotomy should be determined preoperatively based on physical exam, TT/TG ratio, etc.

54.11 Bailout, Rescue, and Salvage Procedures

If the graft fails during the postoperative recovery period, the surgeon can either revise it with a new graft or perform a patellofemoral arthroplasty. Malalignment and maltracking issues should be identified preoperatively and at the time of surgical closure. If they were missed or not addressed appropriately, a work-up to determine the malalignment issue and then a corrective osteotomy or other reconstructive procedure should be undertaken.

Care must be taken to leave adequate native bone in the extensor mechanism when resecting the damaged patella. Err on the side of leaving too much bone as there is not a good bailout to excessive excision of bone.

54.12 Pitfalls

Assess the thickness of the graft and remaining bone with the caliper, and either graft (to increase thickness) or excise additional bone from the allograft (to decrease thickness). Avoid "overstuffing" the patellofemoral joint with a graft that is too thick.

Index

Note: Page numbers set **bold** or *italic* indicate headings or figures, respectively.

Q

R

S

T

U

V

W

Z